DATE DUE

DEC 1 7 2004	
DEC 1 5 2004	
NOV – 4 2005	
DEC 1 4 2005	
MAY – 2 2007	
MAY – 2 2007	
JUL 2 4 2008	
JUL 1 5 2008	
MAY – 5 2009	
APR 2 8 2009	
MAY 1 3 2010	
JUN – 8 2010	
NOV 1 4 2012	

Motor Neuron Disorders

Blue Books of Practical Neurology
(Volumes 1–14 published as BIMR Neurology)

Motor Neuron Disorders

Edited by

Pamela J. Shaw, M.B.B.S., M.D., F.R.C.P.
Head of Academic Neurology Unit and Professor of Neurology, University of
Sheffield; Consultant Neurologist, Royal Hallamshire Hospital, Sheffield,
United Kingdom

and

Michael J. Strong, M.D., F.R.C.P.C.
Professor and Co-chair, Department of Clinical Neurological Sciences, Arthur
Hudson Chair in ALS Research, The University of Western Ontario; Cell
Biology Research Group, Robarts Research Institute, London, Ontario,
Canada

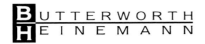

An Imprint of Elsevier Science

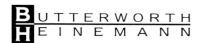

An Imprint of Elsevier Science

The Curtis Center
Independence Square West
Philadelphia, Pennsylvania 19106

NOTICE

Medicine is an ever-changing field. Standard safety precautions must be followed, but as new research and clinical experience broaden our knowledge, changes in treatment and drug therapy may become necessary or appropriate. Readers are advised to check the most current product information provided by the manufacturer of each drug to be administered to verify the recommended dose, the method and duration of administration, and contraindications. It is the responsibility of the licensed prescriber, relying on experience and knowledge of the patient, to determine dosages and the best treatment for each individual patient. Neither the publisher nor the editor assumes any liability for any injury and/or damage to persons or property arising from this publication.

Library of Congress Cataloging-in-Publication Data

Motor neuron disorders / [edited by] Pamela J. Shaw and Michael J. Strong.
     p. ; cm. — (Blue books of practical neurology ; 28)
   Includes index.
   ISBN 0-7506-7442-3
     1. Amyotrophic lateral sclerosis. 2. Motor neurons—Diseases. I. Shaw, Pamela J. II. Strong, Michael J. III. Series.
     [DNLM: 1. Motor Neuron Disease. WE 550 M9192 2003]
   RC406.A24M686 2003
   616.8'3—dc21
                                                                    2003043693

Acquisitions Editor: Susan F. Pioli
Publishing Services Manager: Joan Sinclair
Project Manager: Mary Stermel

Printed in the United States of America

Last digit is the print number: 9   8   7   6   5   4   3   2   1

Contents

Contributing Authors

Peter M. Andersen, M.D., D.M.Sc.
Associate Professor of Clinical Neuroscience, Institute of Clinical Neuroscience, Umeå University; Consultant in Neurology, Umeå University Hospital, Umeå, Sweden

Johanna Anneser, M.D.
Department of Neurology, University of Munich, Munich, Germany

Carmel Armon, M.D., M.H.S.
Professor of Neurology, Loma Linda University School of Medicine; Attending Physician, Department of Neurology, Loma Linda Medical Center; Staff Physician, Department of Neurology, Jerry L. Pettis Memorial Veterans Affairs Medical Center, Loma Linda, California

Gian Domenico Borasio, M.D.
Assistant Professor of Neurology and Palliative Care, University of Munich, Munich, Germany

Peter G.H. Clarke, Ph.D.
Maitre d'Enseignement et de Recherche, Institut de Biologie Cellulaire et de Morphologie, Université de Lausanne, Lausanne, Switzerland

Kay E. Davies, M.A., D.Phil.
Dr. Lee's Professor of Anatomy and Head of Human Anatomy and Genetics Department, University of Oxford, Oxford, United Kingdom

Heather D. Durham, Ph.D.
Professor of Neurology and Neurosurgery, McGill University and the Montreal Neurological Institute, Montreal, Quebec, Canada

Kenneth H. Fischbeck, M.D.
Chief of Neurogenetics Branch, National Institute of Neurological Disorders and Stroke, National Institutes of Health, Bethesda, Maryland

Deborah F. Gelinas, M.D.
Clinical Director, Department of Neurology, Forbes Norris MDA/ALS Center, California Pacific Medical Center, San Francisco, California

Andrew J. Grierson, B.Sc., Ph.D.
Lecturer in Neuroscience, Academic Neurology Unit, University of Sheffield, Sheffield, United Kingdom

Paul G. Ince, BSc., M.D., F.R.C.Path.
Professor of Neuropathology and Head of the Academic Unit of Pathology, Division of Genomic Medicine, University of Sheffield; Honorary Consultant Neuropathologist, Sheffield Teaching Hospitals NHS Trust, Sheffield, United Kingdom

Jean-Pierre Julien, M.D.
Professor of Neurology and Neurosurgery, McGill University; Research Scientist, Centre for Research in Neuroscience, The Research Institute of McGill University Health Centre, Montreal, Quebec, Canada

P. Nigel Leigh, Ph.D., F.R.C.P.
Professor of Clinical Neurology, Institute of Psychiatry and King's MND Care and Research Centre, Guy's, King's and St. Thomas' School of Medicine, London, United Kingdom

Catherine Lomen-Hoerth, M.D., Ph.D.
Assistant Professor of Neurology, University of California, San Francisco, California

Christopher J. McDermott, M.B.Ch.B.
Wellcome Clinical Fellow, Academic Neurology Unit, University of Sheffield, Sheffield, United Kingdom

Robert G. Miller, M.D.
Director, Department of Neurology, Forbes Norris MDA/ALS Center; Chairman, Department of Neurosciences, California Pacific Medical Center, San Francisco, California

Kerry R. Mills, B.Sc., Ph.D., M.B., B.S., F.R.C.P.
Professor of Clinical Neurophysiology, Academic Neurophysiology Unit, Guy's, King's and St. Thomas' School of Medicine, King's College, University of London; Honorary Consultant Clinical Neurophysiologist, King's College and Guy's Hospitals, London, United Kingdom

Erik P. Pioro, M.D., D.Phil., F.R.C.P.C.
Director, Center for ALS and Related Disorders, Department of Neurology, Cleveland Clinic Foundation, Cleveland, Ohio

Serge Przedborski, M.D., Ph.D.
Professor of Neurology and Pathology, Columbia University College of Physicians and Surgeons; Attending Physician, Department of Neurology, Neurological Institute, New York

Wim Robberecht, M.D., Ph.D.
Professor of Neurology, Department of Experimental Neurology and Neuro-chemistry, University of Leuven; Chairman, Department of Neurology, University Hospital Gasthuisberg, Leuven, Belgium

Janice Robertson, Ph.D.
Research Fellow, Department of Neurology, McGill University and Montreal General Hospital Research Institute, Montreal, Quebec, Canada

Lewis P. Rowland, M.D.
Professor of Neurology, Columbia University; Attending Neurologist, Columbia Presbyterian Medical Center-New York Presbyterian Hospital, New York

Pamela J. Shaw, M.B.B.S., M.D., F.R.C.P.
Head of Academic Neurology Unit and Professor of Neurology, University of Sheffield; Consultant Neurologist, Royal Hallamshire Hospital, Sheffield, United Kingdom

Michael J. Strong, M.D., F.R.C.P.C.
Professor and Co-chair, Department of Clinical Neurological Sciences, Arthur Hudson Chair in ALS Research, The University of Western Ontario; Cell Biology Research Group, Robarts Research Institute, London, Ontario, Canada

Charlotte J. Sumner, M.D.
Clinical Fellow, Neurogenetics Branch, National Institute of Neurological Disorders and Stroke, National Institutes of Health, Bethesda, Maryland

Michael Swash, M.D., F.R.C.P., F.R.C.Path.
Professor of Neurology, Department of Neuroscience, Queen Mary, University of London; Consultant Neurologist, Department of Neurology, Royal London Hospital and St. Bartholomew's Hospital, London, United Kingdom

Kevin Talbot, D.Phil., M.B.B.S., M.R.C.P.
MRC/GlaxoSmithKline Clinician Scientist, Department of Human Anatomy and Genetics, University of Oxford; Honorary Consultant Neurologist, Department of Clinical Neurology, Radcliffe Infirmary, Oxford, United Kingdom

Martin R. Turner, M.A., M.B., B.S., M.R.C.P.
Research Fellow, Department of Neurology, Institute of Psychiatry, London, United Kingdom

Philip Van Damme, M.D.
Ph.D. Student, Department of Neurobiology, Katholieke Universiteit Leuven, Campus Gasthuisberg; Neurologist in Training, University Hospital Gasthuisberg, Leuven, Belgium

Ludo Van Den Bosch, Ph.D.
Assistant Professor of Neurobiology, Katholieke Universiteit Leuven, Campus Gasthuisberg, Leuven, Belgium

Weiyan Wen, Ph.D.
Postdoctoral Fellow, Cell Biology Group, The John P. Robarts Research Institute, London, Ontario, Canada

Stephen Wharton, B.Sc., M.B.B.S., M.Sc., M.R.C.Path.
Senior Clinical Lecturer in Neuropathology, Division of Genomic Medicine, University of Sheffield; Honorary Consultant in Neuropathology, Department of Histopathology, Sheffield Teaching Hospitals, Sheffield, United Kingdom

Clare A. Wood-Allum, M.A., B.M.B.S., M.R.C.P.
Wellcome Research Training Fellow, Academic Neurology Unit, University of Sheffield; Honorary Specialist Registrar, Department of Neurology, Royal Hallamshire Hospital, Sheffield, United Kingdom

Wenchang Yang, M.D.
Postdoctoral Research Fellow, Cell Biology Research Group, Robarts Research Institute, London, Ontario, Canada

Series Preface

The *Blue Books of Practical Neurology* denotes the series of monographs previously named the *BIMR Neurology* series, which was itself the successor of the *Modern Trends in Neurology* series. As before, the volumes are intended for use by physicians who grapple with the problems of neurological disorders on a daily basis, be they neurologists, neurologists in training, or those in related fields such as neurosurgery, internal medicine, psychiatry, and rehabilitation medicine.

Our purpose is to produce monographs on topics in clinical neurology in which progress through research has brought about new concepts of patient management. The subject of each book is selected by the Series Editors using two criteria: first, that there has been significant advance in knowledge in that area and, second, that such advances have been incorporated into new ways of managing patients with the disorders in question. This has been the guiding spirit behind each volume, and we expect it to continue. In effect, we emphasize research, both in the clinic and in the experimental laboratory, but principally to the extent that it changes our collective attitudes and practices in caring for those who are neurologically afflicted.

Arthur K. Asbury
Anthony H.V. Schapira
Series Editors

Preface

The first descriptions of amyotrophic lateral sclerosis (ALS) date to the 19th century and include the writings of Aran, Duchenne, and Charcot.[1-4] These seminal papers provided a clear, and little modified, description of the clinical and basic neuropathological aspects of ALS that has remained largely unaltered over the ensuing century and a half with the notable addition of considerable progress in our understanding of the epidemiology and clinical aspects of motor neuron diseases. However, it has been the last decade that has seen the greatest advances in our understanding of the complexity of this disorder as a biological entity. Keeping pace with this burgeoning knowledge base is a considerable challenge even for the most ardent student of motor neuron diseases. As each year passes, the factual basis of our understanding of ALS continues to grow, creating a potential to out-strip our ability to understand it in the context to the disease itself. It has been our hope to develop a text that allows one to have a ready reference in which to place this new information in context.

The text has been laid out in three broad sections, reflecting our view that an understanding of the therapy of ALS must be founded in a solid understanding of the phenomenology of the disease and of its biological characteristics to the extent to which they are known. The first section reviews the clinical, neuropathological, and radiological aspects of ALS and of the related motor neuron diseases. In terms of the latter, it is increasingly evident that lessons learned from the more restricted forms of motor neuron disease, such as the spinal muscular atrophies, have a direct applicability to understanding ALS. Moreover, as the population ages en masse, clinicians will be faced with ever increasing numbers of individuals afflicted with a motor neuron disease and will need to be able to differentiate among the individual variants readily. The classical concept of ALS as a disease of restricted phenotypic expression, with essentially a pure motor neuron degenerative state, is increasingly challenged through clinical and neuropathological studies. The dramatic advances in our ability to image not only the structure of the nervous system, but also of the biochemical characteristics of the brain and spinal cord, similarly have lead to dramatic advances in the diagnosis of ALS.

As this text goes to press, there already will have been significant changes in our understanding of the molecular and biochemical basis of ALS. It is the nature of such texts that information available within the text must be, to some extent, dated. However, there is an increasing recognition that ALS must be a multifactorial disease not only at the clinical and biochemical level, but also at the level of non-neuronal and neuronal involvement. ALS can no longer be viewed as a singular entity but rather as the phenotypic expression of a wide range of cellular perturbations.[5] At the neuropathological level, the hallmark of ALS remains a motor neuron–selective disease process marked by the presence of degenerating motor neurons with a variety of intraneuronal aggregates and with degeneration of the descending supraspinal pathways subserving motor function. However, nonmotor neuronal degeneration also is clearly evident as highlighted by the degenerative changes accompanying the frontotemporal dementia or cognitive impairment observed in increasingly greater numbers of ALS patients. The intricate relationships among the microglia, astrocytes, and degenerating (as well as healthy) motor neurons are undoubtedly a key to the progression or propagation of ALS throughout the nervous system. Once triggered, it seems that the disease may take a life of its own with the potential transfer of neuronal injury via non-neuronal cells. The process of degeneration of motor neurons is itself a mystery. However, there is a convergence of thought suggesting that a cascade of cell death must be triggered and that this cascade recruits participation from a number of key cellular constituents. Mitochondrial damage is evident throughout. There is considerable evidence of oxidative damage, deficiencies in calcium buffering, and alterations in the handling of excitotoxic stimuli. Although this will continue to change, we have provided chapters on each of these areas that will allow an understanding of how perturbations in these realms are of relevance to ALS.

In the end, the preceding chapters are intended to provide a framework on which to understand the therapy of ALS. Whereas one naturally tends to think of such therapy as being specifically directed at the disease process, it is equally critical to recognize that such therapies must also address symptomatic management and impact of the quality of life of the individual afflicted with ALS. The last decade has also taught us that the massive, double-blind, randomized, controlled study may not always address the issues of concern in treating ALS. Novel designs are arising and will be addressed.

The pace of our understanding of ALS has been breathtaking in the last decade, and yet, this is likely only a small fraction of what will transpire in the next decade as the promise of understanding the human genome comes to fruition. The advent of novel molecular and protein analytical techniques suited to the study of the single cell will again change the field. In this text, we hope that the reader will find a welcome home to return to with which to review the basics of the disease as these advances move forward.

REFERENCES

1. Charcot JM, Joffroy A. Deux cas d'atrophie musculaire progressive avec lésions de la substance grise et des faisceaux antérolatéraux de la moelle épinière. *Arch Physiol Norm Pathol* 1869;2:354–744.

2. Aran FA. Recherches sur une maladie non encore décrite du systéme musculaire (atrophie musculaire progressive). *Arch Gén de Méd* 1850;24:5–35.
3. Aran FA. Recherches sur une maladie non encore décrite du systéme musculaire (atrophie musculaire progressive)(2e article-suite et fin). *Arch Gén de Méd* 1850;24:172–214.
4. Duchenne (De Boulogne). Paralysie musculaire progressive de la langue, du voile du palais et des levres; affection non encore décrite comme espèce morbide distincte. *Arch Gen Med* 1860; 16:283–296.
5. Strong MJ. The evidence for ALS as a multisystems disorder of limited phenotypic expression. *Can J Neurol Sci* 2001;28:283–298.

Acknowledgments

Those who treat the patients and their families who suffer with ALS are an incredible lot. It is not a disease for the faint-hearted and not a science that is easily understood. We dedicate this book to those who have allowed us to singularly pursue both those ends, often at an unforeseen cost. These include our spouses (Wendy and Paul), our children who tolerate long hours of absence (Jennifer, James, Alec, and Sophie), and our patients who have taught us immeasurably.

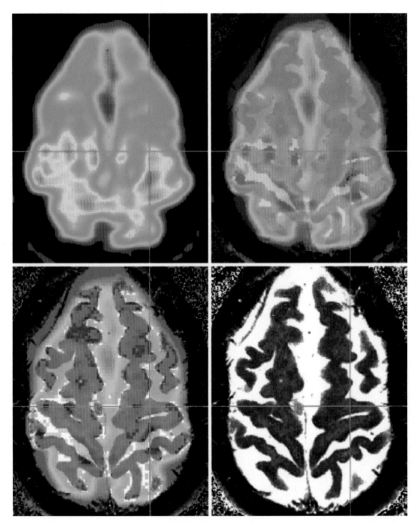

Figure 4.9 Co-registration of transverse positron emission tomography (PET) and magnetic resonance images from a 53-year-old man with amyotrophic lateral sclerosis and frontotemporal dementia reveal prominently diminished metabolism of fluorine-18-fluorodeoxyglucose in motor and premotor regions, as well as cortical atrophy. Blending of the superimposed images from PET only **(upper left)** to magnetic resonance imaging only **(lower right)** allows localization of hypometabolism to frontal regions, especially the superior frontal gyri and parasagittal portions of the precentral gyri. Crossing of planar lines indicates the anterior portion of the left precentral gyrus (primary motor cortex). (Many thanks to Eric LaPresto, CCF, for co-registering the PET and magnetic resonance images.)

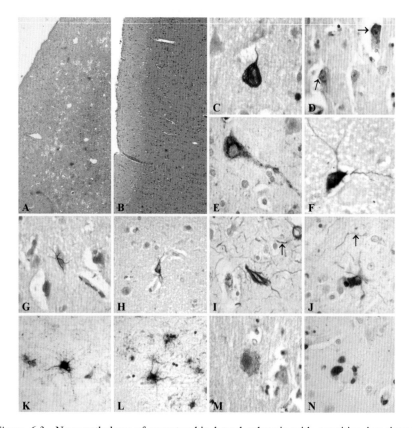

Figure 6.3 Neuropathology of amyotrophic lateral sclerosis with cognitive impairment (ALSci). The features of pathology in ALSci are present in superficial linear spongiosis, tau neuronal, and glial aggregates and extraneuronal inclusions. As observed in a number of the frontotemporal dementias, **(A)** vacuolar changes within the second and third cortical layers (superficial linear spongiosis) is characteristic of patients with ALSci. A similar vacuolization can be observed in cognitively-intact patients with ALS **(B)**, though less often and to a lesser extent. A variety of tau-immunoreactive neuronal, glial, and extraneuronal aggregates are also characteristic of ALSci. Neuronal aggregates are the core feature of ALSci; however, the morphology and immunoreactivity characteristics vary among the varying cortical layers. Gallyas positive filamentous neuronal aggregates are more typically dense, filamentous structures filling the cytoplasm in neurons of the fourth through sixth cortical layers **(C)**, whereas fine, filamentous cellular threads are more typical of the neurons in the immediate subcortical white matter **(G)**. Following dephosphorylation (*Escherichia coli* alkaline phosphatase), **(D)** dense and tufted tau-1 immunoreactive neuronal aggregates are readily observed in layers two through six *(arrows)*. Neurons with immunoreactivity to the monoclonal antibody AT8 (recognizing a tau epitope observed in Alzheimer's disease) were observed in layer two through subcortical white matter **(E, H)**. Rarely, and only in ALSci, tau aggregates immunoreactive to a monoclonal antibody recognizing C-terminus tau hyperphosphorylation (Ser^{396}) were observed **(F)**. Neuritic threads were often observed in the frontal cortex of both ALS and ALSci (Gallyas and AT8 staining, *arrow,* **I** and **J**, respectively). Tau immunoreactive astrocytic aggregates were also characteristic of ALSci (Gallyas and AT8 immunoreactive staining, **K** and **L**, respectively). These were most commonly observed in layers one and six and less often observed in the subcortical white matter. Extraneuronal tau-immunoreactive aggregates are another features of ALSci. Most commonly, these are dense, tau-1 immunoreactive aggregates with poorly defined margins (distinct from corpora amylacea) **(M)** or discrete tau immunoreactive globules **(N)**. **(A, B,** ×10; all other photomicrographs, ×40 before reproduction.)

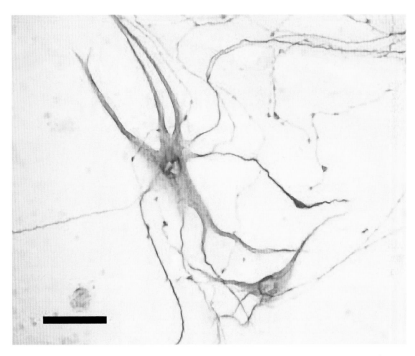

Figure 10.2   Motor neuron culture, stained with the motor neuron marker peripherin (scale bar = 40 micrometers).

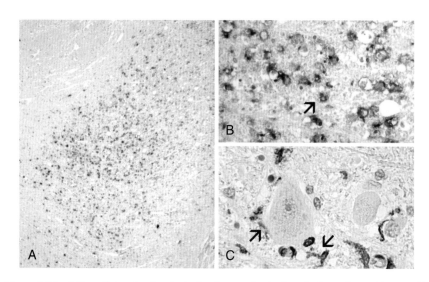

Figure 13.2 Microglial activation in the lumbosacral spinal cord of a patient with sporadic amyotrophic lateral sclerosis. Within regions of degenerating corticospinal tracts **(A)**, microglia proliferation is prominent and can be seen to largely replace the tract (×4, before reproduction). At higher magnification **(B)**, these microglia are seen to have become phagocytotic and are largely responsible for clearing the myelin debris of the degenerating tract (×20, before reproduction). (In both (A) and (C), microglial immunostained with a mouse monoclonal antibody to HLA-DR3 and localized with alkaline phosphatase, giving rise to the red coloration.) In contrast, in the perineuronal milieu **(C)**, activated microglia are seen to cluster around the motor neurons, and to extend processes to the neuronal perikaryon (×40, before reproduction; microglia immunostained with RCA and localized with 3,4-DAB giving rise to the brown coloration). Noteworthy is that normal appearance of the motor neuron, showing no evidence of degeneration at a time when microglial activation, is apparent.

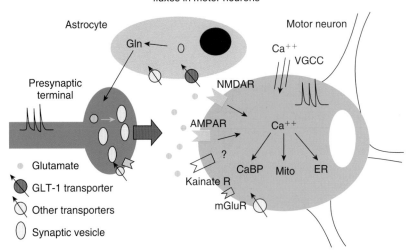

Figure 15.2 Motor neurons are particularly vulnerable to excitotoxicity, particularly by calcium-mediated mechanisms. Excitation by the neurotransmitter, glutamate, results in Ca^{2+} entry through calcium-permeable α-amino-3-hydroxy-5-methyl-4-isoxazole propionic acid (AMPA) receptors, N-methyl-D-aspartate (NMDA) receptors, and voltage-gated calcium channels (VGCCs). Intracellular Ca^{2+} is sequestered by cytosolic calcium-binding protein (CaBP) and transported into mitochondria (Mito) or the endoplasmic reticulum (ER). The role of kainate receptors (kainate R) and metabotropic glutamate receptors (mGluRs) in motor neuron vulnerability is not certain. Glutamate is removed from the synaptic cleft by specific glutamate transporters on astrocytes and also neurons. In astrocytes, glutamate is converted to glutamine (Gl) and recycled to presynaptic nerve terminals.

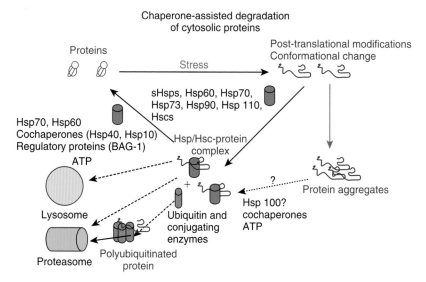

Figure 15.3 The heat shock proteins (Hsps) and heat shock cognate proteins (Hscs) function as molecular chaperones to bind to proteins with altered conformation (through transcriptional errors, genetic mutations or post-translational modifications) to prevent them from forming aggregates in the cell. Under some circumstances, the normal conformation of proteins can be restored in an adenosine triphosphate (ATP)–dependent process involving the cooperative action of chaperones and regulatory proteins. Otherwise, the proteins are targeted to proteasomes, usually following polyubiquitination, but in some cases in a ubiquitin-independent fashion. Lysosomes are the other major organelle for proteolysis in cells. One pathway to lysosomal degradation is chaperone-dependent microautophagy by which Hsp73 delivers proteins to lysosomes.

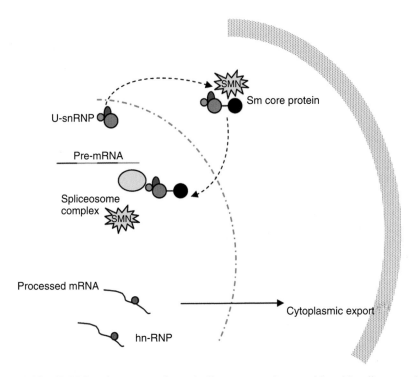

Figure 16.2 SMN functions as a cofactor in Sm core protein assembly with spliceosomal ribonucleoprotein in the cytoplasm. In addition, it appears to have critical nuclear functions in regulating splicing.

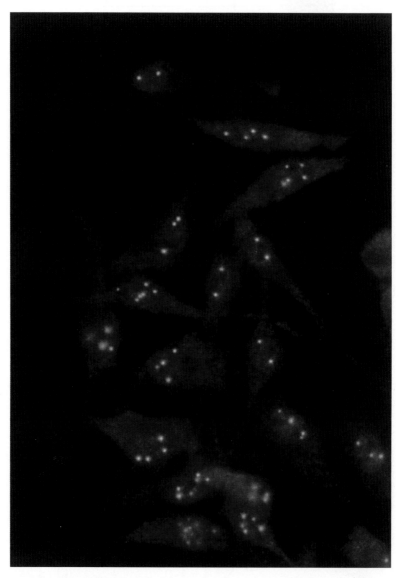

Figure 16.3 Immunostaining of HeLa cells in culture with an antibody directed against the survival motor neuron protein. There is diffuse cytoplasmic staining and punctuate nuclear staining in subnuclear organelles thought to be critical for ribonucleoprotein metabolism. (Courtesy Dr. Kirstie Anderson, Department of Human Anatomy and Genetics, University of Oxford.)

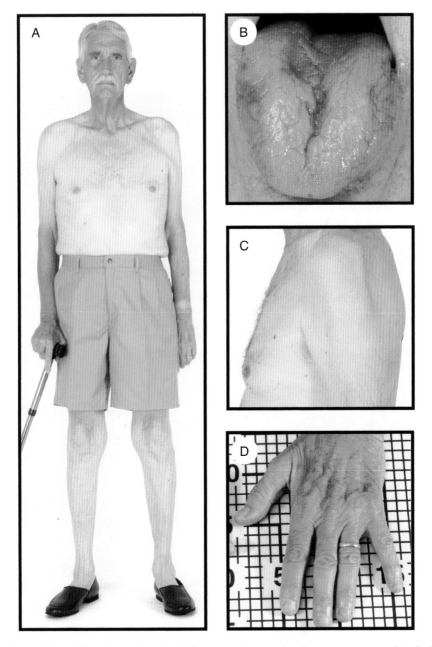

Figure 17.1 This patient with spinobulbar muscular atrophy demonstrates several typical features of the disease: **(A)** mild facial weakness, simian posture of the arms, and wasting of limb muscles; **(B)** atrophy of the tongue with a deep midline furrow; **(C)** weakness and atrophy proximally around the shoulder girdle; and **(D)** distal weakness and atrophy with loss of intrinsic hand muscle bulk, particularly in the first web space. This patient has minimal gynecomastia.

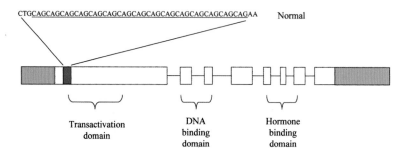

CTGCAGCAGCAGCAGCAGCAGCAGCAGCAGCAGCAGCAGCAGCAGCAGCAGCAGCAGCAGCAGCAGCAGCAGCAGCAGCAGCA
GCAGCAGCAGCAGCAGCAGCAGCAGCAGCAGCAGCAGCAGCAGCAGCAGAA

SBMA

CTGCAGCAGCAGCAGCAGCAGCAGCAGCAGCAGCAGCAGCAGCAGAA   Normal

Transactivation
domain

DNA
binding
domain

Hormone
binding
domain

Androgen receptor gene

Figure 17.2   The functional domains of the androgen receptor gene.

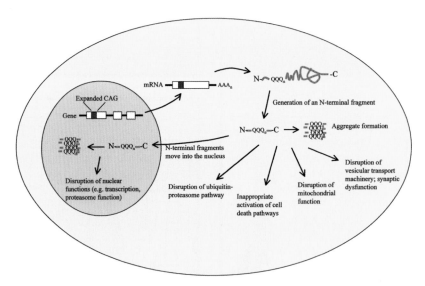

Figure 17.3 Possible mechanisms of spinobulbar muscular atrophy pathogenesis. (Reprinted with permission from Taylor JP, Lieberman AP, Fischbeck KH. Repeat Expansion and Neurological Diseases. In AK Asbury, GM McKhann, WU McDonald, et al (eds), Diseases of the Nervous System (3rd ed). Cambridge: Cambridge University Press, 2002.)

SECTION 1

KEY PRINCIPLES IN THE CLINICAL DIAGNOSIS, PATHOLOGY, AND INVESTIGATION OF MOTOR NEURON DISORDERS

1
Clinical Principles in the Diagnosis of Motor Neuron Disorders

Michael Swash

As with many other diagnostic processes in medicine, the diagnosis of motor neuron disease (MND) (i.e., amyotrophic lateral sclerosis [ALS]) is an exercise in clinical logic. Because the disease is relatively rare, experience of ALS among clinicians is correspondingly often incomplete. Diagnosis depends not only on the clinical features at presentation but also on the ability of the clinician to interpret the relevant features in the patient's history and to elucidate the relevant abnormalities on examination. The latter is a particularly important aspect of diagnosis and requires great clinical skill. In this introductory chapter, the clinical approach to diagnosis is discussed and certain particularly important aspects are emphasized. With the advent of a treatment that slows the progress of the disease, early diagnosis has become more important. If current clinical trials identify a more effective therapy, early diagnosis will become an essential part of good clinical management.

DIAGNOSTIC CRITERIA FOR MOTOR NEURON DISEASE

First, in considering the criteria for diagnosis, we must be clear on the nomenclature. The terms *ALS* and *MND* are often used interchangeably. Although not strictly correct, this is a reasonable compromise that serves to prevent confusion,[1] even though the abbreviation *ALS/MND* is both clumsy and unnecessary. The term *ALS* should properly be used to describe the syndrome first described by Charcot.[2] *MND* has been increasingly used recently to include not only ALS but also the related motor syndromes of progressive bulbar palsy, progressive muscular atrophy, and primary lateral sclerosis (PLS). ALS as described by Charcot accounts for more than 85 percent of all patients with MND. In clinical practice, the term *MND* is used to describe the most common syndrome, ALS.

Diagnostic criteria have been agreed upon in a consensus meeting of an international group of clinicians, under the leadership of the World Federation of Neurology Research Committee on Motor Neuron Diseases. These diagnostic criteria were agreed upon in El Escorial in 1994; these were updated in a subsequent meeting held at Airlie House, in Virginia.[3,4] It is important to realize that these criteria were formulated for use in the clinical trial setting, rather than in clinical practice,[5] but they have influenced clinical thinking because they have inevitably formalized the approach to the clinical and investigational information required for establishing the diagnosis of ALS from other conditions. In principle, these criteria seek to classify patients into categories—definite, probable, and possible ALS—according to the degree of clinical certainty. A fourth category of "not ALS" is used when the diagnosis has been positively excluded.

Definite Amyotrophic Lateral Sclerosis

The diagnosis of definite ALS requires the following features to be demonstrated:

1. The *presence* of the following:
   a. Evidence of *lower motor neuron (LMN) degeneration* by clinical, electrophysiological, or neuropathological examination
   b. Evidence of *upper motor neuron (UMN) degeneration* by clinical examination
   c. *Progressive spread of symptoms or signs* within a region or to other regions, as determined by history or examination
2. The *absence* of the following:
   a. *Electrophysiological or pathological evidence of other disease processes* that might explain the signs of LMN and/or UMN degeneration
   b. *Neuroimaging evidence of other disease processes* that might explain the observed clinical and electrophysiological signs

For a diagnosis of definite ALS, the patient must have UMN and LMN signs in at least three body regions (bulbar, upper limb, thoracic, or lower limb).

The criteria emphasize the importance of the appropriate use of electrophysiological investigation in the assessment of the distribution of LMN involvement, as well as in excluding other disorders, such as motor neuropathy. The following sections explain the different levels of certainty, other than definite ALS, regarding the diagnosis, based on these criteria.

Clinically Probable Amyotrophic Lateral Sclerosis

This category, of less certainty than definite ALS, is defined on clinical evidence alone by UMN and LMN signs in at least two regions with some UMN signs necessarily rostral to the LMN signs.

Clinically Probable: Laboratory-Supported Amyotrophic Lateral Sclerosis

This category requires clinical signs of UMN and LMN dysfunction in only one region, or it is when UMN signs without LMN features are present in one region and LMN signs defined by electromyographic (EMG) criteria are present in at least two limbs, with proper application of neuroimaging and clinical laboratory protocols to exclude other causes. Essentially it allows a diagnosis of probable ALS to be achieved without clinical evidence of involvement of two regions by the addition of EMG data, in the context of normal neuroimaging and other laboratory data.

Clinically Possible Amyotrophic Lateral Sclerosis

When clinical signs of UMN and LMN dysfunction are found in only one region or UMN signs are found alone in two or more regions, or when LMN signs are found rostral to UMN signs and the diagnosis of "clinically probable—laboratory-supported ALS" cannot be proven by clinical evidence alone or in conjunction with electrodiagnostic, neurophysiological, neuroimaging, or clinical laboratory studies, the diagnosis is even less certain. Other diagnoses must be excluded to accept a diagnosis of clinically possible ALS.

VALIDITY OF CONSENSUS CRITERIA FOR DIAGNOSIS OF AMYOTROPHIC LATERAL SCLEROSIS

The interpretation of these criteria in clinical usage in the clinical trial setting has been consistent. However, the criteria are not used routinely in clinical practice. Traynor et al[6] found that 67 percent of patients initially categorized as possible or suspected ALS, using the El Escorial definitions, progressed to definite ALS in the course of their disease. Nonetheless, 10 percent of patients failed to reach the definite category before death intervened, indicating the somewhat artificial nature of these rigorous criteria for defining ALS. The application of the Airlie House revision did not resolve this issue.

CLINICAL DIAGNOSIS IN PRACTICE

In practice, the diagnosis of ALS is made by a process of clinical logic that is defined both by the characteristics of the disease itself and by an intuitive process of decision making in which the clinician weights the clinical evidence according to an experiential model, built up from clinical experience gained over time. This process is common to all clinical diagnostic processes. It has been compared to Boolean logic, because crossings of informational boundaries, in relation to the presence or absence of certain phenomena, assume particular importance. The recognition of certain phenomena occurring together is also an important part of this process. Much depends therefore on the skill and acumen of the clinician in recognizing the presence of the relevant data. This is the point in the diagnostic process at which individual differences in diagnostic accuracy are likely to arise, because the skills involved are not necessarily achieved at the same level by individual clinicians. Although the El Escorial criteria are based on clinical experience and on the standard descriptions of ALS, these criteria rely on the presence of absolute features of UMN and LMN signs in three or more regions. The neurologist, perversely, will not wait for these features to develop before becoming convinced that the diagnosis is ALS, provided that all other possible causes of the syndrome are excluded by appropriate investigation. That is to say, the neurologist relies on a notion of the probability of the diagnosis, based on a combination of positive and negative information. Also important is the recognition that in clinical practice, treatment decisions are necessarily made as early as possible in the course of the disease, in response both to the patient's concerns and to the perceived benefit of starting treatment with riluzole as early as possible.

What Are the Crucial Clinical Data for Diagnosis of Amyotrophic Lateral Sclerosis?

The clinical features used in clinical practice to diagnose ALS include symptoms and signs of UMN and LMN involvement, in the patterns defined in the El Escorial criteria. In practice, even though the experienced clinician's diagnosis is made in relation to less secure clinical features than those spelled out in these research criteria, the diagnosis is relatively rarely incorrect. In the Scottish Motor Neuron Disease database, nonetheless, the diagnosis was incorrect in some 10 percent of cases[7] when reviewed later, and in an American database,[4] a similar rate of incorrect diagnoses was noted, especially when the diagnosis was made very early in the course of the disease. This is clearly important in establishing early treatment, as well as in considering entering a patient into a clinical trial of a putative new therapy. The most frequent missed diagnoses are multiple sclerosis, multifocal motor neuropathy with conduction block, chronic inflammatory demyelinating polyneuropathy and other neuropathies, and Kennedy's syndrome. Atypical, asymmetrical spinal muscular atrophy syndromes may also mimic ALS. PLS and the other related syndromes may also meld into the ALS syndrome as the disorder progresses, causing confusion that is perhaps not strictly of any clinical importance.

Fasciculation of the Tongue

Certain features have overwhelming significance in establishing a diagnosis of ALS. Bilateral fasciculation of the tongue has an approximately 90-percent specificity and sensitivity; unilateral fasciculation of the tongue is a less reliable sign of ALS, because other local causes may result in this phenomenon. Thus unequivocal evidence of fasciculation of the tongue is essential in considering the diagnosis. Fasciculation of the tongue in ALS is almost always accompanied by wasting of the tongue, but not necessarily by tongue weakness, dysarthria, or dysphagia. Fasciculation should be accepted as present only if it is seen when the tongue is at rest in the mouth. Fasciculation of the tongue may be increased when the tongue is protruded or tensed, but if it is seen only when the tongue is not at rest, it should be discounted, because a "fasciculatory contraction" of the tongue is frequent in normal persons. The presence of fasciculation of the tongue can be confirmed by EMG examination of the genioglossus muscle using a needle electrode insertion through the base of the tongue, beneath the jaw, or through the tongue itself.

Fasciculation in Limb Muscles

In many patients, retrospective consideration discloses that fasciculation commenced some months or weeks before the onset of weakness or wasting of muscles. Often this fasciculation is widespread, and sometimes it is of sudden onset. It may be continuous or intermittent, and it may vary in severity from day to day. Sometimes it may interrupt sleep or be apparent to the sleeping partner, even when the patient is unaware of it. There has been controversy concerning the origin of fasciculation in ALS, and many attempts have been made to differentiate fasciculation occurring in ALS from that found in other neurogenic disorders, as well as in normal subjects. For example, Trojaborg and Buchthal[8] considered that fasciculations repeating at slow frequencies (slower than 4 Hz) were characteristic of ALS and termed these slow fasciculations "malignant fasciculation," whereas fasciculations repeating at faster frequencies were not indicative of ALS and were termed "benign fasciculations." In general, though not an absolute phenomenon,[9,10] this distinction has proven useful in EMG work. Fasciculation potentials in ALS are repeated at slower rates than those occurring in normal subjects, because fasciculations in ALS occur in motor units that have been reinnervated, and that therefore fire at slower rates than normal motor units.

More recent work has shown that fasciculations may originate at any point in the motor unit and not solely at the motor neuron soma, as suggested by Denny-Brown and Foley.[11] Fasciculations tend to occur at the motor neuron level in the early stages of ALS, and more peripherally later in the disease, when there are electrically unstable portions of the axon and its branches, following reinnervation and axonal sprouting. Fasciculation occurs in other neurogenic disorders, for example, in peripheral neuropathies, such as the Charcot-Marie-Tooth syndromes, and in the spinal muscular atrophies. In the latter, fasciculations are often not apparent to inspection but become visible after exercise or can be induced by limb hypoxia, such as after the application of a tourniquet or after administration of an anticholinesterase drug. In normal subjects, fasciculation potentials similarly occur commonly after exercise, especially in physically unfit subjects. In normal subjects, fasciculation potentials arise in normal motor units, so they fire faster and are less complex (simple fasciculations) than those in the reinnervated units of muscles damaged by a neurogenic disorder. In ALS, fasciculation potentials are not only more complex in the later stages of the disease, reflecting greater reinnervation and larger motor units, but many may also be recruited voluntarily, indicating that fasciculations arise not in completely denervated motor unit territories, but in motor units damaged by a combination of denervation and reinnervation.[12] They differ fundamentally from fibrillation potentials in that the latter arise in single muscle fibers that have been denervated and are not capable of voluntary recruitment.

Because fasciculation potentials arise in the context of instability of nerve or motor neuron membranes, spontaneous and repetitive firing of the motor unit occurs.[13] Normally the axonal membrane is stable at a membrane potential of about 70 mV, but there are other possible voltages at which temporary membrane stability may be achieved. Bostock and Bergmans[14] have shown that in partial denervation and in certain other nonpathological states, the axonal membrane may show bistability, achieving stability at two points above and below the normal threshold. When this arises, spontaneous firing may occur, generated at the abnormal bistable portion of the axonal membrane, with oscillation between the two points of membrane stability. Recurrent fasciculation potentials may thus be generated.[14,15] In association with fasciculations, other spontaneous neurally generated muscle contractions may occur, including myokymia and cramp.

Myokymia and Cramp

Both myokymia and cramp are frequent and characteristic clinical phenomena in ALS. However, they also occur frequently in normal subjects, in a number of other neuromuscular diseases, especially other neurogenic disorders, and in certain metabolic muscle diseases. The latter includes principally those involving oxidative or energy metabolism such as mitochondrial myopathies and glycogen storage diseases, such as McArdle myophosphorylase deficiency.

Myokymia consists of a painless, rapid, repeated contraction of a group of muscle fibers, representing several motor units firing at a rate of 20 to 40 Hz.[13] In normal subjects, myokymia is especially common in the soleus muscle and in the orbicularis oculi, where it is often a feature of mild hyperventilation associated with anxiety. Cramp is an everyday experience for most people, consisting of the sudden buildup of a painful contraction of the whole muscle or part (at least of several fascicles) of the muscle.

Although it may appear to occur without cause, cramp usually occurs in response to a cutaneous stimulus, especially cold. Cramp is especially common in the calf muscles as a result of getting into a cold bed. It occurs as a particular feature in limbs rendered vulnerable by hypoxic stress when there is vascular impairment in the leg, as well as in neurogenic disorders, such as ALS. In ALS, both myokymia and cramp occur when there is partial denervation and reinnervation, in association with the bistability of the axonal membrane. Cramps, induced by cutaneous stimuli, can be arrested by stimulation of the nerve or the skin overlying the cramped muscle,[14,15] which reduces the motoneuronal excitability and allows the cramp to be inhibited. Similarly mechanical stretching of the cramped muscle will abort the contraction, probably by exciting stretch receptors in the affected muscle. The essential mechanism of cramp in neurogenic disorders is therefore that it is a neurogenic contraction that is stimulus sensitive both in its initiation and in its arrest. In metabolic muscle disease, by contrast, the cramp is induced by the accumulation of lactate or other metabolites, causing failure of the process of muscle relaxation, an energy-dependent process.

Because fasciculation, myokymia, and cramp occur frequently in normal subjects,[13] the occurrence of these phenomena in ALS is important only insofar as they may occur in the early stages of the disease and therefore may be used to indicate the onset of the first features of the disease process. They are important in diagnosis only when they occur in the context of clinical evidence of denervation and reinnervation.[16] A careful EMG examination is often required to be certain of the absence of chronic partial denervation with unstable motor unit potentials, indicating the active denervating process that is so characteristic of ALS. Fasciculations, myokymia, and cramp occurring without these additional features are not in themselves diagnostic features of ALS and most frequently are benign phenomena.

Lower Motor Neuron Signs

Involvement of the LMN is in many ways a hallmark of ALS, but it also occurs with other diseases in which involvement of the LMN occurs, for example, in peripheral neuropathy and in motor nerve root lesions. Therefore we have three issues to consider; First, are there symptoms and signs of LMN involvement; second, is the distribution of these abnormalities commensurate with multiple root lesions, with peripheral neuropathy, or with anterior horn cell disease; and third, is the LMN abnormality consistent with ALS or with another anterior horn cell disease, such as spinal muscular atrophy?

Clinically, LMN signs include weakness, atrophy of the affected muscle, fasciculations, and reduced or absent tendon reflexes. In addition, when there is chronic stable reinnervation, there is often visible irregular recruitment of fascicles of muscle, consisting of reinnervated and enlarged motor units. This "fascicular" pattern of recruitment of an atrophic weakened muscle[16] is characteristically found in spinal muscular atrophy, in chronic relatively nonprogressive peripheral neuropathies, such as one of the Charcot-Marie-Tooth syndromes, or syringomyelia. It may also occur in the distribution of an affected nerve root in spinal cord or cervical root disease. In ALS, by contrast, the neurogenic process is relatively rapidly progressive, and in many patients, the denervating process proceeds too quickly for this reinnervative process to become clinically detectable on clinical examination. There is both EMG and histological evidence that reinnervation in ALS is less efficient than in other neurogenic conditions.[17] This is probably due in part to the rapidity of the denervation process and in part to impairment of the reinnervative capacity as a result of a metabolic abnormality on surviving motor neurons, possibly involving defective axonal transport.

The severity of weakness in ALS depends on the extent of denervation and the effectiveness of any compensatory reinnervation. A further factor is the result of abnormality in the UMN. The role of the UMN lesion in weakness in ALS has so far proven difficult to assess,[16] because of the severity of the LMN disorder in most cases. It is evident that the force generated by a muscle depends on the number of innervated muscle fibers contained within the functional mass of the muscle, the cross-sectional size of the muscle fibers, and their metabolic integrity in force generation. The severity of any LMN lesion is therefore likely to be of major importance as a cause of weakness. This accords with clinical experience in other disorders, such as peripheral neuropathy, motor root lesions, and other anterior horn cell disorders in which there is no UMN lesion, such as spinal muscular atrophy and poliomyelitis.

One additional factor leading to weakness in a debilitating disease such as ALS is the effect of deconditioning of muscle resulting from reduced physical activity. The patient with muscular weakness confined to bed is likely to develop increased weakness. A well-recognized example is the increased weakness that occurs in patients with old polio, spinal muscular atrophy, or muscular dystrophy who are confined to bed after an intercurrent surgical procedure. There may be marked disability when the patient is mobilized, and an exercise program lasting many weeks may be required before recovery is achieved.[16]

Upper Motor Neuron Signs

The recognition of UMN signs in ALS has been a source of controversy for many years. UMN signs are usually recognized by the presence of spasticity, brisk tendon reflexes, and extensor plantar responses. Weakness is also characteristic of UMN lesions but may not be a feature in minor UMN abnormalities. In certain UMN lesions, as in familial spastic paraplegia, spasticity may be very severe, without weakness.

The extensor plantar response is particularly important in the assessment of suspected corticospinal abnormalities. It may be difficult to elicit, especially when there is an associated LMN abnormality in the foot and toe extensor muscles, thus invalidating the response. Indeed, in some peripheral neuropathies, when there is selective weakness of the toe flexors, there may be an apparent extensor toe response. Thus false-positive and false-negative responses may occur in certain clinical situations. However, in suspected ALS, neurologists regard the finding of an extensor plantar response as a sign with high significance in relation to the demonstration of abnormality in the corticospinal pathway. Much depends therefore on careful clinical technique.[18] The response should be sought by deep pressure, almost amounting to the use of a painful stimulus, applied to the lateral aspect of the foot, in a sweeping motion extending from the heel toward the little toe. A medial sweep of the stimulus, usually a key or blunt object, onto the forefoot, beneath the heads of the metatarsals, running across as far as the head of the first metatarsal, is commonly added to the lateral stimulus, but this was not described by Babinski in his original report and is of dubious validity, particularly because if it is applied to the arch of the foot itself, it may form part of a stimulus leading to plantar grasping and thus to flexion of the foot. The Babinski response is itself best considered part of the nociceptive flexion withdrawal response, anatomically termed *extension,* and thus a feature released by the corticospinal lesion. In complete cord lesions, the Babinski response is very active, and in this situation the anterior horn cell pool generating the response is excited by a nonspindle afferent system, applied to neurons that are separated entirely from their supranuclear, corticospinal connections. The Babinski response is a multisynaptic recruitment of a pool of motor neurons disinhibited from supranuclear influences.

Spasticity, unlike the Babinski response, is a spindle-derived response caused by excitation of velocity-dependent primary and secondary sensory endings.

This feature is modulated by cutaneous sensory input, such as the increased excitation that results from cutaneous infection or pressure ulcers or from bladder infection. In ALS, spasticity is usually a relatively minor feature, although in PLS, spasticity predominates and there is no detectable LMN involvement, except perhaps in the later stages of this syndrome. The detection of spasticity involves the presence of muscle and therefore of muscle force. When there is a very marked LMN abnormality, spasticity will be difficult to detect.

In ALS, detection of a corticospinal abnormality often depends on subjective interpretation of the significance of the activity of the tendon reflexes to standard clinical testing with a tendon hammer. This is essentially a matter of clinical experience, and interpretation will vary between observers. In a weak and atrophic muscle with an LMN lesion, the tendon reflexes will be absent, but when there is an associated UMN lesion, the tendon reflex may again be detectable. In this situation (i.e., when there are signs of an LMN lesion), the presence of a tendon reflex suggests that there is also involvement of the UMN. Interpretation of this combination is clinically contentious but important. In essence, the presence of a brisk reflex in a wasted fasciculating muscle is evidence of an associated UMN lesion.

Special Diagnostic Features

A number of features of ALS are of interest but are scientifically unexplained in relation to current concepts on pathogenesis. In most cases, the disease presents with focal involvement before progression occurs and the disease becomes more widespread. Thus there may be wasting and weakness of a hand, a foot, or a shoulder in about 80 percent of cases. Often one limb is involved much more prominently than the opposite side, prompting suggestions that ALS is a myotomal disorder. However, EMG studies, as well as careful clinical observations, clearly show that there is more widespread involvement even at the onset than would initially be suspected from the history alone. The early pattern of progression determines the outcome of the disease.[19]

Bulbar involvement is a presenting feature of the remaining 20 percent. The muscles of respiration are affected when there is cervical involvement; primary involvement of these muscles at the onset of the disease is rare, occurring in fewer than 2 percent of cases, although respiratory failure from muscle weakness is the usual mode of death. The muscles of respiration are innervated by the third, fourth, and fifth cervical segments that supply the diaphragm, together with the thoracic segmental nerves innervating the intercostal muscles, and the lowermost cranial nerves supplying the tongue, palate, and sternomastoid and trapezius muscles. Despite this cervical pattern of innervation, even in patients with the "flail arm" clinical phenotype, in which there is predominant LMN involvement in a cervical distribution, often without prominent UMN features, the respiratory muscles are often relatively spared and life expectancy is long.[20–22] In the more common Charcot form of ALS, however, ventilatory involvement is the rate-limiting feature that determines survival.

In general, it is virtually impossible to separate the effects of LMN and UMN disease on the bulbar muscles; for example, on the tongue or the palate or quality of speech. However, prominent bulbar involvement is associated with released involuntary laughing, crying, and sometimes both. This feature is associated with disconnection of bulbar centers from the frontal and temporal cortical areas controlling mood and emotional expression. Patients with released emotionality also are more likely to show blunting of affect and impaired judgment in tests of frontal executive function, corresponding to degeneration of frontal and temporal cortical neurons with cytoplasmic inclusions and "ubiquitinated" proteinaceous inclusions in surviving cortical neurons.[23–25] These neurons are anterior to the classic motor and premotor cortex but are part of the executive brain and thus are biologically susceptible to the degenerative process. Initial bulbar involvement is more common in women than in men, in a proportion of about 2 : 1, but whether this reflects some hormonally determined susceptibility is not known.

Primary involvement of external ocular muscles is never seen, and indeed, the external ocular muscles are characteristically spared even late in the natural history of the disease. Similarly, the pelvic sphincter muscles function normally throughout the course of the disease, although both EMG and pathological studies show that there is some loss of motor neurons in the Onuf nucleus, which innervates the voluntary striated pelvic floor sphincter muscles. Laryngeal abductor muscles and the cricopharyngeal sphincter also are relatively spared, perhaps reflecting their mainly tonic function.

A proportion of patients show signs of extrapyramidal dysfunction with impaired postural reflexes and thus instability of balance and stance.[26] The pathological correlate of this clinical observation has not been established.

There is no recognized association between the onset of ALS and the overuse of certain muscle groups in work or sport. Although there are many reports of the onset of ALS among prominent sports people, epidemiological studies do not suggest that athleticism is more than a minor factor, if it is at all relevant to the cause of the disease. Similarly, an association of trauma with the onset of ALS is unlikely, and case-control studies have tended to discount any such suggestion.[27]

EARLY AND LATE DIAGNOSIS

When the disease is advanced, diagnosis is relatively easy, but in the early stages of the disease, diagnosis is much more difficult, depending principally on the distribution of LMN and UMN features in the four body regions described in the El Escorial criteria. Most clinicians, however, suspect a diagnosis of ALS when there are signs of both LMN and UMN involvement in the same muscle or a group of muscles in a spinal segment. This particularly applies to the cervical and lumbar segments, although the possibility of spondylosis with cord and root involvement must always be excluded by appropriate clinical investigation. Other disorders such as systemic lupus erythematosus and combined conditions including cerebrovascular disease and spondylotic root disease also need consideration. Multifocal motor neuropathy, discussed elsewhere in this book, is of practical importance because unlike ALS, it responds to treatment, at least in its early stages. Multiple sclerosis is also an important condition to consider in the differential diagnosis. Early diagnosis therefore remains a difficult but important issue in the management of ALS. It is likely that any new therapy would be more effective in terms of delaying disability if applied in the early stages of the disease, before there has been massive loss of UMNs and LMNs.[28,29] The long delay between first symptom and neurological diagnosis, which appears to be a common experience in many countries, is an issue that must be addressed when an effective therapy becomes available.

Weight Loss

Loss of body weight is a sign of poor nutrition, as well as of loss of muscle mass from denervation and disuse. A rapid loss of weight is almost always a sign of malnutrition, due to difficulty swallowing. This is an indication for intervention, first by an assessment by a speech and language therapist and second by barium swallow. Once pooling in the pharynx, or misdirection of swallowed food, has been demonstrated, placement of a percutaneous endoscopic gastrostomy (PEG) should be discussed. In ALS, dysphagia occurs from weakness of the glossal and pharyngeal phases of swallowing, and these are difficult to assess on ordinary clinical examination, hence the importance of careful attention to body weight.

There has been much discussion about placement of PEG in patients with impaired vital capacity. Recommendations published in approved guidelines are arbitrary but are generally accepted as conservative and appropriate. In general, a vital capacity (VC) of less than 50 percent of the predicted value is regarded as conferring increased risk to the procedure of placement of a PEG by conventional means. In practice, however, the VC is often near or at this level when PEG placement is deemed necessary or, more importantly, accepted by the patient. Education before the need arises is clearly of fundamental importance.

Quality of Life

It is a truism that quality of life (QoL) is what a patient says it is, not what an observer judges it to be. People with ALS often claim a good QoL when an observer might think otherwise, but such is the struggle for survival and the determination to keep going, that this view must be respected. An alternative view of this situation is that frontal lobe involvement prevents the patient from fully recognizing the full horror of the situation. Doubtless, some component of each factor is operative. Paradoxically, depression is frequently not far away nonetheless.[30] The stress on caregivers has only recently begun to be studied and is often extreme, both personally and economically.

CLINICAL PRINCIPLES

Clinical principles are few but must be remembered. The *history* is essential in the diagnosis, including descriptions of fasciculations, spasms and cramps, and weakness and wasting. The description of the most essential feature—*progression* of the cardinal features of the disease—is entirely dependent on the history. It is exceptional for there to be any phase of minor improvement in ALS, although some variation in function in individual muscle groups may occur. Once this has been established, the diagnosis rests on firmer ground, provided that no other inconsistent features such as prominent pain, sensory loss, or sphincter involvement become evident as the disease progresses.

The *examination,* as in any neurological disease, is a snapshot of the disease at the time of the assessment. Its distribution and severity, the association with the cardinal features, and the absence of any other inconsistent features can be ascertained at that time.

Investigation is designed to exclude other diseases and therefore includes neuroimaging, a number of biochemical and hematological tests, and an EMG to ascertain the extent of LMN involvement.

FOLLOW-UP

Continued follow-up is essential, not only to reassess the diagnosis as the disease progresses but also to ensure adequate management of developing disabilities. Always be sure to re-examine the patient from time to time. In the event that an effective therapy is found, the establishment of the diagnosis will become both more important and more difficult because the expression of the disease will have been modified by therapy. The current lack of a simple diagnostic test will then become all the more crucial as a requirement for future research.

REFERENCES

1. Swash M, Desai J. Motor neuron disease: classification and nomenclature. Amyotroph Lateral Scler Other Motor Neuron Disord 2000;1:105–112.
2. Charcot JM, Joffroy A. Deux cas d'atrophie musculaire progressive avec lésions de la substance grise et des faisceaux antero-latéraux de la moelle epinière. Arch Physiol Neurol Pathol 1869;2:744.
3. Subcommittee on Motor Neuron Diseases of World Federation of Neurology Research Group on Neuromuscular Diseases. El Escorial "clinical limits of ALS" workshop contributors. El Escorial World Federation of Neurology criteria for the diagnosis of amyotrophic lateral sclerosis. J Neurol Sci 1994;124:96–107.
4. Brooks BR, Miller RG, Swash M, et al. World Federation of Neurology Research Group on Motor Neuron Diseases. El Escorial revisited; revised criteria for the diagnosis of amyotrophic lateral sclerosis. Amyotroph Lateral Scler Other Motor Neuron Disord 2000;1:293–299.
5. Belsh JM. ALS diagnostic criteria of El Escorial revisited: do they meet the needs of clinicians as well as researchers? Amyotroph Lateral Scler Other Motor Neuron Disord 2000;1(suppl 1):S57–S60.
6. Traynor BJ, Codd MB, Corr B, et al. Clinical features of amyotrophic lateral sclerosis according to the El Escorial and Airlie House diagnostic criteria. A population based study. Arch Neurol 2000;57:1171–1176.
7. Chancellor AM, Slattery JM, Fraser H, et al. The prognosis of adult-onset motor neuron disease: a prospective study based on the Scottish Motor Neuron Disease Register. J Neurol 1993;240:339–346.
8. Trojaborg W, Buchthal F. Malignant and benign fasciculation. Acta Neurol Scand 1965;41(suppl 13):251–254.

9. Eisen A, Stewart H. Not-so-benign fasciculation. Ann Neurol 1994;35:375.
10. Reed DM, Kurland LT. Muscle fasciculations in a healthy population. Arch Neurol 1963;9: 363–367.
11. Denny-Brown D, Foley JM. Myokymia and benign fasciculation of muscle. Trans Assoc Am Physicians 1948;61:88–96.
12. De Carvalho M, Swash M. Fasciculation potentials in amyotrophic lateral sclerosis and other neurogenic disorders. Muscle Nerve 1998;21:336–344.
13. Layzer RB. The origin of muscle fasciculations and cramps. Muscle Nerve 1994;17:1243–1249.
14. Bostock H, Bergmans J. Post-tetanic excitability changes and ectopic discharges in a human motor axon. Brain 1994;117:913–928.
15. Baldissera F, Cavalleri P, Dworzak F. Motor neuron "bistability:" a pathogenetic mechanism for cramps and myokymia. Brain 1994;117:929–940.
16. Swash M, Schwartz MS. Neuromuscular Disorders (3rd ed). London: Springer-Verlag, 1997.
17. Wohlfart G. Collateral regeneration from residual motor nerve fibers in amyotrophic lateral sclerosis. Neurology 1957;7:124–134.
18. Van Gijn J. The Babinski Sign—A Centenary. Utrecht: University of Utrecht, 1996.
19. Chiò A, Mora G, Leone M, et al. Early symptom progression rate is related to ALS outcome. A prospective population-based study. Neurology 2002;59:99–103.
20. Katz JS, Wolfe F, Andersson PB, et al. Brachial amyotrophic diplegia. A slowly progressive motor neuron disorder. Neurology 1999;53:1071–1076.
21. Rosenfield H, Chang SW, Jackson CE, et al. Lower extremity amyotrophic diplegia (LAD): a new clinical entity in the spectrum of motor neuron disease. Neurology 2002:58(suppl 3):A411.
22. Hu MTM, Ellis CM, Al-Chalabi, et al. Flail arm syndrome: a distinctive variant of amyotrophic lateral sclerosis. J Neurol Neurosurg Psychiatry 1998;65:950–951.
23. Hudson A. Amyotrophic lateral sclerosis and its association with dementia. Brain 1991;194: 217–247.
24. Neary D, Snowden JS, Northern B, et al. Dementia of frontal lobe type. J Neurol Neurosurg Psychiatry 1988;51:353–361.
25. Neary D, Snowden JS, Mann DM. Cognitive change in motor neurone disease/amyotrophic lateral sclerosis (MND/ALS). J Neurol Sci 2000;180(1–2):15–20.
26. Desai J, Swash M. Extrapyramidal involvement in ALS: backward falls and retropulsion. J Neurol Neurosurg Psychiatry 1999;67:214–216.
27. Kondo K, Tsubaki T. Case control studies of motor neuron disease: association with mechanical trauma. Arch Neurol 1981;38:220–226.
28. Swash M. Early diagnosis of ALS. J Neurol Sci 1998;160:S33-S36.
29. Househam E, Swash M. Diagnostic delay in ALS: what scope for improvement? J Neurol Sci 2000;180:76–81.
30. Peto V, Jenkinson C, Fitzpatrick R, et al, and the ALS-HPS Steering Group. Measuring mental health in amyotrophic lateral sclerosis (ALS): a comparison of the SF-36 Mental Health Index with the Psychological General Well-Being Index. Amyotroph Lateral Scler Other Motor Neuron Disord 2002.

2
Pathology of Motor Neuron Disorders

Stephen Wharton and Paul G. Ince

The disorders discussed in this chapter are characterized by pathologies primarily affecting the motor system within the central nervous system (CNS). For this purpose, we define the motor system to include the following: cortical projection neurons of the motor and premotor cortex, especially the classic upper motor neuron (UMN) "Betz cell" population (Figure 2.1); their axons throughout the hemispheric white matter, internal capsule, pyramids, and ventrolateral spinal tracts (i.e., the direct and indirect corticospinal tracts)[1]; and the lower motor neuron (LMN) pools of the brain stem motor nuclei and the spinal anterior horn (see Figure 2.1). The pathology of these disorders varies anatomically, both in the components of the motor system affected and in their cellular and molecular pathology. This pathological variation is a likely reflection of the variable mechanisms through which the motor system can be selectively damaged. In some cases—for example, those resulting from inherited genetic defects—the etiology is known and an understanding of gene function or the consequences of abnormal gene products is revealing mechanisms linked to cell injury and cell death, and illuminating the selective distribution of degeneration. For example, in the case of amyotrophic lateral sclerosis (ALS), in which some familial cases are caused by mutations in SOD1, the similarity of pathology between familial and sporadic disease is beginning to cast light on the pathogenesis of the more common sporadic form. Although the clinical and pathological manifestations of these disorders are predominantly motor oriented, they also often show pathological involvement of other systems within the CNS, implying a hierarchy of, rather than absolute, selective vulnerability. No classification yet devised satisfactorily accounts for this complexity of genetic, pathological, clinical, and pathophysiological data across this spectrum of disorders. We have therefore chosen to group the disorders into three categories according to the anatomical patterns of disease: (1) predominantly LMN disorders (spinal muscular atrophy [SMA], X-linked spinobulbar muscular atrophy [X-SBMA or Kennedy's disease], postpolio muscular atrophy [PPMA]); (2) mixed UMN and LMN disorders of ALS and variants; (3) predominantly UMN disorders, e.g., hereditary spastic paraparesis (HSP). Where

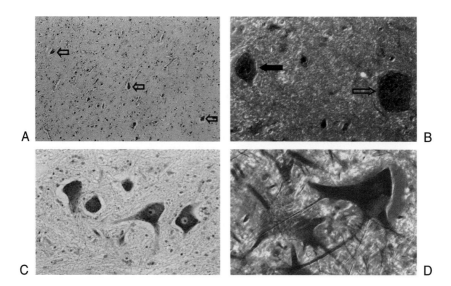

Figure 2.1 (**A**) Normal upper motor neurons (Betz cells) in layer V of the motor cortex *(open arrows)*. (**B**) The neuronal cell body is conspicuously larger than that of adjacent cortical pyramidal neurons and shows a pattern of large dispersed Nissl bodies *(open arrow)* in contrast to the fine peripheral Nissl substance of other pyramidal cell populations *(solid arrowhead)*. (**C**) The lower motor neurons are similar in size, but with a more angulated morphology, and are more densely packed in the ventral horn. (**D**) Major dendrites are more conspicuous than in Betz cells.

we mention primary lateral sclerosis (PLS), we do so in the section on ALS because we regard this syndrome as a relatively pure UMN variant of that disorder.

LOWER MOTOR NEURON DISORDERS

Spinal Muscular Atrophy

Clinical Phenotype

The spinal muscular atrophies are inherited, degenerative disorders that affect LMNs, producing weakness, but are not typically accompanied by UMN or sensory involvement. They may be classified clinically according to age at onset and clinical severity. In SMA-I (Werdnig-Hoffmann disease), onset is usually before 9 months and may present with neonatal hypotonia, so the disease process may begin in utero. Affected infants fail to achieve early motor milestones and are never able to sit. Death from respiratory failure usually occurs within the first 2 years of life. SMA-II, the intermediate or chronic infantile form, has an onset at around 3 to 15 months; these children may sit but do not become ambulant. SMA-III (Kugelberg-Welander disease) has an onset from 1 to 15 years, and these children are able to achieve walking and generally live into adulthood.[2,3] This older group has presented a clinicopathological challenge in terms of their separation from long-duration forms of a pure lower motor variant of ALS. (Also see Chapter 16.)

Genetic Basis of Spinal Muscular Atrophy Types I through III: Pathogenetic Mechanisms

SMA types I through III are inherited as autosomal recessive disorders and are linked to mutations on the long arm of chromosome 5. The region involved contains four genes: the survival motor neuron (SMN) gene; the neuronal apoptosis inhibitory protein (NAIP) gene; p44 encoding a subunit of transcription factor TFIIH; and H4F5. This gene region is duplicated, and it is a mutation of the telomeric SMN gene, SMN1, which gives rise to SMA. Most cases have a homozygous SMN1 deletion, but a minority shows more subtle mutations. SMN1 deletion underlies all three clinical forms, but there is an increase in the copy number of the centromeric SMN gene, SMN2, in milder clinical forms, suggesting a model whereby SMN1 deletion underlies SMA-I, but conversion of SMN1 to SMN2 underlies the milder phenotypes, SMA-II and SMA-III. SMN2 may only be able to partially compensate for loss of activity in the SMN1 locus because SMN2 encodes for an alternatively spliced transcript, due to a C-to-T transition at codon 280 that lacks exon 7.[2,4,5] Identification of these genetic changes has allowed recognition of wider phenotypes associated with SMN mutations including congenital arthrogryposis and congenital cytoplasmic body myopathy.[6,7] An understanding of the function of the SMN protein should illuminate the selective nature of the LMN pathology in SMA. SMN protein is widely expressed in normal tissues, whereas in SMA, its concentration is reduced in proportion to disease severity.[8] In the normal brain and spinal cord, SMN is expressed from early fetal life, consistent with the idea that the pathology begins in utero.[9] SMN protein is strongly expressed in motor neurons, in neuronal populations not clinically affected in SMA, and in non-CNS tissues. Selective motor neuron degeneration in SMA is not accounted for by restricted tissue expression of the SMN gene.

SMN is localized both in the cytoplasm and in nuclei. Nuclear expression of SMN is related to novel structures called *gems* (gemini of coiled bodies) or in coiled bodies (Cajal bodies) with which gems are closely associated, where it binds to proteins involved in RNA metabolism. There is evidence for a role in the assembly and function of spliceosomal complexes, suggesting a role in pre–messenger RNA (mRNA) splicing and possibly other functions in RNA processing. The pathology of SMA may therefore be related to disturbed RNA metabolism, although how this might relate to the selectivity and mechanism of cellular pathology is yet to be determined. Possible mechanisms include loss of SMN function below a threshold required for motor neuron survival, or there may be impairment of a function specific to motor neurons.[2,10–12] Spinal motor neurons show some differences in the morphology of gems and coiled bodies, compared with other cell types. In most cell types, these structures are more numerous in the fetus, where they are separate structures, and they show increasing co-localization with age. In motor neurons, gems and coiled bodies are more numerous in the adult, show earlier co-localization, and form large bodies around the nucleolar perimeter. There are also differences in the nuclear distribution of SMN protein.[13] The possibility is raised therefore that there are unique features of the function of this subcellular organelle system that may underlie the susceptibility of motor neurons to a decrease in SMN levels. SMN has also been implicated in the regulation of apoptosis, a possible mechanism of cell death in SMA. SMN may interact with Bcl-2 to abrogate apoptosis induced by Bax and Fas.[4,14] However, whether the pathogenesis of SMA involves the aberrant regulation of apoptosis, and similarly whether there may be a modulating role for NAIP, have not been ascertained.

Central Nervous System Pathology of Spinal Muscular Atrophy

Autopsy studies of SMA-I have demonstrated loss of motor neurons from the anterior horns of the spinal cord and brain stem motor nuclei (Figure 2.2), with preservation of UMNs and of the corticospinal tracts. Remaining anterior horn

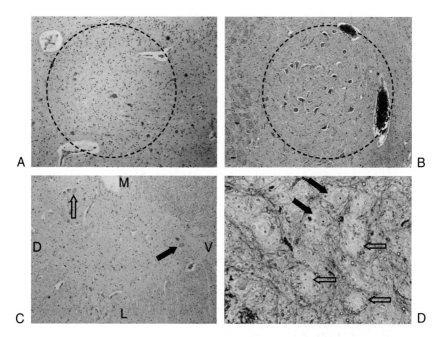

Figure 2.2 Gross depletion of (**A**) motor neurons in spinal muscular atrophy type I (ubiquitin ICC, ×4) contrasts with the (**B**) normal hypoglossal nucleus in the medulla, showing a scattered population of lower motor neurons (H&E, ×4). (**C**) In the spinal ventral horn (ubiquitin ICC, ×4), there are only two surviving motor neurons *(solid arrow),* one of which shows "chromatolytic" swelling. The neurons of the Clarke's column (spinocerebellar nucleus) show good cell preservation, although a swollen neuron is present *(clear arrow)* (D = dorsal; L = lateral; M = medial; V = ventral). (**D**) In the lumbar ventral horn (Luxol fast blue, ×20), two surviving normal motor neurons are present *(solid arrows),* together with frequent "empty beds" in which motor neurons have been destroyed *(clear arrows).*

motor neurons show swelling (ballooned neurons) and loss of Nissl substance reminiscent of chromatolysis (Figure 2.3). Occasional neurons appear atrophic or show neuronophagia, surrounded by microglia. "Empty beds," in which the neuron has been lost leaving a space surrounded by glial fibers, are described (see Figure 2.2). The anterior horns show astrocytic gliosis, most conspicuous at the gray-white matter junction. As expected from the profound anterior horn cell loss, there is a loss of myelinated axons from anterior nerve roots. Heterotopic motor neurons and bundles of astroglia have also been described in anterior nerve roots but are probably not a specific pathology. Motor neurons of the trigeminal, facial, hypoglossal, and nucleus ambiguus nerve nuclei show similar changes. Ballooned neurons may also be observed within the thoracic nucleus (Clarke's nucleus) of the spinal cord, in the ventrolateral region of the thalamus and with nodules of Nageotte in dorsal root ganglia.[3,15–20] Therefore though clinically a disease of the LMN, the pathology of SMA can be a multisystem disorder. Extraocular muscle involvement is not a clinical feature, but motor neurons of the extraocular muscle nuclei may show chromatolysis.[21] Onuf's nucleus in the sacral spinal cord is preserved, although occasional chromatolytic neurons occur.[22,23] The neuropathology of Kugelberg-Welander disease (SMA-III) has been less well studied. The disease is characterized by loss of anterior horn cells and anterior horn gliosis. Remaining motor neurons appear small and pyknotic. UMNs and corticospinal tracts appear unaffected.[24]

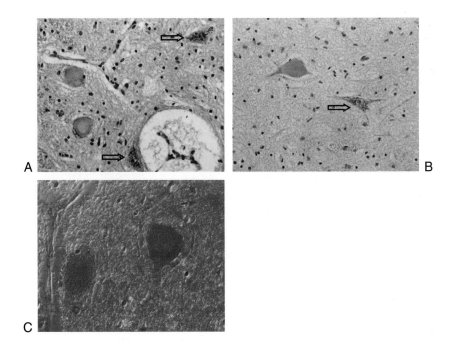

Figure 2.3 (**A**) Two "chromatolytic" swollen neurons in the hypoglossal nucleus in spinal muscular atrophy type I (H&E, ×20) contrast with two normal-appearing lower motor neurons *(clear arrows)*. These swollen neurons show (**B**) a diffuse low-intensity immunoreactivity for ubiquitin (ubiquitin ICC, ×20), compared with a normal negatively staining neuron *(clear arrow),* and (**C**) no discrete inclusion bodies (ubiquitin ICC, ×40).

The ballooned neurons seen in Werdnig-Hoffmann disease resemble chromatolytic neurons, a hypertrophic change that neurons undergo in response to axonal damage. However, more detailed analyses of ballooned neurons reveal differences from the chromatolytic neurons of the axon reaction. Ultrastructural studies have demonstrated a loose accumulation of intermediate filaments at the periphery of the neuron with an accumulation of mitochondria, vesicles, and lysosomes in the center. Incarcerated synaptic boutons are seen within the cytoplasm at the cell periphery.[17,25] These ultrastructural abnormalities are accompanied by abnormal protein expression. Ballooned neurons show a loss of membrane synaptophysin but increased cytoplasmic expression.[26] In normal neurons, neurofilaments become phosphorylated within the axonal compartment. Ballooned neurons, however, demonstrate phosphorylated neurofilaments within the perikaryon. In chromatolysis, phosphorylated neurofilament staining is diffuse, whereas in the ballooned neurons of SMA, it appears as a band around the periphery of the cytoplasm, corresponding to the site of filament accumulation seen by electron microscopy. There is an abnormal pattern of diffuse ubiquitin staining (see Figure 2.3), particularly in the central perikaryon, in contrast to the inclusions observed in ALS.[2,15,17,21,25,27] There are also changes in the distribution of certain enzymes and in patterns of glycosylation.[25] Abnormal phosphorylation and glycosylation of neurofilament proteins may imply that defects in neurofilament assembly and function are involved in the pathogenesis of this disorder.

A number of studies have addressed the potential role of apoptosis in neuronal cell death in SMA. Studies using the TUNEL staining method report variable results in anterior horn motor neurons,[18,20] but positive results are also reported in the ventrolateral thalamic nucleus. Ultrastructural changes supportive of apoptosis including loss of Bcl-2 expression and strong p53 expression are also reported in motor neurons.[20] The number of TUNEL-positive motor neurons is low in the positive studies, as might be expected in a slowly progressive disorder. TUNEL positivity was also observed in microglia and was interpreted as phagocytosis of DNA from apoptotic cells.[20] A high proportion of TUNEL-positive anterior horn neurons have been reported, accompanied by neuronal loss, in 12-week-old fetal SMA spinal cord.[28] Autopsy studies are limited by the necessity of looking at endstage disease in SMA, and TUNEL staining, though reflecting DNA damage, does not appear to be specific to apoptosis.[29] The potential function of SMN and NAIPs may suggest a central role for dysregulation of apoptosis in the pathogenesis of SMA, but given the evidence for the function of SMN in RNA metabolism, other pathogenetic mechanisms may be pre-eminent. The importance of apoptosis and of apoptosis-regulatory mechanisms in SMA therefore remains to be determined.

Muscle Pathology in Spinal Muscular Atrophy

The muscle biopsy in SMA-III shows appearances typical of chronic neurogenic atrophy, with small angular fibers, small group atrophy, and fiber typing grouping indicative of reinnervation. These changes are accompanied by secondary myopathic changes that may correlate with a raised serum creatine kinase level.[24,30] These appearances differ somewhat from those seen in

SMA-I and SMA-II, in which skeletal muscle shows large groups of atrophic fibers that may involve whole fascicles (Figure 2.4). The atrophic fibers are small and rounded, rather than angulated, and may be of type I or II, usually distributed in a normal checkerboard pattern. Fewer fibers of normal or hypertrophic size are scattered among the atrophic groups, and these are most commonly of type I in myofibrillar adenosine triphosphatase (ATPase) preparations.[2,30] Immunohistochemical studies have demonstrated widespread expression of neural cell adhesion molecule (NCAM) on small and large muscle fibers in SMA-I, whereas in SMA-III, only the small fibers are NCAM positive. NCAM is expressed in developing muscle, but not in adult innervated muscle. It is re-expressed on denervation. In SMA-I, the NCAM positivity supports the interpretation that the small fibers are denervated. It has been further suggested that NCAM positivity on large fibers indicates unstable innervation and predicts ongoing denervation.[31]

Many of the small skeletal muscle fibers in SMA-I have an immature appearance, because they have central nuclei and ultrastructural morphology similar to myotubes.[16] Satellite cells in SMA-I are increased, but their ultrastructure is quiescent. The failure of these satellite cells to activate or cooperate with growing fibers may reflect immaturity. Increased numbers of type 2c fibers[32] may reflect immaturity or may represent fiber-type switching. The hypothesis of muscle fiber immaturity in SMA-I is further supported by expression of fetal isoforms of muscle proteins. Embryonic, fetal, and adult isoforms of slow and fast myosin heavy chains are sequentially expressed in development. In SMA-I, a prenatal type of myosin heavy chain was found in only a few small fibers, in contrast to widespread expression in normal 20-week-old fetal muscle.[33] However, more extensive antibody panels suggest expression of fetal isoforms of myosin heavy chain in SMA-I muscle. The large fibers express slow myosin, consistent with their type 1 histochemistry. Atrophic fibers may express either fast or slow myosin and express prenatal myosin isoforms, particularly in type 2 fibers. Although denervation affects both fiber types, the predominance of type 1 in the large fiber population suggests preservation of slow twitch fibers. The proportion of type 2 atrophic fibers increases with the age of the patient. Whereas fiber type switching occurs in reinnervation, the increasing proportion of type 2 fibers may be directly caused by denervation. Thus maintenance of type 1 differentiation is innervation dependent, so denervated type 1 fibers synthesize fast myosin and switch to a type 2 phenotype.[34] The immaturity of fibers in SMA may arise from prenatal onset of denervation, which slows fiber

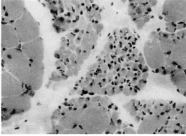

Figure 2.4 Muscle biopsy in a case of spinal muscular atrophy type I showing a fascicle uniformly composed of atrophic rounded fibers.

maturation. Muscle fibers in SMA-I show other abnormalities. Type 1 hypertrophic and type 2 atrophic fibers show abnormal accumulation of desmin and titin.[34] Apoptotic bodies may be found in SMA muscle by electron microscopy.[16] There is strong expression of the proapoptotic oncoprotein Bax in SMA muscle, but little or no expression of Bcl-2, Bcl-x, ICE, and Apo 1/Fas. In both SMA-I and SMA-II, most fibers express Bax, but in SMA-III, it appears confined to atrophic fibers. This pattern is similar to that for NCAM staining, suggesting that unstable innervation may contribute to apoptosis.[35] The presence of fiber immaturity and muscle cell apoptosis in SMA may result in secondary motor neuron degeneration through loss of their peripheral targets,[16] but, as discussed earlier, the ballooned neurons in the anterior horns in SMA-I show differences from chromatolytic neurons of the axon reaction and do not necessarily indicate that neuronal damage occurs secondary to a distal axonal or target tissue effect. More importantly, the CNS pathology is also found in nonmotor systems, and it is more likely that neuronal degeneration occurs as a primary event.

The SMN gene is expressed in skeletal muscle,[5,36] and it remains possible that effects of the mutation within skeletal muscle may contribute to the pathogenesis of SMA. A contributory role for primary muscle pathology is supported by coculture studies of SMA muscle with rat embryonic spinal neurons. Degeneration and apoptosis occurs in the muscle and in the motor neurons, triggered by contact between axon and muscle in excess of cultures using muscle from normal or disease controls.[37,38]

X-Linked Spinobulbar Muscular Atrophy (Kennedy's Disease)

Clinical Phenotype

X-linked spinal and bulbar muscular atrophy (X-SBMA), eponymously known as Kennedy's disease, is a motor system degeneration of males, with clinical onset most commonly in the third to fifth decades. LMN weakness affects limb and bulbar muscles with slow progression. The neurological manifestations are associated with gynecomastia, as well as late reduction in fertility, severe oligospermia, and testicular atrophy. Carrier females, heterozygous for the gene mutation, do not show clinical manifestations,[39] but investigation of such individuals has suggested subclinical neuromuscular involvement.[40] Although the neurological symptoms are predominantly motor, the objective presence of sensory loss in some cases, and electrophysiological evidence of sural axonal neuropathy suggest that the pathology is not restricted to the motor system. (Also see Chapter 17.)

Genetics of X-Linked Spinobulbar Muscular Atrophy
and Molecular Pathogenesis

X-SBMA results from a mutation in the androgen receptor gene on chromosome Xq11-q12. Point mutations in the DNA-binding and steroid-binding regions of the androgen receptor lead to the androgen insensitivity syndrome. In contrast, X-SBMA is due to an expansion of a CAG trinucleotide repeat in exon 1 of the gene.[41] The CAG repeat length in normal individuals ranges from about 11 to 33 repeats, and in X-SBMA, the repeat size is roughly doubled to a range of about 40 to 62 repeats, encoding an expanded polyglutamine tract. Thus X-SBMA belongs to the group of diseases characterized by CAG expansion including Huntington's disease, dentatorubral-pallidoluysian atrophy (DRPLA), and several forms of the hereditary spinocerebellar ataxias. There are variable reports of correlation between the size of the CAG repeat in X-SBMA and the clinical phenotype. A significant correlation between the size of trinucleotide repeat and the standardized disability scores, in addition to an inverse correlation with age at clinical onset, has been demonstrated.[42] However, other studies report a poor correlation with age at onset or clinical manifestations,[39] and a family in which the CAG repeat length was constant showed considerable phenotypical variability.[43]

The androgen receptor is widely expressed in the perikarya and nuclei of neurons in the CNS, including motor neurons, cerebral cortex, hippocampus, basal ganglia, thalamus, Purkinje cells, and dorsal root ganglia. Androgens appear to have a role in motor neuron growth, development, and regeneration. There is little expression in glia.[44–46] Expression of the receptor is also seen in non-neural tissues including testis, scrotal skin, and muscle, but not liver, spleen, and kidney. Given this widespread expression in the CNS, the selectivity of this disease is not explained simply by the distribution of the protein. RNA studies have confirmed that mRNA with the expanded repeat code is expressed in the sensory system,[47] whereas in situ hybridization studies have suggested that there may be a specific reduction in androgen receptor mRNA in motor neurons in X-SBMA.[48]

The mechanism by which the mutation in the androgen receptor leads to neurodegeneration remains unclear, but a number of candidate mechanisms have been suggested. Polyglutamine tracts are susceptible to conformational change and aggregation as β-pleated sheets, and it is possible that interaction with the polyglutamine-rich regions of other transcription factors may lead to altered activity. The expanded polyglutamine tract may also alter processing of the androgen receptor protein, because it may form a better substrate for transglutaminase activity. The mutation may also lead to partial loss of function with decreased transactivation activity and possible effects on the neuronal cytoskeleton.[45,49,50] Morphological studies have shown the tendency for trinucleotide repeat expansion to induce aggregation. This process is represented pathologically by the formation of intranuclear inclusions (INIs) in X-SBMA measuring 1 to 5 μm in diameter (Figure 2.5). These inclusions are usually single and heavily ubiquitinated. They stain with antibodies that recognize epitopes in the 20 to 21 amino acids, forming the N-terminal of the androgen receptor, implying that epitopes in the remainder of the molecule are masked or that the aggregated protein is truncated. The inclusions occur in surviving neurons of affected groups, but not in those neurons of unaffected systems, implying that they may play a role in the pathogenesis of the neurodegeneration.[44] INIs are also seen in non-neural tissue including kidney, heart, testis, and scrotal skin, but not liver, spleen, or muscle.[51] INIs have also been described in other CAG repeat diseases and appear to be a common event. INIs generally contain the mutated protein, are ubiquitinated, and occur in affected neuronal groups.[52] The ultrastructure is of granular and filamentous components that are not membrane

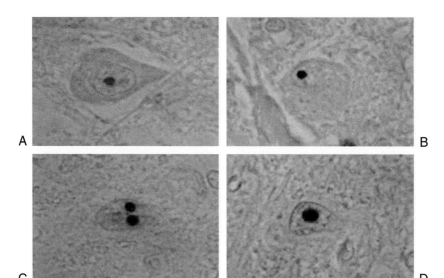

Figure 2.5 Immunohistochemistry of the AR protein in nuclear inclusions in the central nervous system of patients with spinobulbar muscular atrophy. AR staining is observed in motor neurons of the **(A, B)** medulla oblongata and the **(C, D)** pons. (A and B are stained with PG-21, and C and D are stained with AR[N-20].) (Reprinted with permission from Li M, Nakagomi Y, Kobayashi Y, et al. Non-neural nuclear inclusions of androgen receptor protein in spinal and bulbar muscular atrophy. Am J Pathol 1998;153:695–701.)

bound. INIs in X-SBMA differ in not having a filamentous component.[44] Their role in pathogenesis remains uncertain, and whether they are protective or cyto-pathic is unclear. Immunohistochemistry shows that they contain transcription factors such as TATA-binding protein, CREB, and CREB-binding protein, which contain glutamine-rich domains. The inclusions also appear to sequester chaperone proteins such as heat shock protein (Hsp40 and Hsp70). INI formation may therefore be associated with perturbations of nuclear function and gene transcription.

Central Nervous System Pathology: Motor System

The brunt of the pathology of X-SBMA is borne by the LMNs. Autopsy studies have demonstrated severe loss of anterior horn motor neurons at all levels of the spinal cord, as well as of motor neurons from the motor nuclei of cranial nerves (CNs) V, VII, XI, and XII. There is preservation of motor neurons in the nuclei of CNs III, IV, and VI, supplying the extraocular muscles. Motor neuron loss is accompanied by loss of axons from the ventral motor roots of the spinal cord. In contrast to the profound involvement of LMNs, there is no degeneration of the pyramidal tract and the motor cortex appears preserved, in keeping with the lack of pyramidal signs.[40,53–55] A quantitative study has demonstrated additional loss of small neurons from the intermediate zone of the spinal gray matter, which appears more severe than in ALS.[56] Remaining anterior horn cells may show simple atrophy, but no chromatolysis, suggesting that the degeneration is a primary perikaryal event, rather than a retrograde axonal degeneration.[40] Immunohistochemical studies, in contrast to ALS, do not reveal ubiquitinated inclusions (UBIs) and neurofilament phosphorylation patterns appear unperturbed.[57,58]

Central Nervous System Pathology: Extramotor Systems

In the spinal cord, the intermediolateral neurons and Clarke's nucleus are preserved.[40,55] Cerebral atrophy in computed tomography images, in addition to neuropsychological impairment of long-term memory and selective attention, is described.[43] In one case, a presenile dementia developed, characterized by personality change, behavioral disturbance, and progression to memory loss with global cognitive impairment.[58] Neuropathological examination revealed the typical LMN pathology of X-SBMA, together with subcortical frontal gliosis, not associated with overt cortical pathology. The hippocampus showed neuronal depletion, gliosis, and microglial reaction, affecting in particular the pyramidal layer of the CA1 region. Gliosis and microglial reaction were also observed in the subthalamic nucleus, thalamus, and caudate. There is therefore evidence that at least in some cases, the selectivity for LMNs is relative and that other parts of the nervous system may be involved.

Sensory Pathology

Although most patients do not have sensory clinical features, pathological studies in X-SBMA demonstrate that there is a sensory central and peripheral axonopathy, more marked distally.[40,47] Sural nerve biopsy shows loss of myelinated nerve fibers, particularly larger diameter fibers, which is evidence of axonal atrophy and degeneration, as well as an increase in segmental demyelination and remyelination.[39,40,43,47,59] These changes are independent of the presence of diabetes mellitus. There is also evidence of central sensory involvement. Dorsal root ganglion neurons are preserved, but there is a decrease in large-diameter axons and an increase in small-diameter axons. Myelinated fibers are lost from the fasciculus gracilis without gliosis, particularly in more rostral segments.[58] Medullary neurons within the nucleus gracilis and cuneatus appear preserved. It has been suggested that these changes result from dysfunction of sensory neurons without cell loss, but whether the mechanism is the same as that leading to the profound loss of motor neurons remains undetermined.

Muscle Pathology

Muscle biopsies from patients with X-SBMA reveal severe chronic denervation with fiber-type grouping indicative of reinnervation. The presence of nuclear clusters is a reflection of severe fiber atrophy.[40,43,54,60] Myopathic changes may also be present with occasional necrotic fibers, presumably accounting for the raised serum creatine kinase level that may be observed in X-SBMA. Subtle pathological changes have also been observed in the muscle of a carrier female, consisting of moderate type 2 fiber predominance, with increased variation in myofiber size.[61]

Testicular Pathology

The testis in X-SBMA shows arrested spermatogenesis, and in some cases, tubules are hyalinized in association with hyperplasia of Leydig cells.[54,55] Primary testicular failure appears to be the basis of severe oligospermia.

Poliomyelitis and the Postpolio Syndrome

Clinical Phenotype

Paralytic poliomyelitis is an acute disease in which viral infection is associated with destruction of anterior horn cells. Patients with a history of paralytic poliomyelitis may develop a late deterioration in their neurological status after 30 or 40 years of neurological stability. Within this syndrome, some authors distinguish as a separate entity late deterioration, which occurs because of increasing infirmity due to age or intercurrent illness, which impairs the capacity to compensate for a fixed postpolio neurological deficit. This differs from the development of new progressive weakness, atrophy, and often fatigue, in specific muscle groups, so-called progressive PPMA. The clinical features are reviewed elsewhere,[62,63] and an interesting perspective is provided by the account of Halstead.[64] Although sometimes misdiagnosed as ALS, PPMA is focal and more slowly progressive than is characteristic for that disorder; a mean yearly loss of neurological function of 1 percent has been measured on neurological assessment scales.[65]

Pathology of Acute Poliomyelitis

The poliovirus is an enterovirus of the Picornaviridae family that is transmitted by the fecal-oral route. The virus multiplies in the alimentary tract, a viremia ensues, and the virus may enter the CNS by a hematogenous route or via peripheral nerves. The receptor for poliovirus, hPVR, has been characterized and is a member of the immunoglobulin gene superfamily.[66] In the CNS, the virus replicates in neurons, especially motor neurons, causing neuronal destruction. The well-described pathology of acute poliomyelitis is that of an acute lytic viral infection.[61,65,67,68] In the immediate phase, postinfection motor neurons show chromatolysis and perinuclear chromatin aggregation before inflammation appears, changes suggested to represent apoptosis.[65] Inclusion bodies may develop but are not prominent. The cellular inflammatory response may be intense, including perivascular and meningeal lymphocytic infiltrates. Hypertrophic microglia are seen, and dying neurons undergo neuronophagia (Figure

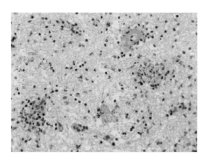

Figure 2.6 Motor neurons within the anterior horn of the spinal cord undergoing neuronophagia in a case of acute poliomyelitis.

2.6). Neuronophagia is no longer observed after the first several days, and the phase of neuronal degeneration is brief. Surviving chromatolytic neurons may recover morphological normality in less than a month. In severe cases, there is hemorrhagic necrosis of the spinal anterior horns. The distribution of pathology within the spinal cord is patchy and asymmetrical, with the severity of pathology correlating with patterns of clinical weakness. Although the spinal cord and medulla bear the brunt of the pathology, infection is not limited to motor neurons and pathology may be widespread, particularly in the brain stem, the thalamus, and the hypothalamus. The cerebral cortex is relatively spared, with the exception of the motor cortex.

Pathology of Postpolio Muscular Atrophy

The pathology of PPMA, a slow progressive motor neuron degeneration, contrasts with the lytic destructive picture of acute poliomyelitis. During the stable postpolio period, the spinal cord shows anterior horn atrophy with neuronal loss accompanied by gliosis. Anterior horn cells are said to show an increase in lipofuscin and loss of Nissl substance, but no inclusion bodies can be identified. Even many years after the acute infection, there is persistent inflammation with perivascular lymphocytes and plasma cells, along with some parenchymal and meningeal lymphocytes, mainly T cells.[69,70] Spinal white matter shows little pathology, but there may be some attenuation of myelin and fiber loss from dorsal root entry zones. There is little evidence of corticospinal tract involvement, implying that there is no secondary descending tract degeneration following anterior horn cell loss.[71] In cases of PPMA, the spinal cord pathology is similar to that seen in the stable late postpolio state. In addition, occasional chromatolytic neurons have been described,[70] implying ongoing anterior horn cell pathology. These authors also comment on the presence of axonal spheroids, but because they are common in the spinal cord of normal elderly subjects, this is unlikely to be disease specific. In contrast to ALS, the LMNs of the spinal cord in PPMA have not shown any evidence of ubiquitinated intraneuronal inclusions.[72]

Muscle Pathology in Postpolio Muscular Atrophy

Muscle biopsies taken from patients with postpolio syndrome have been studied in some detail. The muscle shows evidence of denervation and reinnervation with large groups of fibers of the same histochemical fiber type and sometimes group atrophy. Some of these muscles also show secondary myopathic changes. Chronic denervation changes in muscles not affected during the acute illness phase provide further evidence that the pathology may be more widespread than clinically suspected. In PPMA, but not in stable patients with late postpolio, isolated angulated esterase-positive fibers are present, suggesting ongoing denervation. Occasional small perimysial and perivascular lymphocytic infiltrates may also be present. These infiltrates consist of CD8[+] and CD4[+] T cells and occur in association with class I major histocompatibility complex (MHC) expression on muscle fibers.[65,73,74] Changes in PPMA muscle reminiscent of inclusion body myositis (i.e., the presence of rimmed vacuoles with Congo red–positive amyloid deposits and immunohistochemical positivity for β-APP and ubiquitin) have been reported in addition to neurogenic features.[75]

Pathogenesis of Postpolio Muscular Atrophy

Based on the pathological findings, it has been suggested that the pathogenesis of PPMA relates to new neuronal degeneration. The presence of isolated angulated muscle fibers implies new denervation and is not seen in stable patients with late postpolio. It has been suggested that isolated fiber atrophy indicates the death of individual nerve terminals, rather than of whole motor units, a conclusion supported by electrophysiological studies. The presence of normal-size muscle fibers that are positive for NCAM is further evidence of recent denervation. The hypothesis is proposed that acute poliomyelitis is followed by extensive attempted reinnervation of muscle fibers by the remaining anterior horn neurons as a compensatory mechanism. These neurons therefore maintain enlarged motor units and may be further "stressed" by ongoing denervation and reinnervation. Under chronic metabolic stress or in the face of new insults, they may not be able to maintain distal axonal sprouts, resulting in individual fiber denervation.[65,73] Impaired neuromuscular transmission has been described in PPMA. This hypothesis explains many of the clinical and pathological features of the postpolio syndrome, but other factors may also operate.[65] There are myopathic fibers with "moth-eaten" changes in enzyme histochemistry preparations, which show impaired energy metabolism by phosphorus-31 magnetic resonance imaging spectroscopy, and which may be relevant to fatigue in the postpolio syndrome. Inflammatory cell infiltrates may persist in the spinal cord and skeletal muscle, and there is some evidence for viral persistence, so immunological factors may also be involved. The significance of poliovirus persistence and its potential role in the postpolio syndrome remain to be determined.

MIXED UPPER AND LOWER MOTOR NEURON DISORDERS

Amyotrophic Lateral Sclerosis

We use the term *ALS* to encompass the disorder also known in the traditional U.K. nomenclature as "motor neurone disease." We also recognize that this

diagnostic label should be regarded as encompassing a range of clinicopathological syndromes that include clinical presentation as apparently pure LMN
(progressive muscular atrophy [PMA] and progressive bulbar palsy) or UMN
(PLS) phenotypes, and which may evolve into combined UMN/LMN disease
(ALS).[76] Recent molecular evidence suggests that these syndromes share a
common pathogenesis and are best reviewed together. The pathology of this
group of disorders has been described many times,[1,19,77,78] and there is little to
add to these accounts of the classic anatomical pathology in the CNS and skeletal muscle. This section focuses on three issues: (1) evidence for a common
molecular pathology among the syndromes of ALS, PMA, and PLS in the
context of neuronal inclusion bodies; (2) a review of the evidence for ALS as
a multisystem disorder; and (3) a review of published accounts of the molecular pathology of familial ALS (FALS), especially cases related to mutations in
the gene encoding SOD1.

Molecular Pathology of Amyotrophic Lateral Sclerosis and Related Disorders: Inclusion Bodies and Intermediate Filaments

The literature on motor neuron inclusion bodies in ALS is difficult to assimilate and encompasses a confusing plethora of nomenclature and interpretations.
This problem arises from the unsatisfactory conflation of different concepts
arising from studies that refer to inclusions on the basis of tinctorial properties
(e.g., "eosinophilic inclusions" or "basophilic inclusions"), or from those that
use inappropriate terms borrowed from other diseases in which inclusions occur
(e.g., "spinal Lewy bodies" or "Lewy-like hyaline inclusions"), or those that
involve the uncritical application of pathophysiological theory to bias morphological interpretation, for example, the myth that ubiquitinated motor neuron
inclusion bodies in sporadic ALS are immunoreactive for SOD1.

In our practical experience of ALS, three distinct types of inclusion bodies
have been encountered, although a fourth inclusion morphology is illustrated
in papers on SOD1 FALS, usually termed "Lewy-like hyaline inclusions" and
"astrocytic hyaline inclusions." The three that are usually encountered are
Bunina bodies,[79] ubiquinated inclusions,[80,81] and neurofilament-rich, "hyaline
conglomerate inclusions" (HCIs).[1,82–84] Any other nomenclature encountered in
the literature can usually be assigned to one of these categories. Ambiguity
arises over terms such as "Lewy-like hyaline inclusion" or "hyaline inclusion"
often because the published studies do not include information from a sufficiently comprehensive panel of antibodies. Scientific journals should expect a
uniform minimum standard for publication of pathological studies in ALS,
which must include both ubiquitin and neurofilament antibodies. The present
literature on inclusion bodies across the spectrum of SOD1 FALS mutations is
difficult to interpret because of such failings (see the following sections).

Bunina Bodies

These bodies were originally described in 1962 as small eosinophilic bodies,
often with a rather refractile angular morphology, which are associated with the

cell body of spinal motor neurons in ALS. They are present in both sporadic and familial cases and are reported to be present in up to 85 percent of cases.[85] More recently, they have been described in cerebral neurons including Betz cells, the subthalamic nucleus, and the brain stem reticular formation.[86,87] Bunina bodies are immunoreactive for the protein cystatin C[88] and show ultra-structural properties, suggesting a lysosomal origin.[89,90] These structures do not appear to be directly related to the UBIs of ALS, described in the following section.

Ubiquitinated Inclusions

These structures were first described in 1988 and can be reliably demonstrated only by ubiquitin immunocytochemistry.[80,81,91–94] They show a variable morphology and are divided into two broad groups.[76,95] The first and most frequent of these is the "skein" (Figure 2.7A). This appearance consists of variable numbers of filamentous profiles within the cell soma and proximal dendrites. There may be as few as only one or two of these filaments, so the appearances are difficult to evaluate with certainty. In our experience, if there is a typical clinical history and a strong clinical certainty to the diagnosis, even infrequent small filaments are a reliable diagnostic finding when associated with spinal motor neuron loss. Such appearances are not encountered in other disorders or in normal spinal tissue from later life except in very rare examples. These skeins have no discernible morphological counterpart in sections stained by conventional means (e.g., hematoxylin-eosin [H&E] stains).

The second morphology encountered is of more compact and rounded structures (Figure 2.7B). They often show a minor degree of irregularity around the periphery that on closer inspection is satisfactorily interpreted as filamentous material identical to skeins. Thus these inclusions appear to be composed of the same material as skeins, and it is not unusual to find either intermediate morphologies (Figure 2.8) or individuals whose motor neurons contain both skeins and compact UBIs. Ultrastructural data support this conclusion and suggest that the inclusions are composed of straight filaments of about 10 micrometers in diameter. Complete certainty about these interpretations is hampered by the lack

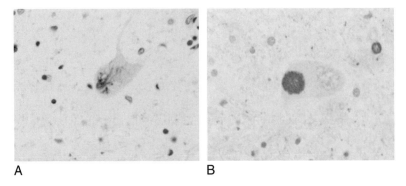

A   B

Figure 2.7 Ubiquitinated inclusions with lower motor neurons from patients with amyotrophic lateral sclerosis show either a skein (**A**) or compact (**B**) morphology.

of a specific protein marker for either type of UBI. Multiple published studies have used an exhaustive range of antibodies to a wide range of cytoplasmic proteins without consistent success.[95,96] There are various claims in the literature that UBIs stain with antibodies to neurofilaments or to SOD1,[97] but these are not substantiated in the authors' series of 100 cases of ALS and variants. It is possible that the filamentous protein within UBIs that has been tagged with ubiquitin is sufficiently modified or damaged as to be unrecognizable by conventional antibodies, but it is probably more likely that we do not yet know what the protein is and have not used appropriate immunocytochemical markers. The hunt for the identity of this enigmatic filament is a key goal for ALS research. In contrast to skeins, the compact variant of the UBI is not infrequently visible in H&E-stained sections as a rounded body with variable tinctorial characteristics spanning from basophilic, through amphophilic, to eosinophilic.[97] There may also be a peripheral halo, which then gives these inclusions a likeness to the Lewy bodies that characterize the α-synucleinopathies (e.g., Parkinson's disease). Unfortunately, papers referring to "Lewy body–like" inclusions in ALS still appear in the literature. In our opinion, this is regrettable and confusing. Several groups have confirmed that there is no evidence that ALS is associated with any accumulation of α-synuclein in the CNS, and the name "Lewy-like" (or similar terms) should be avoided.[98]

UBIs are almost universal in ALS and its variants. They are the most specific molecular marker for the disease and form the basis on which it has been proposed that a number of disorders should be regarded as part of a disease spectrum resulting in various clinicopathological syndromes.[76] This aspect is discussed further. In one series, only 4 of 100 patients with motor system disease (i.e., 94% prevalence) did not have such lesions if the other disorders covered in this chapter are excluded.[99] Two of these UBI-negative patients had pure LMN disorders in whom the possibility of SMA or some other non-ALS LMN degeneration is considered likely. The other two patients had relatively limited anatomical sampling of the spinal cord in whom there was subtotal loss of ventral horn cells.

This illustrates the difficulty of demonstrating neuronal inclusion bodies when the susceptible population of cells has been virtually obliterated in the tissue available for study. No widely accepted protocol for sampling the CNS to exclude UBIs has been published. We recommend sampling both limb enlargements at two or more segmental levels, together with levels of the thoracic cord, and medulla/pons (at the levels of the hypoglossal and motor nuclei

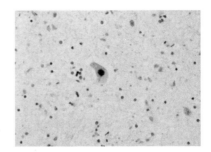

Figure 2.8 An intermediate form of UBI showing a compact lesion with filamentous edges.

of CNs V and VII), before accepting the absence of UBIs in any case examined. It is additionally useful to examine a ribbon of serial sections at the spinal levels sampled.

Neurofilament Inclusions: Hyaline Conglomerates, Spheroids

The HCI is an argyrophilic inclusion in the perikaryon and proximal dendrites, most commonly encountered in motor neurons of the spinal cord. The lesions are reactive to neurofilament antibodies that detect both phosphorylated and nonphosphorylated epitopes of heavy- and medium-chain neurofilament proteins (e.g., SMI31 and SMI32). In H&E or Nissl stains, they are visible as large hyaline concretions of variable morphology displacing the nucleus and Nissl bodies (Figure 2.9). In our experience of more than 100 patients, these inclusions were present in only 3 individuals with otherwise clinicopathologically typical ALS. Two of these cases had an I113T point mutation in the SOD1 gene.[83] The other was an apparently sporadic case unrelated to SOD1. Many other authors have described these lesions,[82,91,100–102] which show ultrastructural features of bundles and aggregates of 10- to 15-μm filaments with additional mixed components of cytoplasmic organelles.[103] They have been described in non-ALS neurological patients and in controls, so they do not have the specificity for ALS that seems to apply to the UBI.[91] The rarity of this lesion in ALS is supported by the data of Chou,[82] who observed HCIs in only 2 of 82 autopsied cases of ALS. Another single case report describes argyrophilic inclusions in rapidly progressive sporadic ALS, which were immunoreactive for ubiquitin but not for neurofilament antibodies.[104]

HCIs are probably closely related to another morphological feature of the spinal ventral horn, which are termed *spheroids* and *globules*.[105] These comprise fusiform enlargements of the axons and proximal dendrites. Using either immunocytochemistry or electron microscopy, we can see that these lesions are similar to HCIs, suggesting that similar cytoskeletal dysfunction underlies both types of inclusions. It is suggested that spheroids are immunoreactive both to neurofilament heavy and to peripherin, the latter of which was not observed in UBIs.[106] Like HCIs, these lesions are not specific to ALS, because they are almost universally present in the aging spinal cord irrespective of disease status. Previous claims that they are more frequent or abundant in ALS remain unconfirmed.[57,91,107]

A third abnormality of neurofilament metabolism that manifests in pathological material is diffuse change in the phosphorylation state of the perikaryal cytoskeleton. Several authors have drawn attention to the increased intensity of staining for phosphorylated neurofilament epitopes in the cell body of motor neurons in ALS.[57,107–109] These observations are confirmed in a series of cases by one of us (P.G.I.),[98] which showed an increased proportion of LMN perikarya that stained intensely for phosphorylated neurofilament compared with control cases (25% versus 4%).

The most difficult aspect of the ALS literature to assimilate with current observations is the concept of the "hyaline inclusion."[100,110–112] All of these early reports were of familial disease and predated any genetic screening (e.g., for SOD1 mutations) or immunocytochemistry. The concept of hyaline inclusions

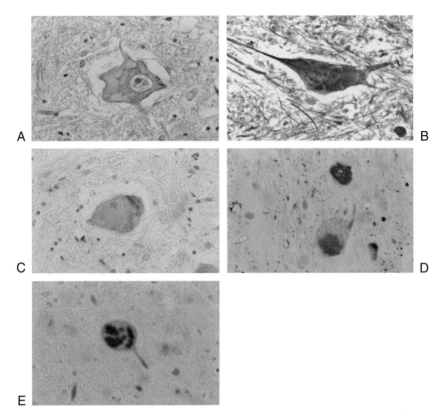

Figure 2.9 Hyaline conglomerate inclusions appear (**A**) as glassy irregular areas of cytoplasm (cresyl fast violet) and (**B**) as argyrophilic structures (Palmgren). They are (**C**) variably and often weakly immunoreactive for ubiquitin, but they are strongly reactive to both (**D**) phosphorylated (SMI31) and (**E**) nonphosphorylated (SMI32) neurofilament epitopes.

survives in the literature beyond the threshold of modern molecular pathology and the literature is cited[1] to argue that such lesions are strongly decorated by ubiquitin antibodies and variably by those to neurofilaments.[80,81,113–115] This nomenclature therefore has likely been used variably to describe compact UBIs, HCIs, and the hyaline concentric bodies, which are frequently encountered in the literature relating to FALS due to mutations in the SOD1 gene and in mouse transgene models of SOD1 FALS (see later discussion).

Amyotrophic Lateral Sclerosis as a Multisystem Disorder

The evidence that ALS is a multisystem disorder is now overwhelming. This concept has two discrete aspects. The first concerns the implication of a common molecular pathology, characterized morphologically by the UBI. This lesion is encountered in a spectrum of disorders spanning LMN degeneration (PMA), through combined UMN/LMN degeneration (ALS), pure UMN degeneration (PLS), and dementia. The latter syndrome may present as a combination of motor neuron disease with dementia or as a pure dementia syndrome. Numerous publications now document cerebral degeneration characterized by cerebral UBI pathology, in the absence of changes of ALS, with clinical and anatomical features either of typical frontotemporal dementia (FTD) or primary progressive aphasia (PPA), both examples of so-called *lobar atrophies*. The second concerns the evidence that even in typical ALS, there is molecular pathological evidence for widespread involvement of extramotor regions of the CNS.

The Spectrum of Amyotrophic Lateral Sclerosis–Related Disorders

We have previously proposed that ALS is characterized by UBI pathology as a morphological expression of a specific molecular phenotype, and that this is analogous to the pathologies that underlie the spectrum of α-synucleinopathies (Parkinson's disease, dementia with Lewy bodies, pure autonomic failure), or tauopathies (Alzheimer's disease, argyrophilic grain disease, and so on).[76,98] UBIs are near universal in ALS. Where they are not found, there is an unresolved issue of the extent to which severely degenerated spinal segments should be sampled before accepting their absence. In essence, the argument is that these are intraneuronal lesions and by definition are not demonstrable when the susceptible population of neurons has been destroyed. We have recently shown that UBIs are also a consistent finding in PMA spinal cord,[99] and that half of these patients with PMA have clinically unsuspected corticospinal tract pathology at autopsy. Similarly, in PLS, UBIs are frequent in the motor and premotor cortex and may be found in the hippocampal dentate granule cells (Figure 2.10).[116] Two cases of PLS reported in the modern pathological literature showed occasional UBIs in spinal motor neurons in the absence of LMN degeneration.[116,117] It is well established that ALS-dementia (some degree of cognitive decline) affects about 5 percent of patients with ALS at some stage of the disease.[118–127] Patients with ALS-dementia have both the characteristic motor system UBIs of ALS, together with cerebral pathology comprising small globular UBIs of the dentate granule cells, and a variable component of neocortical ubiquitinated neurites and small neuronal UBIs.[123,126,128–130] Such UBI pathology has also been reported in the striatum of ALS-dementia,[131] although it has been argued that the changes in this region are a manifestation of normal aging.[132] Finally this cerebral pathology of UBIs can be found in a subset of patients presenting with a pure dementia syndrome.[133] These patients fall clinicopathologically into two groups. Most show typical features of frontotemporal dementia[133] and some reported cases have included the spinal cord in which occasional LMN UBIs were demonstrated.[134] A second smaller group presents as primary progressive aphasia and shows a population of UBIs and neuritic pathology predominantly affecting cerebral cortical regions involved in speech pathways.[127,135]

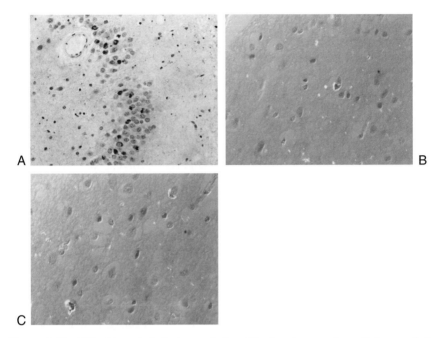

Figure 2.10 Ubiquitinated inclusions of the (**A**) dentate granule cell layer of the hippocampus and the (**B, C**) frontotemporal neocortex in amyotrophic lateral sclerosis associated with dementia.

Multisystem Disease in Amyotrophic Lateral Sclerosis

The classic accounts of ALS include reference to subtle pathology in nonmotor regions of the CNS such as the thalamus.[77] There is also extensive literature on spinal dorsal column degeneration, which is reported to be present in up to 70 percent of cases at autopsy.[118,136–138] The emphasis in some of this early literature on familial disease does not appear to be substantiated in that dorsal column pallor is also frequent in sporadic cases. Peripheral sensory nerve morphology is affected in ALS.[139,140] There is also evidence in the literature on degeneration of the spinocerebellar pathway,[141,142] both in terms of cell loss from the thoracic nucleus of Clarke and in terms of pallor of ascending spinocerebellar pathways.[1,77,143]

There is a Japanese literature on the neuropathology of patients who were maintained by long-term ventilatory support in a severe "locked-in" state.[144–148] These reports document widespread CNS degeneration of many regions not classically involved in the disease at earlier stages, including oculomotor nuclei, brain stem reticular formation, periaqueductal gray matter, red nucleus, globus pallidus, subthalamic nucleus, thalamus, substantia nigra, and cerebellar dentate nucleus. Thus the degenerative process that characterizes ALS is only relatively selective for the motor system, and in most patients, the evolution of motor dysfunction is lethal before the development of overt pathology in other CNS regions. In some cases, this more widespread pathology occurs spontaneously without prolonged ventilatory support.[149,150]

Much of this literature on extramotor pathology predates molecular pathology using markers such as ubiquitin. Where immunocytochemistry has been used, there is emerging evidence of regular involvement of structures like the substantia nigra in patients with ALS-dementia,[151,152] and the extramotor cortex in ALS.[129]

Molecular and Cellular Pathology of SOD1 Familial Amyotrophic Lateral Sclerosis

Both the literature and our personal experience of six cases highlights the similarity of SOD1 FALS to sporadic ALS.[83,153] Many older reports have suggested that posterior column or spinocerebellar tract involvement is more frequent in FALS,[100,118] but this is not so in our series of cases in which posterior column pallor was present in at least 20 percent of all sporadic cases. All the intraneuronal inclusion bodies described earlier have been observed in FALS. There is no clear picture of whether each specific mutation in the SOD1 gene is associated with UBIs or HCIs, but there is some suggestion that this may be so for some mutations. HCIs have been described in three mutations: A4V,[83,84,154] I113T,[83,155] and H48Q.[156] Another familial case was reported using illustrations typical of HCIs, but there was no information about SOD1 gene analysis.[157] In contrast, there are six mutations reported in which UBIs appear to be observed: A4T,[158] E100G,[153] L126S,[159] H48Q[156] (as noted earlier, this case had both UBIs and HCIs), D101N,[160] and del125–126.[161,162] Two more case reports of other mutations (H46A and V118L) have been published in which neuronal inclusions were not identified.[144,163] In one patient,[163] the investigators had access only to a small amount of spinal tissue; the second patient[144] was of "locked-in" ALS maintained with ventilatory support and in which there was almost total loss of LMNs. These two cases illustrate the difficulty of detecting neuronal inclusions in cases with severe depletion of the target neuronal population.

Two SOD1 mutations appear to be associated with relative preservation of the corticospinal tract: A4V[164] and D101N.[160]

There are now up to 100 ALS-associated mutations in the SOD1 gene, and it is likely to be a considerable time before a clear picture emerges in the literature about the consistency of molecular pathology in each of these variants. If there are consistent patterns between different mutations, either it may indicate differing pathogenetic pathways between different mutations or it may indicate that the mutations tend to occur against different genetic backgrounds that act to modify disease expression.

The literature on SOD1 transgenic mice has emphasized the occurrence of morphological evidence of SOD1 accumulation in affected tissues. A number of reports claim that anti-SOD1 antibodies similarly decorate "Lewy-like hyaline inclusions" in human FALS.[154,165–171] This is the one circumstance in the pathology of ALS in which this term may have utility (though not validity because this lesion is not reactive for α-synuclein). The morphology and immunoreactivity of these lesions in the human material reported in the literature is rather different than that of UBIs in that they are distinctly hyaline rather than fibrillary, rounded, and show a concentric pattern with an apparently more dense core. The prominence of immunoreactivity to SOD1 in these lesions is emphasized, and most authors make it clear that they are not skein or compact types of UBI. One report suggests that they may also occur in sporadic patients.[172] However, our experience suggests that these lesions are not prominent in a survey of autopsy material from sporadic ALS cases in which no SOD1 immunoreactive lesions were identified. In the published work, the specificity of the antibodies used is often not well described and it is possible that uncharacterized cross-reactivities may arise with some reagents. Alternatively, SOD1 immunoreactivity in the inclusions of FALS may not be a universal phenomenon.

Astrocytic hyaline inclusions are also described in both human FALS and animal models of SOD1 FALS.[167,168,170,171,173–175] In the mouse models of FALS, these lesions are often more prominent than in neurons. It is possible that the pathology observed in the animal models is modified, relative to human disease, by the increased copy number of the transgenes expressed, resulting in an abnormal excess of mutant protein compared with human patients.

UPPER MOTOR NEURON DISORDERS

Hereditary Spastic Paraparesis

Clinical Phenotypes

HSP, or Strümpell-Lorrain syndrome, may be defined as a heterogeneous group of hereditary CNS disorders characterized by slowly progressive spastic paraparesis as the cardinal clinical manifestation.[176] It may occur in a pure form, or it may be complicated by a variety of additional clinical manifestations.[177] Pure HSP is divided into types I or II based on age at onset, with a cutoff at 35 years of age. Late-onset type II HSP shows a greater prevalence of pyramidal weakness, sensory abnormalities, and urinary symptoms.[178] In addition to clinical heterogeneity, there is genetic heterogeneity with autosomal dominant, autosomal recessive, and X-linked forms of inheritance. A number of genes and linkage sites have been identified and a genetic classification of HSP is emerging.[177,179,180] The extent to which clinical and genetic heterogeneity is reflected in pathological heterogeneity remains to be defined. Detailed neuropathological findings have been reported in relatively few cases, possibly because life expectancy is little reduced and patients usually die at home or in nursing care.[176] Furthermore, because genetic characterization has only recently emerged, few of the patients in whom pathology is reported have been genetically defined. (See Chapter 18.)

Central Nervous System Pathology: Spinal Cord

The core neuropathological features of HSP were first described by Strümpell and confirmed in a series of reports.[181–184] The spinal cord shows pallor of the lateral and, more variably, the anterior corticospinal tracts with loss of axons

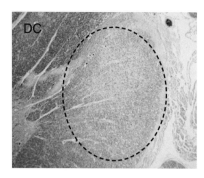

Figure 2.11 Hereditary spastic paraparesis: Lower thoracic spinal cord section stained for myelin; pallor of the lateral corticospinal tract *(open circle)* contrasted with normal myelin of the dorsal column *(DC).*

and myelin, which is most marked distally in the lumbar region. There is also pallor of the dorsal column, affecting the fasciculus gracilis, but there is sparing of the more laterally placed fasciculus cuneatus, most marked in the cervical cord (Figure 2.11). Involvement of the spinocerebellar tracts is described in approximately half of cases. Loss of Betz cells from the motor cortex is reported in some cases,[185] but the anterior horn motor neurons are usually normal. Degeneration has occasionally been described in neurons of the dorsal nucleus of Clarke. A consistent finding in these reports is more severe involvement of the distal part of the corticospinal tracts and dorsal columns, so the most marked changes are in the lumbar and cervical cord, respectively. This has led to the suggestion that degeneration occurs as a dying back neuropathy, affecting the most distal part of these long axons first. The pathogenesis of this degeneration is unclear, and the involvement of different genes, encoding proteins of varying function, in different genetic subtypes of HSP indicates that there may be varying molecular pathways to similar long-tract degeneration.[186] Based on the functions of some of the products of genes mutated in HSP, suggested mechanisms include impaired tract development (L1CAM), impaired interaction of axons and glia (proteolipid protein), and impaired mitochondrial function (paraplegin). Mutation of the spastin gene accounts for 40% of autosomal dominant HSP and has been implicated in microtubule regulation, suggesting an impairment of cytoskeletal function in such cases.[187]

Central Nervous System Pathology of Hereditary Spastic Paraparesis: Cerebral Pathology

In many neuropathological reports of pure HSP, cerebral structures, with the exception of Betz cells, are said to be uninvolved. However, subclinical involvement of other parts of the nervous system is often identified in cases of so-called pure HSP,[188] suggesting that the distinction between pure and complicated HSP is not clear-cut. In particular, there is emerging recognition of cognitive impairment on neuropsychological testing, particularly in cases of HSP associated with a spastin gene mutation.[189–191] The neuropathological substrate of cognitive impairment currently remains poorly defined. Ferrer et al[192] studied a case of HSP in which progressive spastic paraparesis was associated with the later development of severe mental impairment. In addition to the typical spinal cord changes of HSP, the authors described prefrontal atrophy and loss of frontal white matter associated with atrophy of deep gray nuclei. Histological examination demonstrated a loss of neurons in the atrophic cortex including loss of calbindin$_{D-28k}$–immunoreactive neurons and parvalbumin-immunoreactive dendrites. White et al[193] described the neuropathological findings in a case of HSP associated with a spastin mutation who developed dementia. Two other family members also had cognitive decline. The spinal cord changes were typical of HSP. In addition, the hippocampus revealed gross neuronal depletion from the pyramidal sector, with frequent tau-immunoreactive neurofibrillary tangles but without plaques. Ballooned neurons in the limbic cortex and neocortex labeled with tau, but not ubiquitin, and tau-positive glial inclusions were identified. The substantia nigra revealed neuronal loss with α-synuclein–immunoreactive Lewy body formation. The cerebral findings in this case were not typical of known tauopathies, but whether such neurodegenerative cerebral pathology is common to cases of spastin-associated HSP with cognitive impairment is unclear.

Muscle Pathology in Hereditary Spastic Paraparesis

In autosomal recessive forms of HSP associated with mutation in the paraplegin gene on chromosome 16, muscle biopsies have shown ragged red fibers. Scattered muscle fibers show negative histochemical reaction for cytochrome oxidase but preserved or elevated succinate dehydrogenase activity and peripheral accumulation of mitochondria. These changes, which are typical of oxidative phosphorylation defects in muscle, support a role for impairment of oxidative phosphorylation in the pathogenesis of paraplegin mutation–associated HSP.[186,194,195]

Examination of skeletal muscle in autosomal dominant HSP linked to chromosome 8q did not reveal pathological changes, suggesting that mitochondrial changes seen in paraplegin mutations are not a common factor in all HSP cases.[196] Skeletal muscle has not been widely surveyed in other types of HSP.

Acknowledgments

This work was supported by the Medical Research Council and the ALS Association of the United States of America.

REFERENCES

1. Chou SM. Pathology of Motor System Disorder. In PN Leigh, M Swash (eds), Motor Neuron Disease: Biology and Management. London: Springer-Verlag, 1995;53–92.
2. Schmalbruch H, Haase G. Spinal muscular atrophy: present state. Brain Pathol 2001;11:231–247.
3. Osawa M, Shishikura K. Werdnig-Hoffmann Disease and Variants. In JMBV de Jong, P Vinken, RPM Bruyn, et al (eds), Handbook of Clinical Neurology. Amsterdam: Elsevier, 1991;51–80.
4. Biros I, Forrest S. Spinal muscular atrophy: untangling the knot? J Med Genet 1999;36:1–8.
5. Lefebvre S, Burgle Reboullet S, Clermont O, et al. Identification and characterization of a spinal muscular atrophy–determining gene. Cell 1995;80:1–5.

6. Bingham PM, Shen N, Rennert H, et al. Arthrogryposis is due to infantile neuronal degeneration associated with deletion of the SMNT gene. Neurology 1997;49:848–851.
7. Vajsav J, Balslev T, Ray PN, et al. Congenital cytoplasmic body myopathy with survival motor neuron gene deletion or Werdnig-Hoffmann disease. Neurology 1998;51:873–875.
8. Lefebvre S, Burlet P, Liu Q, et al. Correlation between severity and SMN protein level in spinal muscular atrophy. Nature Genet 1997;16:265–269.
9. Tizzano E, Cabot C, Baiget M. Cell-specific survival motor neuron gene expression during human development of the central nervous system. Implications for the pathogenesis of spinal muscular atrophy. Am J Pathol 1998;153:355–361.
10. Terns MP, Terns RM. Macromolecular complexes: SMN—the master assembler. Current Biol 2001;11:R862–R864.
11. Jablonka S, Rossoll W, Schrank B, et al. The role of SMN in spinal muscular atrophy. J Neurol 2000;247:I37–I42.
12. Sendtner M. Molecular mechanisms in spinal muscular atrophy: models and perspectives. Current Opin Neurol 2001;14:629–634.
13. Young PJ, Le TT, Dunckley M, et al. Nuclear gems and Cajal (coiled) bodies in fetal tissues: nucleolar distribution of the spinal muscular atrophy protein, SMN. Exp Cell Res 2001;265:252–261.
14. Iwahashi H, Eguchi Y, Yasuhara N, et al. Synergistic anti-apoptotic activity between Bcl-2 and SMN implicated in spinal muscular atrophy. Nature 1997;390:413–417.
15. Lippa CF, Smith TW. Chromatolytic neurons in Werdnig-Hoffman disease contain phosphorylated neurofilaments. Acta Neuropathol 1988;77:91–94.
16. Fidzianska A, Goebel HH, Warlo I. Acute infantile spinal muscular atrophy. Brain 1990;113:433–445.
17. Murayama S, Bouldin TW, Suzuki K. Immunocytochemical and ultrastructural studies of Werdnig-Hoffman disease. Acta Neuropathol 1991;81:408–417.
18. Hayashi M, Arai N, Murakami T, et al. A study of cell death in Werdnig-Hoffmann disease brain. Neurosci Lett 1998;243:117–120.
19. Lowe J, Leigh P. Disorders of Movement and Systems Degeneration. In D Graham, P Lantos P (eds), Greenfield's Neuropathology (7th ed). London: Arnold, 2002;325–420.
20. Simic G, Seso-Simic D, Lucassen PJ, et al. Ultrastructural analysis and TUNEL demonstrate motor neuron apoptosis in Werdnig-Hoffmann disease. J Neuropathol Exp Neurol 2000;59:398–407.
21. Kato S, Hirano A. Ubiquitin and phosphorylated neurofilament epitopes in ballooned neurons of the extraocular muscle nuclei in a case of Werdnig-Hoffmann disease. Acta Neuropathol 1990;80:334–337.
22. Iwata M, Hirano A. Sparing of the Onufrowicz nucleus in sacral anterior horn lesions. Ann Neurol 1978;4:245–249.
23. Sung JH, Mastri AR. Spinal autonomic neurons in Werdnig-Hoffmann disease, mannosidosis, and Hurler's syndrome: distribution of autonomic neurons in the sacral spinal cord. J Neuropathol Exp Neurol 1980;39:441–451.
24. Zierz S, Zerres K. Wohlfart-Kugelberg-Welander Disease. In JMBV de Jong, P Vinken P, RPM Bruyn, et al (eds), Handbook of Clinical Neurology. Amsterdam: Elsevier, 1991;81–96.
25. Chou SM, Wang HS. Aberrant glycosylation/phosphorylation in chromatolytic motoneurons of Werdnig-Hoffmann disease. J Neurol Sci 1997;152:198–209.
26. Ikemoto A, Hirano A, Matsumoto S, et al. Synaptophysin expression in the anterior horn of Werdnig-Hoffmann disease. J Neurol Sci 1996;136:94–100.
27. Sobue G, Hashizume Y, Yasuda T. Phosphorylated high molecular weight neurofilament protein in lower motor neurons in ALS and other neurodegenerative diseases involving the ventral horns. Acta Neuropathol 1990;79:402–408.
28. Soler-Botija C, Ferrer I, Gich I, et al. Neuronal death is enhanced and begins during fetal development in type I spinal muscular atrophy spinal cord. Brain 2002;125:1624–1634.
29. Grasl-Kraupp B, Ruttkay-Nedecky B, Koudelka H, et al. In situ detection of fragmented DNA (TUNEL assay) fails to discriminate among apoptosis, necrosis and autolytic cell death: a cautionary note. Hepatology 1995;21:1465–1468.
30. Anderson J. Spinal Muscular Atrophy. In G Gresham (ed), Current Histopathology: Atlas of Skeletal Muscle Pathology. Lancaster: MTP Press, 1985;45–52.
31. Walsh F, Moore S, Lake B. Cell adhesion molecule N-CAM is expressed by denervated myofibers in Werdnig-Hoffmann and Kugelberg-Welander type spinal muscular atrophies. J Neurol Neurosurg Psychiatry 1987;50:439–442.
32. Saito Y. Muscle fibre type differentiation and satellite cell population in Werdnig-Hoffmann disease. J Neurol Sci 1985;68:75–87.

33. Swachak J, Benoff B, Sher J, et al. Werdnig-Hoffmann disease: myosin isoform expression is not arrested at prenatal stage of development. J Neurol Sci 1990;95:183–192.
34. Soussi-Yanicostas N, Hamida BC, Bejaoui K, et al. Evolution of muscle specific proteins in Werdnig-Hoffmann's disease. J Neurol Sci 1992;109:111–120.
35. Tews DS, Goebel HH. Apoptosis-related proteins in skeletal muscle fibers of spinal muscular atrophy. J Neuropathol Exp Neurol 1997;56:150–156.
36. Williams BY, Vinnakota S, Sawyer CA, et al. Differential subcellular localization of the survival motor neuron protein in spinal cord and skeletal muscle. Biochem Biophys Res Commun 1999;254:10–14.
37. Guettier-Sigrist S, Hugel B, Coupin G, et al. Possible pathogenetic role of muscle cell dysfunction in motor neuron death in spinal muscular atrophy. Muscle Nerve 2002;25:700–708.
38. Braun S, Croizal B, Lagrange M-C, et al. Constitutive muscular abnormalities in culture in spinal muscular atrophy. Lancet 1995;345:694–695.
39. Amato A. Kennedy disease: a clinicopathologic correlation with mutations in the androgen receptor gene. Neurology 1993;43:791–794.
40. Sobue G, Hashizume Y, Mukai E, et al. X-linked recessive bulbospinal neuronopathy—a clinicopathological study. Brain 1989;112:209–232.
41. La Spada A, Wilson E, Lubahn D, et al. Androgen receptor gene mutations in x-linked spinal and bulbar muscular atrophy. Nature 1991:77–79.
42. Dogu M, Sobue G, Mukai E, et al. Severity of X-linked recessive bulbospinal neuronopathy correlates with size of the tandem CAG repeat in the androgen receptor gene. Ann Neurol 1992;32:707–710.
43. Guidetti D. X-linked bulbar and spinal muscular atrophy, or Kennedy disease: clinical, neurophysiological, neuropathological, neuropsychological and molecular study of a large family. J Neurol Sci 1996;135:140–148.
44. Li M, Nakagomi Y, Kobayashi Y, et al. Non-neural nuclear inclusions of androgen receptor protein in spinal and bulbar muscular atrophy. Am J Pathol 1998;153:695–701.
45. MacLean H, Warne G, Zajac J. Spinal and bulbar muscular atrophy: androgen receptor dysfunction caused by trinucleotide repeat expansion. J Neurol Sci 1996;135:149–157.
46. Clancy A, Bonsall R, Micheal R. Immunohistochemical labeling of androgen receptors in brain of monkey and rat. Life Sci 1992;50:409–417.
47. Li M, Sobue G, Doyu M, et al. Primary sensory neurons in X-linked recessive bulbospinal neuronopathy: histopathology and androgen receptor gene expression. Muscle Nerve 1995:301–308.
48. Nakamura M, Mita S, Matuura T, et al. The reduction of androgen receptor mRNA in motoneurons of X-linked spinal and bulbar muscular atrophy. J Neurol Sci 1997;150:161–165.
49. Brooks BP, Fischbeck KH. Spinal and bulbar muscular atrophy: a trinucleotide-repeat expansion neurodegenerative disease. Trends Neurosci 1995;18:459–461.
50. Gallo J. Kennedy's disease: a triplet repeat disorder or a motor neuron disease. Brain Res Bull 2001;56:209–214.
51. Li M, Miwa S, Kobayashi Y, et al. Nuclear inclusions of the androgen receptor protein in spinal and bulbar muscular atrophy. Ann Neurol 1998;44:249–254.
52. Yamada M. Pathology of CAG repeat diseases. Neuropathology 2000;20:319–325.
53. Kennedy R, Alter M, Sung JH. Progressive proximal spinal and bulbar muscular atrophy of late onset: a sex linked recessive trait. Neurology 1968;18:671–680.
54. Arbizu T, Santamaria J, Gomez JM, et al. A family with adult spinal and bulbar muscular atrophy, X-linked inheritance and associated testicular failure. J Neurol Sci 1983;59:371–382.
55. Nagashima T, Seko K, Hirose K, et al. Familial bulbo-spinal muscular atrophy associated with testicular atrophy and sensory neuropathy (Kennedy-Alter-Sung syndrome). Autopsy case report of two brothers. J Neurol Sci 1988;87:141–152.
56. Terao S, Sobue G, Hashizume Y, et al. Disease-specific patterns of neuronal loss in the spinal ventral horn in amyotrophic lateral sclerosis, multiple system atrophy and X-linked bulbospinal neuronopathy, with special reference to the loss of small neurons in the intermediate zone. J Neurol 1994;241:196–203.
57. Sobue G, Hashizume Y, Yasuda T, et al. Phosphorylated high molecular weight neurofilament protein in lower neurons in amyotrophic lateral sclerosis and other neurodegenerative diseases involving ventral horn cells. Acta Neuropathol 1990;79:402–408.
58. Shaw PJ, Thagesen H, Tomkins J, et al. Kennedy's disease: new molecular pathological and clinical features. Neurology 1998;51:252–255.
59. Wilde J, Moss T, Thrush D. X-linked bulbospinal neuronopathy: a family study of 3 patients. J Neurol Neurosurg Psychiatry 1987;50:279–284.

60. Harding AE, et al. X-linked recessive bulbospinal neuropathy: a report of ten cases. J Neurol Neurosurg Psychiatry 1982;45:1012–1019.
61. Sobue G, Doyu M, Kachi T, et al. Subclinical phenotypic expressions in heterozygous females of X-linked recessive bulbospinal neuropathy. J Neurol Sci 1993;117:74–78.
62. Mulder DW. The Postpolio Syndrome. In JMBV de Jong, P Vinken, RPM Bruyn, et al (eds), Handbook of Clinical Neurology. Amsterdam: Elsevier, 1991;35–40.
63. Kidd D, Williams AJ, Howard RS. Poliomyelitis. Postgrad Med J 1996;72:641–647.
64. Halstead L. Post-polio syndrome. Sci Am 1998;278:42–47.
65. Dalakas M. Pathogenetic mechanisms of post-polio syndrome: morphological, electrophysiological, virological and immunological correlations. Ann N Y Acad Sci 1995;753:167–185.
66. Ohka S, Nomoto A. Recent insights into poliovirus pathogenesis. Trends Micro 2001;9:501–506.
67. Love S, Wiley C. Viral Diseases. In D Graham, P Lantos (eds), Greenfield's Neuropathology (7th ed). London: Arnold, 2002;1–105.
68. Bodian D. Histopathologic basis of diseased findings in poliomyelitis. Am J Med 1949;6:563–578.
69. Kaminski HJ, Tresser N, Hogan RE, et al. Spinal cord histopathology in long-term survivors of poliomyelitis. Muscle Nerve 1995;18:1208–1209.
70. Pezeshkpour GH, Dalakas MC. Long-term changes in the spinal cords of patients with old poliomyelitis—signs of continuous disease activity. Arch Neurol 1988;45:505–508.
71. Fishman PS. Late-convalescent poliomyelitis. Arch Neurol 1987;44:98–100.
72. Ito H, Hirano A. Comparative study of spinal cord ubiquitin expression in post-poliomyelitis and sporadic amyotrophic lateral sclerosis. Acta Neuropathol 1994;87:425–429.
73. Dalakas MC, Elder G, Hallett M, et al. A long-term follow-up study of patients with post-poliomyelitis neuromuscular symptoms. N Engl J Med 1986;314:959–961.
74. Dalakas MC. Morphologic changes in the muscles of patients with post-poliomyelitis neuromuscular symptoms. Neurology 1988;38:99–104.
75. Semino-Mora C, Dalakas MC. Rimmed vacuoles with β-amyloid and ubiquitinated filamentous deposits in the muscles of patients with long-standing denervation (post-poliomyelitis muscular atrophy): similarities with inclusion body myositis. Hum Pathol 1998;29:1128–1133.
76. Ince PG, Lowe J, Shaw PJ. Amyotrophic lateral sclerosis: current issues in classification, pathogenesis and molecular pathology. Neuropathol Appl Neurobiol 1998;24:104–117.
77. Brownell B, Oppenheimer DR, Hughes JT. The central nervous system in motor neurone disease. J Neurol Neurosurg Psychiatry 1970;33:338–357.
78. Martin JE, Swash M. The Pathology of Motor Neuron Disease. In PN Leigh, M Swash (eds), Motor Neuron Disease: Biology and Management. London: Springer-Verlag, 1995;93–118.
79. Bunina TL. Intracellular inclusions in familial amyotrophic lateral sclerosis. Zh Neuropathol Pskyat 1962;62:1293–1299.
80. Leigh PN, Anderton BH, Dodson A, et al. Ubiquitin deposits in anterior horn cells in motor neuron disease. Neurosci Lett 1988;93:197–203.
81. Lowe J, Lennox G, Jefferson D, et al. A filamentous inclusion body within anterior horn neurons in motor neuron disease defined by immunocytochemical localization of ubiquitin. Neurosci Lett 1988;93:203–210.
82. Chou SM. Pathognomy of Intraneuronal Inclusions in ALS. In T Tsubaki, Y Toyokura (eds), Amyotrophic Lateral Sclerosis. Tokyo, Baltimore: Tokyo University Press and University Park Press; 1979;135–177.
83. Ince PG, Tomkins J, Slade JY, et al. Amyotrophic lateral sclerosis associated with genetic abnormalities in the gene encoding superoxide dismutase: molecular pathology of five new cases and comparison with 73 sporadic cases and previous reports. J Neuropathol Exp Neurol 1998;57:895–904.
84. Rouleau GA, Clark AW, Rooke K, et al. SOD1 mutation is associated with accumulation of neurofilaments in amyotrophic lateral sclerosis. Ann Neurol 1996;39:128–131.
85. Piao Y-S, Wakabayashi K, Kakita A, et al. Neuropathology with clinical correlations of sporadic amyotrophic lateral sclerosis: 102 autopsy cases examined between 1962 and 2000. Brain Pathol 2003;12:10–22.
86. Sasaki K, Iwata M. Ultrastructural study of Betz cells in the primary motor cortex of the human brain. J Anat 2001;199:699–708.
87. Kusaka H. Neuropathology of the motor neuron disease—Bunina body. Clin Neurol 1999;39:65–66.
88. Okamoto K, Hirai S, Amari M, et al. Bunina bodies in amyotrophic lateral sclerosis immuno-stained with rabbit antiserum. Neurosci Lett 1993;162:125–128.

89. Sasaki S, Maruyama S. Ultrastructural study of Bunina bodies in the anterior horn neurons of patients with amyotrophic lateral sclerosis. Neurosci Lett 1993;154:117–120.
90. Tomonaga M, Saito M, Yoshimura M, et al. Ultrastructure of the Bunina bodies in anterior horn cells of amyotrophic lateral sclerosis. Acta Neuropathol 1978;42:81–86.
91. Leigh PN, Dodson A, Swash M, et al. Cytoskeletal abnormalities in motor neuron disease: an immunocytochemical study. Brain 1989;112:521–535.
92. Leigh PN, Whitwell H, Garofalo O, et al. Ubiquitin-immunoreactive intraneuronal inclusions in amyotrophic lateral sclerosis: morphology, distribution and specificity. Brain 1991;114:775–788.
93. Love S, Saitoh T, Quijada S, et al. Alz-50, ubiquitin and tau immunoreactivity of neurofibrillary tangles, Pick bodies and Lewy bodies. J Neuropathol Exp Neurol 1988;47:393–405.
94. Lowe J, Blanchard A, Morrell K, et al. Ubiquitin is a common factor in intermediate filament inclusion bodies of diverse type in man, including those of Parkinson's disease, Pick's disease and Alzheimer's disease as well as Rosenthal fibers in cerebellar astrocytomas, cytoplasmic inclusion bodies in muscle and Mallory bodies in alcoholic liver disease. J Pathol 1988;155:9–15.
95. Lowe J. New pathological findings in amyotrophic lateral sclerosis. J Neurol Sci 1994; 124(suppl):38–51.
96. Mather K, Martin JE, Swash M, et al. Histochemical and immunocytochemical study of ubiquitinated neuronal inclusions in amyotrophic lateral sclerosis. Neuropathol Appl Neurobiol 1993;19:141–145.
97. Sasaki S, Toi S, Shirata A, et al. Immunohistochemical and ultrastructural study of basophilic inclusions in adult-onset motor neuron disease. Acta Neuropathol 2001;102:200–206.
98. Ince PG. Neuropathology. In RJ Brown, V Meininger, M Swash (eds), Amyotrophic Lateral Sclerosis. London: Martin Dunitz, 2000;83–112.
99. Ince P, Evans J, Forster G, et al. Corticospinal tract degeneration in the progressive muscular atrophy variant of ALS. Neurology 2003;60:1252–1258.
100. Hirano A, Kurland LT, Sayre GP. Familial amyotrophic lateral sclerosis: a subgroup characterized by posterior and spinocerebellar tract involvement and hyaline inclusions. Arch Neurol 1967;16:232–243.
101. Schochet JS, Hardmann JM, Ladewig PP, Earle KM. Intraneuronal conglomerates in sporadic motor neuron disease. Arch Neurol 1969;20:548–553.
102. Kondo A, Iwaki T, Tateishi J, et al. Accumulation of neurofilaments in a sporadic case of amyotrophic lateral sclerosis. Jpn J Psychiatry Neurol 1986;40:677–684.
103. Hirano A, Donnefeld H, Sasaki S, Nakano I. Fine structural observations on neurofilamentous changes in amyotrophic lateral sclerosis. J Neuropathol Exp Neurol 1984;43:461–470.
104. Katayama S, Watanabe C, Kohriyama T, et al. Gallyas-positive argyrophilic and ubiquitinated filamentous inclusions in rapidly progressive motor neuron disease: Immunohistochemical and electron microscopic studies. Acta Neuropathol 2000;100:221–227.
105. Carpenter S. Proximal axonal enlargement in motor neuron disease. Neurology 1968;18:841–851.
106. Wong N, He B, Strong M. Characterization of neuronal intermediate filament protein expression in cervical spinal neurons in sporadic amyotrophic lateral sclerosis. J Neuropathol Exp Neurol 2000;59:972–982.
107. Mannetto V, Sternberger NH, Perry G, et al. Phosphorylation of neurofilaments is altered in amyotrophic lateral sclerosis. J Neuropathol Exp Neurol 1988;47:642–653.
108. Munoz DG, Greene C, Perl DP, Selkoe DJ. Accumulation of phosphorylated neurofilaments in anterior horn motoneurons of amyotrophic lateral sclerosis patients. J Neuropathol Exp Neurol 1988;47:9–18.
109. Arima K, Ogawa M, Sunohara N, et al. Immunohistochemical and ultrastructural characterization of ubiquitinated eosinophilic fibrillary neuronal inclusions in sporadic amyotrophic lateral sclerosis. Acta Neuropathol 1998;96:75–85.
110. Takahashi K, Nakamura H, Okada E. Hereditary amyotrophic lateral sclerosis. Arch Neurol 1972;27:292–299.
111. Tanaka S, Yase Y, Yoshimasu H. Familial amyotrophic lateral sclerosis. Ultrastructural study of intraneuronal hyaline inclusion material. Adv Neurol Sci 1980;24:386–387.
112. Metcalf C, Hirano A. Clinicopathological studies of a family with amyotrophic lateral sclerosis. Arch Neurol 1971;24:518–523.
113. Sasaki S, Yamane K, Sakuma H, Murayama S. Sporadic motor neuron disease with Lewy body–like hyaline inclusions. Acta Neuropathol 1989;78:555–560.
114. Murayama S, Mori H, Ihara Y, et al. Immunocytochemical and ultrastructural studies of lower motor neurons in ALS. Ann Neurol 1990;27:137–148.

115. Murayama S, Ookawa Y, Mori H, et al. Immunocytochemical and ultrastructural study of Lewy body–like inclusions in familial amyotrophic lateral sclerosis. Acta Neuropathol 1989;78:143–152.
116. Konagaya M, Sakai M, Matsuoka Y, et al. Upper motor neuron predominant degeneration with frontal and temporal lobe atrophy. Acta Neuropathol 1998;96:532–536.
117. Watanabe R, Iino M, Honda M, et al. Primary lateral sclerosis. Neuropathology 1997;17:220–224.
118. Hudson AJ. Amyotrophic lateral sclerosis and its association with dementia, parkinsonism and other neurological disorders: a review. Brain 1981;104:217–247.
119. Wilkstrom J, Paetau A, Palo J, et al. Classic amyotrophic lateral sclerosis with dementia. Arch Neurol 1982;39:681–683.
120. Mitsuyama Y. Presenile dementia with motor neuron disease in Japan: clinicopathological review of 26 cases. J Neurol Neurosurg Psychiatry 1984;47:953–959.
121. Mitsuyama Y. Presenile dementia with motor neuron disease. Dement Geriatr Cogn Disord 1993;4:137–142.
122. Mitsuyama Y, Kogoh H, Ata K. Progressive dementia with motor neuron disease: an additional case report and neuropathological review of 20 cases in Japan. Eur Arch Psychiatry Neurol Sci 1985;235:1–8.
123. Neary D, Snowden JS, Mann DMA, et al. Frontal lobe dementia and motor neurone disease. J Neurol Neurosurg Psychiatry 1990;53:23–32.
124. Morita K, Kaiya H, Ikeda T, Namba M. Presenile dementia combined with amyotrophy: a review of 34 Japanese cases. Arch Gerontol Geriatr 1987;6:263–277.
125. Gallassi R, Montaga P, Ciardulli C, et al. Cognitive impairment in motor neuron disease. Acta Neurol Scand 1985;71:480–484.
126. Peavy GM, Herzog AG, Rubin NP, Mesulam MM. Neuropsychological aspects of dementia of motor neuron disease: a report of two cases. Neurology 1992;42:1004–1008.
127. Caselli RJ, Windebank AJ, Petersen RC, Komori T. Rapidly progressive aphasic dementia and motor neuron disease. Ann Neurol 1993;33:200–207.
128. Wightman G, Anderson VER, Martin J, et al. Hippocampal and neocortical ubiquitin-immunoreactive inclusions in amyotrophic lateral sclerosis with dementia. Neurosci Lett 1992;139:269–277.
129. Okamoto K, Hirai S, Yamazaki Y, et al. New ubiquitin-positive intraneuronal inclusions in the extra-motor cortices in patients with amyotrophic lateral sclerosis. Neurosci Lett 1991;129:233–236.
130. Brun A, Englund B, Gustafson L, et al. Consensus on clinical and neuropathological criteria for frontotemporal dementia. J Neurol Neurosurg Psychiatry 1994;57:416–418.
131. Kawashima T, Kikuchi H, Takita M, et al. Skein-like inclusions in the neostriatum from a case of amyotrophic lateral sclerosis with dementia. Acta Neuropathol 1998;96:541–545.
132. Kawashima T, Furuta A, Doh-ura K, et al. Ubiquitin-immunoreactive skein-like inclusions in the neostriatum are not restricted to amyotrophic lateral sclerosis, but are rather aging-related structures. Acta Neuropathol 2000;100:43–49.
133. Cooper P, Jackson M, Lennox G, et al. Tau, ubiquitin, and αB crystallin immunohistochemistry define the principal causes of degenerative frontotemporal dementia. Arch Neurol 1995;52:1011–1015.
134. Holton L, Révész T, Crooks R, Scaravilli F. Evidence for pathological involvement of the spinal cord in motor neuron disease-inclusion dementia. Acta Neuropathol 2002;103:221–227.
135. Tsuchiya K, Ozawa E, Fukushima J, et al. Rapidly progressive aphasia and motor neuron disease: a clinical, radiological and pathological study of an autopsy case with circumscribed lobar atrophy. Acta Neuropathol 2000;99:81–87.
136. Castaigne P, Lhermitte F, Cambier J, et al. Étude neuropathologique de 61 observations de sclérose latérale amyotrophique: discussion nosologique. Rev Neurol 1972;127:401–414.
137. Iwata M, Hirano A. Current Problems in the Pathology of Amyotrophic Lateral Sclerosis. In HM Zimmerman (ed), Progress in Neuropathology. New York: Raven Press, 1979;277–298.
138. Lawyer TJ, Netsky MG. Amyotrophic lateral sclerosis: a clinicopathological study of 53 cases. Arch Neurol Psychiatry 1953;69:171–192.
139. Dyck PJ, Stevens JC, Mulder DW, Espinosa RE. Frequency of nerve fiber degeneration of peripheral and sensory neurons in amyotrophic lateral sclerosis. Neurology 1975;25:781–785.
140. Bradley WG, Good P, Rasool CG, Adelman LS. Morphometric and biochemical studies of peripheral nerves in amyotrophic lateral sclerosis. Ann Neurol 1983;14:267–277.
141. Averback P, Crocker P. Regular involvement of Clarke's nucleus in sporadic amyotrophic lateral sclerosis. Arch Neurol 1982;39:155–156.
142. Swash M, Leader M, Brown A, Swettenham KW. Focal loss of anterior horn cells in the cervical cord in motor neuron disease. Brain 1986;109:939–952.

143. Takasu T, Mizutani T, Sakamaki S, et al. An autopsy case of sporadic amyotrophic lateral sclerosis with degeneration of the spinocerebellar tracts and the posterior columns. Ann Rep Neurodeg Dis Res Committee in Japan 1985;94–100.
144. Shimizu T, Kawata A, Kato S, et al. Autonomic failure in ALS with a novel SOD1 mutation. Neurology 2000;54:1534–1537.
145. Tabuchi T, Takahashi K, Tanaka F. Familial ALS with ophthalmoplegia. Clin Neurol 1983;23:278–287.
146. Mizutani T, Sakamaki S, Tsuchiya N, et al. Amyotrophic lateral sclerosis with ophthalmoplegia and multisystem degeneration in patients on long term use of respirators. Acta Neuropathol 1992;84:372–377.
147. Hayashi H, Kato S. Total manifestations of amyotrophic lateral sclerosis (ALS) in the totally locked-in state. J Neurol Sci 1989;93:19–35.
148. Akiyama K, Tsutusumi H, Onoda N, et al. An autopsy case of sporadic amyotrophic lateral sclerosis with sensory disturbances and ophthalmoplegia. Rinsho Byori 1987;5:921–927.
149. Sudo S, Fukutani Y, Matsubara R, et al. Motor neuron disease with dementia combined with degeneration of striatonigral and pallidoluysian systems. Acta Neuropathol 2002;103:521–525.
150. Machida Y, Tsuchiya K, Anno M, et al. Sporadic amyotrophic lateral sclerosis with multiple system degeneration: a report of an autopsy case without respirator administration. Acta Neuropathol 1999;98:512–515.
151. Su M, Yoshida Y, Ishiguro H, Hirota K. Nigral degeneration in a case of amyotrophic lateral sclerosis. Evidence of Lewy body–like and skein inclusions in the pigmented neurons. Clin Neuropathol 1999;18:293–300.
152. Al-Sarraj S, Maekawa S, Kibble M, et al. Ubiquitin only intraneuronal inclusion in the substantia nigra is a characteristic feature of motor neurone disease with dementia. Neuropathol Appl Neurobiol 2002;28:120–128.
153. Ince PG, Shaw PJ, Slade JY, et al. Familial amyotrophic lateral sclerosis with a mutation in exon 4 of the Cu/Zn superoxide dismutase gene: pathological and immunocytochemical changes. Acta Neuropathol 1996;92:395–403.
154. Chou SM, Wang HS, Taniguchi A. Role of SOD1 and nitric oxide/cyclic GMP cascade on neurofilament aggregation in ALS/MND. J Neurol Sci 1996;139(suppl):16–26.
155. Kokubo Y, Kuzahara S, Narita Y, et al. Accumulation of neurofilaments and SOD1-immunoreactive products in a patient with familial amyotrophic lateral sclerosis with I113T SOD1 mutation. Arch Neurol 1999;56:1506–1508.
156. Shaw CE, Enayat ZE, Powell JF, et al. Familial amyotrophic lateral sclerosis: molecular pathology of a patient with a SOD1 mutation. Neurology 1997;49:1612–1616.
157. Sasaki S, Yamane K, Sakuma H, Iwata M. An unusual case of familial amyotrophic lateral sclerosis with extensive involvement and neuronal cytoplasmic inclusions. Neuropathol Appl Neurobiol 2000;26:398–402.
158. Takahashi H, Makifuchi T, Nakano R, et al. Familial amyotrophic lateral sclerosis with a mutation in the Cu/Zn superoxide dismutase gene. Acta Neuropathol 1994;88:185–188.
159. Takehisa Y, Ujike H, Ishizu H, et al. Familial amyotrophic lateral sclerosis with a novel Leu126Ser mutation in the copper/zinc superoxide dismutase gene showing mild clinical features and Lewy body–like hyaline inclusions. Arch Neurol 2001;58:736–740.
160. Cervenakova L, Protas I, Hirano A, et al. Progressive muscular atrophy variant of familial amyotrophic lateral sclerosis (PMA/ALS). J Neurol Sci 2000;177:124–130.
161. Kedekawa J, Fujimura H, Ogawa Y, et al. A clinicopathological study of a patient with familial amyotrophic lateral sclerosis associated with a two base pair deletion in the copper/zinc superoxide dismutase (SOD1) gene. Acta Neuropathol 1997;94:617–622.
162. Kato S, Shimoda M, Watanabe Y, et al. Familial amyotrophic lateral sclerosis with a two base pair deletion in superoxide dismutase 1 gene: multisystem degeneration with intracytoplasmic hyaline inclusions in astrocytes. J Neuropathol Exp Neurol 1996;55:1089–1101.
163. Ohi T, Saita K, Takechi S, et al. Clinical features and neuropathological findings of familial amyotrophic lateral sclerosis with a His46Arg mutation in Cu/Zn superoxide dismutase. J Neurol Sci 2002;197:73–78.
164. Cudkowicz ME, McKenna-Yasek D, Chen C, et al. Limited corticospinal tract involvement in amyotrophic lateral sclerosis subjects with the A4V mutation in the copper/zinc superoxide dismutase gene. Ann Neurol 1998;43:703–710.
165. Shibata N, Hirano A, Kobayashi M, et al. Cu/Zn superoxide dismutase–like immunoreactivity in Lewy body–like inclusions of sporadic amyotrophic lateral sclerosis. Neurosci Lett 1994;179:149–152.

166. Shibata N, Hirano A, Kobayashi M, et al. Intense superoxide dismutase-1 immunoreactivity in intracytoplasmic hyaline inclusions of familial amyotrophic lateral sclerosis with posterior column involvement. J Neuropathol Exp Neurol 1996;55:481–490.
167. Bruijn L, Becher M, Lee M, et al. ALS-linked SOD1 mutant G85R mediates damage to astrocytes and promotes rapidly progressive disease with SOD1-containing inclusions. Neuron 1997;18: 327–338.
168. Bruijn L, MK H, Kato S, et al. Aggregation and motor neuron toxicity of an ALS-linked SOD1 mutant independent from wild-type SOD1. Science 1998;281:1851–1854.
169. Sasaki S, Ohsawa Y, Yamane K, et al. Familial amyotrophic lateral sclerosis with widespread vacuolation and hyaline inclusions. Neurology 1998;51:871–873.
170. Watanabe M, Dykes-Hoberg M, Cullota V, et al. Histological evidence of protein aggregation in mutant SOD1 transgenic mice and in amyotrophic lateral sclerosis neural tissues. Neurobiol Dis 2001;8:933–941.
171. Shibata N, Hirano A, Kobayashi M, et al. Presence of Cu/Zn superoxide dismutase (SOD) immunoreactivity in neuronal hyaline inclusions in spinal cords from mice carrying a transgene for Gly93Ala mutant human Cu/Zn SOD. Acta Neuropathol 1998;95:136–142.
172. Matsumoto S, Kusaka H, Ito H, et al. Sporadic amyotrophic lateral sclerosis with dementia and Cu/Zn superoxide dismutase–positive Lewy body–like inclusions. Clin Neuropathol 1996;15: 41–46.
173. Kato S, Horiuchi S, Nakashima K, et al. Astrocytic hyaline inclusions contain advanced glycation end products in familial amyotrophic lateral sclerosis with superoxide dismutase 1 gene mutation: immunohistochemical and immunoelectron microscopical analyses. Acta Neuropathol 1999;97: 260–266.
174. Kato S, Nakashima K, Horiuchi S, et al. Formation of advanced glycation end-product–modified superoxide dismutase-1 (SOD1) is one of the mechanisms responsible for inclusions common to familial amyotrophic lateral sclerosis patients with SOD1 gene mutation, and transgenic mice expressing human SOD1 gene mutation. Neuropathology 2001;21:67–81.
175. Shibata N. Transgenic mouse model for familial amyotrophic lateral sclerosis with superoxide dismutase-1 mutation. Neuropathology 2001;21:82–92.
176. Bruyn RPM, Scheltens P. Hereditary Spastic Paraparesis (Strümpell-Lorrain). In JMBV de Jong, P Vinken, RPM Bruyn, Klawans H (eds), Handbook of Clinical Neurology. Amsterdam: Elsevier, 1991;301–318.
177. McDermott CJ, White K, Bushby K, Shaw PJ. Hereditary spastic paraparesis: a review of new developments. J Neurol Neurosurg Psychiatry 2000;69:150–160.
178. Harding AE. Hereditary "pure" spastic paraplegia: a clinical and genetic study of 22 families. J Neurol Neurosurg Psychiatry 1981;44:871–883.
179. Fink JK, Heiman-Patterson T, Bird TD, et al. Hereditary spastic paraplegia: advances in genetic research. Hereditary Spastic Paraplegia Working Group. Neurology 1996;46:1507–1515.
180. Figlewicz D, Bird TD. "Pure" hereditary spastic paraplegias. Neurology 1999;53:5–7.
181. Sack GH Jr, Huether CA, Garg N. Familial spastic paraplegia—clinical and pathologic studies in a large kindred. Johns Hopkins Med J 1978;143:117–121.
182. Strümpell A. Ueber eine bestimmte Form der primaren combinierten Systemerkrankung des Ruckenmarks. Arch Psychiatry Nervenkr 1886;17:217–238.
183. Schwartz G. Hereditary (familial) spastic paraplegia. Arch Neurol Psychiatry 1952;68:655–682.
184. Behan W, Maia M. Strümpell's familial spastic paraplegia: genetics and neuropathology. J Neurol Neurosurg Psychiatry 1974;37:8–20.
185. Schwartz G, Liu C. Hereditary (familial) spastic paraplegia: further clinical and pathologic observations. Arch Neurol Psychiatry 1956;75:144–162.
186. Casari G, Rugarli E. Molecular basis of inherited spastic paraplegias. Curr Opin Genet Dev 2001;11:336–342.
187. Errico A, Ballabio A, Rugarli EI. Spastin, the protein mutated in autosomal dominant hereditary spastic paraplegia, is involved in microtubule dynamics. Hum Mol Genet 2002;11:153–163.
188. Tedeshi G, Alloca S, DiConstanzo A, et al. Multisystem involvement of the central nervous system in Strümpell's disease. J Neurol 1991;103:55–60.
189. Byrne PC, McMonagle P, Webb S, et al. Age-related cognitive decline in hereditary spastic paraparesis linked to chromosome 2p. Neurology 2000;1:1510–1517.
190. McMonagle P, Byrne PC, Fitzgerald B, et al. Phenotype of AD-HSP due to mutations in the SPAST gene: comparison with AD-HSP without mutations. Neurology 2000;55:1794–1800.
191. Webb S, Coleman D, Byrne PC, et al. Autosomal dominant hereditary spastic paraparesis with cognitive loss linked to chromosome 2p. Brain 1998;121:601–609.

192. Ferrer I, Olive M, Rivera R, et al. Hereditary spastic paraparesis with dementia, amyotrophy and peripheral neuropathy. A neuropathological study. Neuropathol Appl Neurobiol 1995;21:255–261.
193. White KD, Ince PG, Lusher ME, et al. Clinical and pathologic findings in hereditary spastic paraparesis with spastin mutation. Neurology 2000;55:89–94.
194. Casari G, De Fusco M, Ciarmatori S, et al. Spastic paraplegia and OXPHOS impairment caused by mutations in paraplegin, a nuclear-encoded mitochondrial metalloprotease. Cell 1998;93: 973–983.
195. McDermott CJ, Dayaratne RK, Tomkins J, et al. Paraplegin gene analysis in hereditary spastic paraparesis (HSP) pedigrees in north east England. Neurology 2001;56:467–471.
196. Hedera P, DiMauro S, Bonilla E, et al. Phenotypic analysis of autosomal dominant hereditary spastic paraplegia linked to chromosome 8q. Neurology 1999;1:44–49.

3
Neurophysiological Investigation of Motor Neuron Disorders

Kerry R. Mills

In the absence of a definitive marker for idiopathic amyotrophic lateral sclerosis (ALS), electrophysiology forms the cornerstone of diagnosis. As the prognosis for ALS is so poor, the clinical neurophysiologist bears a heavy responsibility in differentiating ALS from other conditions that can mimic it, such as cervical myelopathy, radiculopathy, and multifocal motor neuropathy with focal conduction block. Neurophysiological techniques are also of use in the other motor neuron disorders to be described such as familial ALS (FALS), primary lateral sclerosis (PLS), progressive bulbar palsy, spinal muscular atrophy (SMA), and the postpolio syndrome.

A variety of electrophysiological techniques are available: Sensory nerve conduction studies assess the integrity of dorsal root ganglia and peripheral sensory axons; motor nerve conduction studies assess peripheral motor axons from the spinal motor neuron distally; central motor conduction studies using magnetic brain stimulation assess the corticospinal pathways; and electromyography (EMG) can detect fasciculations and signs of acute or chronic lower motor neuron (LMN) degeneration in the muscles, even in those that are clinically unaffected. Techniques are available for studying not only limb muscles but also bulbar muscles and the diaphragm.

With the advent of possible treatments for ALS and the trial of a number of agents,[1] the question of using neurophysiological parameters as measures of outcome also must be addressed. Although muscle force in this context is probably the most relevant parameter to measure, the need for quantitative assessments unaffected by the voluntary effort of the patient remains. Serial studies that give useful indicators of the number of surviving motor units in a muscle[2-6] and the serial assessment of corticospinal conduction[7] are two such measures currently being considered.

The available techniques are described in the following sections, as are the findings in motor neuron diseases (MNDs). A neurophysiological diagnostic strategy to differentiate as accurately as possible ALS from its mimics is offered. In addition, one of the cardinal clinical features of ALS is deterioration over time and repeated neurophysiological investigations are often required to verify the diagnosis.

NERVE CONDUCTION STUDIES

Motor Nerve Conduction

Motor nerve conduction studies are important in the investigation of MNDs for a number a reasons. First, it is important to exclude generalized or focal peripheral neuropathy, radiculopathy, or plexopathy. Second, it is important to exclude multifocal motor neuropathy with focal conduction block because this can closely simulate ALS but has a much better prognosis.[8–13] Third, some motor nerve conduction parameters correlate with the clinical state of the patient and may therefore be useful in follow-up.

Technically, the easiest nerves to study are the median and the ulnar nerves in the upper limb and the common peroneal and posterior tibial nerves in the lower limb. Surface recording electrodes are placed over the relevant muscles: abductor pollicis brevis (APB) for the median, abductor digiti minimi (ADM) or the first dorsal interosseous (FDI) for the ulnar, extensor digitorum brevis for the common peroneal, and abductor hallucis for the posterior tibial. Supramaximal stimulation of the peripheral nerve evokes a maximal compound muscle action potential (CMAP), or M wave. The magnitude, best measured as the initial negative peak amplitude or area of the CMAP, reflects the volume of excitable muscle tissue accessible from nerve stimulation. CMAP amplitude may be reduced by axon loss, conduction block in the nerve trunk or its distal branches, neuromuscular block, or indeed conduction block at the muscle fiber membrane. Normal values for CMAP amplitude are wide, are related to age and sex, and are dependent on the habitual use of the muscle. As a rule of thumb, CMAP amplitudes in intrinsic hand muscles of less than 5 millivolts are usually abnormal. Thus in ALS, CMAP amplitude may be small and is approximately correlated with the degree of wasting of the muscle; interestingly, it is correlated in a curvilinear fashion with muscle strength as estimated with the Medical Research Council scale.[14] Of course, CMAP amplitude reflects the combined effects of denervation and reinnervation and so may remain within the normal range even when EMG shows signs of acute denervation and chronic reinnervation. Serial studies of CMAP amplitude in patients with ALS have been tried as a measure of deterioration. For this to be valid, knowledge of the variability of these measurements over time is required, in addition to the interobserver variability. Such available studies[15–18] indicate that at least 10-percent variability can be expected on repeated measurements, and thus a change in CMAP amplitude of at least this figure is required to indicate true deterioration with some degree of certainty. Repeated measurements taken on patients, however, do show the expected decline over time.[6]

The latency from distal stimulation, say, at the wrist, in upper limb nerves, also termed the *terminal* or *distal motor latency* (DML), is the time consumed in conduction down the nerve trunk, conduction along the fine intramuscular nerve terminal branches, neuromuscular transmission, and the initiation of action potentials in the postsynaptic muscle membrane. Proximal stimulation at, say, the elbow involves the same processes but adds conduction in the elbow to wrist segment. Subtraction of the two latencies therefore merely reflects this conduction time, and division into the distance yields motor conduction velocity (MCV). It should be pointed out that because latency is measured from the first deflection from the baseline, the actual velocity measured is that of the fastest conducting fiber in the nerve. In ALS, DML and MCV remain almost normal, never falling beyond 70 percent of the upper or lower limit of normal.[19–23] This is because the primary abnormality is axon loss, rather than peripheral nerve demyelination, and the loss does not preferentially affect a particular fiber population. Only if the fastest conducting motor fibers degenerate will there be a reduction in MCV.

Motor nerve conduction can also be assessed in more proximal nerve segments: Ulnar nerve fibers can be supramaximally stimulated in the axilla, the Erb's point (over the brachial plexus), and at the exit foramen of the eighth cervical root (Figure 3.1).[24] This becomes particularly important when searching for conduction block.[9] Proximal studies in the median nerve are also possible, but the problem of volume-conducted responses from ulnar-innervated hand muscles is more serious. It is not possible to stimulate the median nerve above the elbow without also exciting the ulnar nerve. Recordings from the APB are therefore contaminated by responses from the nearby ulnar-innervated thenar flexor muscles and the FDI. The reverse is not true because the ADM is relatively isolated and is less contaminated by median CMAPs. Proximal stimulation is best conducted with a high-voltage electrical stimulator[24,25] because it is important to verify that the response is indeed maximal. Magnetic stimulation over the vertebral column also excites the motor roots at their exit foramina, but even in healthy individuals, it is not possible to guarantee maximal stimulation.[25] If magnetic stimulus intensity is increased, then the point of nerve excitation moves distally and falsely short values are obtained. In healthy subjects, the conduction velocity in distal nerve segments is slightly slower than that in proximal nerve segments, presumably because axons are thinner distally. This proximal distal MCV gradient is usually maintained in ALS, compared with acquired neuropathies in which it may be reversed. The definition of *conduction block* (see later discussion) requires a reduction of CMAP amplitude of 50 percent when comparing adjacent distal and proximal stimulation sites. In ALS, the response to proximal stimulation is often markedly less than that with wrist stimulation, but there is a gradual change in amplitude as stimulation proceeds proximally. In contrast, in multifocal motor neuropathy, there is a step change in amplitude, which is useful in diagnosis (see Figure 3.1).

Proximal stimulation of lower limb nerves is technically less satisfactory. Lumbar roots can be stimulated electrically or magnetically,[26–28] but ensuring a maximal stimulus, which is required for the diagnosis of conduction block, is difficult and the exact site of stimulation is not well defined.

F-Wave Studies

When a peripheral nerve is stimulated, impulses propagate in both directions. The antidromically directed impulses in motor nerves invade the spinal motor

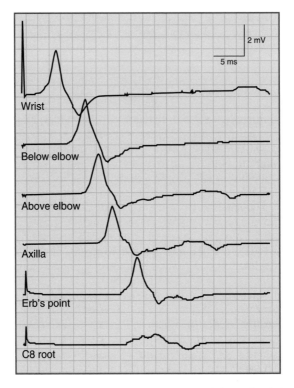

Figure 3.1 Compound muscle action potentials recorded from the right abductor digiti minimi muscle in a patient with multifocal motor neuropathy with focal conduction block. The ulnar nerve has been stimulated supramaximally at six points from the wrist up to the C8 root. Motor conduction velocity is normal in all segments, but there is a focal conduction block in the segment between the C8 root exit foramen and the Erb's point. F waves at normal latency can be seen in the traces from the wrist, above the elbow and axilla.

neuron cell bodies, and in some cases, there is re-excitation and impulses propagate again down the motor axon to the muscle. This results in F waves recorded in hand muscles after wrist stimulation at about 30 milliseconds after the initial direct response. F waves are important because they assess motor conduction over the whole pathway from spinal motor neuron to muscle. They are particularly effective in disclosing a general slowing of conduction but are less good when there is a focal abnormality of conduction.[16] F-wave latency is related to height, particularly in lower limb nerves. In ALS, F waves may be marginally prolonged or absent.[20,21,29] The slight slowing of conduction is explicable in terms of the dropout of fast-conducting motor fibers; the delay in F waves, prolongation of DML, and reduction in MCV are proportionate when conduction distance is taken into account. Absence of F waves in ALS is seen occasionally, presumably because the subpopulation of motor neurons capable of producing F responses has degenerated. Absence of an F response is also seen in multifocal motor neuropathy, but clearly this finding in isolation cannot be taken as definitive evidence of block.

Sensory Nerve Conduction

Sensory conduction studies are performed by electrically stimulating a peripheral sensory nerve and then recording the nerve action potentials from the same nerve either proximally (orthodromic conduction) or distally (antidromic conduction). Averaging the response over a number of trials is necessary to reduce noise. The sural, medial plantar, and median; ulnar (from digital nerve stimulation); and radial nerves are the most useful. The amplitude of a sensory nerve action potential (SNAP) is approximately related to the number of sensory axons in the nerve and to the synchrony with which action potentials reach the recording electrode. Thus in peripheral neuropathies caused by axonal loss or demyelination, SNAPs are reduced in amplitude or absent. The amplitude of SNAPs also declines with age, and this clearly must be considered during interpretation.

Sensory nerve function is usually reported to be normal in ALS, but in practical terms, sensory nerve conduction studies should be performed to exclude peripheral neuropathy, multiple mononeuropathy, and lumbar radiculopathy. However, a point to remember is that patients who are relatively immobile or wheelchair bound may develop pressure palsies with a sensory component. Thus carpal tunnel syndrome from wheelchair propulsion or heavily leaning on sticks,[30] ulnar neuropathy at the elbow from the use of crutches and other walking aids, and common peroneal nerve lesions at the fibular head from poorly fitting footdrop prostheses are all encountered with some regularity. Clearly, the finding of abnormal sensory conduction must be interpreted in the clinical context.

Although SNAPs in nerves not prone to pressure palsies are usually well preserved in ALS, there are reports of a decline in sensory nerve function if serial studies are performed.[30–32] However, amplitudes tend to remain within the normal range. Somatosensory evoked potentials are also reportedly abnormal in ALS,[31,33–37] and a number of pathological studies suggest that ALS is not a pure motor syndrome. This may be important for studies of pathogenesis but is not useful from the purely diagnostic viewpoint.

REPETITIVE NERVE STIMULATION

A decrement in the CMAP during repetitive nerve stimulation at 1 Hz or 3 Hz has been reported in up to half of patients with ALS.[38] The decrement is usually less than 10 percent, but as in myasthenia, the decrement is maximal after four or five stimuli, disappears after a brief period of exercise, and reappears 2 minutes later. Single fiber abnormalities may also be evident.[39] Both effects are thought to be due to the insecurity of impulse transmission in the new nerve sprouts involved in intramuscular reinnervation. It is unusual for these effects to cause diagnostic confusion with neuromuscular junction abnormalities, however, because in these conditions, acute and chronic denervation do not occur. It has been suggested that the decrement found in ALS may be used in combination with other clinical and neurophysiological parameters to assess prognosis.[38]

CENTRAL MOTOR CONDUCTION STUDIES

Magnetic stimulation of the brain excites the motor cortex and causes a descending volley of impulses in the corticospinal tract, which in turn causes spinal motor neurons to discharge. Motor evoked potentials can be recorded in most human muscles.[7] A number of parameters of central conduction are of interest in motor neuron disorders.

First, the threshold of excitation can be measured.[40,41] A major difference between central motor conduction studies and peripheral nerve conduction is the variability of responses obtained from brain stimulation. Even when all conditions are held as constant as possible, responses to brain stimulation may vary by an order of magnitude in amplitude. Defining the threshold for motor cortex activation therefore is done on a statistical basis. A technique has been developed that allows threshold to be determined to the nearest 1 percent of stimulator output, which involves giving shocks of first increasing and then decreasing intensities until, by a bracketing process, a value is reached at which responses are obtained on 50 percent of trials.[40] In healthy subjects, threshold determined by this method in the relaxed hand muscle varies between 36 and 65 percent of maximal stimulator output. The test-retest variability of the technique indicates that changes of greater than 13 percent are significant over a 3-month period. In ALS, the most common finding is for threshold to be raised or for no response to be obtained. Threshold also varies with the evolution of the disease. In early patients in whom no upper motor neuron (UMN) signs are evident, threshold may be lower than normal.[41,42] Later in the evolution, and especially when UMN signs are present, threshold is usually raised.

Second, the conduction time from cortex to muscle can be measured, which allows calculation of the central motor conduction time (CMCT). The latency of a muscle response is dependent on whether the muscle is active voluntarily. In the relaxed state, the latency is about 2 to 3 ms longer than if the muscle is activated. Most authors measure CMCT with the muscle slightly activated voluntarily. CMCT is estimated by subtracting from the cortex-muscle latency an estimate of the peripheral conduction time. This can be done in two ways: First, the latency of the direct response to root stimulation can be subtracted, or second, the F-wave latency can be used to estimate the peripheral conduction time from motor neuron to muscle. The two methods can be combined to give a conduction time in the most proximal motor root from spinal motor neuron to root exit. Normal values for CMCT to a variety of muscles are available.[7] In ALS, CMCT to hand muscles is most often normal.[23,43–45] About 15 to 20 percent of patients show prolongation of CMCT, but this is usually modest, being no more than 4 to 5 ms. Marked prolongation of CMCT is rarely found in idiopathic ALS and if found in a suspected case should lead to a consideration of other diagnoses such as multiple sclerosis, FALS or PLS.

The diagnosis of ALS can be helped by using transcranial magnetic stimulation to measure CMCT to bulbar muscles.[46] In 30 patients with ALS, only 2 of whom had clinical evidence of UMN involvement of the cranial nerves, 17 and 15 had central motor conduction abnormalities to the orofacial muscles and to the tongue, respectively. The abnormality was predominantly an absent response, although five patients showed a modestly prolonged CMCT.

A number of other more complex measurements can be made of central motor excitability. When the brain is stimulated, the cortex goes though a cycle of changes in excitability, first inhibition then excitation. Intracortical inhibition can be measured by giving pairs of cortical shocks. If the first (conditioning) shock is submaximal and the second (test) shock is above threshold, then the test response is attenuated by prior conditioning at intervals of 1 to 5 ms. This phenomenon probably reflects γ-aminobutyric acid–transmitting (GABAergic) intracortical inhibitory circuits.[47–52] Second, if the patient is asked to maintain a voluntary contraction of the muscle while the brain is stimulated, there is a pause in the ongoing voluntary EMG activity, which may last for 150 to 200 ms depending on the stimulus intensity. The origin of this inhibition is complex but involves both intracortical and spinal inhibitory circuits.[53–57] Abnormalities of both intracortical inhibition and the duration of the silent period have been found in ALS.[58–61] It appears that on average the degree of intracortical inhibition is less than normal (Figure 3.2), and the silent period is shorter than normal, leading to the suggestion that there may be a state of cortical hyperexcitability in ALS, possibly related to glutamate excitotoxicity.

ELECTROMYOGRAPHY

Standard EMG aims to detect spontaneous activity in the muscle and to examine the size, configuration, and firing rate of motor units during voluntary activity. The distribution of such changes, whether in a nerve, root, or more generalized distribution, gives important clues to the diagnosis. In the context of ALS, it is clearly important to examine clinically unaffected muscles, all four limbs, and muscles innervated by cranial nerves. It is better, if possible, to avoid muscles commonly involved as a result of coincidental entrapment neuropathies.

Spontaneous Activity

Fibrillations (Figure 3.3) represent the spontaneous discharge of single muscle fibers that have been rendered hyperexcitable by acute denervation. Fibrillations are also found occasionally in muscle diseases, for example, polymyositis. Positive sharp waves have the same significance as fibrillations being generated when the action potential in a spontaneously active fiber propagates away from the needle electrode. In the context of ALS, the finding of fibrillations or positive sharp waves is strong evidence of an acute neurogenic process affecting the muscle sampled; that is, of an LMN component. The degree of fibrillation

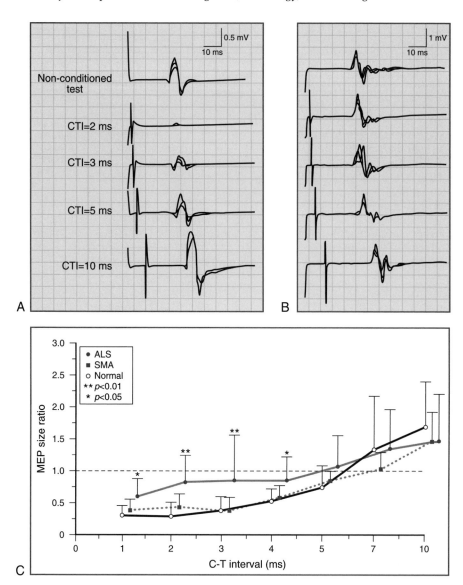

Figure 3.2   The effect of a subthreshold conditioning magnetic stimulus on the responses in abductor pollicis brevis to a suprathreshold test stimulus applied 1 to 10ms later. Results from a healthy subject (**A**) and from a patient with amyotrophic lateral sclerosis (ALS) (**B**) are shown. (**C**) The mean (±SD) ratios of the conditioned to the unconditioned response amplitudes in groups of patients with ALS and spinal muscular atrophy are shown. (Reprinted with permission from Yokota T, Yoshino A, Inaba A, Saito Y. Double cortical stimulation in amyotrophic lateral sclerosis. J Neurol Neurosurg Psychiatry 1996;61:596–600.)

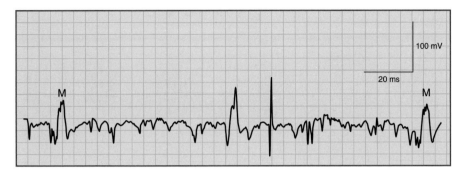

Figure 3.3 Electromyographic recording from the extensor digitorum communis muscle in a patient with amyotrophic lateral sclerosis. Profuse fibrillations and positive sharp waves are seen, indicating an acute neurogenic abnormality. In addition, a small highly polyphasic motor unit potential *(M)* is seen. This appearance indicates early reinnervation.

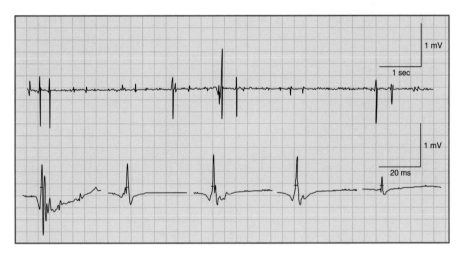

Figure 3.4 Fasciculations in amyotrophic lateral sclerosis recorded with an electromyography needle in the tibialis anterior muscle. Above is a 10-second continuous record. Below, on an expanded time scale, are the wave forms of fasciculations; the third and fourth wave forms show the same fasciculation with an unstable component.

may be used qualitatively to provide an assessment of the rate of progression of the disease. Muscles that show solely fibrillation but little in the way of chronic neurogenic change suggest a rapid progression, whereas muscles showing little fibrillation and marked chronic neurogenic change suggest active reinnervation is occurring and therefore a slower evolution.

Fasciculations represent the spontaneous discharge of a single motor unit or part thereof (Figure 3.4); fasciculations are found in MNDs, polyneuropathy, radiculopathy, and occasionally hyperthyroidism. Fasciculations are usually regarded as not being under voluntary control, but there is still some debate about this. It may be that if fasciculations reflect dying motor units, then there may a

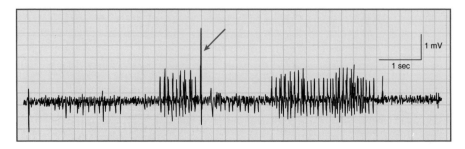

Figure 3.5   Spontaneous electromyographic activity recorded from the tongue of a patient with amyotrophic lateral sclerosis. The patient was unable to relax the tongue completely and rhythmic motor unit activity is seen. A fasciculation *(arrow)* clearly larger than the early recruited voluntary motor units fires just singly, rather than in a rhythmic fashion.

stage during which they remain under voluntary control. More important is to differentiate fasciculations from motor units discharging because the patient is poorly relaxed. Voluntary motor units in this context always fire as a short train of fairly regularly discharging potentials, at about 6 to 10 Hz (Figure 3.5). Fasciculations occur as single discharges at an irregular frequency of at most 1 hertz but often much less frequently. Early recruited motor units are usually small and have relatively simple wave forms, whereas fasciculations tend to be large and often have complex and unstable wave forms (see Figure 3.4).

There is some debate concerning the site of origin of fasciculations.[62–66] They occur in conditions affecting the motor neuron or the proximal motor axon and yet appear to be generated in the intramuscular nerve terminals. Cutting the peripheral nerve to a fasciculating muscle reduces but does not abolish the fasciculation, proving that they do not originate in the proximal axon or motor neuron soma. Careful recordings of many fasciculations, including the F response of a fasciculation[62] and its response to peripheral nerve stimulation, indicate that fasciculations originate in the terminal arborizations of the nerve fibers supplying the motor unit. Indeed, there is evidence of multiple generators of the same fasciculation within the terminal arborization. More recently, techniques to assess the biophysical properties of human axons in vivo have been used to study ALS.[67,68] In some patients, there appears to be an instability of the nerve membrane, making it more likely spontaneously to generate an impulse and hence a fasciculation. There are some reports of fasciculations that may be of central origin. Magnetic stimulation at weak strengths can evoke single motor unit discharges; occasionally in ALS, fasciculations, clearly different than the earliest recruited voluntary units, can also be evoked by magnetic stimuli.[64,65] It has been suggested that these fasciculations, which tend to have simpler wave forms, could arise in the central nervous system.

Differentiating benign fasciculations from those associated with more serious disease is occasionally difficult; no electrophysiological parameters can reliably differentiate the two in a given patient.[69] However, it should be appreciated that benign fasciculations are not associated with denervation and tend to be limited to the distal lower limb, especially the gastrocnemius muscle. Malignant fasciculations tend to be associated with progressive weakness and signs of denervation on EMG. Clearly, if doubt exists whether fasciculations are benign or malignant, then repeated EMG after an interval will be required.

Fasciculations can also be recorded with surface electrodes, and by using a multichannel system (such as an electroencephalographic machine), one can record from multiple muscles and decide on the frequency and distribution of such spontaneous muscle activity.[70,71]

Other forms of spontaneous activity are occasionally encountered in ALS and include complex repetitive discharges and doublet fasciculations. The former characteristically has an abrupt onset and offset, and the frequency of discharge tends to be constant. Complex discharges can be prolonged (many minutes) or brief. The wave form of each complex is remarkably constant, and individual components show very low jitter; these characteristics indicate that the discharge arises from ephaptic transmission among a group of denervated muscle fibers. Doublet fasciculations in which the same wave form is repeated after a short (4- to 5-ms) interval are seen in ALS and neuromyotonia, although in the latter, there is usually no associated neurogenic change on EMG.

Electromyography of Voluntary Activity

The electrical activity associated with voluntary action gives information about the structure of motor units. Activity is assessed when the patient makes a modest contraction thereby recruiting a few motor units, the wave forms of which can be examined, and when the patient performs a maximal contraction thereby recruiting many motor units, which gives rise to an interference pattern.

The processes of denervation and reinnervation are inferred from EMG findings. In ALS, death of motor neurons will lead to degeneration of motor axons and acute denervation of muscle fibers, which will be evident as fibrillations. Surviving fine intramuscular nerves now sprout to reinnervate the denervated fibers. The immature nerve sprouts conduct impulses insecurely and with reduced velocity. Hence, satellite potentials occur after the motor unit potential (MUP) associated with the reinnervating motor unit. In addition, because of insecure transmission, there may be variations in the shape of successive MUPs; single fiber EMG may show blocking, and repetitive nerve stimulation may give rise to decrements.[72] Eventually, the collateral nerve spouts mature and conduct normally giving rise now to MUPs with increased amplitudes and durations.

The amplitude, configuration, and duration of MUPs aid the differentiation of myopathy, early reinnervation, and chronic reinnervation. In myopathy, MUPs are small, polyphasic, and short in duration. In early reinnervation, MUPs show complex wave forms of normal amplitude but prolonged duration, often with satellite potentials. In chronic denervation with reinnervation, MUPs are large and relatively simple in wave form but are of prolonged duration.

When a motor unit is first recruited, it begins to fire at about 10 hertz, and this rate is modulated upward as more force is required. When the number of motor units is reduced, for example, in ALS, the drive from the central nervous system causes motor units to fire faster, at up to 25 hertz. Electromyographers are skilled at listening to the EMG signal during maximal voluntary activation of the muscle and detecting this high firing rate even when single motor units cannot be distinguished in the interference pattern. In UMN weakness, motor unit firing rates tend to be lower than normal, but this feature is not reliable for diagnosis, being easily confused with poor volition. Whereas a normal motor unit may have amplitude in the range of 1 to 5 mV, in chronic reinnervation, motor units can reach amplitudes of up to 25 mV, sometimes referred to as "giant" motor units. Clearly, there is a limit to the degree of reinnervation that can take place, but it has been estimated that up to 50 percent of motor neurons may be lost before there is detectable loss of strength in the muscle.[73]

Quantitative Electromyography

Quantification of the EMG signal is usually not required for diagnostic purposes but may be useful in documenting change or response to treatment. The parameters of early recruited motor units can be measured by isolating the units during weak voluntary contractions and then using delayed triggering to display and average the MUP. Conventionally 20 such MUPs are isolated and the amplitude, duration, and number of phases are determined. The technique suffers from the drawback that the sample of motor units is biased toward the low threshold units and often the onset and offset of the potential are difficult to define. Normal values for amplitude and duration are available for a number of muscles.[74]

The recruitment pattern may be quantified in a number of ways. The simplest is to use the turns/amplitude technique in which the number of turns, or changes, in the direction of the signal per second and the amplitude change between each turn are measured automatically with a computer. In muscle disease, there are increased turns per second with small mean amplitudes, whereas with chronic neurogenic disease, there are a reduced number of turns of larger amplitude. The number of turns per second and the mean amplitude depend on the force of contraction, but having the patient produce a known fraction of the maximal force of the muscle can control this.

In the macro-EMG technique a specialized needle is used to record from a single muscle fiber, and then the signal derived from the whole motor unit is extracted by averaging the signal derived from the shaft of the needle.[39,75-82] The resulting averaged MUP is a reflection of the whole motor unit, rather than a subset of its fibers, as is obtained from conventional concentric needle EMG. The technique can also be used to estimate fiber density, which is the number of fibers belonging to a single unit within the pickup area of the single fiber needle. Clearly if there is fiber type grouping as would be expected in partial reinnervation, then fiber density will be increased.

Motor Unit Counting Techniques

A basic piece of information that would be useful in the serial study of ALS is how many functioning motor units remained in the muscle. A number of techniques are available for this.[3-6,83-89] Basically, surface recordings are made from a muscle and the motor nerve is stimulated electrically at just threshold intensity so only one motor unit is activated. This is recognized by its constant wave form and its all-or-none response. The intensity is gradually increased so the second, third, and each subsequent motor unit is recruited individually. Usually, no more than about five motor units can be discerned by this method. Knowing the average amplitude of the single motor units and the amplitude of the maximal CMAP, one can calculate an estimate of the total number of motor units contributing activity. This technique has been used to follow the decline in motor unit numbers in patients with ALS[3–6,87] and to investigate the postpolio syndrome.[90]

PROTOCOL FOR INVESTIGATING PATIENTS WITH SUSPECTED AMYOTROPHIC LATERAL SCLEROSIS

The approach to the diagnosis of a patient with suspected ALS is dictated by the clinical situation and a consideration of the alternative possibilities (Table 3.1), but a number of core investigations should be conducted in all patients. The need for further testing is confirmed by the results of these tests and the clinical signs. To make a confident diagnosis of ALS, the clinical neurophysiologist must do the following:

1. Prove that sensory nerve function is normal, or if not normal, that it is explicable by some coincidental factor such as entrapment neuropathy. As a minimum, the sural, median, and ulnar SNAPs on one side should be measured.
2. Prove that the motor conduction in upper and lower limbs is normal or near normal. As a minimum, the posterior tibial and ulnar nerves, including measurement of CMAP amplitude, conduction velocity, and F-wave latency, on one side should be examined.
3. If warranted by the clinical situation (e.g., lack of any UMN signs, asymmetrical upper limb onset, weakness without wasting of muscles, or absence of F waves on motor testing), a search for conduction block should be instituted, including the proximal segments of upper limb nerves.
4. Establish evidence of an LMN lesion in a widespread distribution; that is, not explicable in terms of a single nerve, root, or plexus lesion. This usually involves sampling at least two muscles in the most affected limb, at least one

Table 3.1 Conditions that may cause diagnostic confusion with amyotrophic lateral sclerosis

---

Cervical or lumbar radiculopathy ± myelopathy
Multifocal motor neuropathy with conduction block
Peripheral neuropathy: especially chronic inflammatory demyelinating neuropathy
Spinal muscular atrophy
Primary lateral sclerosis
Polymyositis
Myasthenia gravis
Syringomyelia
Hyperthyroidism

---

muscle in the other limbs, and at least one muscle innervated by a cranial nerve (e.g., tongue, sternomastoid, or trapezius). In the clinical context, it is more important to establish evidence of denervation or fasciculation in a clinically unaffected muscle than one that is clearly wasted. It makes sense to examine a clinically affected muscle first to establish that it indeed has a neurogenic abnormality and then to examine clinically less or unaffected muscles in other limbs to establish the distribution of abnormality.

5. Attempt to provide evidence of a UMN lesion by demonstrating prolongation of the CMCT to upper and/or lower limb muscles and/or bulbar muscles or a lack of response to maximal brain stimulation.

FAMILIAL AMYOTROPHIC LATERAL SCLEROSIS

It is now generally accepted that some 5 percent of ALS cases are familial. Twenty percent of these familial cases have been found to have mutations of the copper/zinc superoxide dismutase gene; many mutations have now been reported. In terms of nerve conduction studies and EMG, the findings are indistinguishable from idiopathic ALS.

Central motor conduction studies have been reported in patients with FALS with the D90A mutation.[91] Thirty homozygous patients from nine families had the characteristic phenotype featuring wasting, weakness, fasciculations, and hyperreflexia initially affecting the legs but over 4 to 6 years affecting the arms and then bulbar muscles. Central motor conduction was performed in seven of these patients and was found to be abnormal in all. In those patients in whom a response was obtained, CMCT was markedly prolonged to both upper and lower limb muscles. Interestingly, single motor unit studies have shown that the delayed response to magnetic stimulation is preceded by a period of inhibition, suggesting that fast-conducting corticomotoneuronal connections had been lost, but slower conducting connections were preserved.[92] This contrasts with idiopathic ALS in which there is desynchronization in the fast-conducting corticospinal fibers but only minimal delay.[65] In other patients with FALS without the D90A mutation, CMCT and corticomotor threshold are normal.[7]

PRIMARY LATERAL SCLEROSIS

The nosological identity of this condition and its relationship to ALS remain uncertain, but most authorities regard it as one end of a spectrum in which UMN abnormalities predominate. Typically, it presents as a slowly progressive spinobulbar spasticity without LMN findings either clinically or on EMG.[93] There are some reports of PLS evolving over many years into a syndrome resembling ALS. On EMG, however, infrequent fasciculations may be seen and occasional fibrillations, even though the time course of the condition is much slower than ALS.[94] Brown et al[95] (1992) have reported central motor conduction studies in seven patients with PLS. In four patients, CMAPs could not be obtained, but in the remaining three, CMCT was markedly prolonged, much beyond the range found in idiopathic ALS. This adds some credence to the notion that PLS, which differs in its clinical and pathological characteristics from ALS, is a nosological entity.

X-LINKED BULBOSPINAL NEURONOPATHY (KENNEDY'S DISEASE)

This condition tends to have an earlier age at onset than ALS but can occasionally cause diagnostic confusion if the clinical picture is not characteristic. It presents as a slowly progressive symmetrical LMN syndrome affecting bulbar and limb muscles, associated in some patients with testicular atrophy and gynecomastia (see Chapter 17). EMG findings are similar to ALS, although bulbar abnormalities predominate in Kennedy's disease, especially facial and tongue denervation and fasciculation.[96] Motor nerve conduction studies are usually normal, apart from small CMAPs in wasted muscles, but more than half the patients have reduced or absent SNAPs[97] or delayed somatosensory evoked potentials.[98] CMCT in contrast is normal.[99]

SPINAL MUSCULAR ATROPHY

The infantile and childhood spinal muscular atrophies are autosomal recessive conditions classified in terms of age at onset (see Chapter 16). The rapidly progressive type I (Werdnig-Hoffmann disease) presents at or soon after birth. The early childhood variant (type II) presents at 6 to 18 months, and type III presents later, after 18 months. EMG is useful in these cases to confirm the neurogenic abnormality by the presence of fibrillations. Fasciculations are seen but are less frequent than in ALS.

Adult forms of SMA may have predominantly proximal weakness when the principal differential diagnosis is muscular dystrophy, usually easily differentiated on EMG. Distal symmetrical forms of adult-onset SMA may cause confusion with ALS because both show chronic neurogenic change, fibrillations, and fasciculations on EMG, but of course, UMN signs are lacking. The degree of reinnervation and hence the size of MUPs is usually greater in SMA than ALS and the incidence of fibrillations and fasciculations is less, but in the individual patient when the length of history is short, the only solution is to reexamine the patient after a period looking for UMN signs or marked deterioration in the LMN component. In these conditions, motor and sensory nerve conduction studies are usually normal. Central motor conduction studies are normal in adult-onset SMA.[99-102]

MULTIFOCAL MOTOR NEUROPATHY WITH FOCAL CONDUCTION BLOCK

Multifocal motor neuropathy with conduction block is characterized by a slowly progressive, asymmetrical, predominantly upper limb distal weakness, without sensory abnormalities. A clear pointer to the condition is the presence of a normal CMAP in a muscle that shows no wasting but is weak. Focal fasciculations and preserved tendon reflexes are also features.[13] Differentiation on clinical grounds from ALS and distal SMA can be difficult. Neurophysiologically, there are multiple motor conduction blocks at "non-usual" sites, with normal MCV and preserved SNAPs. Indeed, sensory nerve function is normal in the same nerve segment showing motor block. Fasciculations or neuromyotonia may be prominent in the weak muscles. The cause of motor conduction block in this condition is not known for certain. Although a demyelinating process is often assumed and there is some pathological data to support this,[103] the rapidity of the response to intravenous immunoglobulin precludes remyelination as a mechanism. The condition may in fact be a focal channelopathy that could account for the conduction block and its rapid reversal.

The motor conduction block is often in the forearm or more proximal segments of upper limb nerves. The criteria for the definition of conduction block are still being debated. The problem arises because temporal dispersion caused simply by demyelination can lead to a large drop in CMAP amplitude even when there is no block. Temporal dispersion causes an increase in the duration of the CMAP, and so definitions of block include both amplitude and duration criteria. Most investigators would accept a decrease in amplitude of 50 percent when comparing the usual adjacent stimulation sites with an increase in duration of the CMAP of less than 20 percent as definite evidence of block. With these strict criteria, some blocks are probably being missed. If, however, the affected nerve is accessible to stimulate over short segments (2 to 3 cm), then a focal fall in amplitude of 10 percent is good evidence for conduction block. Proximal electrical stimulation at the Erb's point and the motor roots improves the diagnosis of multifocal motor neuropathy. For example, of eight patients with the condition, four had a conduction block that was limited to the proximal nerve segments.[9] An example is seen in Figure 3.1.

EMG in patients with early multifocal motor neuropathy is usually normal in clinically unaffected muscles. Affected muscles show the EMG signs of conduction block, that is, a reduced recruitment pattern of motor units of normal configuration. As the block persists, however, there must be secondary axonal loss and fibrillation and signs of chronic neurogenic change appear. In some long-standing cases, the clinical and EMG signs can be indistinguishable from distal SMA.

HEREDITARY SPASTIC PARAPARESIS

The hereditary spastic parapareses (HSP) form a heterogeneous group with a variety of modes of inheritance. The so-called "pure" form of HSP is characterized by slowly progressive spastic paraparesis with pyramidal signs in the lower limbs, with about 25 percent of patients eventually developing upper limb hyperreflexia. Many cases are associated to variable degrees with other neurological abnormalities including mental retardation, cerebellar ataxia, pigmentary retinopathy, optic atrophy, and sensory neuropathy (see Chapter 18).

Nerve conduction studies and EMG results are usually normal in HSP, except in cases in which there is an associated peripheral neuropathy or neuronopathy. Motor nerve function remains normal, but SNAPs may be small or absent. EMG reveals signs only attributable to the UMN lesion, that is, normal motor units in a reduced recruitment pattern having normal wave forms but a reduced firing rate.

Central motor conduction studies in HSP tend to show delayed or absent responses in the lower limbs with normal responses in the upper limbs.[104] A study of ten patients with the "pure" form of HSP examined central motor conduction to small hand muscles and found modestly increased CMCT in two patients.[105] Central motor conduction using the electrical scalp stimulation method in 11 patients with "pure" HSP found all patients had delayed or reduced responses in leg muscles, but only 2 patients had abnormal central conduction to intrinsic hand muscles.[106] Similarly, using magnetic stimulation, 83 percent of patients had abnormal lower limb responses but only 32 percent had abnormal upper limb responses.[107] Of a family that was clearly not "pure" HSP in having evidence of an associated sensory neuropathy, all had very prolonged CMCTs to both upper and lower limb muscles.

Sporadic cases of HSP can be confused with tropical spastic paraparesis. In these cases, a slowly progressive paraparesis beginning in middle life associated with high titers of antibodies against human T-lymphotropic virus type 1 (HTLV-1) in serum and cerebrospinal fluid is seen. The brunt of the disability falls on the lower limbs, with the upper limbs often being normal or having mild pyramidal signs. Central motor conduction studies in a small series of patients found normal responses in the upper limbs and delayed responses in the lower limbs, suggesting that the pyramidal tract involvement was limited to the thoracic cord.[108] A larger series of 18 HTLV-1—positive Jamaican patients showed prolonged CMCTs to both upper and lower limb muscles, but the prolongation was more marked in the lower limbs. Furthermore, the degree of CMCT abnormality correlated with disease progression.[109]

POSTPOLIO SYNDROME

The development of new symptoms decades after an attack of poliomyelitis is referred to as the *postpolio syndrome*. New symptoms may include weakness and wasting or fatigue of limb or respiratory muscles.[110] The pathogenesis of these new symptoms has been successfully investigated using quantitative EMG techniques, particularly macro-EMG[111–114] and motor unit counting.[90,115] It appears that after the initial insult to the spinal motor neurons, there is intramuscular reinnervation, which may result in complete functional recovery but which will be evident to the EMG technician as larger motor units corresponding to the fiber-type grouping seen on muscle biopsy. As the aging process continues, there is progressive loss of spinal motor neurons, occurring in all subjects healthy or otherwise. In the patients with polio, this further loss of motor neurons leads to further denervation and reinnervation until a threshold is reached beyond which a single motor neuron is unable to support all the muscle fibers it is innervating. Further loss of motor neurons now leads to progressive weakness and wasting. Clearly, muscles weakened by the initial attack will be the first to develop new weakness, but muscles that were initially clinically unaffected may now become weak.[116]

The question about whether patients with postpolio syndrome who often complain of fatigue also have a defect in neuromuscular transmission is still unsettled.[117] Single fiber EMG does in some patients demonstrate increased jitter,[118] but these may reflect insecurity of transmission in newly sprouting intramuscular axons.

EMG in postpolio syndrome reveals marked chronic reinnervation changes with large MUPs of long duration. Fibrillations and fasciculations, however, may also be seen in a small proportion of patients.[90] Motor nerve conduction studies show small CMAPs in clinically wasted muscles and slight reductions in conduction velocity dependent on the loss of fast-conducting axons. Sensory nerve conduction is normal.

REFERENCES

1. Bensimon G, Lacomblez L, Meininger V. A controlled trial of riluzole in amyotrophic lateral sclerosis. N Engl J Med 1994;330:585–591.
2. Bromberg M. Electrodiagnostic studies in clinical trials for motor neuron disease. J Clin Neurophysiol 1998;15:117–128.
3. Armon C, Brandstater ME. Motor unit number estimate-based rates of progression of ALS predict patient survival. Muscle Nerve 1999;22:1571–1575.
4. Felice KJ. A longitudinal study comparing thenar motor unit number estimates to other quantitative tests in patients with amyotrophic lateral sclerosis. Muscle Nerve 1997;20:179–185.
5. Olney RK, Yuen EC, Engstrom JW. Statistical motor unit number estimation: reproducibility and sources of error in patients with amyotrophic lateral sclerosis. Muscle Nerve 2000;23:193–197.
6. Yuen EC, Olney RK. Longitudinal study of fiber density and motor unit number estimate in patients with amyotrophic lateral sclerosis. Neurology 1997;49:573–578.
7. Mills K. Magnetic Stimulation of the Human Nervous System. Oxford: Oxford University Press, 1999.
8. Bentes C, de Carvalho M, Evangelista T, Sales-Luis ML. Multifocal motor neuropathy mimicking motor neuron disease: nine cases. J Neurol Sci 1999;169:76–79.
9. Jaspert A, Claus D, Grehl H, Neundorfer B. Multifocal motor neuropathy: clinical and electrophysiological findings. J Neurol 1996;243:684–692.
10. Bouche P, Moulonguet A, Younes-Chennoufi AB, et al. Multifocal motor neuropathy with conduction block: a study of 24 patients. J Neurol Neurosurg Psychiatry 1995;59:38–44.
11. Lange DJ, Trojaborg W, Latov N, et al. Multifocal motor neuropathy with conduction block: is it a distinct clinical entity? Neurology 1992;42:497–505.
12. Parry GJ, Clarke S. Multifocal acquired demyelinating neuropathy masquerading as motor neuron disease. Muscle Nerve 1988;11:103–107.
13. Roth G, Rohr J, Magistris MR, Ochsner F. Motor neuropathy with proximal multifocal persistent conduction block, fasciculations and myokymia. Evolution to tetraplegia. Eur Neurol 1986;25:416–423.
14. Mills KR. Wasting, weakness and the MRC scale in the first dorsal interosseous muscle. J Neurol Neurosurg Psychiatry 1997;62:541–542.
15. de Carvalho M, Lopes A, Scotto M, Swash M. Reproducibility of neurophysiological and myometric measurement in the ulnar nerve-abductor digiti minimi system. Muscle Nerve 2001;24:1391–1395.
16. Kimura J. Facts, fallacies, and fancies of nerve conduction studies: twenty-first annual Edward H. Lambert Lecture. Muscle Nerve 1997;20:777–787.
17. Tjon ATAM, Lemkes HH, van der Kamp-Huyts AJ, van Dijk JG. Large electrodes improve nerve conduction repeatability in controls as well as in patients with diabetic neuropathy. Muscle Nerve 1996;19:689–695.

18. Bleasel AF, Tuck RR. Variability of repeated nerve conduction studies. Electroencephalogr Clin Neurophysiol 1991;81:417–420.
19. de Carvalho M, Swash M. Nerve conduction studies in amyotrophic lateral sclerosis. Muscle Nerve 2000;23:344–352.
20. Argyropoulos CJ, Panayiotopoulos CP, Scarpalezos S. F- and M-wave conduction velocity in amyotrophic lateral sclerosis. Muscle Nerve 1978;1:479–485.
21. Cornblath DR, Kuncl RW, Mellits ED, et al. Nerve conduction studies in amyotrophic lateral sclerosis. Muscle Nerve 1992;15:1111–1115.
22. Thacker AK, Misra S, Katiyar BC. Nerve conduction studies in upper limbs of patients with cervical spondylosis and motor neurone disease. Acta Neurol Scand 1988;78:45–48.
23. Mills K, Nithi K. Peripheral and central motor conduction in amyotrophic lateral sclerosis. J Neurol Sci 1998;159:82–87.
24. Mills KR, Murray NM. Electrical stimulation over the human vertebral column: which neural elements are excited? Electroencephalogr Clin Neurophysiol 1986;63:582–589.
25. Mills KR, McLeod C, Sheffy J, Loh L. The optimal current direction for excitation of human cervical motor roots with a double coil magnetic stimulator. Electroencephalogr Clin Neurophysiol 1993;89:138–144.
26. Ugawa Y, Rothwell JC, Day BL, et al. Magnetic stimulation over the spinal enlargements. J Neurol Neurosurg Psychiatry 1989;52:1025–1032.
27. Maccabee PJ, Lipitz ME, Desudchit T, et al. A new method using neuromagnetic stimulation to measure conduction time within the cauda equina. Electroencephalogr Clin Neurophysiol 1996;101:153–166.
28. Ertekin C, Nejat RS, Sirin H, et al. Comparison of magnetic coil stimulation and needle electrical stimulation in the diagnosis of lumbosacral radiculopathy. Clin Neurol Neurosurg 1994;96:124–129.
29. Albizzati MG, Bassi S, Passerini D, Crespi V. F-wave velocity in motor neurone disease. Acta Neurol Scand 1976;54:269–277.
30. Schulte-Mattler WJ, Jakob M, Zierz S. Focal sensory nerve abnormalities in patients with amyotrophic lateral sclerosis. J Neurol Sci 1999;162:189–193.
31. Theys PA, Peeters E, Robberecht W. Evolution of motor and sensory deficits in amyotrophic lateral sclerosis estimated by neurophysiological techniques. J Neurol 1999;246:438–442.
32. Gregory R, Mills K, Donaghy M. Progressive sensory nerve dysfunction in amyotrophic lateral sclerosis: a prospective clinical and neurophysiological study. J Neurol 1993;240:309–314.
33. Zanette G, Tinazzi M, Polo A, Rizzuto N. Motor neuron disease with pyramidal tract dysfunction involves the cortical generators of the early somatosensory evoked potential to tibial nerve stimulation. Neurology 1996;47:932–938.
34. Radtke RA, Erwin A, Erwin CW. Abnormal sensory evoked potentials in amyotrophic lateral sclerosis. Neurology 1986;36:796–801.
35. Georgesco M, Salerno A, Camu W. Somatosensory evoked potentials elicited by stimulation of lower-limb nerves in amyotrophic lateral sclerosis. Electroencephalogr Clin Neurophysiol 1997;104:333–342.
36. Dasheiff RM, Drake ME, Brendle A, Erwin CW. Abnormal somatosensory evoked potentials in amyotrophic lateral sclerosis. Electroencephalogr Clin Neurophysiol 1985;60:306–311.
37. Cosi V, Poloni M, Mazzini L, Callieco R. Somatosensory evoked potentials in amyotrophic lateral sclerosis. J Neurol Neurosurg Psychiatry 1984;47:857–861.
38. Daube J. Electrophysiologic studies in diagnosis and prognosis of motor neuron diseases. Neurol Clin 1985;3:473–493.
39. Stalberg E. Use of single fiber EMG and macro EMG in study of reinnervation. Muscle Nerve 1990;13:804–813.
40. Mills KR, Nithi KA. Corticomotor threshold to magnetic stimulation: normal values and repeatability. Muscle Nerve 1997;20:570–576.
41. Mills KR, Nithi KA. Corticomotor threshold is reduced in early idiopathic amyotrophic lateral sclerosis. Muscle Nerve 1997;20:1137–1141.
42. Eisen A, Pant B, Stewart H. Cortical excitability in amyotrophic lateral sclerosis: a clue to pathogenesis. Can J Neurol Sci 1993;20:11–16.
43. Claus D, Brunholzl C, Kerling FP, Henschel S. Transcranial magnetic stimulation as a diagnostic and prognostic test in amyotrophic lateral sclerosis. J Neurol Sci 1995;129:30–34.
44. Eisen A, Shytbel W, Murphy K, Hoirch M. Cortical magnetic stimulation in amyotrophic lateral sclerosis. Muscle Nerve 1990;13:146–151.

45. Ingram DA, Swash M. Central motor conduction is abnormal in motor neuron disease. J Neurol Neurosurg Psychiatry 1987;50:159–166.
46. Urban P, Vogt T, Hopf H. Corticobulbar tract involvement in amyotrophic lateral sclerosis: a transcranial magnetic stimulation study. Brain 1998;121:1099–1108.
47. Mavroudakis N, Caroyer JM, Brunko E, Zegers de Beyl D. Effects of vigabatrin on motor potentials evoked with magnetic stimulation. Electroencephalogr Clin Neurophysiol 1997;105:124–127.
48. Inghilleri M, Berardelli A, Marchetti P, Manfredi M. Effects of diazepam, baclofen and thiopental on the silent period evoked by transcranial magnetic stimulation in humans. Exp Brain Res 1996;109:467–472.
49. Nihei K, McKee A, Kowall N. GABAergic local circuit neurons degenerate in the motor cortex of amyotrophic lateral sclerosis patients. Soc Neurosci Abstracts 1992;18:1249.
50. Ziemann U, Lonnecker S, Paulus W. Inhibition of human motor cortex by ethanol. A transcranial magnetic stimulation study. Brain 1995;118:1437–1446.
51. Ziemann U, Lonnecker S, Steinhoff BJ, Paulus W. Effects of antiepileptic drugs on motor cortex excitability in humans: a transcranial magnetic stimulation study. Ann Neurol 1996;40:367–378.
52. Ziemann U, Lonnecker S, Steinhoff BJ, Paulus W. The effect of lorazepam on the motor cortical excitability in man. Exp Brain Res 1996;109:127–135.
53. Cantello R, Gianelli M, Civardi C, Mutani R. Magnetic brain stimulation: the silent period after the motor evoked potential. Neurology 1992;42:1951–1959.
54. Haug BA, Schonle PW, Knobloch C, Kohne M. Silent period measurement revives as a valuable diagnostic tool with transcranial magnetic stimulation. Electroencephalogr Clin Neurophysiol 1992;85:158–160.
55. Inghilleri M, Berardelli A, Cruccu G, Manfredi M. Silent period evoked by transcranial stimulation of the human cortex and cervico-medullary junctions. J Physiol 1993;466:521–534.
56. Nakamura H, Kitagawa H, Kawaguchi Y, et al. Intracortical facilitation and inhibition after paired magnetic stimulation in humans under anesthesia. Neurosci Lett 1995;199:155–157.
57. Triggs WJ, Cros D, Macdonell RA, et al. Cortical and spinal motor excitability during the transcranial magnetic stimulation silent period in humans. Brain Res 1993;628:39–48.
58. Yokota T, Yoshino A, Inaba A, Saito Y. Double cortical stimulation in amyotrophic lateral sclerosis. J Neurol Neurosurg Psychiatry 1996;61:596–600.
59. Ziemann U, Winter M, Reimers CD, et al. Impaired motor cortex inhibition in patients with amyotrophic lateral sclerosis. Evidence from paired transcranial magnetic stimulation. Neurology 1997;49:1292–1298.
60. Desiato MT, Caramia MD. Towards a neurophysiological marker of amyotrophic lateral sclerosis as revealed by changes in cortical excitability. Electroencephalogr Clin Neurophysiol 1997;105:1–7.
61. Prout AJ, Eisen AA. The cortical silent period and amyotrophic lateral sclerosis. Muscle Nerve 1994;17:217–223.
62. Conradi S, Grimby L, Lundemo G. Pathophysiology of fasciculations in ALS as studied by electromyography of single motor units. Muscle Nerve 1982;5:202–208.
63. Roth G. The origin of fasciculation. Ann Neurol 1982;12:542–547.
64. Kaji R, Kohara N, Kimura J. Fasciculations evoked by magnetic cortical stimulation in patients with ALS. Ann Neurol 1993;43:A257.
65. Mills KR. Motor neuron disease. Studies of the corticospinal excitation of single motor neurons by magnetic brain stimulation. Brain 1995;118:971–982.
66. Wettstein A. The origin of fasciculations in motoneuron diseases. Ann Neurol 1979;5:295–300.
67. Mogyoros I, Kiernan MC, Burke D, Bostock H. Strength-duration properties of sensory and motor axons in amyotrophic lateral sclerosis. Brain 1998;121:851–859.
68. Mogyoros I, Kiernan MC, Burke D, Bostock H. Ischemic resistance of cutaneous afferents and motor axons in patients with amyotrophic lateral sclerosis. Muscle Nerve 1998;21:1692–1700.
69. Trojaborg W, Buchthal F. Malignant and benign fasciculations. Acta Neurol Scand 1965;41:251–254.
70. Hjorth RJ, Walsh JC, Willison RG. The distribution and frequency of spontaneous fasciculation. J Neurol Sci 1973;18:469–474.
71. Howard RS, Murray NMF. Surface EMG in the recording of fasciculations. Muscle Nerve 1992;15:1240–1245.
72. Maselli R, Wollman R, Leung C. Neuromuscular transmission in amyotrophic lateral sclerosis. Muscle nerve 1993;16:1193–1203.
73. Carleton M, Brown W. Changes in motor unit populations in motor neuron disease. J Neurol Neurosurg Psychiatry 1979;42:42–51.

74. Nandedkar S, Stalberg E, Sanders D. Quantitative EMG. In D Dumitru, AA Amato, MJ Zwarts (eds), Electrodiagnostic Medicine (2nd ed). Philadelphia: Hanley and Belfus, 2002;293–356.

75. Vogt T, Nix WA. Functional properties of motor units in motor neuron diseases and neuropathies. Electroencephalogr Clin Neurophysiol 1997;105:328–332.

76. Tackmann W, Vogel P. Fiber density, amplitudes of macro-EMG motor unit potentials and conventional EMG recordings from the anterior tibial muscle in patients with amyotrophic lateral sclerosis. A study on 51 cases. J Neurol 1988;235:149–154.

77. Stalberg E. Macroelectromyography in reinnervation. Muscle Nerve 1982;5:S135–S138.

78. Stalberg E. Macro EMG, a new recording technique. J Neurol Neurosurg Psychiatry 1980;43:475–482.

79. Guiloff RJ, Modarres-Sadeghi H. Voluntary activation and fiber density of fasciculations in motor neuron disease. Ann Neurol 1992;31:416–424.

80. Gan R, Jabre JF. The spectrum of concentric macro EMG correlations, part II: patients with diseases of muscle and nerve. Muscle Nerve 1992;15:1085–1088.

81. Dengler R, Konstanzer A, Kuther G, et al. Amyotrophic lateral sclerosis: macro-EMG and twitch forces of single motor units. Muscle Nerve 1990;13:545–550.

82. de Koning P, Wieneke GH, van der Most van Spijk D, et al. Estimation of the number of motor units based on macro-EMG. J Neurol Neurosurg Psychiatry 1988;51:403–411.

83. Bromberg MB, Forshew DA, Nau KL, et al. Motor unit number estimation, isometric strength, and electromyographic measures in amyotrophic lateral sclerosis. Muscle Nerve 1993;16: 1213–1219.

84. Bromberg MB, Larson WL. Relationships between motor-unit number estimates and isometric strength in distal muscles in ALS/MND. J Neurol Sci 1996;139(suppl):38–42.

85. Daube JR. Estimating the number of motor units in a muscle. J Clin Neurophysiol 1995;12: 585–594.

86. Fang J, Shahani BT, Graupe D. Motor unit number estimation by spatial-temporal summation of single motor unit potentials. Muscle Nerve 1997;20:461–468.

87. Felice KJ. Thenar motor unit number estimates using the multiple point stimulation technique: reproducibility studies in ALS patients and normal subjects. Muscle Nerve 1995;18:1412–1416.

88. McComas AJ. Motor unit estimation: anxieties and achievements. Muscle Nerve 1995;18:369–379.

89. Olney RK, Lomen-Hoerth C. Motor unit number estimation (MUNE): how may it contribute to the diagnosis of ALS? Amyotroph Lateral Scler Other Motor Neuron Disord 2000;1(suppl 2):S41–S44.

90. McComas AJ, Quartly C, Griggs RC. Early and late losses of motor units after poliomyelitis. Brain 1997;120:1415–1421.

91. Andersen PM, Forsgren L, Binzer M, et al. Autosomal recessive adult-onset amyotrophic lateral sclerosis associated with homozygosity for Asp90Ala CuZn-superoxide dismutase mutation. A clinical and genealogical study of 36 patients. Brain 1996;119:1153–1172.

92. Weber M, Eisen A, Stewart HG, Andersen PM. Preserved slow conducting corticomotoneuronal projections in amyotrophic lateral sclerosis with autosomal recessive D90A CuZn-superoxide dismutase mutation. Brain 2000;123:1505–1515.

93. Pringle CE, Hudson AJ, Munoz DG, et al. Primary lateral sclerosis. Clinical features, neuropathology and diagnostic criteria. Brain 1992;115:495–520.

94. Kuipers-Upmeijer J, de Jager AE, Hew JM, et al. Primary lateral sclerosis: clinical, neurophysiological, and magnetic resonance findings. J Neurol Neurosurg Psychiatry 2001;71:615–620.

95. Brown WF, Ebers GC, Hudson AJ, et al. Motor-evoked responses in primary lateral sclerosis. Muscle Nerve 1992;15:626–629.

96. Meriggioli MN, Rowin J, Sanders DB. Distinguishing clinical and electrodiagnostic features of X-linked bulbospinal neuronopathy. Muscle Nerve 1999;22:1693–1697.

97. Trojaborg W, Wulff CH. X-linked recessive bulbospinal neuronopathy (Kennedy's syndrome): a neurophysiological study. Acta Neurol Scand 1994;89:214–219.

98. Kachi T, Sobue G, Sobue I. Central motor and sensory conduction in X-linked recessive bulbospinal neuronopathy. J Neurol Neurosurg Psychiatry 1992;55:394–397.

99. Weber M, Eisen A. Assessment of upper and lower motor neurons in Kennedy's disease: implications for corticomotoneuronal PSTH studies. Muscle Nerve 1999;22:299–306.

100. Misra UK, Kalita J. Central motor conduction in Hirayama disease. Electroencephalogr Clin Neurophysiol 1995;97:73–76.

101. Hefter H, Heidenreich F, Benecke R. Electrophysiological characterization of the X-linked recessive bulbospinal neuronopathy (XRBSN). Electromyogr Clin Neurophysiol 1991;31:451–460.

102. Imai T, Matsuya M, Matsumoto H, et al. Preservation of central motor conduction in patients with spinal muscular atrophy type II. Brain Dev 1995;17:432–435.
103. Kaji R, Oka N, Tsuji T, et al. Pathological findings at the site of conduction block in multifocal motor neuropathy. Ann Neurol 1993;33:152–158.
104. Polo JM, Calleja J, Combarros O, Berciano J. Hereditary "pure" spastic paraplegia: a study of nine families. J Neurol Neurosurg Psychiatry 1993;56:175–181.
105. Claus D, Waddy HM, Harding AE, et al. Hereditary motor and sensory neuropathies and hereditary spastic paraplegia: a magnetic stimulation study. Ann Neurol 1990;28:43–49.
106. Pelosi L, Lanzillo B, Perretti A, et al. Motor and somatosensory evoked potentials in hereditary spastic paraplegia. J Neurol Neurosurg Psychiatry 1991;54:1099–1102.
107. Schady W, Dick JP, Sheard A, Crampton S. Central motor conduction studies in hereditary spastic paraplegia. J Neurol Neurosurg Psychiatry 1991;54:775–779.
108. Tomita I, Shibayama K, Matsuo H, et al. Central motor conduction time in patients with HTLV-1 associated myelopathy. Acta Neurol Scand 1989;79:419–427.
109. Young RE, Morgan OS, Forster A. Motor pathway analysis in HAM/TSP using magnetic stimulation and F-waves. Can J Neurol Sci 1998;25:48–54.
110. Dalakas MC. The post-polio syndrome as an evolved clinical entity. Definition and clinical description. Ann N Y Acad Sci 1995;753:68–80.
111. Stalberg E, Grimby G. Dynamic electromyography and muscle biopsy changes in a 4-year follow-up: study of patients with a history of polio. Muscle Nerve 1995;18:699–707.
112. Trojan DA, Gendron D, Cashman NR. Electrophysiology and electrodiagnosis of the post-polio motor unit. Orthopedics 1991;14:1353–1361.
113. Rodriquez AA, Agre JC, Harmon RL, et al. Electromyographic and neuromuscular variables in post-polio subjects. Arch Phys Med Rehabil 1995;76:989–993.
114. Rodriquez AA, Agre JC, Franke TM. Electromyographic and neuromuscular variables in unstable postpolio subjects, stable postpolio subjects, and control subjects. Arch Phys Med Rehabil 1997;78:986–991.
115. McComas AJ, Galea V, de Bruin H. Motor unit populations in healthy and diseased muscles. Phys Ther 1993;73:868–877.
116. Luciano CA, Sivakumar K, Spector SA, Dalakas MC. Electrophysiologic and histologic studies in clinically unaffected muscles of patients with prior paralytic poliomyelitis. Muscle Nerve 1996;19:1413–1420.
117. Sunnerhagen KS, Grimby G. Muscular effects in late polio. Acta Physiol Scand 2001;171:335–340.
118. Einarsson G. Muscle adaptation and disability in late poliomyelitis. Scand J Rehabil Med Suppl 1991;25:1–76.

4
Neuroimaging in Motor Neuron Disorders

Erik P. Pioro

The clinical evaluation of a patient with suspected amyotrophic lateral sclerosis (ALS) or motor neuron disease (MND) should include neuroimaging to identify treatable conditions mimicking ALS. This remains the most important use of neuroimaging in such patients, and magnetic resonance imaging (MRI) is the most widely used technique. In "El Escorial Revisited: Revised Criteria for the Diagnosis of Amyotrophic Lateral Sclerosis," the World Federation of Neurology (WFN) recommends neuroimaging studies "to rule out structural lesions that may explain the observed signs and symptoms" in all patients with possible or probable ALS.[1] Table 4.1 lists some of the structural lesions detected by neuroimaging that would be inconsistent with a diagnosis of ALS. The WFN revised criteria state that neuroimaging is not essential for "patients with clinically definite ALS with bulbar or pseudobulbar involvement." This reflects the unlikelihood that structural lesions could produce a clinical picture of definite ALS, as defined by the El Escorial criteria, for example, combined upper motor neuron (UMN) and lower motor neuron (LMN) deficits at three of bulbar, cervical, thoracic, and lumbar levels.[1]

Separate from identifying look-alike conditions, however, neuroimaging reveals changes in ALS and MND that are increasingly being recognized as specific and potentially diagnostic. The most widely recognized neuroimaging modalities are related to MRI, although the nuclear medicine techniques of positron emission tomography (PET) and single photon emission computed tomography (SPECT) have provided significant insights into UMN dysfunction in ALS. This chapter focuses on how magnetic resonance–based and nuclear medicine–based techniques have been useful in (1) identifying pathologies producing MND-like clinical features, (2) revealing lesions of the motor pathway that support the diagnosis of MND, and (3) providing novel information about MND per se. Not only do these techniques have the potential to assist in the accurate and timely diagnosis of ALS and other MNDs, but they may provide insights into disease mechanisms and potential for therapeutic intervention.

73

Table 4.1   Neuroimaging features inconsistent with the diagnosis of amyotrophic lateral sclerosis[a]

Significant bony abnormalities visible on plain x-ray films of the skull or spinal canal that might explain the clinical findings

Significant abnormalities of head or spinal cord magnetic resonance imaging that suggest intraparenchymal or extraparenchymal processes not confined to the corticospinal tract

Significant abnormalities of spinal cord myelography with or without computed tomography (CT) or on CT alone suggesting the lesions previously noted

Significant abnormalities on spinal cord angiography suggesting arteriovenous malformations

---

Reprinted with permission from Brooks BR, Miller RG, Swash M, Munsat TL. El Escorial revisited: revised criteria for the diagnosis of amyotrophic lateral sclerosis. Amyotroph Lateral Scler Other Motor Neuron Disord 2000;1:293–299.

[a]Or confounding the interpretation of diagnostic or clinical trial results.

IDENTIFYING MOTOR NEURON DISEASE LOOK-ALIKES

Various intracranial and intraspinal structural lesions can mimic MND by producing varying amounts of UMN and LMN dysfunction in a focal, multifocal, or generalized distribution. The clinician's prudent use of MRI (or computed tomography [CT]) in evaluating individuals with symptoms and signs of ALS is to hopefully identify treatable or curable conditions. In addition to limiting the differential diagnosis, recognizing clinical features that are "typical" or "atypical" of ALS helps the clinician to select the most relevant neuraxial region or regions to be imaged (Table 4.2). Unless the diagnosis of ALS is definite, patients suspected of having ALS should undergo well-performed neuroimaging studies (preferably MRI) of the cervical spinal cord and usually the brain.

The spinal cord is the most common site of pathology mimicking MND, especially at the cervical level. The responsible lesions are most often compressive, causing myelopathy with or without radiculopathy. These arise from degenerative disc disease, bony and ligamentous hypertrophy, or tumor. In the absence of neck or limb pain, such structural pathology may elude diagnosis until neuroimaging is performed. An MRI of the cervical spine revealed severe spondylotic stenosis in a man initially thought to have primary lateral sclerosis (PLS), a purely UMN disorder (Figure 4.1). Less common spinal cord lesions resulting in predominantly UMN deficits include demyelination, inflammation, and ischemia. If bulbar signs exist, a search must be made for lesions at more rostral central nervous system (CNS) levels, including the cervicomedullary junction (Figure 4.2).

Promptly identifying treatable causes of ALS-like symptoms will not only maximize the chances of successful therapy but also minimize the emotional toll of diagnostic uncertainty. It is important to remember, however, that pathology mimicking ALS does not exclude the coexistence of bona fide ALS. For example, cervical spondylotic radiculomyelopathy from spinal stenosis and early ALS—both more common in older individuals—can produce similar findings. Lack of improvement and clinical progression in a patient after

Table 4.2   Clinical features of amyotrophic lateral sclerosis resulting from look-alike conditions

Clinical feature	Region of CNS to image	Responsible non-ALS pathology
Typical		
Unilateral	Brain	Inflammation (e.g., MS, transverse myelitis)
	Spinal cord (cervical/ thoracic)	Ischemia (e.g., stroke)
		Mass (e.g., tumor, vascular malformation)
		Radiculopathies (cervical, lumbosacral)
UMN-predominant or pure UMN	Brain	Demyelinating disease (e.g., MS)
	Spinal cord (cervical/ thoracic)	Ischemia (e.g., strokes)
		Parasagittal mass (e.g., meningioma, vascular malformation)
		Retroviral myelopathy
		Spondylotic myelopathy
		SCD of the spinal cord
Bulbar onset	Brain stem; base of skull	Chiari I malformation
		Demyelinating disease (e.g., MS) in brain stem
		Mass (e.g., tumor, vascular malformation) in brain stem; at foramen magnum
		Syringobulbia, ischemia, for example, brain stem
Atypical		
Sensory loss and/or pain	Spinal cord (e.g., cervical)	Radiculopathy, radiculomyelopathy
		Syringomyelia
Dementia	Brain	Prion disease (e.g., Creutzfeldt-Jakob disease)
Bladder involvement	Spinal cord (e.g., thoracolumbar)	Demyelination (e.g., MS)
		Inflammation (e.g., transverse myelitis)
		Mass (e.g., tumor, vascular malformation)
Recovering ± relapsing	Brain Spinal cord	MS (relapsing-remitting form)

ALS = amyotrophic lateral sclerosis; CNS = central nervous system; MS = multiple sclerosis; SCD = subacute combined degeneration; UMN = upper motor neuron.

decompressive laminectomies reveal the true nature of the underlying neurodegenerative pathology.

MAGNETIC RESONANCE IMAGING ABNORMALITIES

Hyperintensity of the Corticospinal Tract

The increasing use of MRI at 1.5 teslas to examine the CNS of patients with MND has resulted in greater detection of parenchymal pathology that was not visible on CT. The most characteristic neuroimaging finding in ALS is a hyperintense (increased) signal along the corticospinal tract (CST) (or pyramidal

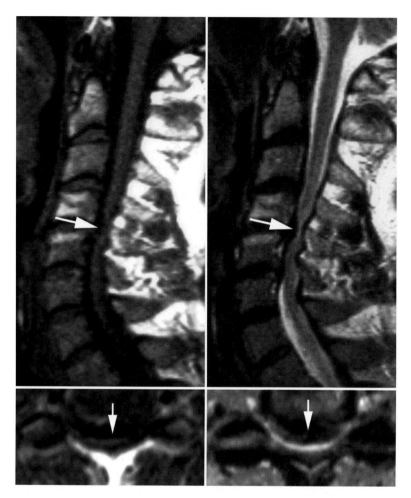

Figure 4.1   Severe compression of the cervical spinal cord is identified on T1- (**left,** *arrows*) and T2- (**right,** *arrows*) weighted magnetic resonance images in a 47-year-old man who had been experiencing progressive gait difficulty for 7 years. Cervical spondylosis, worst at the C4–5 intervertebral level, seen in sagittal (**upper,** *arrows*) and transverse (**lower,** *arrows*) planes, results in ribbon-thin compression of the spinal cord. The patient was thought to have primary lateral sclerosis, a pure upper motor neuron disease, until relatively acute deterioration of handwriting prompted the taking of the magnetic resonance image.

tract) on T2-weighted, proton-density–weighted, and fluid-attenuated inversion-recovery (FLAIR)–weighted MRI. This abnormality, which is bilaterally symmetrical and more frequently detected in the cerebrum than in the spinal cord, probably represents wallerian degeneration of the CST, although only one study has examined this with postmortem pathological correlation.[2] Although not pathognomonic, the occurrence of prominent CST hyperintensity in the appropriate clinical setting helps confirm the diagnosis of ALS.

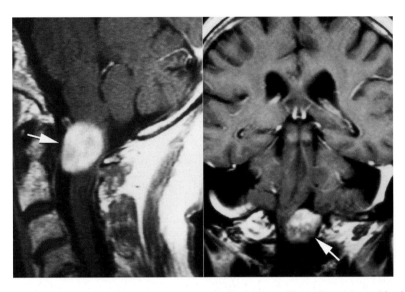

Figure 4.2 Limb spasticity and weakness accompanied by unilateral tongue atrophy in a 63-year-old woman was found to result from a gadolinium-enhancing meningioma of the foramen magnum *(arrows)*. Sagittal **(left)** and coronal **(right)** T1-weighted views reveal severe compression and displacement of the spinomedullary junction.

Intracranial

There have been numerous reports of subcortical white matter hyperintensities in the brain of patients with ALS.[3–13] Intracranial CST hyperintensity has been demonstrated by T2-weighted and proton-density–weighted MRI from its origin beneath the cortical layer (centered on the primary motor cortex), through the centrum semiovale, posterior limb of the internal capsule, and in the ventral brain stem (Figure 4.3). A combined neuroimaging and pathological study showed that the hyperintensity corresponded to demyelination and degeneration of large-caliber CST fibers.[2] This may provide insights into the pathogenesis of the degeneration. Hyperintensity of the CST is most easily identified in the internal capsules and cerebral peduncles (Figures 4.3 and 4.4) but is rarely seen in the lower brain stem.

Depending on the study, the reported frequency of such CST hyperintensity in patients with ALS ranges from 17 to 100 percent (median 40%).[9] Similar changes have been observed in other forms of motor neuron degeneration,[9] including PLS, familial ALS, and juvenile-onset ALS.[14] The wide range of occurrence may reflect a referral bias in the patient population studied or it may represent technical limitation of detection. However, CST hyperintensity possibly may occur in a specific subset of patients with MND. Compared with patients with no MRI abnormality, patients included in the subset tend to more often be female, younger, have prominent UMN features (e.g., spasticity, hyperreflexia, Babinski reflex), and a more rapid initial decline, though not necessarily a shorter duration of disease. However, after analysis of pooled data from

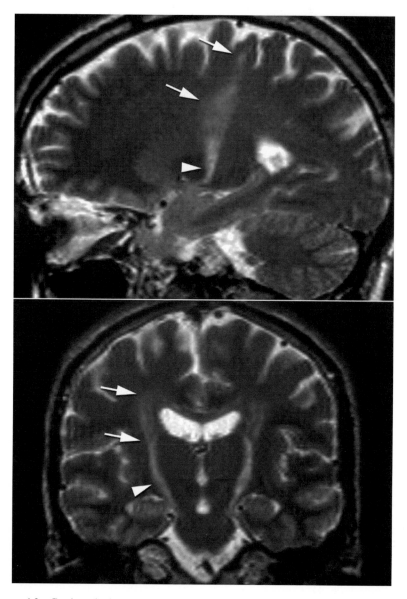

Figure 4.3 Corticospinal tract hyperintensity in a 35-year-old man with upper motor neuron–predominant amyotrophic lateral sclerosis is noted on T2-weighted sagittal **(top)** and coronal **(bottom)** magnetic resonance brain images. This can be followed from the subcortical white matter rostrally *(arrows)* to the internal capsule caudally *(arrowheads).*

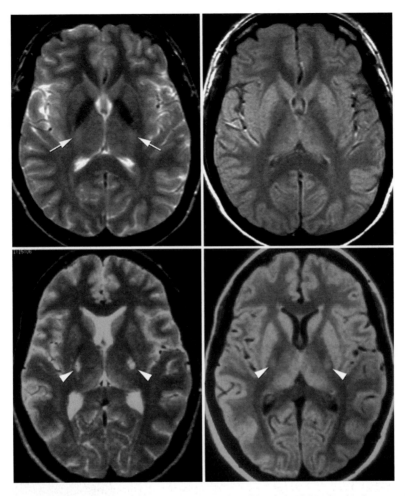

Figure 4.4 Healthy individuals occasionally have a faint hyperintensity in the posterior third of the posterior limb of the internal capsule on T2-weighted (**top left,** *arrowheads*) but not on proton-density–weighted (**top right**) magnetic resonance imaging. This is in contrast to the intense hyperintensity in a patient with amyotrophic lateral sclerosis visible on both T2-weighted (**bottom left**) and proton-density–weighted (**bottom right**) sequences *(arrows).*

published descriptions (*t* test assuming unequal variances), no statistically significant differences were noted between the two groups for all of these features except age.[9] Patients with ALS with CST hyperintensities were significantly ($p < 0.001$) younger (50.7 ± 11.0 years, mean $\pm$ SD, n = 42) than those without such MRI abnormalities (59.0 ± 10.7 years, n = 74). Although this may be due to ascertainment bias because younger patients with ALS tend to have brain MRI obtained more readily, it may represent a patient subgroup with earlier onset disease.

However, between 53 and 76 percent (median 57%) of normal individuals are reported to have a small area of hyperintensity in the posterior limb of the internal capsule detected by T2-weighted MRI[4,8,9,15] (see Figure 4.4). This is a circumscribed, faint hyperintensity that does not extend beyond the internal capsule and cerebral peduncle levels. It probably results from the large-diameter myelinated axons of the normal CST in this location.[2] In contrast to the CST hyperintensity in patients with ALS, the increased signal in healthy individuals is visible on T2-weighted and FLAIR[5] sequences but not on proton-density MRI[8,9,15] (see Figure 4.4). Although more time consuming than FLAIR sequences, the higher specificity of proton-density–weighted MRI makes it the preferred sequence to supplement T2-weighted images when confirming abnormal CST hyperintensity.

Intracranial areas away from the CST have also been reported to have hyperintense signals on T2-weighted and proton-density–weighted MRI in some patients with ALS. One of these is the middle third of the corpus callosum.[5,7] Postmortem studies of the brain of patients with ALS have revealed a discrete bundle of degenerated fibers in this region,[16] likely representing homotopic fiber connections between the precentral gyri. Another non-CST region with reported hyperintensities is the premotor frontal white matter, where punctate lesions were found in 9 (28%) of 32 patients with MND.[12] Although the relationship of these lesions to the disease process is not known, the authors suggested this represented degeneration of afferent fibers to the anterior frontal cortex.

If CST hyperintensity on T2-weighted MRI is correlated with prominent UMN signs, patients with PLS, an MND prominently affecting only UMNs, would be expected to frequently demonstrate this change. However, one MRI study that compared 8 patients with PLS to 31 patients with ALS did not reveal this, despite 7 patients with PLS showing marked spasticity and hyperreflexia.[17] The number of patients with no hyperintensity or mild or moderate hyperintensity (as defined by the authors) was essentially the same in both groups and marked CST hyperintensity was detected only in patients with ALS (10%). In another study of ten patients with PLS, only one showed an increased T2-weighted signal in the posterior limb of the internal capsule extending into the corona radiata.[18] Hereditary spastic paraparesis (HSP) is a neurodegenerative condition producing prominent UMN signs, with autosomal dominant, autosomal recessive, and sex-linked inheritance. The "pure" or "uncomplicated" form usually has no significant changes except spinal cord atrophy (as discussed later). However, some forms of HSP that are "complicated" because they are accompanied by other neurological abnormalities, such as optic neuropathy, mental retardation, dementia, or cerebellar ataxia, have been found to have extensive hyperintensities in the periventricular white matter that extend beyond the CST. An X-linked form of HSP accompanied by mental retardation, cerebellar ataxia, and tremor was found to have bilateral posterior periventricular white matter lesions.[19]

In addition to CST hyperintensities on T2-weighted MRI, T1-related hyperintensities have been reported by one group in up to 67 percent (14/21) of patients with ALS.[20] Unlike T2-related changes, however, those in T1-weighted images were only infrequently observed intracranially along the CST (36%). The T1-related hyperintense signal was found primarily in the anterolateral columns of the spinal cord and not dorsolaterally where the CST is situated.

Because no postmortem tissue analysis was performed, the authors could only speculate that the hyperintensity arose from an accumulation of lipid-laden macrophages, neurofilaments, and toxic metals. Of the five patients with T1-weighted CST hyperintensities intracranially, two (40%) had overlapping T2-related abnormalities.[20] A more subtle change in the T1-weighted appearance of the intracranial CST has been reported by others. Whereas CST fibers in the posterior limb of the internal capsule normally appear slightly hypointense relative to surrounding brain parenchyma, this region in patients with ALS often appears isointense, suggesting a relative hyperintensity.[21] It is of interest that one of the causes of the hyperintense signal on T1-weighted images are free radicals,[22] which have been implicated in the pathogenesis of ALS.[23]

FLAIR sequences have been reported to increase detection of brain lesions in various neurological diseases.[24,25] Because of technical limitations probably related to cerebrospinal fluid (CSF) pulsation, lesions in the brain stem are poorly visualized on FLAIR imaging.[25] A study of 31 patients with ALS and 33 healthy individuals compared the ability of FLAIR, T2-weighted, proton-density–weighted, and T1-weighted sequences to detect cortical and subcortical abnormalities.[21] Signal changes were graded visually by two blinded observers, based on surrounding brain tissue, as isointense, mild, or distinct. FLAIR appeared to be superior to T2-weighted and proton-density–weighted sequences at detecting hyperintensity in patients with ALS at the rostral extent of the CST, that is, at precentral gyrus and centrum semiovale levels (Figure 4.5). On the other hand, at caudal levels of the CST, beginning at the internal

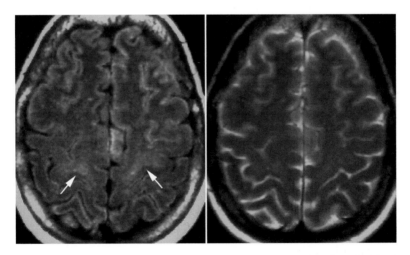

Figure 4.5 Hyperintensity of the corticospinal tract at the level of the subcortical precentral gyrus in a 66-year-old patient with amyotrophic lateral sclerosis is more evident on the fluid-attenuated inversion-recovery sequence (**left**, *arrows*) than in the accompanying T2-weighted transverse magnetic resonance image (**right**). (Adapted with permission from Hecht MJ, Fellner F, Fellner C, et al. MRI-FLAIR images of the head show corticospinal tract alterations in ALS patients more frequently than T2-, T1- and proton-density–weighted images. J Neurol Sci 2001;186:37–44.)

capsule, FLAIR sequences revealed nonspecific hyperintensity (mild or distinct) that was seen even in control individuals.[21] A quantitative analysis was also applied to the CST region to derive a contrast-to-noise ratio (CNR), which was found to be higher in FLAIR images than in all other sequences. The presence of hyperintensity on FLAIR did not correlate with the extent of UMN dysfunction, El Escorial classification, or duration of disease. When scans were separated by site of onset, however, patients with spinal-onset ALS had significant correlation of El Escorial criteria to hyperintensity in the subcortical precentral gyrus ($r = 0.461$; $p < 0.05$). Follow-up MRI in 17 of the original patients 15.7 ± 3.0 months after the initial evaluation showed no significant change in CST hyperintensity visually. However, there was a significant increase in quantitative FLAIR CNR values of the subcortical precentral gyrus region between the first (4.57 ± 1.5) and second (6.03 ± 1.6) examinations ($p = 0.002$). This did not correlate with clinical parameters, although there was progression in the extent of UMN signs and El Escorial scoring.

Spinal Cord

T2-related hyperintensity of the CST is detected less frequently in the spinal cord (dorsolateral columns) than intracranially, either because of technical limitations of detection or a true regional difference in pathology. It has been reported in only 16 patients with ALS, most of whom also had intracranial hyperintensities.[5,9,11,20] As with intracranial CST hyperintensities, those in the spinal cord probably result from axonal degeneration and demyelination.[2]

As mentioned, T1-weighted hyperintensity has been described in the anterolateral columns of the spinal cord in some patients with ALS, although it may not involve the dorsolaterally situated CST. No definite relationship was observed between the T1-related spinal cord hyperintensities and clinical features such as symptom duration or severity of UMN signs. It will be notable if other groups report similar T1-weighted hyperintensities in the brain or spinal cord of patients with ALS.

Hypointensity of the Neocortex

The neocortical gray matter has a hypointense (diminished) signal on T2-weighted and FLAIR MRI in the brains of some patients with ALS. With T2-weighted sequences, 12 to 93 percent (median, 52%) of patients with ALS are reported to have a bilateral ribbon-like hypointensity of the cortical margin in the precentral gyrus and occasionally in the postcentral gyrus.[5,6,9,10,13,20,21,26,27] The bandlike hypointense signal in transversely oriented images near the vertex is rather obvious because of the hyperintense signal of CSF in adjacent sulci (Figure 4.6). Unlike hyperintensity of the CST, hypointensity of the neocortex is better visualized on T2-weighted images and not FLAIR images.[21,26] Follow-up imaging of patients with ALS demonstrated an increase in neocortical hypointensity on T2-weighted MRI from 12 percent to 35 percent ($p < 0.05$) after approximately 16 months.[26] Its cellular basis is uncertain, but it reflects a

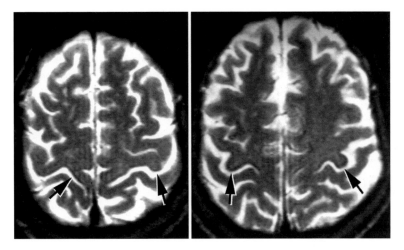

Figure 4.6 Two transverse T2-weighted images near the vertex reveal a thin bandlike hypointensity along the posterior margin of the precentral gyrus (primary motor cortex) in a 54-year-old man with amyotrophic lateral sclerosis *(arrows)*. Note that the subcortical white matter of this gyrus is faintly hyperintense relative to white matter in adjacent gyri.

shortening of the T2. One postmortem study revealed iron-laden astrocytes and macrophages in the precentral cortex of such brains.[28] Because oxidative stress and nitrosyl groups also shorten T2,[29] it is attractive to suggest that this contributes to the signal change in the neocortex. The same report indicated 4 (27%) of 15 patients with ALS had combined cortical hypointensity and CST hyperintensity.[28] We have observed this combined change in approximately 20 percent of patients with ALS (see Figure 4.6).

However, the fact that this MRI abnormality occurs in some patients with other neurodegenerative diseases[9] and even in healthy individuals[5,10,30] limits its specificity. Nonetheless, a diminished signal in the primary motor cortex on T2-weighted MRI scans of patients presenting with features of ALS is supportive of the diagnosis, especially when occurring with hyperintensity of the CST.

Atrophy of Central Nervous System and Muscle

Brain and spinal cord atrophy are generally not prominent in ALS. However, few studies have carefully compared its frequency by MRI in patients and age-matched controls. Most, but not all, report some degree of atrophy in patients with MND.[9,31–36] This is consistent with postmortem analyses that have revealed varying degrees of atrophy.[16] Discrepancies in findings between these studies may relate, in part, to the analytical methodologies used and the presence or absence of overt dementia.

Brain Atrophy

A prospective CT and MRI study of 22 patients with ALS documented the sequential appearance of cerebral atrophy in the following hemispheric regions, from earliest to latest: frontal and anterior temporal lobes, precentral gyrus (primary motor cortex), postcentral gyrus (primary sensory cortex), cingular gyrus, and corpus callosum.[35] The severity of cerebral atrophy did not correlate with presence of dementia (n = 3) or disease duration or severity. However, patients with early respiratory failure and severe ophthalmoplegia developed marked frontotemporal atrophy most rapidly, whereas three patients surviving 10 to 20 years without ventilator support had no atrophy. Atrophy of the brain stem tegmentum was also obvious in the five patients with prominent ophthalmoplegia.

A subsequent MRI study of clinically nondemented patients with sporadic ALS (n = 11) and PLS (n = 8), compared with 49 healthy individuals, revealed significant atrophy of the cortex (premotor, primary motor, supplementary motor) and related white matter regions only in the PLS group.[37] Although patients with ALS had prominent reduction in frontal subcortical white matter, cortical surface area was the same as in the controls. This was believed to represent degeneration of axons projecting to the frontal cortex from elsewhere, consistent with subtle frontal lobe dysfunction (word fluency, judgment, and attention problems), which can occur in ALS. In contrast, a study of 12 nondemented patients with ALS (7 definite and 5 probable by El Escorial criteria) revealed atrophy of the precentral gyrus in all except one with probable ALS.[13]

A case report of four patients with long-standing juvenile familial ALS (mean duration, 27 years) and overt dementia demonstrated moderately severe atrophy of the cerebrum and brain stem in one patient undergoing MRI (symptomatic for 21 years).[32] A planimetric MRI study of 74 consecutive patients with sporadic ALS revealed significant cerebral atrophy in the subgroup with neuropsychological impairment (n = 45) compared with the subgroup with intact short-term memory and normal frontal lobe function.[31] Another study of 26 patients with ALS documented frontal atrophy only in the subgroup (n = 14) with cognitive impairment.[33] Therefore pooling ALS patients with and without neuropsychological impairment may account for conflicting results in other earlier studies of cerebral atrophy.

Automated volumetric analysis of cerebral gray and white matter in 16 patients with ALS and 8 normal controls revealed focal atrophy in the premotor (Brodmann's areas 8, 9, and 10) but not the motor cortex of patients with ALS. Despite the lack of cortical atrophy in the precentral gyrus, the underlying white matter along the CST was atrophic in patients with bulbar- but not limb-onset ALS.[36] This suggests that axonal degeneration occurs as a "dying back" process, at least in some patients with bulbar-onset ALS.

MRI changes in PLS have been found to be primarily cortical atrophy rather than CST hyperintensity,[17,18] although the latter also occurs.[17,38] Imaging in nine patients with PLS revealed "conspicuous" atrophy in the cortical and subcortical portions of the precentral (frontal) regions.[18] This was seen most clearly in T1-weighted parasagittal images with reduction to approximately 75 percent of normal. Of note, there was also prominent atrophy in all patients of the parieto-occipital area.[18] Another study of 39 patients with MND, which included 8 with PLS, found cortical atrophy in 29 (74%). Of these patients 16 (14%) had atrophy restricted to the parietal region (including the superior temporal gyrus), and most of these (n = 14) had ALS. In contrast, atrophy of the central region (with or without parietal atrophy) was observed in eight patients, five of whom had PLS (63%).[17] Of interest, central atrophy occurred more frequently in PLS than did hyperintensity of the CST. Degeneration of the parietospinal tract was implicated as the cause of parietal atrophy, although there was no explanation for the regional atrophy differences in ALS versus PLS. In a case report, serial MRI of a patient with PLS over an 8.5-year period revealed brain atrophy that progressed from the pericentral and premotor cortices to include the superior parietal cortex and more extensive portions of the premotor and prefrontal cortices (Figure 4.7).

The corpus callosum has also been found on parasagittal MRI to be atrophic in some types of MNDs. Of 25 right-handed patients with ALS and 25 age- and sex-matched right-handed control subjects who consecutively underwent T1-weighted MRI, 5 patients had severe atrophy of the anterior fourth of the corpus callosum. Only these patients had cognitive decline and psychiatric symptoms.[34] A patient with PLS was found over an 8.5-year follow-up to have progressive thinning of his corpus callosum, especially in the posterior portion of the midbody, whereas genu, rostrum, and splenium were spared.[39] This is the region where postmortem studies in ALS revealed degeneration of fiber bundles,[16] which are probably homotopic fiber connections between the precentral gyri. Patients with "complicated" HSP have been reported to have atrophy of the corpus callosum. An autosomal recessive form of HSP with linkage to chromosome 15q, which has associated mental retardation and cerebellar ataxia, had prominent thinning of the entire corpus callosum.[40,41]

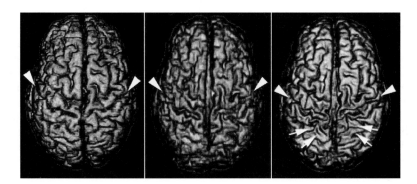

Figure 4.7 Cortical surface renderings from three-dimensional magnetic resonance imaging of a patient with primary lateral sclerosis at baseline (**left**), approximately 5 years (**middle**), and 8.5 years (**right**) later. There is progressive atrophy in the paracentral cortex (*arrowheads* indicate the central sulcus) until it is apparent in the superior parietal region in the most recent scan (*double arrows*). (Adapted with permission from Smith CD. Serial MRI findings in a case of primary lateral sclerosis. Neurology 2002;58:647–649.)

Spinal Cord Atrophy

Spinal cord anatomy is much better visualized with MRI than CT, but its resolution is still limited on 1.5-teslas magnets. MRI has rarely documented spinal cord atrophy in ALS. A 51-year-old woman with bulbar-onset ALS and prominent UMN signs was found to have mild atrophy of the cervical spinal cord,[42] although this was relatively minor. The most dramatic spinal cord atrophy has been demonstrated in patients with benign focal amyotrophy (monomelic amyotrophy), a slowly progressive focal MND primarily affecting the lower cervical cord in young individuals.[43,44] It is known by several names including juvenile muscular atrophy of the distal upper limb, monomelic amyotrophy, or Hirayama disease. The presence of spinal cord atrophy in such patients would favor this relatively benign condition over early stages of juvenile-onset ALS. Prominent spinal cord atrophy has been described in some forms of "uncomplicated" HSP likely because of the extensive axonal degeneration that occurs in this condition. An autosomal dominant form linked to chromosome 8q resulted in marked thinning of the cervical and thoracic spinal cords.[45]

Muscle Atrophy

Although only a few MRI studies of skeletal muscle in patients with ALS have been performed, they provide an objective and quantitative approach to assessing muscle that is independent of patient effort.[46,47] T1-weighted MRI (at 0.5 and 1.0 tesla) of tongue musculature in 16 patients with ALS revealed reduction in size up to two thirds of control in 14 patients (88%).[47] Characteristic changes were noted in the shape and position of the patients' tongues such that they became less curvilinear and more rectangular, retracting away from the incisors and palate. In addition, there was disorganization of the normal tongue internal structure, and 12 patients (75%) had increased T1-signal intensity, suggestive of fatty or fibrotic tissue replacement. Although no correlative data were presented, the authors suggested that the MRI changes were more frequent and severe than clinically suspected.

A quantitative MRI comparison of T2 relaxation time in the tibialis anterior muscle of 11 patients with ALS and the compound muscle action potential (CMAP) from this muscle or maximal voluntary isometric contraction (MVIC) on foot dorsiflexion revealed a strong negative correlation ($r < -0.8; p \leq 0.01$) between the imaging and electrodiagnostic parameters.[46] In addition, the change in muscle T2 relaxation time correlated inversely with the change in CMAP as the disease progressed. Because sensitivity and reliability of such findings has not been determined, the clinical utility of muscle MRI in ALS is unknown.

UNCONVENTIONAL MAGNETIC RESONANCE SEQUENCES

A number of magnetic resonance–based modalities are being explored as imaging techniques to study the UMN of patients with ALS, although experience with them is limited. These include diffusion-weighted imaging (DWI) or diffusion tensor imaging (DTI), functional MRI (fMRI), and magnetization transfer imaging (MTI). Because there is no readily available objective test of UMN dysfunction in ALS—in contrast to electromyography, which reveals the LMN involvement—a clinically accessible and sensitive magnetic resonance technique to detect cortical and CST abnormalities would be very useful. All the aforementioned imaging techniques are possible on clinically available 1.5-teslas magnets, although resolution and acquisition times can be improved on higher field strength magnets (e.g., 3 teslas). There is much to be learned about how useful each of these modalities will be in assisting with diagnosis and furthering our understanding of ALS. Because only an abbreviated introduction is given here for each of these methodologies, the interested reader is referred to specific articles dealing with the techniques for details.

Diffusion-Weighted Imaging

DWI is based on visualizing the random movement of water molecules in and among various tissue components in health and in disease.[48] The extent of such movement, or "diffusion coefficient," is restricted by normal tissue structures, such as neurons, neuroglia, and axons. The "apparent diffusion coefficient" (ADC) is the quantitative measure of diffusion in a single direction. The presence or absence of directionality influences the ADC because water molecules prefer to move along the direction of structured material (e.g., axon fibers) rather than across it. This directionality of diffusion can be quantified by an anisotropy value, which is the ratio of "diffusivity parallel to" versus "perpendicular to" the fibers. For example, axon fibers result in ADC values that are higher along their length and less across it with correspondingly high diffusion anisotropy. In contrast, areas with little or no directionality (e.g., cortex) result in low ADC values and low diffusion anisotropy. Therefore various pathologies (e.g., edema, demyelination, wallerian degeneration) can alter the ADC and anisotropy, resulting in regional changes in image appearance.

In a study of 18 patients with ALS, 20 healthy controls, and 25 neurological controls (strokes), no differences were noted in the ADC perpendicular to the CST in the posterior limb of the internal capsule. However, in five patients who had discrete paraventricular lesions, ADC of this region was increased in all directions and anisotropy was therefore lost. This suggested that the pathology in the paraventricular region was different than that in the internal capsule.[49]

Though useful, a single ADC does not represent what occurs in a three-dimensional biological situation in which diffusion occurs in multiple directions. The development of rapid echo planar imaging (EPI) made it possible to acquire images with a range of diffusion weighting in multiple directions (DTI) within a practical time frame.[50] It allows directionally independent diffusion measures (mean diffusivity) and determination of the anisotropy of diffusion, that is, the directional dependence. For example, high mean diffusivity implies a less restricted environment (e.g., cortex), whereas a low mean diffusivity implies a more restricted environment (e.g., white matter tracts). Images can be generated representative of these variations, allowing visualization of myelinated fiber tracts (Figure 4.8).

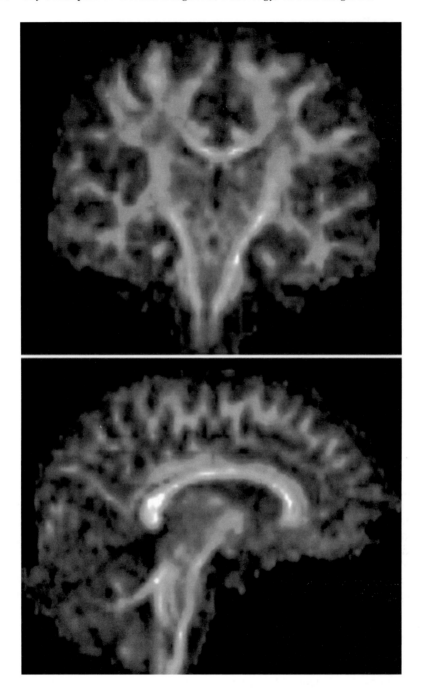

Figure 4.8 Fractional anisotropy data from a 39-year-old healthy individual that has been reformatted into coronal **(top)** and sagittal **(bottom)** planes from the original 60-slice data set acquired axially as 2.5-millimeter thick contiguous slices. Reconstruction of fiber-tract trajectories ("tractography") clearly delineates individual white matter tracts and distinguishes them from gray matter because of differences in relative anisotropy. (Reprinted with permission from Jones DK, Williams SC, Gasston D, et al. Isotropic resolution diffusion tensor imaging with whole brain acquisition in a clinically acceptable time. Hum Brain Mapp 2002;15:216–230.)

The first DTI study in ALS examined 22 patients (11 limb onset and 11 bulbar onset) compared with 20 healthy, age-matched controls.[51] Coronal images centered to include the posterior limb of the internal capsule revealed significantly increased mean diffusivity along the CSTs of patients compared with controls (p = 0.001). Fractional anisotropy, which is the degree of directionality of diffusion within a single voxel, was reduced along the CST of all patients ($p = 0.02$) and correlated with measures of disease severity ($r = 0.63; p = 0.003$) and UMN involvement ($r = -0.55; p \leq 0.01$). This was due to significant reductions in patients with bulbar-onset and not limb-onset ALS. Of interest, none of the patients with both increased diffusivity and reduced anisotropy had CST hyperintensities. However, there was significant overlap between patient and control values, suggesting the technique may not be useful for early diagnosis of individual patients. Longitudinal studies of mean diffusivity and fraction anisotropy in patients are required to determine the usefulness of DTI in studying disease course and drug response in ALS.

Functional Imaging

Activation of cortical neurons results in increased regional blood flow, which in turn results in a relative decrease of blood deoxyhemoglobin locally. This occurs because the increased blood flow is not matched by increased oxygen extraction. Because deoxyhemoglobin is paramagnetic, differences in the magnetic field characteristics of it and oxyhemoglobin at activated areas result in increased signal intensity on fMRI.[52]

Only one group has reported fMRI studies in patients with ALS.[53] Using standard motor paradigms (e.g., index-thumb opposition), a preliminary report found activation of cortical regions outside the normal primary motor area, including bilateral supplementary motor areas (SMAs), premotor, and sensory cortices. This expanded somatotopic representation is similar to what has been reported in earlier PET studies of patients with ALS (see later discussion) and was especially enlarged when UMN signs were prominent. Whether this increased "output zone" is due to loss of inhibitory cortical interneurons or inhibitory pyramidal cell axon collaterals or whether it represents the recruitment of motor neurons in less affected regions that compensate for dysfunctional ones in degenerating areas is unclear. However, an unexpected observation was the alteration of cortical activation following sensory stimulation of the hand and foot of patients with ALS compared with controls. Mechanical stimulation of the hand (palm) or foot (sole), as in a Babinski response, resulted in diminished activation of sensorimotor cortex.[53] This suggests somatosensory dysfunction at the CNS level, which could explain the not uncommon sensory complaints of patients with ALS who have normal peripheral sensory nerve function. Depending on the reproducibility of these findings, the combination of cortical activation that is increased with motor paradigms and decreased with sensory stimulation may provide a marker of cortical dysfunction in ALS. However, whether these changes occur early enough that they may be diagnostic markers is not known. In addition, it is not known whether such changes could be used as surrogates for neuronal recovery in therapeutic trials.

Cortical reorganization was examined in 11 patients with ALS compared with 13 healthy volunteers who used a simple handgrip force transducer to squeeze at 10 percent of their own maximal voluntary contraction force.[54] Cluster analysis of fMRI data were performed after transformation of anatomical and functional images into standardized (Talairach) space. Patients demonstrated activation of motor cortex more anteriorly than controls, including the premotor area and an enhancement of SMA activation with a shift toward the pre-SMA. The results were interpreted as indicating recruitment of related motor areas usually involved in planning and initiation of movement when primary motor areas degenerate.

Magnetization Transfer Imaging

Cross-relaxation between free ("mobile") water protons and restricted protons in macromolecules is the basis of MTI. This technique serves to enhance contrast or itself provide a novel contrast mechanism that allows quantification of structural or biochemical changes in certain pathological states.[55] MTI shows significant promise in the study of CNS lesions in multiple sclerosis, but its use in ALS has been very limited.

Magnetization transfer measurements were performed in the brains of patients with ALS (n = 9) and control subjects (n = 9).[56] Magnetization transfer ratios (MTRs) of a 3-millimeter-diameter circular region were obtained from the posterior third of the posterior limb of the internal capsule (location of CST) as well as widespread gray and white matter areas. Only the region of the CST in the posterior limb of the internal capsule revealed MTR values 20 percent lower in patients compared with controls ($p < 0.0007$). This decrease was proposed to represent degeneration of the CST. Of note, all patients had MTRs below the normal mean, although only three (33%) had T2-weighted CST hyperintensity in this location. This suggests that the use of MTRs may be able to detect earlier stages of CST degeneration. However, no relationships were observed between MTRs and ALS scores, duration of illness, or signal intensity on T2-weighted images.

A subsequent study, in contrast, found MTR to be reduced by only 2.6 percent in CST-related but not non-CST–related white matter of ten patients with ALS compared with 17 age-matched controls.[57] This mean difference was statistically significant ($p < 0.02$) because of the small variance, even though the difference was small. However, individual MTR values of patients (8/10) and controls (15/17) overlapped extensively in the same 95 percent confidence interval, indicating limited usefulness for diagnosis. There was a significant correlation with UMN dysfunction ($r = 0.61$; $p < 0.005$), as revealed by maximum rate of finger and foot tapping.

RADIOLABELED TRACER IMAGING

PET and SPECT are nuclear medicine techniques that have been used to assess cerebral blood flow (CBF) and neuronal metabolism in various disease states, including ALS.[9,58,59] Patients with MND, particularly ALS, have decreased CBF and diminished neuronal metabolism, primarily in sensorimotor regions. CBF abnormalities in extramotor regions have also been detected by PET and SPECT in some patients with ALS with clinical or subclinical dementia. The use of newer radiolabeled tracers that identify specific neuronal or glial populations may provide unique insights into MND degeneration and even pathogenesis. Although these nuclear medicine techniques have been used primarily for research purposes, they may assist in the clinical diagnosis of MND, especially with the development of specific tracers and in cases associated with dementia.

Positron Emission Tomography

Results from PET studies in patients with ALS have been somewhat inconsistent, at least in part because of differences in technique and analysis of statistical data.[9,58–63] Various radiolabeled isotopes have been used: fluorine-18-fluorodeoxyglucose (^{18}F-FDG) and [^{18}F]6-fluorodopa (^{18}F-dopa) for measurements while the subject is at rest, and oxygen-15–labeled gas (^{15}O) or [^{15}O]carbon dioxide ($C^{15}O_2$) primarily for studies while the subject performs certain motor tasks. The latter studies have provided information on the dynamic state of brain activation in ALS and revealed abnormalities when measurements at rest were normal. More recently, ligands targeting neuronal receptors have been used in an attempt to document cell loss or other changes expected in ALS.

Positron Emission Tomography Studies at Rest

In general, nondemented patients with ALS at rest appear to have at least a trend toward diminished brain glucose metabolism in the sensorimotor cortex and basal ganglia.[58] Patients who are demented or have neuropsychological dysfunction of frontal lobes have more significant FDG hypometabolism in frontal (superior and inferior) and temporal (superior and mesial) cortical regions.[64] Such anatomical localization of the hypometabolism is accomplished when PET and MRI images from the same individual are co-registered (Figure 4.9). The regional distribution of hypometabolism in patients with ALS and dementia is opposite that of patients with Alzheimer dementia (low in parietal cortex and normal in frontal lobes). The association of ALS with parkinsonism (e.g., Guamanian ALS) prompted 6-fluorodopa PET studies in patients with sporadic

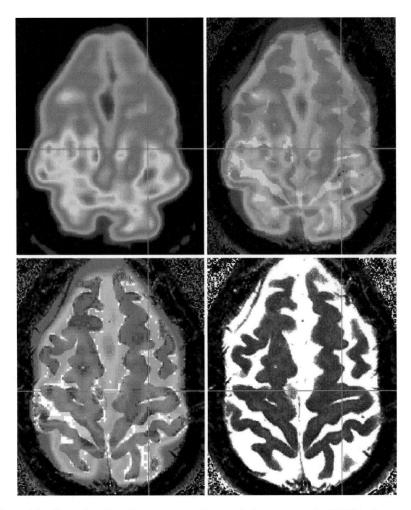

Figure 4.9 Co-registration of transverse positron emission tomography (PET) and magnetic resonance images from a 53-year-old man with amyotrophic lateral sclerosis and frontotemporal dementia reveal prominently diminished metabolism of fluorine-18-fluorodeoxyglucose in motor and premotor regions, as well as cortical atrophy. Blending of the superimposed images from PET only **(upper left)** to magnetic resonance imaging only **(lower right)** allows localization of hypometabolism to frontal regions, especially the superior frontal gyri and parasagittal portions of the precentral gyri. Crossing of planar lines indicates the anterior portion of the left precentral gyrus (primary motor cortex). See color insert. (Many thanks to Eric LaPresto, CCF, for co-registering the PET and magnetic resonance images.)

ALS.[62] Compared with age-matched controls, striatal 6-fluorodopa uptake progressively decreased as the ALS progressed.

Positron Emission Tomography Studies with Activation

Results of PET studies using ^{15}O and $C^{15}O_2$ to measure regional CBF (rCBF) and oxygen metabolic rate in patients with ALS making freely selected joystick movements suggested cortical reorganization and abnormal recruitment of non–primary motor areas as a result of motor neuron loss.[60] Stereotyped movements in patients with ALS revealed impaired activation in frontal lobe regions, suggesting underlying frontal lobe cognitive deficits even though none were clinically demented. Similar activation PET studies of five patients with LMN-predominant ALS have uncovered cortical dysfunction (anterior insular cortex) even when no abnormalities were detectable at rest.[61] Abnormal activation of this perisylvian area was thought to reflect recruitment of an accessory sensorimotor area in response to limb weakness. Verbal fluency and testing of executive frontal lobe function have identified other extramotor neuronal deficits, especially along a thalamofrontal association pathway in some patients with ALS.[63]

Novel Positron Emission Tomography Tracers

Novel radiolabeled ligands are beginning to be used in ALS in an attempt to identify changes in number or functioning of motor neurons and neuroglia. The γ-aminobutyric acid (GABA$_a$) ligand carbon-11-flumazenil (^{11}C-FMZ) binds to GABA receptors localized to cortical pyramidal neurons. A study of 17 nondemented patients with definite or probable ALS and 17 controls found significantly reduced ($p < 0.001$) FMZ volumes of distribution (which correlate closely with receptor density) in several motor and extramotor cortical regions.[65] These include prefrontal, premotor, motor, parietal, and visual association cortices ($p < 0.001$) and relative reductions in other regions, including the Broca area of the right temporal cortex.

The 5-hydroxytryptamine (5-HT) PET ligand specific for 1A receptors (5-HT$_{1A}$), ^{11}C-WAY100635 binds to the axon hillock of motor neurons in the cortex (pyramidal), brain stem, and spinal cord.[66] A preliminary study found approximately 39 percent (range, 33% to 57%; $p < 0.0001$) less global cerebral binding of ^{11}C-WAY100635 in patients with ALS (n = 6) than in healthy, age-matched controls (n = 8).[67] There was no regional cortical variation or correlation between loss of binding and disability. This preliminary study was unable to determine whether the loss of binding represents a downregulation of 5-HT$_{1A}$ receptors or loss of the neurons containing them.

Microglia become activated and hypertrophic as neurons and axons degenerate, and they have been implicated in the propagation of the degeneration. The PET ligand ^{11}C-PK11195 binds to peripheral benzodiazepine receptors and reportedly identifies activated microglia, as has been demonstrated in Alzheimer disease even early in the course of disease.[68] Therefore it may be a useful marker for cortical and subcortical degeneration in ALS, possibly in early disease.

Single Photon Emission Computed Tomography

Unlike PET studies, SPECT studies do not measure CBF, although values in ALS are usually expressed relative to blood flow in regions not believed to be affected, such as the cerebellum.[9,33] The potential clinical usefulness of SPECT over PET arises from several differences: more widely available machines and familiarity of technique, less complex technical support, less expensive, and more stable radiochemicals (iodine-123-iodoamphetamine; technetium-99m-hexamethylpropyleneamine oxime; iodine-123-*N*-[3-iodopropen-2-yl]-2β-car-bomethoxy-3β[4-chlorophenyl]-tropane [^{123}I-IPT]).

Most studies have revealed regional cerebral hypoperfusion in motor and pre-motor areas of many patients with ALS. Those with superimposed dementia have more widespread hypoperfusion, including regions anterior and often inferior to the primary motor cortex. As with PET studies at rest, SPECT abnormalities were not found in patients with LMN-predominant ALS. A pilot radioligand study examined whether patients with ALS and no signs of parkinsonism have presynaptic nigrostriatal dopaminergic deficits detectable by SPECT. Using the cocaine analog ^{123}I-IPT, which selectively binds to the dopamine transporter located on dopaminergic nerve terminals, striatal IPT binding was found to be significantly reduced ($p < 0.01$) in the ALS group (n = 18) compared with age-matched controls (n = 11).[69] Striatal IPT uptake values overlapped between groups, with 12 of 18 patients having values more than 1 SD below the control mean. There was no correlation between uptake values and site of disease onset, age of patient, or duration of the disease. These data suggest that that nigrostriatal dopaminergic neurons are subclinically affected in a subset of patients with sporadic ALS.

PROTON MAGNETIC RESONANCE SPECTROSCOPY

Proton magnetic resonance spectroscopy (^{1}H-MRS) allows noninvasive in vivo measurement of certain proton-containing, nonwater metabolites, which may be altered in various diseases.[70] Of these metabolites, *N*-acetyl (NA) groups, e.g., *N*-acetylaspartate (NAA) and *N*-acetylaspartylglutamate (NAAG) are the most easily detected and are found only in neurons, at least in the mature CNS. In the cerebrum, most of the NA groups are composed of NAA, whereas in the brain stem, the proportion of NAAG increases. Therefore NAA has been used as a surrogate marker of neuronal (including axonal and dendritic) health, at least in the cerebrum. Two other easily identified metabolites in the CNS are choline (Cho), a lipid component in cell membranes that does not appear to be significantly altered in ALS,[71–75] at least in the cortex,[76] and creatine-phospho-creatine (Cr), compounds involved in energy metabolism with a relatively evenly distribution in the brain, which have been used to normalize signal from the other metabolites. Therefore decreased NAA/Cr or NAA/Cho resonance intensity is consistent with neuronal loss or dysfunction, as shown in a patient with UMN-predominant ALS (Figure 4.10). A stereological study estimating the total number of neurons in the neocortex and motor cortex of eight patients with ALS and nine controls found no differences between groups.[77] This

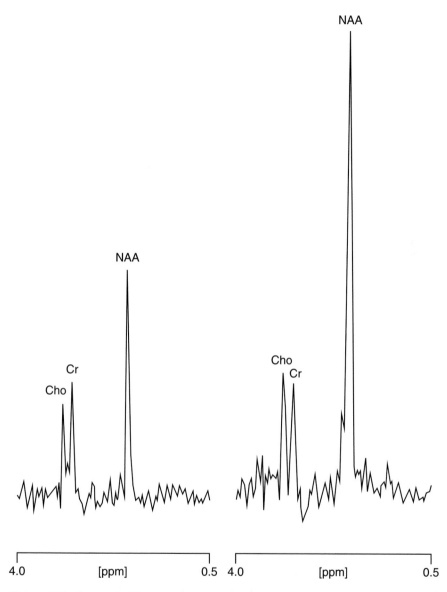

Figure 4.10 Long echo time proton magnetic resonance spectroscopy of the precentral gyrus (primary motor cortex) shows an *N*-acetylaspartate *(NAA)* signal that is lower, relative to creatine *(Cr),* in a patient with upper motor neuron–predominant amyotrophic lateral sclerosis **(left)** than in a healthy age-matched volunteer **(right)**. Both the Cr and choline *(Cho)* signal intensities remain relatively constant. ppm = parts per million. (Adapted with permission from Pioro EP, Antel JP, Cashman NR, Arnold DL. Detection of cortical neuron loss in motor neuron disease by proton magnetic resonance spectroscopic imaging in vivo. Neurology 1994;44:1933–1938.)

suggests that NAA changes in ALS are not simply a reflection of neuronal loss but likely represent neuronal dysfunction or shrinkage.

One of the goals of ^{1}H-MRS in ALS, therefore, has been to assess objectively and quantitatively the existence and degree of UMN dysfunction or degeneration in vivo. Most ^{1}H-MRS studies of ALS have used a long echo time (TE), usually TE 136 milliseconds or TE 272 milliseconds, which reveals three major metabolites normally found in CNS: NA groups, Cho, and Cr.[78] Some ALS ^{1}H-MRS studies have employed short TE sequences (e.g., 40 milliseconds or less) because they reveal additional metabolites with short T2 times, including *myo*-inositol (mI), glutamate (Glu), and glutamine (Gln), which are of potential interest in ALS.[72,79–82]

Pericentral Neocortex

Patients with MND were first reported to have ^{1}H-MRS evidence of neuronal degeneration or loss in the neocortex and subjacent white matter if clinical LMN changes were accompanied by definite UMN signs (classic ALS) or *probable UMN signs* (ALS-PUMNS) but not if present in isolation (progressive spinal muscular atrophy [PSMA]).[71] Compared with healthy controls, NAA/Cr values from the primary sensorimotor cortex were decreased most significantly in patients with classic ALS, followed by those with ALS-PUMNS (Figure 4.11). Because long TE spectra were obtained simultaneously from multiple voxels, or volume elements (i.e., ^{1}H-MRS imaging), data could be analyzed from multiple cortical regions. This revealed a gradient of improving NAA/Cr ratios as distance increased from the precentral and postcentral gyri until values were no different than those of controls in the superior frontal gyrus, anteriorly. This relatively widespread distribution of putative neuronal abnormality is consistent with the extensive cortical origin of the primate CST. Evidence that decreased NAA/Cr is a marker of UMN pathology (of the corticomotoneuron, at least) and included the following: proportionately lower ratios as severity of UMN signs increased (classic ALS versus ALS-PUMNS) and normal ratios when no UMN signs exist (PSMA); and continued decline of NAA/Cr ratios in the primary motor and precentral cortices of a patient with ALS-PUMNS who underwent a second ^{1}H-MRS after 8 months of clinical deterioration.

Subsequent ^{1}H-MRS studies—mostly single voxel—of the motor cortex in patients with ALS have confirmed a reduction of NAA signal, relative either to Cr, Cho, Cho + Cr (as a ratio)[72,74,81–89] or to internal water (as relative concentration).[13,75,85,90] The ^{1}H-MRS studies published after 1994 have used the El Escorial WFN criteria to group patients based on certainty of diagnosis.[91] Most studies have reported concordant results despite differences in hardware (acquisition parameters) and software (postprocessing).[78] These will have to be resolved if multicenter clinical trials will incorporate ^{1}H-MRS as a noninvasive technique to monitor the effects of investigational treatments on cerebral metabolites.

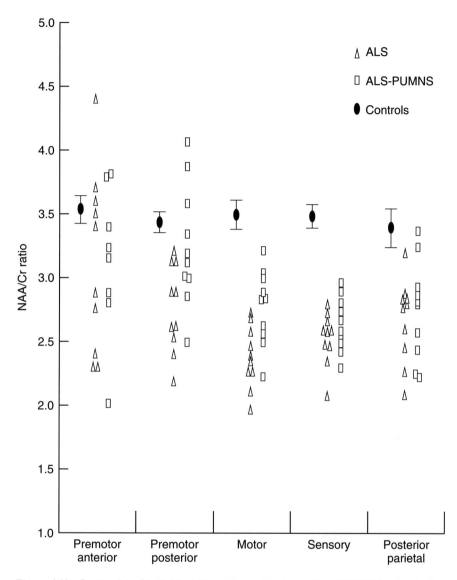

Figure 4.11 Scatterplot of individual *N*-acetylaspartate-to-creatine (NAA/Cr) ratios in five cortical regions of patients with classic amyotrophic lateral sclerosis (ALS) (*triangle,* n = 12) and with ALS with probable upper motor neuron signs (*square,* n = 12). Compared to the means (±SEM) from healthy age-matched controls (n = 10), statistically significant (*p* < .05) decreases occur in the primary motor and primary sensory cortices of all patients. NAA/Cr ratios remain significantly lower in the posterior portion of the premotor cortex and posterior parietal cortex of the ALS group only and are in the normal range in more anterior regions. Statistical analysis was by Wilcoxon rank sum test. (Data used with permission from Pioro EP, Antel JP, Cashman NR, Arnold DL. Detection of cortical neuron loss in motor neuron disease by proton magnetic resonance spectroscopic imaging in vivo. Neurology 1994;44:1936.)

Single-Voxel Proton Magnetic Resonance Spectroscopy

Long and short TE acquisitions were used in a single-voxel ^{1}H-MRS study of the precentral gyrus in 33 patients with MND, as defined by El Escorial criteria[91] and 24 healthy controls.[81] NAA/Cr and NAA/Cho ratios were both significantly lower in patients, especially in the subgroup with definite ALS. Both Cho/Cr and mI/Cr ratios were increased, but only in the latter subgroup. Nine patients who underwent follow-up scans for up to 2 years revealed progressive reduction primarily in the NAA/Cho ratio. This decrease was most dramatic in patients with the most normal ratios on initial investigation, such as one patient initially thought to have a pure LMN syndrome (suspected ALS) but who subsequently developed UMN signs. Because the Cho/Cr ratio was found to be elevated in the suspected and especially definite ALS groups, however, the progressive decline in the NAA/Cho ratio may not have resulted only from a loss of NAA per se, but also because of increasing Cho signal. Increased Cho/Cr ratios could result from similar causes, as discussed earlier. A subsequent study using long TE (272 milliseconds) by the same group[85] on 70 patients with ALS compared with 48 healthy control subjects helped to clarify the initial observations. First, it confirmed the previous findings that the NAA/Cho and NAA/Cr ratios were reduced in all El Escorial subgroups ($p < 0.001$) and the Cho/Cr ratio was increased in patients with definite ALS ($p < 0.05$). The metabolite ratio changes corresponded to the lateralization of clinical symptoms and were weakly correlated with disease duration and disease severity. In 16 patients with follow-up scanning over a mean ($\pm$ SD) of 12.1 ± 8.7 months, the NAA/Cho ratio dropped by 9.1 percent ($p < 0.01$), and the Cho/Cr ratio increased by 7.0 percent ($p < 0.01$). These changes of metabolite ratios were significantly correlated with progression of disease severity. Second, when absolute metabolite concentrations were obtained in 30 patients and 15 controls by using the unsuppressed water signal as an internal reference, NAA ($p < 0.001$) and Cr ($p < 0.05$) were reduced in motor cortices of patients, whereas Cho concentrations remained unchanged. The importance of these absolute concentration findings is that NAA/Cr ratios may be underestimating the degree of reduction of NAA because the Cr concentration may also be decreasing. Rather, the NAA/Cho ratios were suggested as most appropriate to detect motor cortex degeneration by single-volume ^{1}H-MRS.

Another study used short and long TE (STEAM) ^{1}H-MRS and the unsuppressed water signal to measure metabolite concentrations in the precentral gyrus.[13] The mean concentration of NAA was decreased ($p < 0.001$) in 12 patients with definite or probable ALS compared with 10 age-matched healthy control subjects, and Cho or Cr concentrations were unaltered. NAA concentration in primary motor cortex correlated weakly with Norris scale scores ($r = 0.30$; $p < 0.0001$) but not with the ALS Functional Rating Scale score or disease duration. In addition, the patients with hypointense signal in the primary motor cortex (n = 7) had lower NAA ($p < 0.009$) than those without (n = 5).

A single-volume short TE (20 milliseconds, STEAM) ^{1}H-MRS study determined concentrations of metabolites in the motor cortex of 20 ALS patients and 14 age-matched controls[92] by using LC model, which fits in vivo data with an in vitro basis set of reference metabolites.[93] NAA content in patients with ALS compared with controls was reduced in the motor cortex by 7.7 percent ($p =$

0.015). The degree of reduction of NAA was related to the severity of UMN abnormalities. This group used the same techniques to expand their studies of motor and extramotor cortices of 18 patients with ALS and 12 healthy volunteers.[27] Concentrations for metabolites NA, Cr, Cho, Glu, Gln, and mI were determined in the left precentral and cuneus (occipital) gyri. In addition, T2-weighted signal intensities of the precentral gyrus were assessed qualitatively in a blinded fashion. No difference in metabolite concentrations between groups was observed for the cuneus gyrus. For the precentral gyrus, the ALS group had significantly decreased NA and Glu but increased Cho and mI. The metabolite changes significantly correlated with the severity of clinical UMN signs and were greater in the subset of patients with ALS with precentral gyrus signal changes on imaging. In particular, the increased mI concentration was associated with cortical hypointensity on fast spin-echo MRI scans.

A single-volume study compared the ability of ^{1}H-MRS and conventional MRI to detect abnormalities of the UMN in 43 patients with MND (ALS, ALS-PUMNS, PLS, LMN–predominant MND) and 14 control subjects.[86] MRI scans were evaluated blindly for CST hyperintensity and dilation of the central sulcus, an indicator of motor cortex atrophy. Mean ratios of NAA/Cr from the right or the left motor cortex of control subjects and patients with ALS and PLS were significantly different ($p < 0.05$), and a cutoff value of 2.5 was deemed optimal. By this criterion, NAA/Cr values were abnormal in 79 percent (15/19) of patients with ALS and ALS-PUMNS, 67 percent (12/18) of patients with PLS, 17 percent (1/6) of patients with non-UMN disorders, and 7 percent (1/14) of control subjects. In contrast, CST hyperintensity, central sulcus enlargement, or both were found in only 43 percent of the ALS and ALS-PUMNS group, 24 percent of the PLS group, and 7 percent of the control group. Using these criteria, the receiver operating characteristic curves illustrated that ^{1}H-MRS of the motor cortex was more sensitive and more specific than standard MRI findings in detecting UMN disease (Figure 4.12).

In contrast, another single-voxel long TE (136 milliseconds) ^{1}H-MRS study revealed no significant reductions of NAA/Cr or NAA/Cho ratio in the parasagittal primary motor cortex and subcortex of 19 patients with ALS compared with 8 healthy age-matched control subjects.[74] However, the patients with bulbar-onset ALS (n = 8) had lower NAA/Cr ratios than those with limb-onset (n = 8) disease. This is somewhat curious because placement of the 4-milliliter volume of interest was in the parasagittal subcortical white matter through which lower extremity and not bulbar-projecting CST fibers would be expected to traverse. Significant correlations were observed between NAA/Cr reduction and the Hillel ALS Severity Scale[94] ($r = 0.63$; $p = 0.01$) but not the degree of UMN dysfunction, as assessed by a modified Ashworth Spasticity Scale and a reflex scale (unvalidated) devised by the authors. A follow-up study by the same authors[90] examined the absolute concentrations of NAA, Cr, and Cho in the subcortical white matter of the motor region in 16 patients with MND (8 with bulbar onset and 8 with limb onset) and 8 healthy, age-matched controls. Metabolite concentrations were determined using the water signal as an internal standard. In contrast to the findings of reduced metabolite concentrations described earlier,[25,85,92] no differences were found in the concentrations of NAA, Cr, or Cho in the motor region of the total MND group compared with controls. In addition, no differences were found in NAA concentrations in the

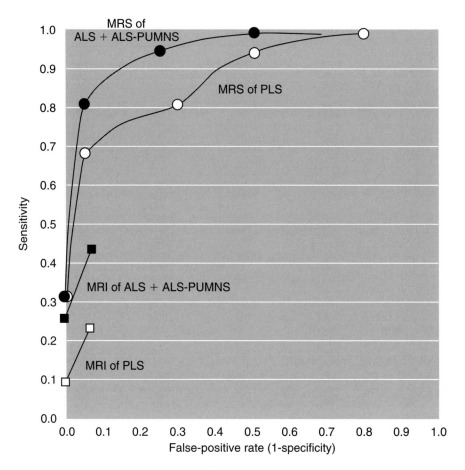

Figure 4.12 Receiver operating characteristic curves for proton magnetic resonance spectroscopy (^{1}H-MRS) and magnetic resonance imaging (MRI) data obtained in the combined group of amyotrophic lateral sclerosis (ALS) alone *(ALS)* and ALS with probable upper motor neuron signs *(ALS-PUMNS)* and the primary lateral sclerosis *(PLS)* group. The curves demonstrate that ^{1}H-MRS has greater accuracy in detecting upper motor neuron (UMN) abnormalities in the former than in the latter. In addition, at the specificity rates of 93 and 100 percent, ^{1}H-MRS is more sensitive than MRI in the detection of UMN abnormalities in both groups. (Reprinted with permission from Chan S, Shungu DC, Douglas-Akinwande A, et al. Motor neuron diseases: comparison of single-voxel proton MR spectroscopy of the motor cortex with MR imaging of the brain. Radiology 1999;212:767.)

bulbar-onset group compared with the limb-onset group. Rather, the concentration of Cr was significantly higher in the subcortical white matter of the bulbar-onset group ($p = 0.04$), possibly as a result of gliosis in the motor region. These results suggested that Cr concentration may not remain stable in MND and its elevation would result in an apparent reduction of the NAA/Cr ratio.

In a prospective study of cognitive decline in ALS, single-voxel short TE (TE 20 milliseconds, STEAM) ^{1}H-MRS was performed at 4 teslas in each of the anterior cingulate and right primary motor cortex of patients (n = 13) and spouse control subjects (n = 5).[87] At the initial scan, bulbar-onset (n = 5) but not limb-onset (n = 8) ALS patients showed significantly decreased NAA/Cr ratios in cingulate ($p < 0.05$) and motor ($p < 0.001$) cortices. On repeat study 6 months later, six limb-onset patients now showed significant reductions of NAA/Cr ratio ($p < 0.05$) in the same regions. Decreased NAA/Cr ratios indicating neuronal dysfunction or loss were present in the anterior cingulate gyrus early in the course of cognitive impairment and correlated with its appearance.

Nine patients with Kennedy's disease (KD), an X-linked spinobulbar neuronopathy without clinical UMN signs, were examined by long TE (272 milliseconds, PRESS) single-voxel ^{1}H-MRS.[88] Compared with 17 male, age-matched, healthy control subjects, there were significant reductions in the motor cortex of NAA/Cho ($p = 0.04$) and NAA/Cr ($p = 0.03$) ratios. This result was surprising considering that absence of UMN signs is an important clinical finding in KD, although the reduction mainly resulted from decreased metabolite ratios in three patients. Changes in metabolite ratios did not correlate with the elevated number of trinucleotide cytosine-adenine-guanine (CAG) repeats normally observed in KD. The decreased metabolite ratios were interpreted to represent subclinical involvement of the motor region in a subset of patients, although there was no correlation with the trinucleotide repeat length. A subsequent study of 10 patients with KD (only one apparently common to both studies) and 12 healthy volunteers using short TE (15 milliseconds, STEAM) ^{1}H-MRS and LC model postprocessing[93] found no significant reduction of NAA/Cr in the motor cortex.[82] During acquisition of spectra, metabolite nulling was used to detect the presence of macromolecular resonances that may represent pathological proteins. This is of interest because polyglutamine, which is encoded by the expanded CAG repeat, accumulates in nuclear inclusion bodies of patients with KD.[95] Macromolecules at 0.9 parts per million were significantly elevated ($p < 0.04$) in patients and there was a slight negative correlation of the CAG repeat number ($r = -0.488$; $p < 0.03$) with NAA/Cr but not NAA concentration. This implies a link between neuronal integrity and a genetic abnormality. In addition, there was elevation in the motor cortex of the mI concentration ($p < 0.03$) but not mI ratios, suggesting neuroglial alteration. This is of interest particularly if it occurs in the absence of detectable neuronal dysfunction.

Multivoxel Proton Magnetic Resonance Spectroscopy

A multislice, multivoxel ^{1}H-MRS imaging analysis of frontoparietal cortex and subcortical CST pathways revealed regional decreases of NAA/(Cho + Cr) ratios in ten patients with definite or probable ALS compared with nine normal subjects.[84] Reductions in this ratio were significant ($p = 0.02$) in motor cortex (19%) and the subcortical CST (corona radiata and posterior limb of the internal capsule; 16%) but not in frontal cortex, parietal cortex, medial gray matter, or anterior internal capsule. A significant positive correlation was noted between the cortical NAA/(Cho + Cr) ratios and maximum finger-tap rate ($r = 0.80$; $p = 0.01$), a sensitive test of UMN function. These results further suggest that decreased cortical NAA signal is an objective and quantifiable surrogate marker of corticomotoneuron loss in ALS. The same data were reanalyzed with improved techniques, which included automated curve fitting (to obtain metabolite concentrations) and tissue-volume correction (to co-register MRI and MRS imaging for better localization).[76] The results were essentially the same as in the original report with two important exceptions. A 23 percent reduction of absolute NAA signal was confirmed in the motor cortex of patients with ALS ($p = 0.004$) but not in the posterior limb of the internal capsule. Rather, the absolute Cho signal was increased in the latter region by 20 percent ($p = 0.02$) and not elsewhere. This suggests the decreased NAA/(Cho + Cr) ratio in the original study was not the result of an absolute reduction in NAA. The increased Cho signal in the posterior limb of the internal capsule also correlated positively with increased UMN impairment ($r = 0.68$; $p < 0.05$). Release of choline phosphoglycerides following cell membrane damage from demyelination or increased lipid turnover from neuroglial proliferation could increase the Cho signal.

^{1}H-MRS has been used to examine the potential effects of pharmacotherapies on the brain of patients with ALS. The first drug whose effect has been examined is riluzole (Rilutek), a glutamate antagonist that prolongs survival and time to tracheostomy in patients with ALS.[96] After 3 weeks of standard riluzole therapy in 11 patients, NAA/Cr in the precentral gyrus increased from 2.14 ± 0.26 to 2.27 ± 0.24 ($p = 0.04$), whereas, in 12 untreated patients it decreased from 2.17 ± 0.20 to 2.08 ± 0.20 ($p = 0.099$).[89] The change in NAA/Cr between the treated and untreated groups was 0.22 ± 0.095 ($p = 0.008$). There was no correlation between the degree of NAA/Cr increase and age, sex, duration of treatment or disease, the presence of probable or definite UMN signs, bulbar features, or pretreatment NAA/Cr. The explanation of the increased NAA/Cr in the riluzole-treated patients, which did not persist, is unclear but may reflect at least temporary preservation of neuronal functioning and health in ALS. However, another study did not detect any effect of riluzole treatment for 2 weeks on NAA concentration in the precentral gyrus, although it is unclear how many patients were examined for this effect.[92]

Brain Stem

Only a few ^{1}H-MRS studies have examined the brain stem in patients with ALS[73,79,80,92] or KD.[82,88] This region of the brain is especially problematic to examine by ^{1}H-MRS in vivo for several reasons, including technical limitations and patient movement. However, it may be a particularly rewarding region to study in ALS because neuronal (and axonal) degeneration is prominent in the brain stem, particularly the medulla oblongata, even before more rostral regions are affected.[16]

A long TE study at 3 teslas of the upper medulla and pontine tegmentum (4.3-milliliter voxel) in 12 patients revealed significantly decreased NA/Cr ratios compared with 17 healthy controls.[73] Patients with severe spasticity or prominent bulbar weakness had the lowest NA/Cr ratios, whereas those with mostly LMN limb weakness had near-normal values.

A short TE (40 milliseconds, PRESS) study at 1.5 teslas of the medulla oblongata (2.0-milliliter voxel) revealed 17 percent lower NA/Cr ($p = 0.03$) and 55 percent higher Glu + Gln/Cr ($p = 0.02$) in ten patients compared with seven healthy individuals[80] (Figure 4.13). The reduced NA/Cr ratio is consistent with

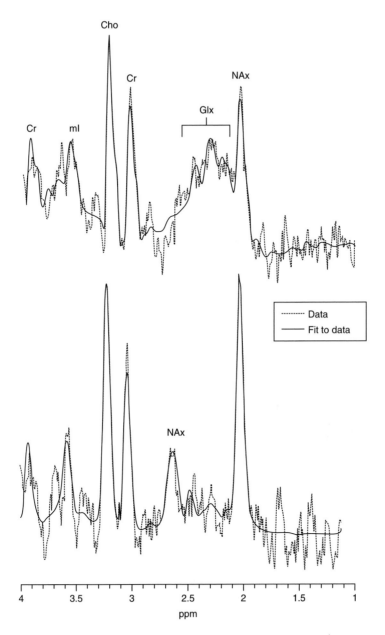

Figure 4.13 Short echo time proton magnetic resonance spectroscopy (^{1}H-MRS) spectra from the medulla of a patient with amyotrophic lateral sclerosis (ALS) **(top)** and an age-matched healthy individual **(bottom)**, demonstrating the fitted metabolite peaks: Cho = choline; Cr = creatine-phosphocreatine; Glx = glutamate + glutamine; NAx = *N*-acetylaspartate + *N*-acetylaspartylglutamate; mI = *myo*-inositol. Compared to the healthy control, the spectrum from the patient with ALS has lower NAx and higher Glx signals. Resonant frequencies of the chemical species are expressed in parts per million *(ppm)*. (Adapted from Pioro EP, Majors AW, Mitsumoto H, et al. ^{1}H-MRS evidence of neurodegeneration and excess glutamate + glutamine in ALS medulla. Neurology 1999;53:71–79.)

the neural pathology that occurs in lower cranial nerve nuclei and corticospinal (pyramidal) tracts in ALS.[16] Whether the increased Glu + Gln signal was primary or secondary to the neuronal (and axonal) degeneration, however, could not be determined in this cross-sectional study. Nonetheless, an inverse correlation was observed between bulbar symptoms, assessed by the validated ALS Functional Rating Scale, and the Glu + Gln/Cr ratio ($r = -0.68$; $p = 0.03$). These findings provide in vivo evidence of disturbed Glu metabolism in the medulla of patients with ALS, which parallels bulbar dysfunction. Data acquisition in the brain stem with multivoxel ^{1}H-MRS will provide more region-specific information and may improve clinicopathological correlations. A preliminary study of the upper medulla and pontine tegmentum at 1.5 teslas using short TE (STEAM TE = 20 milliseconds) found NAA concentration reduced by 21.5 percent ($p = 0.035$) in patients with ALS compared with controls, but no differences in concentration of Glu + Gln.[92]

SUMMARY

The primary purpose of neuroimaging in the workup of a patient suspected of having MND is to exclude other conditions that may resemble or mimic it. These include diseases affecting primarily the spinal cord, where lesions can result in dysfunction of the UMN, LMN, or both. In addition, some intracranial pathologies can produce UMN-predominant forms of MND. However, more specific changes on routine MRI can be seen in some patients with MND or ALS that, in the proper clinical context, help confirm the diagnosis. Hyperintensity of the CST primarily along its intracranial course is occasionally detected on T2-weighted, proton-density–weighted and FLAIR images. This change is thought to represent wallerian degeneration of the CST and can rarely be detected in the lateral columns of the cervical spinal cord. Hypointensity of the primary motor cortex can be sometimes seen on T2-weighted and even on FLAIR images and may represent accumulation of iron in neuroglia or free radicals. These more specific MRI changes occur in the minority of patients with MND, particularly in those with prominent UMN involvement. Whether these patients represent a subtype of MND remains to be determined. Atrophy in brain, spinal cord, or muscle detected by MRI reflects advanced degeneration of these structures. Of interest, cortical atrophy and not CST hyperintensity appears more prominently in patients with PLS, including in parietal regions. Unconventional or nontraditional MRI sequences have been recently used in patients with MND and ALS, although experience with them has been limited to only a few reports. DWI and DTI may be sensitive sequences to detect CST degeneration, even before T2-weighted hyperintensities are visible. fMRI has shown activation beyond the primary motor areas, as had been previously shown with PET, although the mechanism is unclear. Unexpectedly, sensory cortex activation after tactile stimulation of hand or foot was much lower in patients with ALS compared with controls, suggesting neurodegeneration in nonmotor regions. MTI may also reveal CST degeneration in patients before hyperintensities are detected on T2-weighted MRI, although overlap with control values may limit its clinical usefulness. The nuclear medicine techniques of PET and SPECT have demonstrated decreased neuronal metabolism and CBF, respectively, in patients with MND. This is especially true for patients with ALS and frontotemporal dementia. The most promising application of PET and possibly SPECT relates to using novel radioligands that can identify specific aspects of the neurodegeneration occurring in MND. ^{1}H-MRS can noninvasively detect metabolites in specific brain regions that represent the health of neurons and neuroglia. Several studies have shown significant reductions in the neuronal marker NAA in motor-related regions of the brains of patients with ALS and UMN-predominant MND. This appears to correlate with the degree of UMN dysfunction and reveals abnormalities better than MRI or transcranial magnetic stimulation. A few studies have also evaluated markers of neuroglia and glutamate metabolism. The challenge with ^{1}H-MRS remains to standardize acquisition parameters and postprocessing of data if this technique is to be useful in monitoring surrogate markers of disease progression or stabilization in multicenter therapeutic trials.

REFERENCES

1. Brooks BR, Miller RG, Swash M, Munsat TL. El Escorial revisited: revised criteria for the diagnosis of amyotrophic lateral sclerosis. Amyotroph Lateral Scler Other Motor Neuron Disord 2000;1:293–299.
2. Yagishita A, Nakano I, Oda M, Hirano A. Location of the corticospinal tract in the internal capsule at MR imaging. Radiology 1994;191:455–460.
3. Goodin DS, Rowley HA, Olney RK. Magnetic resonance imaging in amyotrophic lateral sclerosis. Ann Neurol 1988;23:418–420.
4. Abe K, Fujimura H, Kobayashi Y, et al. Degeneration of the pyramidal tracts in patients with amyotrophic lateral sclerosis. A premortem and postmortem magnetic resonance imaging study. J Neuroimag 1997;7:208–212.
5. Thorpe JW, Moseley IF, Hawkes CH, et al. Brain and spinal cord MRI in motor neuron disease. J Neurol Neurosurg Psychiatrry 1996;61:314–317.
6. Waragai M, Takaya Y, Hayashi M. Serial MRI and SPECT in amyotrophic lateral sclerosis: a case report. J Neurol Sci 1997;148:117–120.
7. Van Zandijcke M, Casselman J. Involvement of corpus callosum in amyotrophic lateral sclerosis shown by MRI. Neuroradiology 1995;37:287–288.
8. Hofmann E, Ochs G, Pelzl A, Warmuth-Metz M. The corticospinal tract in amyotrophic lateral sclerosis: an MRI study. Neuroradiology 1998;40:71–75.
9. Mitsumoto H, Chad DC, Pioro EP. Neuroimaging. Amyotrophic Lateral Sclerosis. Philadelphia: Oxford University Press, 1998;134–150.
10. Fazekas G, Kleinert G, Schmidt R, et al. Magnetic resonance tomography of the brain in amyotrophic lateral sclerosis. Wien Medizin Wochensch 1996;146:204–206.
11. Waragai M. MRI and clinical features in amyotrophic lateral sclerosis. Neuroradiology 1997;39:847–851.
12. Andreadou E, Sgouropoulos P, Varelas PGA, Papgeorgiou C. Subcortical frontal lesions on MRI in patients with motor neurone disease. Neuroradiology 1998;40:298–302.
13. Sarchielli P, Pelliccioli GP, Tarducci R, et al. Magnetic resonance imaging and ^{1}H-magnetic resonance spectroscopy in amyotrophic lateral sclerosis. Neuroradiology 2001;43:189–197.
14. Midani H, Truwit CL, Parry GJ. MRI in juvenile ALS: a patient report. Neurology 1998;50:1879–1881.
15. Guermazi A. Is high signal intensity in the corticospinal tract a sign of degeneration [letter]? AJNR Am J Neuroradiol 1996;17:801–802.
16. Brownell B, Oppenheimer DR, Hughes JT. The central nervous system in motor neurone disease. J Neurol Neurosurg Psychiatrry 1970;33:338–357.
17. Peretti-Viton P, Azulay JP, Trefouret S, et al. MRI of the intracranial corticospinal tracts in amyotrophic and primary lateral sclerosis. Neuroradiology 1999;41:744–749.

18. Kuipers-Upmeijer J, de Jager AE, Hew JM, et al. Primary lateral sclerosis: clinical, neurophysiological, and magnetic resonance findings. J Neurol Neurosurg Psychiatry 2001;71:615–620.
19. Gutmann DH, Fischbeck KH, Kamholz J. Complicated hereditary spastic paraparesis with cerebral white matter lesions. Am J Med Genet 1990;36:251–257.
20. Waragai M, Shinotoh H, Hayashi M, Hattori T. High signal intensity on T1 weighted MRI of the anterolateral column of the spinal cord in amyotrophic lateral sclerosis. J Neurol Neurosurg Psychiatry 1997;62:88–91.
21. Hecht MJ, Fellner F, Fellner C, et al. MRI-FLAIR images of the head show corticospinal tract alterations in ALS patients more frequently than T2-, T1- and proton-density–weighted images. J Neurol Sci 2001;186:37–44.
22. de Kerviler E, Cuenod CA, Clement O, et al. What is bright on T1 MRI scans? J Radiol 1998;79:117–126.
23. Mitsumoto H, Chad DC, Pioro EP. Excitotoxicity and Oxidative Damage. Amyotrophic Lateral Sclerosis. Philadelphia: Oxford University Press, 1998;197–225.
24. Hajnal JV, Bryant DJ, Kasuboski L, et al. Use of fluid attenuated inversion recovery (FLAIR) pulse sequences in MRI of the brain. J Comput Assist Tomogr 1992;16:841–844.
25. Okuda T, Korogi Y, Shigematsu Y, et al. Brain lesions: when should fluid-attenuated inversion-recovery sequences be used in MR evaluation? Radiology 1999;212:793–798.
26. Hecht MJ, Fellner F, Fellner C, et al. Hyperintense and hypointense MRI signals of the precentral gyrus and corticospinal tract in ALS: a follow-up examination including FLAIR images. J Neurol Sci 2002;199:59–65.
27. Bowen BC, Pattany PM, Bradley WG, et al. MR imaging and localized proton spectroscopy of the precentral gyrus in amyotrophic lateral sclerosis. AJNR Am J Neuroradiol 2000;21:647–658.
28. Oba H, Araki T, Ohtomo K, et al. Amyotrophic lateral sclerosis: T2 shortening in motor cortex at MR imaging. Radiology 1993;189:843–846.
29. Noseworthy MD, Bray TM. Effect of oxidative stress on brain damage detected by MRI and in vivo ^{31}P-NMR. Free Radic Biol Med 1998;24:942–951.
30. Iwasaki Y, Ikeda K, Shiojima T, et al. Clinical significance of hypointensity in the motor cortex on T2-weighted images. Neurology 1994;44:1181.
31. Frank B, Haas J, Heinze HJ, et al. Relation of neuropsychological and magnetic resonance findings in amyotrophic lateral sclerosis: evidence for subgroups. Clin Neurol Neurosurg 1997;99:79–86.
32. Otero Siliceo E, Arriada-Mendicoa N, Balderrama J. Juvenile familial amyotrophic lateral sclerosis: four cases with long survival. Develop Med Child Neurol 1998;40:425–428.
33. Abe K, Fujimura H, Toyooka K, et al. Cognitive function in amyotrophic lateral sclerosis. J Neurol Sci 1997;148:95–100.
34. Yamauchi H, Fukuyama H, Ouchi Y, et al. Corpus callosum atrophy in amyotrophic lateral sclerosis. J Neurol Sci 1995;134:189–196.
35. Kato S, Hayashi H, Yagishita A. Involvement of the frontotemporal lobe and limbic system in amyotrophic lateral sclerosis: as assessed by serial computed tomography and magnetic resonance imaging. J Neurol Sci 1993;116:52–58.
36. Ellis CM, Suckling J, Amaro EJ, et al. Volumetric analysis reveals corticospinal tract degeneration and extramotor involvement in ALS. Neurology 2001;57:1571–1578.
37. Kiernan JA, Hudson AJ. Frontal lobe atrophy in motor neuron diseases. Brain 1994;117:747–757.
38. Marti-Fabregas J, Pujol J. Selective involvement of the pyramidal tract on magnetic resonance imaging in primary lateral sclerosis. Neurology 1990;40:1799–1800.
39. Smith CD. Serial MRI findings in a case of primary lateral sclerosis. Neurology 2002;58:647–649.
40. Teive HA, Iwamoto FM, Della Coletta MV, et al. Hereditary spastic paraplegia associated with thin corpus callosum. Arq Neuropsiquiatry 2001;59(3-B):790–792.
41. Nakamura A, Izumi K, Umehara F, et al. Familial spastic paraplegia with mental impairment and thin corpus callosum. J Neurol Sci 1995;131:35–42.
42. Friedman DP, Tartaglino LM. Amyotrophic lateral sclerosis: hyperintensity of the corticospinal tracts on MR images of the spinal cord. Am J Radiol 1993;160:604–606.
43. Biondi A, Dormont D, Weitzner IJ, et al. MR imaging of the cervical cord in juvenile amyotrophy of distal upper extremity. AJNR Am J Neuroradiol 1989;10:263–268.
44. Kira J, Ochi H. Juvenile muscular atrophy of the distal upper limb (Hirayama disease) associated with atopy. J Neurol Neurosurg Psychiatry 2001;70:798–801.
45. Hedera P, DiMauro S, Bonilla E, et al. Phenotypic analysis of autosomal dominant hereditary spastic paraplegia linked to chromosome 8q. Neurology 1999;53:44–50.

46. Bryan WW, Reisch JS, McDonald G, et al. Magnetic resonance imaging of muscle in amyotrophic lateral sclerosis. Neurology 1998;51:110–113.
47. Cha CH, Patten BM. Amyotrophic lateral sclerosis: abnormalities of the tongue on magnetic resonance imaging. Ann Neurol 1989;25:468–472.
48. LeBihan D, Breton E, Aubin ML. MR imaging of intravoxel incoherent motions: application to diffusion and perfusion in neurologic disorders. Radiology 1986;161:401–407.
49. Segawa F, Kishibayashi J, Kamada K, et al. MRI of paraventricular white matter lesions in amyotrophic lateral sclerosis—analysis by diffusion-weighted images. Brain Nerve 1994;46: 835–840.
50. Basser PJ, Mattiello J, Le Bihan D. MR diffusion tensor spectroscopy and imaging. Biophys J 1994;66:259–267.
51. Ellis CM, Simmons A, Jones DK, et al. Diffusion tensor MRI assesses corticospinal tract damage in ALS. Neurology 1999;53:1051–1058.
52. Ogawa S, Menon RS, Kim SG, Ugurbil K. On the characteristics of functional magnetic resonance imaging of the brain. Annu Rev Biophys Biomol Struct 1998;27:447–474.
53. Brooks BR, Bushara K, Khan A, et al. Functional magnetic resonance imaging (fMRI) clinical studies in ALS—paradigms, problems and promises. Amyotroph Lateral Scler Other Motor Neuron Disord 2000;1(suppl 2):S23–S32.
54. Konrad C, Henningsen H, Bremer J, et al. Pattern of cortical reorganization in amyotrophic lateral sclerosis: a functional magnetic resonance imaging study. Exp Brain Res 2002;143:51–56.
55. Finelli DA. Magnetization Transfer in Neuroimaging. MRI Clinics of North America. Philadelphia: WB Saunders, 1998;31–52.
56. Kato Y, Matsumura K, Kinosada Y, et al. Detection of pyramidal tract lesions in amyotrophic lateral sclerosis with magnetization-transfer measurements. AJNR Am J Neuroradiol 1997;18:1541–1547.
57. Tanabe JL, Vermathen M, Miller R, et al. Reduced MTR in the corticospinal tract and normal T2 in amyotrophic lateral sclerosis. Magn Reson Med 1998;16:1163–1169.
58. Hoffman JM, Mazziotta JC, Hawk TC, Sumida R. Cerebral glucose utilization in motor neuron disease. Arch Neurol 1992;49:849–854.
59. Tanaka M, Kondo S, Hirai S, et al. Cerebral blood flow and oxygen metabolism in progressive dementia associated with amyotrophic lateral sclerosis. J Neurol Sci 1993;120:22–28.
60. Kew JJ, Leigh PN, Playford ED, et al. Cortical function in amyotrophic lateral sclerosis. A positron emission tomography study. Brain 1993;116(pt 3):655–680.
61. Kew JJ, Brooks DJ, Passingham RE, et al. Cortical function in progressive lower motor neuron disorders and amyotrophic lateral sclerosis: a comparative PET study. Neurology 1994;44: 1101–1110.
62. Takahashi H, Snow BJ, Bhatt MH, et al. Evidence for a dopaminergic deficit in sporadic amyotrophic lateral sclerosis on positron emission scanning. Lancet 1993;342:1016–1018.
63. Abrahams S, Goldstein LH, Kew JJ, et al. Frontal lobe dysfunction in amyotrophic lateral sclerosis. A PET study. Brain 1996;119(pt 6):2105–2120.
64. Levine RL, Brooks BR, Matthews CG, et al. Frontotemporal hypometabolism in amyotrophic lateral sclerosis–dementia complex. J Neuroimaging 1993;3:234–241.
65. Lloyd CM, Richardson MP, Brooks DJ, et al. Extramotor involvement in ALS: PET studies with the GABA(A) ligand [(11)C]flumazenil. Brain 2000;123(pt 11):2289–2296.
66. Azmitia EC, Gannon PJ, Kheck NM, Whitaker-Azmitia PM. Cellular localization of the 5-HT1A receptor in primate brain neurons and glial cells. Neuropsychopharmacology 1996;14:35–46.
67. Turner MR, Rabiner E, Grasby P, et al. [^{11}C]-WAY100635 PET-A potential in vivo marker for ALS [abstract]. Amyotroph Lateral Scler Other Motor Neuron Disord 2001;2(suppl 2):122–123.
68. Cagnin A, Brooks DJ, Kennedy AM, et al. In-vivo measurement of activated microglia in dementia. Lancet 2001;358:461–467.
69. Borasio GD, Linke R, Schwarz J, et al. Dopaminergic deficit in amyotrophic lateral sclerosis assessed with [I-123] IPT single photon emission computed tomography. J Neurol Neurosurg Psychiatry 1998;65:263–265.
70. Castillo M, Kwock L, Mukherji SK. Clinical applications of proton MR spectroscopy. AJNR Am J Neuroradiol 1996;17:1–15.
71. Pioro EP, Antel JP, Cashman NR, Arnold DL. Detection of cortical neuron loss in motor neuron disease by proton magnetic resonance spectroscopic imaging in vivo. Neurology 1994;44:1933–1938.
72. Jones AP, Gunawardena WJ, Coutinho CMA, et al. Preliminary results of proton magnetic resonance spectroscopy in motor neurone disease (amyotrophic lateral sclerosis). J Neurol Sci 1995;129(suppl):85–89.

73. Cwik VA, Hanstock C, Allen PS, Martin WRW. Estimation of brainstem neuronal loss in ALS with in vivo proton MR spectroscopy. Neurology 1998;50:72–77.
74. Ellis CM, Simmons A, Andrews C, et al. A proton magnetic resonance spectroscopic study in ALS: correlation with clinical findings. Neurology 1998;51:1104–1109.
75. Gredal O, Rosenbaum S, Topp S, et al. Quantification of brain metabolites in amyotrophic lateral sclerosis by localized proton magnetic resonance spectroscopy. Neurology 1997;48:878–881.
76. Schuff N, Rooney WD, Miller R, et al. Reanalysis of multislice (1)H MRSI in amyotrophic lateral sclerosis. Magn Reson Med 2001;45:513–516.
77. Gredal O, Pakkenberg H, Karlsborg M, Pakkenberg B. Unchanged total number of neurons in motor cortex and neocortex in amyotrophic lateral sclerosis: a stereological study. J Neurosci Methods 2000;95:171–176.
78. Pioro EP. Proton magnetic resonance spectroscopy (^{1}H-MRS) in ALS. Amyotroph Lateral Scler Other Motor Neuron Disord 2000;1(suppl 2):S7–S6.
79. Pioro EP. MR spectroscopy in amyotrophic lateral sclerosis/motor neuron disease. J Neurol Sci 1997;152(suppl 1):S49–S53.
80. Pioro EP, Majors AW, Mitsumoto H, et al. ^{1}H-MRS evidence of neurodegeneration and excess glutamate + glutamine in ALS medulla. Neurology 1999;53:71–79.
81. Block W, Karitzky J, Traber F, et al. Proton magnetic resonance spectroscopy of the primary motor cortex in patients with motor neuron disease: subgroup analysis and follow-up measurements. Arch Neurol 1998;55:931–936.
82. Mader I, Karitzky J, Klose U, et al. Proton MRS in Kennedy disease: absolute metabolite and macromolecular concentrations. J Magn Reson Imaging 2002;16:160–167.
83. Giroud M, Walker P, Bernard D, et al. Reduced brain *N*-acetyl-aspartate in frontal lobes suggests neuronal loss in patients with amyotrophic lateral sclerosis. Neurol Res 1996;18:241–243.
84. Rooney WD, Miller RG, Gelinas D, et al. Decreased N-acetylaspartate in motor cortex and corticospinal tract in ALS. Neurology 1998;50:1800–1805.
85. Pohl C, Block W, Karitzky J, et al. Proton magnetic resonance spectroscopy of the motor cortex in 70 patients with amyotrophic lateral sclerosis. Arch Neurol 2001;58:729–735.
86. Chan S, Shungu DC, Douglas-Akinwande A, et al. Motor neuron diseases: comparison of single-voxel proton MR spectroscopy of the motor cortex with MR imaging of the brain. Radiology 1999;212:763–769.
87. Strong MJ, Grace GM, Orange JB, et al. A prospective study of cognitive impairment in ALS. Neurology 1999;53:1665–1670.
88. Karitzky J, Block W, Mellies JK, et al. Proton magnetic resonance spectroscopy in Kennedy syndrome. Arch Neurol 1999;56:1465–1471.
89. Kalra S, Cashman NR, Genge A, Arnold DL. Recovery of *N*-acetylaspartate in corticomotor neurons of patients with ALS after riluzole therapy. Neuroreport 1998;9:1757–1761.
90. Ellis CM, Simmons A, Glover A, et al. Quantitative proton magnetic resonance spectroscopy of the subcortical white matter in motor neuron disease. Amyotroph Lateral Scler Other Motor Neuron Disord 2000;1:123–129.
91. Brooks BR. El Escorial World Federation of Neurology criteria for the diagnosis of amyotrophic lateral sclerosis. J Neurol Sci 1994;124(suppl):96–107.
92. Bradley WG, Bowen BC, Pattany PM, Rotta F. [1]H-magnetic resonance spectroscopy in amyotrophic lateral sclerosis. J Neurol Sci 1999;169:84–86.
93. Provencher SW. Estimation of metabolite concentrations from localized in vivo proton NMR spectra. Magn Reson Med 1993;30:672–679.
94. Hillel AD, Miller RM, Yorkston K, et al. Amyotrophic lateral sclerosis severity scale. Neuroepidemiology 1989;8:142–150.
95. Fischbeck KH. Polyglutamine expansion neurodegenerative disease. Brain Res Bull 2001;56:161–163.
96. Lacomblez L, Bensimon G, Leigh PN, et al. Dose-ranging study of riluzole in amyotrophic lateral sclerosis. Amyotrophic Lateral Sclerosis/Riluzole Study Group II. Lancet 1996;347:1425–1431.

SECTION 2

AMYOTROPHIC LATERAL SCLEROSIS/MOTOR NEURON DISEASE

5
Clinical Aspects of Sporadic Amyotrophic Lateral Sclerosis/Motor Neuron Disease

Lewis R. Rowland

NAMING NAMES

The goal of this chapter is to describe the clinical features of sporadic motor neuron disease (MND) without intruding on other chapters devoted to differential diagnosis, epidemiology, genetics, and pathology. The diverse clinical features have led to a language of ambiguities, and when language is unclear, so is thought. For the purposes of this chapter, I rely on definitions proposed often in the past[1-3] and only slightly modified by scientific advances of the past decade.[4]

Motor Neuron Diseases (Plural)

MNDs make up a group of diseases in which the primary disorder is thought to involve the motor neuron, as defined by clinical observations, electromyography (EMG), and postmortem pathology. Whether the primary disorder arises within the motor neuron, an "autonomous" cellular process, is uncertain. Alternatively, pathology within glial cells or some other non-neuronal mechanism could affect the motor neuron secondarily and the disorder would be "nonautonomous."

MNDs are heterogeneous in etiology, encompassing acquired disorders such as viral diseases (poliomyelitis) or neuronal damage after radiotherapy for cancer, as well as hereditary diseases caused by different mutations (including amyotrophic lateral sclerosis [ALS], childhood spinal muscular atrophy [SMA], and adolescent-onset spinobulbar muscular atrophy) and cryptogenic disorders that include sporadic MND (singular), which is defined next.

Motor Neuron Disease (Singular)

Use of the hybrid acronym "ALS/MND" is a confession that two very different meanings are implied in different parts of the world. In the United Kingdom, *MND* is now used not only for ALS itself but also for conditions considered variants of ALS (progressive bulbar palsy [PBP] and progressive muscular atrophy). In the United States, however, *ALS* has been used in both senses— for all the variants and for the specific syndrome defined by the combination of both upper motor neuron (UMN) and lower motor neuron (LMN) signs. The British usage is less ambiguous because it restricts ALS to one particular form, whereas U.S. custom accepts this but also accepts the umbrella term. According to the El Escorial criteria, described later, the variants (PBP, adult-onset progressive SMA [PSMA], and primary lateral sclerosis [PLS]) are all listed as forms of "suspected ALS."

ALS itself is heterogeneous in origin because some cases are familial and heritable and others are sporadic. Among the sporadic cases, heterogeneity is suggested by extreme differences in duration and by the number of different associated conditions. The number of causes of sporadic ALS is not known.

It was long thought that the condition is restricted to motor neurons because of their "selective vulnerability" to some noxious agent. Now, the increasing attention to frontotemporal dementia (FTD) and parkinsonism in patients with ALS—with attendant pathology in the hemispheres and substantia nigra and the presence of neuronal inclusions throughout—many students consider ALS a multisystem disorder.[5–7] In addition to the clinical and neuropathological evidence, imaging has contributed to this view.[8] Rarely, the findings of ALS may be seen with sensory neuropathy.[9] Even so, the condition can still be regarded as one primarily affecting the motor neuron, which accounts for the essential clinical manifestations in almost all patients.

Amyotrophic Lateral Sclerosis (Specific Usage)

In terms of histopathology, ALS is not only diagnosed but also defined by the presence of abnormalities in the motor neurons (both upper and lower) and the corticospinal tracts. In living patients, there must be LMN signs (weakness and visible atrophy of skeletal muscle, usually but not always with visible fasciculation). For formal definition, there ought to be UMN signs as well (overactive tendon reflexes, Hoffmann sign, Babinski sign, and clonus).

ALS is familial and autosomal dominant in about 5 percent of cases. The clinical features are essentially the same except for a younger age at onset in heritable forms. In familial ALS (FALS) resulting from some SOD1 mutations, there may be only LMN signs, but the diagnosis is validated either by finding UMN signs in other family members or by identifying the mutation.[10]

Amyotrophic Lateral Sclerosis with Probable Upper Motor Neuron Signs

In a purely LMN disease, the tendon reflexes should be lost. In some patients, however, overt UMN signs are lacking, but involvement of the corticospinal tracts is implied by the incongruous presence of active tendon jerks in limbs

Table 5.1   Autopsy findings in clinical syndromes of motor neuron diseases: spinal muscular atrophy and amyotrophic lateral sclerosis

	Degeneration of pyramidal tracts			
Clinical	*Brownell, Oppenheimer, and Hughes*[11]	*Lawyer and Netsky*[12]	*Leung*[19]	*Total (%)*
Lower motor neuron alone	11/17[a]	6/8	8/12	25/37 (67.6)
Lower motor neuron plus upper motor neuron	16/18	45/45	50/53	111/116 (95.7)
Total	27/35	51/53	58/65	136/153 (88.8)

[a]Number abnormal/number studied.

with weak, wasted, and twitching muscles. In the past, this combination was regarded as "virtually pathognomonic" of ALS. With the discovery of motor neuropathies in the mid-1980s, a new term appeared—*predominantly LMN disorders*—leaving it undecided whether the condition was one of the peripheral nervous system, the central nervous system (CNS), or both.

In ALS itself, the condition can be manifest clinically as one of only the LMNs, but at autopsy, the corticospinal tracts may be involved, as actually occurs in most (but not all) patients with adult-onset PSMA (Table 5.1).[11–16] If that is true, it ought to be true of what we called "ALS with probable UMN signs (ALS-PUMNS)."[17] In fact, this view has been supported by magnetic resonance spectroscopy[18] and new postmortem studies.[16,19]

In the original El Escorial criteria, described later, active tendon jerks in limbs with signs of denervation were not listed as "UMN signs." That was the main reason for devising the neologism "ALS-PUMNS." In the revised El Escorial criteria, however, this combination is accepted as a UMN sign, largely eliminating the need for a designation of ALS-PUMNS.

Uncertainty, however, still beclouds this issue because patients with multifocal motor neuropathy (MMN), which is defined by electrophysiological signs of peripheral neuropathy, may show brisk tendon jerks in affected limbs, a finding that links it to ALS/MND. In fact, all four autopsy studies recorded thus far have shown disease of the motor neurons, not just the peripheral nerves. At least in these few patients, the disorder may affect both the central and the peripheral nervous system. The pathophysiology need not be restricted to one or the other, that is, the central or the peripheral nervous system, because both may be affected together. Similarly, patients with the Guillain-Barré polyneuropathy may have hyperactive tendon jerks, a discrepancy also attributed to CNS involvement.[20]

Amyotrophy

Amyotrophy implies LMN dysfunction. It has been used clinically as a shorthand description of a combination of weakness, wasting, and visible fasciculation—or even fasciculation alone. This usage is buttressed if there are changes of denervation in the EMG.

Progressive Spinal Muscular Atrophy

In theory, PSMA should be a disease in which both clinical findings and post-mortem histopathology are limited to the LMN. In the childhood forms, this is true, but those conditions are hereditable and differ from the sporadic syndromes of later onset. When PSMA begins in adulthood, postmortem examination proves that it is ALS in most cases because the corticospinal tracts are affected along with the LMNs. In making this diagnosis clinically, one must exclude MMN, a treatable condition.[21,22] In this chapter, *PSMA* is used to designate the adult form. *SMA* is already in widespread use for the childhood form.

Progressive Bulbar Palsy

PBP denotes a condition in which symptoms of dysarthria and dysphagia accompany signs of LMN disease of the tongue (wasting and fasciculation) and weakness of the soft palate and upper pharynx. However, almost all patients with this combination of symptoms and signs already have visible fasciculations of limbs and trunk, or there are UMN signs in the limbs; that is, the syndrome is generalized, not restricted to the medulla, and it is therefore ALS. Similarly, autopsy shows that the LMN disease extends beyond the medulla and pathology is likely to be found in the corticospinal tract. The term and concept are therefore of limited value. *Bulbar onset,* however, may imply a more rapidly progressive form of ALS than *spinal onset.*

Pseudobulbar Palsy

Dysarthria and dysphagia may be seen without LMN signs if there are UMN signs in limb muscles. A clue to the UMN disorder is given by the presence of emotional lability, with readily induced laughing and crying. Although patients and physicians often consider this a manifestation of depression, there is a disconnection between the emotional state and the motor act, as though corticobulbar tract pathology has released the reflex performance of laughing or crying from inhibitory controls, just as tendon reflexes are released and exaggerated. Patients with this syndrome perform less well on psychological tests of frontal lobe function.[23,24]

Pseudobulbar palsy may be seen after bilateral lesions of the corticospinal tracts that are caused by strokes or multiple sclerosis; in these two diseases, LMN signs are not seen. In ALS, remarkably, pseudobulbar palsy and true bulbar palsy may be seen in the same patient.

Motor Neuronopathy

Motor neuronopathy is yet another term with two meanings. Some use it for syndromes attributed to the disease of the anterior horn cell body (in parallel with *sensory neuronopathies,* which are attributed to disease of the posterior root ganglion cells). We have used it to denote disorders in which there are only LMN signs clinically and electrodiagnostic studies do not determine whether the condition is primarily one of the perikaryon or the peripheral nerve.[25]

El Escorial Criteria

In 1994,[26] an international committee of ALS experts published a classification system that defined criteria for "definite," "probable," "possible," and "suspected" ALS. The criteria were intended to provide clinically uniform groups of patients "for clinical research purposes and therapeutic trials," not for daily use in patient care. Nevertheless, these criteria have become standards and are popular with clinicians (and editors).

However, the criteria are not flawless. For instance, the diagnosis of definite ALS requires the presence of both UMN and LMN signs in three body regions. One of those regions could be the thorax or abdomen, but it is difficult to identify UMN signs there. Therefore, combined UMN and LMN signs must be evident in the arms, legs, and head, a requirement that puts undue emphasis on the snout, pharyngeal, and jaw reflexes.

Also, it is unhelpful to inform patients that they have *probable* or *possible* ALS when the diagnosis is really unarguable. Even *suspected* ALS can be a definite diagnosis. If an adult shows fasciculation in the tongue and limbs with no abnormality in nerve conduction studies, that can be taken as the PSMA form of ALS. The criteria can seem needlessly complex for clinical diagnosis.[27]

Even when the El Escorial criteria are used only for clinical trials, there may be problems. Traynor et al[28] pointed out that 67 percent of patients who were in the possible and suspected groups at the time of diagnosis later converted to probable or definite ALS and then became eligible for trials, but 10 percent of the patients died of ALS without meeting criteria for a therapeutic trial. They found that later revisions of the criteria did not improve diagnosis.[29,30]

WHO GETS SPORADIC AMYOTROPHIC LATERAL SCLEROSIS/MOTOR NEURON DISEASE?

Sex

In most series of patients, men outnumber women in a ratio of about 1.4 : 1.0. Eisen and Krieger[31] found that the male preponderance was especially pronounced when symptoms started before 45 years of age; gradually the difference narrowed, and by age 70, women were affected as often as men. The mean age at onset of symptoms is significantly younger in men than in women, a difference that might imply hormonal influences.

Age

ALS is an age-related disorder. Starting at about age 40, the incidence increases with each decade until age 80. After that, it may decrease somewhat. The implications of this fundamental fact are not clear, but accumulation of a toxic intraneuronal product could be a factor. For instance, the finding of neuronal inclusions is almost universal. Ubiquitinated skeins and/or Bunina bodies are found in many surviving neurons. Determination of the content of these structures might give clues to pathogenesis and treatment. The duration or rate of progression is partly age related: The younger the age at onset, the longer the duration. The rate of progression seems to be more rapid in older patients.

Only 10 percent of cases begin before age 40, and 5 percent before age 30. There is no consistent difference in age at onset of familial and sporadic cases, but there may be more young-onset cases in the inherited form. Sporadic ALS almost never begins before age 20. In patients whose symptoms start before age 20, there is likely to be debate about whether the condition is really ALS.[32,33]

Genetic Susceptibility

Why only a few people get ALS has never been explained. Presumably, susceptibility genes make the individual vulnerable to some environmental agent. Current views therefore invoke both heredity and the environment.

Some people with apparently sporadic ALS carry a mutant SOD1 gene for FALS even though neither of their parents is symptomatic or shows the mutation; the affected individual is therefore considered to have a new mutation. In different series, this kind of FALS accounts for about 2 percent of all cases of sporadic ALS.[34,35] That number is expected to rise as more FALS genes are identified.

With completion of the human genome project, susceptibility factors are expected to be easier to identify. One is an abnormal copy number (one or three) of the survival motor neuron-1 (SMN1) gene, which is affected in childhood SMA.[36] Deletions of the SMN1 gene itself, however, do not predispose to ALS.[37] Deletions of the SMN2 gene may play a role in prognosis but not susceptibility.[38] Similarly, a mutation in the gene for the ciliary neurotrophic factor (CNTF) may be a modifier gene that affects the age at onset in both sporadic ALS and FALS.[39] Apolipoprotein E-4 does not affect the age at onset of ALS.[40]

Scarmeas et al[41] found that patients with ALS tended to have been slim all their lives, and more of them than controls were varsity athletes in high school or college, but past studies were inconsistent on this point. Others had earlier noted the unusual prevalence of athletes with ALS.[42,43] Longstreth et al[44] summarized the evidence that hard labor has been a risk factor in several epidemiological studies. However, we have not noted an unusual prevalence of laborers in our urban ALS center. An alternative explanation for the prominence of athletes is that slimness and athletic talent could be nonspecific genetic markers of susceptibility to ALS; that is, the genetic basis of athletic prowess could parallel the genetic contribution to sporadic ALS. Similarly, many clinicians believe that most patients with ALS are nice people, which might be either a genetic or an acquired risk factor.[45]

Other occupations have not been consistently incriminated, and the role of trauma has been the source of controversy. Most experienced clinicians have seen some striking examples of ALS beginning in a limb still in a cast from a fractured bone. (Dr. Armon considers the epidemiology of ALS in Chapter 7.)[46]

As for possible environmental causes of MNDs, viral diseases are discussed later. The motor neuron disorder that follows radiotherapy is the clearest current example, and technical advances have reduced the frequency of this complication. In earlier times, lead intoxication could induce a syndrome that was clinically identical to ALS. Exposure had to be severe and the condition was largely restricted to those in exposed occupations, workers in lead mines, smelters, or battery manufacturers. The last well-documented case was recorded in 1976, and it was completely reversed by chelation therapy.[47] Whether mercury intoxication actually ever caused an MND is uncertain.

Clusters from Guam to the Gulf War

During World War II, the renowned neuropathologist Harry M. Zimmerman was stationed in a U.S. Navy hospital on the island of Guam. Doing routine autopsies on indigenous people, he noted an unusual frequency of ALS. He called this to the attention of authorities, and formal epidemiological studies corroborated his suspicions; the incidence of ALS on that remote island was 50 times higher than anywhere else in the world. A similar area of high incidence was found later in the Kii peninsula of Japan.

Despite intense investigation by several groups of talented neurologists (Donald Mulder, Wigbert Wiederholt, Douglas Galasko, and Leon Thal), neuropathologists (Asao Hirano), epidemiologists (Leonard Kurland), geneticists (Gerald Schellenberg), and a group headed by Nobelist Carleton Gajdusek, the high incidence has not been explained. In the most recent survey, the incidence of ALS had fallen to a level about the same as elsewhere. The incidence of the parkinsonism-dementia complex is still high, and as the population ages, Alzheimer's disease manifestations increase (Mariana dementia).[48] Plato et al[49] has assiduously maintained a registry of patients and controls for 40 years, concluding that relatives of patients are at a greater risk than relatives of controls, but there is no clear genetic pattern. The great medical analyst and writer Oliver Sacks has written about the mystery.[50]

As an explanation, inheritance came and went—and came back again. The decline in the frequency of ALS implicates an environmental factor. A local plant cycad was incriminated and exonerated, but Cox and Sacks[51] brought it back with a theory that flying squirrels eat the plant and were then consumed by people, thus transmitting the toxin.

In parallel with the declining frequency of ALS in Guam, the companion diseases, parkinsonism and dementia, have also decreased in frequency and start at a later age. The disappearance of the epidemic implies that the environment has changed in 50 years, removing the cause in the process.

Other clusters have been equally impervious to analysis or have simply been dismissed as a statistical fluke. "Epidemics" at a football stadium, an Air Force Base, an area dominated by petrochemical industries, or one with magnetic fields have all be examined for naught. Now we hear reports that military personnel in the Gulf War are at special risk, but a year after public announcement, the data have not yet been published in a peer-reviewed journal. We still cannot predict who will get ALS, except in FALS where the mutation is known.

CLINICAL MANIFESTATIONS OF SPORADIC AMYOTROPHIC LATERAL SCLEROSIS/MOTOR NEURON DISEASE: AMYOTROPHIC LATERAL SCLEROSIS, PROGRESSIVE SPINAL MUSCULAR ATROPHY, AND PROGRESSIVE BULBAR PALSY

Duration and Rate of Progression: Prognostic Predictors

The rate of progression seems to be set at the onset,[52] which may be one reason why the interval from symptom onset to diagnosis has prognostic value: The shorter the time, the more aggressive the disease.[53] Progression is linear;[54] plateaus are unusual and acceleration of progress is equally unusual. The bibrachial ("person-in-a-barrel") form of ALS seems to be associated with longer survival,[55,56] as does the lower half analogy, bilateral leg weakness.[57] The syndrome restricted to proximal arms has been called the *Vulpian-Bernhardt form of ALS,*[58] or the *flail arm syndrome.*[59]

In almost all series, bulbar onset is associated with shorter survival. Chancellor et al[60] also linked shorter duration to bulbar onset, which they found was more common in older patients, especially women. Years ago, Mulder and Howard[61] wrote that 20 percent of patients at the Mayo Clinic survived for more than 5 years. Twenty-five years later, with presumably better management, del Aguila et al[53] found a 5-year survival of only 7 percent in the area near Seattle. They did not, however, compare SMA with ALS, and some variation is to be expected in different locales at different times. In Scotland,[60] 28 percent of patients lived more than 5 years. The reason survival estimates vary so much is not clear.

Younger age at onset is more likely to imply longer duration than older age at onset.[31,62] Similarly, a shorter interval from onset of symptoms to the time of diagnosis is predictive of shorter survival time, perhaps because more rapid progression propels the patient to see a neurologist promptly.[63,64]

Purely LMN forms may progress more slowly. As emphasized especially by Norris, adult-onset SMA may be survived for 10 or 20 years, or more.[65,66] The longest documented survival in the Norris series was 39 years. His views about longevity in ALS have been substantiated in a prospective series of patients with purely LMN syndromes beginning between 1985 and 2000.[67,68] The mean duration of symptoms was 14 years, with a range of 4 to 35 years. The mean age at onset was 45 years. In Italy, the 5-year survival was 67 percent for PMA and 18 percent for ALS.[69] Even in FALS, LMN syndromes may fare better; one such patient lived 47 years after symptom onset.[70] A related disorder is the syndrome of distal SMA, which may last 40 years.[71,72] On the other hand, PSMA may also progress rapidly, whether sporadic[16] or familial.[73]

Amyotrophic Lateral Sclerosis, Progressive Spinal Muscular Atrophy, and Progressive Bulbar Palsy: Clinical Manifestations

Symptoms and Signs

Limb onset of symptoms accounts for 75 percent of patients, compared with 21 percent for bulbar onset, according to a compilation of data from five series by Swash[74] (Table 5.2).

Bulbar Symptoms and Signs

Cranial symptoms include dysarthria, dysphagia, or less commonly, difficulty chewing. Dysphagia may be preceded by taking longer to eat meals or by increasingly frequent episodes of momentary choking. The corresponding signs of bulbar palsy are fasciculation and atrophy of the tongue and dysarthria. The pharyngeal reflex may be depressed or absent (LMN) or exaggerated (UMN). In a mixture of UMN and LMN signs, overt emotional lability could be evident, with difficulty controlling laughing and crying. Other UMN signs of the head include the snout and jaw reflexes, and repetitive movements of the tongue may be slow. There is an audible difference between the slurred speech of bulbar palsy and the high-pitched, dysprosodic, strangulated speech of pseudobulbar palsy.

Limb Symptoms and Signs

If symptoms begin in the arms, there may be difficulty lifting objects overhead. In the hands, problems would be evident by difficulty writing, doing buttons (especially the top button of a shirt or using one hand to button the other cuff), using dining utensils, turning keys, turning door knobs, or continuing a skilled

Table 5.2 Early symptoms of amyotrophic lateral sclerosis/motor neuron disease in 2517 patients

	Percent of patients	
	Range	*Mean*
Limb onset	63–81	74.2
Bulbar onset	19–25	19.4
Two legs	0–20	7.8
Two arms	0–9	4.6
One leg	12–40	25.4
One arm	11–44	30.6
Arm and leg	0–4	1.6

Modified with permission from Swash M. Clinical Features and Diagnosis of Amyotrophic Lateral Sclerosis. In RH Brown Jr, V Meininger, M Swash (eds), Amyotrophic Lateral Sclerosis. London: Martin Dunitz, 2000;3–30.

activity such as sewing, crocheting, playing a musical instrument, or using a keyboard for typing. These symptoms would inevitably imply the finding of LMN signs—weakness, atrophy, and fasciculation—in proximal arm muscles and the hands. UMN pathology alone would be unlikely to cause arm or hand symptoms.

Gait disorder, in contrast, can be due to either UMN or LMN disorders. In LMN pathology, footdrop may be an early symptom and sign. In UMN disorders, a spastic gait is likely to be present. In either case, the syndrome may be grossly asymmetrical or even unilateral for months.

Despite the conventional term *spastic paraparesis,* UMN disorders may spare strength. Instead, repetitive movements are slowed—tapping or turning the hand rapidly, or tapping the toes of one foot repeatedly, as in a dance. Tendon reflexes may be increased and accompanied by Hoffmann and Babinski signs, which are still reliable guides to corticospinal tract malfunction. If tendon reflexes are still active in limbs with atrophic twitching muscles, that is a reliable clue to the diagnosis of ALS.

Symptoms begin in the limbs in about 75 percent of patients, and bulbar onset accounts for less than a quarter (see Table 5.2). Other common symptoms include cramps and weight loss, both undoubtedly more common than those listed in Table 5.2. Cramps seem to be more common in denervated muscles and the weight loss may be caused by the combination of early dysphagia and atrophy of limb and trunk muscles. Although fasciculation is uncommonly noted by the patients before a physician calls attention to the twitching, it is seen in more than half the patients, up to 95 percent in some series, and more often in the hands and arms than the legs or tongue. Symmetrical twitching and atrophy of the tongue are almost diagnostic of MND by themselves, and even more so if there are also limb signs (regardless of El Escorial criteria).

Spared Functions

Some functions are spared. For instance, it is exceptional to encounter urinary incontinence or other autonomic dysfunction. Similarly, eye movements are rarely involved but ophthalmoplegia[75] and nystagmus have been documented.[76] Physiological studies track abnormalities of oculomotor function to the frontal lobes.[77] Ophthalmoplegia has been seen in patients living for a long time on long-term mechanical ventilation.[78] The search for autonomic dysfunction has usually been fruitless or conflicting,[79] but it has long been recognized that patients with ALS seem to be resistant to bed sores and some chemical alteration of the skin has been implied.[80]

Course of Amyotrophic Lateral Sclerosis/Motor Neuron Disease

The progression of symptoms is ordinarily steady, without abrupt exacerbations or remissions. Gradually, walking is impaired more seriously and the aids needed progress from canes to walkers to wheelchairs, punctuated sometimes by falls and fractures. Loss of hand use leads to increasing dependency in activities of daily living. Loss of swallowing leads to problems of nutrition that can be managed by percutaneous gastrostomy for feeding. Loss of speech can be ameliorated at first by speech augmentation and synthesizers; ultimately, the patient may be locked in, able to understand speech but without means to respond other than by blinking or eye movements.

This smooth course is occasionally disrupted by explosive respiratory failure.[81] Sometimes, hypercapnic coma is the first symptom of previously undiagnosed ALS and the first indication for medical care. Or the patient may be in a more advanced stage of recognized ALS, but respiratory failure is precipitated by aspiration or pneumonia. This kind of emergency may lead to intubation, tracheostomy, and long-term mechanical ventilation. That is why it is important for every patient to understand—well in advance—that this major decision will have to be confronted some day, whether to live as long as possible on long-term ventilation or to be kept comfortable at the end. Advance directives that emphasize this problem are available,[82] as are guidelines for respiratory care.[83–85]

Physicians caring for patients are faced with the dilemma of keeping hope alive and dismissing hope by frank discussions that are needed to permit truly informed consent in decision making. When ALS services are organized, 88 percent of patients have advance directives, but nevertheless experience discomfort in the terminal stages.[86,87] Symptoms include dyspnea, pain, and insomnia.

Mood Disturbances

This grim outlook raises two additional specters: depression and suicide. Many health workers concerned with ALS assume that most patients are suffering a clinical depression and prescribe appropriate medication. However, formal studies indicate that only about 20 percent of all patients are depressed.[88,89] Others have found higher rates, depending on the definition of depression.[90]

As for suicide, ALS figures prominently in public discussions and made the front pages with the publication of a paper from the Netherlands, stating that 17 percent of patients with ALS chose euthanasia and 3 percent chose assisted suicide.[91] These high figures challenged my own belief that the rise of hospice services would diminish the need for physician-assisted death,[92] because we assume that effective hospice care is available in that advanced country. In the accompanying editorial, Ganzini and Block[93] described experience in Oregon, where 5 percent of ALS deaths involved physician-assisted suicide, in contrast to only 0.4 percent of cancer deaths. Depression seemed not to play a role in that choice, but hopelessness did. Spirituality may be important in decisions about tracheostomy.[94] The unique depredations of ALS put it in a special category among lethal diseases; suicide could be the choice of any rational person who has full knowledge of the prognosis for the patient and the burden imposed on the family and immediate caregivers by long-term mechanical ventilation.[95] Yet some opt to live as long as possible. That difference is the essence of patient autonomy.

RELATED SYNDROMES

Primary Lateral Sclerosis

In theory, PLS ought to be a syndrome restricted to the UMN. The fundamental problem is the obverse of that in the SMA, which can be a purely LMN syndrome in life but may show involvement of corticospinal tracts at autopsy. In PLS, purely UMN syndromes in life can show anterior horn cell pathology in postmortem examination. Also, a purely UMN syndrome may prevail for more than 20 years before LMN signs appear.[96]

The concept of PLS depends on seven autopsies described in English-language journals since 1977[97–99] and one available only in Japanese[100] but cited in English.[99] In these patients, the LMNs were spared in postmortem examination and there were no LMN signs in life. Strictly speaking, the clinical diagnosis should not be made if there are any LMN signs clinically or in the EMG.[101,102] Symptoms usually begin after age 40, but a few cases have been recorded in children. Among the symptoms and signs are emotional lability and pseudobulbar palsy. Because there are so few autopsy-proven cases, clinical variations are not known with certainty; for instance, some observers consider urinary symptoms to be incompatible with the diagnosis, but we have seen bladder disturbance in otherwise clinically typical cases.

The major disability, however, is the spastic gait disorder. There may be no evident weakness on manual muscle testing, but alternative movements are slowed, tendon jerks are overactive, and there are Hoffmann and Babinski signs, often with clonus. Another constant feature is slow progression, much slower than ALS.[103] Gastaut et al[104] recorded survival for at least 28 years without LMN signs. Pringle et al[102] required absence of LMN signs for at least 3 years before making the diagnosis, but patients will be seen before that time and they must be told a diagnosis and informed that the prognosis of PLS is much better than that of ALS. Pseudobulbar dysarthria may be prominent and may progress to complete anarthria, the Foix-Cavany-Marie syndrome.[99,105,106]

Diagnosis requires exclusion of cervical cord compression or myelopathy, multiple sclerosis, and other cord diseases. Imaging is therefore essential and documentation of UMN involvement increasingly relies on magnetic stimulation to assess central conduction and magnetic resonance spectroscopy to evaluate the motor cortex. Repeated studies may show the evolution of pathology.[107,108] A high signal in affected corticospinal tracts can be useful in making the clinical diagnosis, but similar appearance in the cervical cord may be confused with myelomalacia and cervical spondylotic myelopathy.[109]

PLS may sometimes be paraneoplastic with breast or lung cancers. Monoclonal gammopathy and human immunodeficiency virus (HIV) infection are other associations. Adrenoleukodystrophy and late-onset Friedreich's ataxia may be limited to pyramidal tract signs. PLS is sometimes accompanied by dementia, and it was seen with Lewy body disease in one case. In other words, PLS can be regarded as a clinical syndrome of diverse etiology. Because there is no biological marker in life, the diagnosis can be made with certainty only by postmortem examination and even that may be difficult.[98] Oral treatment with baclofen or tizanidine has not been effective in my hands.

PLS may be a form of MND, but we should be careful in basing theories on clinical observations, especially when the diagnosis is applied to syndromes that include LMN signs and therefore qualify for a clinical diagnosis of ALS, even without prolonged observation or autopsy.[110,111] If there are minimal LMN signs,[112] the term *UMN-dominant ALS*[98] might be appropriate, but that would be ALS, not PLS. That term might also be considered for patients with clinically pure UMN syndromes with evidence of denervation in the EMG. Whether such disorders also have a prognosis less lethal than that of ALS also remains to be seen.

Amyotrophic Lateral Sclerosis–Parkinsonism

Guam is not the only place where ALS and parkinsonism are seen together. Many clinicians have recorded individuals or families in whom the two conditions have occurred together, sometimes with dementia, too. The association is uncommon, but there have been so many of these reports that it is difficult to think the associations are purely chance occurrences.[113] In some individual cases, there may be a chance association of ALS with typical Lewy body Parkinson disease, but in others, the findings suggest "inclusion body MND," a concept that includes both conditions, as described later.

Simultaneous onset of symptoms of ALS and parkinsonism may favor a common pathogenesis.[114] Years ago, we used the label "Brait-Fahn-Schwarz syndrome" for the combination, an eponym that has been used by no one else.[115] In one formal epidemiological study,[116] dementia was significantly more common in first-degree relatives of people with ALS and there was a trend in that direction for parkinsonian symptoms, but it did not reach significance; the findings raised the possibility of "shared genetic susceptibility." Another group, however, found no increase of age-related neurodegenerative diseases in relatives of ALS probands.[117] One additional link between parkinsonism and ALS is provided by histopathology because ubiquitin-inclusions can be found in the substantia nigra of patients with MND, even when there has been no clinically evident dementia or parkinsonism.[118]

Amyotrophic Lateral Sclerosis-Dementia-Parkinsonism

It has long been recognized that dementia is seen in 5 to 10 percent of all patients with ALS. As recently as 1994, diverse pathologies were found in these patients, including Alzheimer's disease, Huntington's disease, Pick's disease, or no specific pathology.[119] Even dementia pugilistica has been adduced.[120] Concepts changed, however, in the mid-1980s and 1990s with three observations: the 1987 recognition of frontal dementia;[121–126] the 1994 mapping of autosomal dominant FTD to chromosome 17;[127] and then the 1998 demonstration of tau mutations in some chromosome 17–linked families.[128–131] Remarkably, dementia is rarely, if ever, seen in FALS with SOD1 mutations.[132]

In 1997, Al-Shahi et al[133] found 14 patients with overt dementia among 104 autopsy-proven cases of ALS. Among the 14 patients, 8 had frontotemporal atrophy, 5 had Alzheimer changes, and one had cerebral Buerger's disease. FTD is now thought to account for about 20 percent of patients with symptom onset before age 65, making it the second most common form of dementia, and it has a special relation to ALS.[134,135]

It is said that ALS occurs in about 15 percent of patients with FTD, but this is probably a gross understatement. Lomen-Hoerth, Anderson, and Miller[136] examined 35 patients in a clinic for patients with sporadic FTD: 5 met criteria for definite ALS; 5 had prominent fasciculations; and 2 had EMG evidence of denervation in one limb. The total was therefore almost 36 percent, and there may have been more because 6 patients had dysphagia, with normal limb EMG.

They then evaluated cognitive function in patients with ALS who had no gross evidence of dementia and found impaired function on word generation tests in 33 percent, and when patients were given neuropsychological tests, nearly all of those with word generation abnormalities and 25 percent of those who had performed normally in the word tests showed evidence of FTD.[137] Cognitive abnormalities were found in neuropsychological tests in 40 percent, and imaging suggested FTD in 57 percent.[138] Cognitive abnormalities have also been found in measures of oculomotor function, which depends on the integrity of the frontal lobe.[139] These neuropsychological reports are the latest among many evaluations of cognitive function in patients with ALS who are not overtly demented.[140–143] But cognition may be impaired for other reasons: Nocturnal hypoventilation is common in ALS and can lead to sleepiness during the day; if noninvasive positive pressure ventilation is applied, test scores assessing cognition improve.[144]

The clinical hallmark of the frontotemporal syndromes is that behavioral abnormalities precede the dementia.[145] Among the symptoms are social misconduct, hyperorality, gluttony, and akinesia in the absence of severe amnesia or perceptual problems. Other symptoms are called stereotypical behavior, altered eating preferences, and disinhibited behavior. A consensus panel posited three major categories of cognitive decline: FTD, progressive nonfluent aphasia, and semantic dementia.[146] Either the dementia or the MND may come first.[147]

Men predominate in a ratio of 4:1. About half is familial, and among them, 90 percent are inherited in autosomal dominant pattern.[148] About 10 percent show signs of ALS, and 5 percent, parkinsonism. Dementia may be more likely in patients with bulbar palsy and amyotrophy rather than those with corticospinal and corticobulbar features.[149] But ALS and FTD are also related pathologically. Ubiquitinated inclusions are characteristic of both ALS and FTD; dementia may correlate with the number and distribution of inclusions.[150] It has therefore been suggested that the dementia syndrome could be called "FTD/MND."[149,151] Nevertheless, not all patients with both ALS and dementia show the typical pathology.[152,153] In addition, when ALS is combined with dementia but not parkinsonism, the pathology may include the hippocampus but not the neostriatum.[154]

In the Manchester series about 15 percent of the cases of FTD were associated with tau mutations.[155] Poorkaj et al[156] found no tau mutations in sporadic FTD, but half the cases were familial and 10 percent of the familial cases were attributed to tau mutations. Among those showing tau pathology, mutations were found in 33 percent. The non–tau cases provided evidence of genetic heterogeneity, and there was also allelic heterogeneity because a father and son had the same mutation; the father had FTD and the son had corticobasal degeneration.[157] In the Netherlands, tau mutations were found in 17.8 percent of all patients with FTD, and 43 percent of those who had a family history of affected relatives.[158] Tau mutations have also been found in progressive supranuclear palsy, and familial FTD has been mapped to sites other than chromosome 17.[159]

Prion Disease and Amyotrophy

The clinical features of MND with dementia may also be seen with prion diseases, especially with Creutzfeldt-Jakob disease (CJD) but also the others. Before 1967, when CJD was first transmitted to chimpanzees, the diseases were defined largely by neuropathology, which was not precise. After Salazar et al[160] had transmitted the disease, they reportedly failed to transmit ALS with dementia. In fact, however, they did transmit 2 of 33 cases, which they regarded as insignificant because the pair was "atypical."[160] Later, however, a third case was transmitted, making the rate of transmission 10 percent, which hardly seems insignificant. Then Worrall et al[161] found 50 cases in the literature in which the diagnosis of prion disease was unequivocal and there was clinical or EMG evidence of amyotrophy. Possible cases continue to be reported.[162] In an EMG study of prion diseases, most abnormalities indicated peripheral neuropathy, but one patient showed evidence of LMN disease, and at autopsy, the corticospinal tracts were involved.[163]

Monomelic Amyotrophy (Hirayama Syndrome)

Most of the reports of this condition have come from Japan where it was first described, but others have been identified everywhere and in all ethnic groups. It is only rarely familial, but one set of brothers was affected.[164] The manifestations consistently affect a young adult, almost always a man about age 20 who notes weakness of one arm and hand, with fasciculation and cramps. Symptoms progress for a year or so and then cease. Only rarely is the other arm involved and there are no UMN signs. Magnetic resonance imaging (MRI) scan is usually normal but may show evidence of cord atrophy and anterior displacement of the cord when the neck is flexed and extended.[165–167]

However, not all investigators agree with that mechanical observation[168,169] and surgical decompression is not recommended. Use of a cervical collar has not been controlled for evaluation of EMG changes.[170] The condition is benign and only one autopsy is cited, showing necrosis, shrinkage and loss of anterior horn cells, and gliosis; an ischemic lesion was suggested.[171] Other investigators believe it is a disorder of the motor neurons, but there is no explanation for the restrictions—one arm, age about 20 years, and always men. There is no evident external trauma or clear relationship to physical labor or contact sports. The picture is so typical that it can be readily diagnosed, but it is mandatory to observe for at least a year to be certain that progression terminates and that UMN signs do not appear. Whether a similar disorder can affect the legs is uncertain.[172,173]

Reversible Amyotrophic Lateral Sclerosis

Reversible amyotrophic lateral sclerosis is so rare that it borders on the miraculous. But there have been reports of ten patients with convincing findings of ALS that disappeared.[174–176] One was 18 years old; the others were between ages 39 and 74 years. All had widespread fasciculation; three had Babinski signs and four others had overactive tendon jerks. Only one lasted more than 2 years. Conduction studies have not shown peripheral neuropathy or plexopathy. The nature of the disorder is therefore unknown, but some kind of myelopathy seems likely, perhaps a viral infection. In one subject, the syndrome followed bacille Calmette-Guérin (BCG) treatment of bladder cancer, possibly a hypersensitivity reaction.[177] Cerebrospinal fluid (CSF) studies in the chronic phase have not shown evidence of inflammation. However, delayed and persistent LMN signs may follow myelitis or poliomyelitis,[178] and some may be attributed to MMN.[179]

Benign Fasciculation and Cramps (Syndrome of Denny-Brown and Foley)

Another form of motor neuron disorder may be related to reversible ALS. It was first described in 1948 by Derek Denny-Brown and Joseph Foley.[180] The syndrome of benign fasciculation comprises muscle twitching and often cramps, with no other abnormality on EMG or nerve conduction studies or CSF examination and no UMN signs. Many experienced neurologists believe that these symptoms may herald the onset of ALS.[181] It would also make sense if that were true. If ALS can start with symptoms in limbs or bulbar regions, and if symptoms can be dominantly UMN or LMN, why cannot fasciculations and cramps be the first manifestations? In fact, however, ALS almost never starts that way; there is only one recorded case in which it happened.[182] Many normal people say they have experienced muscle twitches,[183] and spontaneous potentials can appear in the EMG of asymptomatic people.[184] A follow-up study of patients diagnosed with benign fasciculation at the Mayo Clinic found that none of them had developed ALS.[185] The contrary view arises from patient reports that they noticed fasciculation long before the onset of limb weakness. But the patients were not actually examined at that time to exclude weakness and atrophy or EMG abnormalities that would have established the diagnosis of ALS.[186] Perhaps, like transient ALS, the syndrome of Denny-Brown and Foley is a kind of viral inflammation of the spinal cord.

Juvenile Amyotrophic Lateral Sclerosis, Fazio-Londe Syndrome, and Madras Motor Neuron Disease

Juvenile onset of ALS is almost always familial and autosomal recessive. If an isolated child or adolescent has appropriate manifestations, it can be reasonably suspected of being a new mutation of a familial disorder. That is also true of the form with primarily bulbar manifestations, the Fazio-Londe syndrome.[187,188]

In India, especially in Madras and Bangalore, a motor cranial neuropathy is encountered; it involves cranial nerves VII to XII, differing from Fazio-Londe syndrome in that hearing is often affected.[189]

Multifocal Motor Neuropathy

MMN is a peripheral neuropathy; it was first identified and defined by the presence of conduction block. Histological changes in peripheral nerves include demyelination (including the sensory sural nerve), sometimes with tomaculous changes. In one patient, deposits of immunoglobulins were found at the node of Ranvier.[190] In mice, gamma globulins from patients blocked conduction in nerve terminals.[191] The autoimmune basis of the disorder was deduced from the presence of ganglioside antibodies in many patients and then by therapeutic responses to immunotherapy, especially now with intravenous immune globulin (IVIG) therapy.[192,193] However, the concept of neuropathy has been expanded to include cases that show no block, but slowing or other abnormalities of motor conduction and nevertheless respond to IVIG therapy.[194–196]

The relationship of motor neuropathy to ALS involves clinical features and postmortem examination. Clinically, it is the only peripheral neuropathy that is purely motor in terms of clinical symptoms and signs. Except for the neuropathy of amyloidosis, MMN is the only one in which about 50 percent of reported cases show visible fasciculation and it is the only neuropathy in which about half of the reported cases show active tendon jerks in limbs with weak, wasted, and fasciculating muscles.

Remarkably, there have only been four published autopsies of patients with MMN with conduction block.[197–200] Although all four showed pathological changes in peripheral nerves or nerve roots, all four also showed loss of motor neurons. Bunina bodies or ubiquitinated inclusions were present in all three cases so examined. Two showed changes in the corticospinal tracts. In one report,[200] central conduction velocity was prolonged in 3 of 12 patients with MMN. In addition to the central lesions, autopsy also showed histopathological changes in peripheral nerves or plexus nerves. We can conclude that there is sometimes mixed pathology, simultaneously affecting motor neurons and peripheral nerves, not necessarily one or the other.

In some patients with the same clinical syndrome of motor neuropathy—except for progression to death—postmortem examination shows inflammatory demyelinating neuropathy[201] and axonal radiculopathy, with chromatolysis of motor neurons.[202]

Human Immunodeficiency Virus and Amyotrophic Lateral Sclerosis/Motor Neuron Disease

For years, there has been interest in the possibility that ALS could be caused by a virus, but there has been little clinical evidence to support that view. Debates and doubt challenge the theory that infectious prion disease could be responsible and there have been only a few cases of human T-lymphotrophic virus type 1 (HTLV-1) infection with features of ALS.[203] In 2000 therefore, it was something of a sensation when there were reports of HIV-positive patients who had UMN and LMN signs that were reversed by treatment with either nucleoside anti-HIV agents or protease inhibitors.[204–206] The disorder differed clinically from ALS in rapidity of progression, CSF pleocytosis, and in two patients, changes in the spinal cord on MRI. Because the patients recovered, there were no autopsies. In three similar cases, however, antiretroviral therapy failed.[207–210] Therefore there seem to be two kinds of motor neuron disorders in HIV-positive people: one suggesting a subacute viral myelitis that may respond to antiviral therapy; and the second, ALS of the usual lethal variety.[207] Whether being HIV positive is a risk factor for ALS itself is still uncertain.

There have been only five autopsies on HIV-positive patients who had both UMN and LMN signs in life.[207,211–213] None of them had a typical clinical course or typical findings of ALS (Table 5.3).

Transgenic mice carrying the HIV-1 genome develop either a vacuolar myelopathy[214] or an axonal neuropathy,[215] but with no histological evidence of MND. Reverse-transcriptase enzyme activity has been in the blood of people with ALS.[216] Of 59 patients with ALS, 34 (59%) tested positive, compared with 29 (5%) of 58 controls. There was no reverse-transcriptase activity, however, for HIV-1, HIV-2, or HTLV-1 or HTLV-2. Instead, the evidence pointed to some other—unknown—retrovirus.

Table 5.3   Autopsies in human immunodeficiency virus–positive people with amyotrophic lateral sclerosis–like manifestations

Reference	*Diagnosis*	*Clinical features*
Behar, Wiley, and McCutchan[211]	Myeloradiculopathy; CMV; chromatolysis of anterior horn cells	Diffuse fasciculation; Babinski signs, normal sensation, but retinitis, urinary incontinence; CSF pleocytosis; duration, 7 weeks
Galassi et al[209]	Loss and atrophy anterior horn cells; gliosis; no CST pathology	Clinically and pathologically, SMA; died 3 months after onset despite zidovudine therapy
Sher[213]	Vacuolar myelopathy plus loss of anterior horn cells and gliosis	30-year-old man; both UMN and LMN signs, dementia; died 3 months after onset
Simpson et al[210]	Loss of anterior horn cells; degeneration of CST, lymphocytes	Both UMN and LMN signs, IgM monoclonal gammopathy, anti-asialo-G_{M1} 1:3200; zidovudine therapy 4 years after onset
Verma et al[212]	"Myelopathy" plus loss of anterior roots, but anterior horn cells normal	Pure LMN signs, improved; died of opportunistic infections 2 years after onset

CMV = cytomegalovirus; CSF = cerebrospinal fluid; CST = corticospinal tract; LMN = lower motor neuron; SMA = spinal muscular atrophy; UMN = upper motor neuron.

Paraneoplastic Motor Neuron Disease

In 1948, Denny-Brown[217] and Wyburn-Mason[218] independently described sensory neuropathy in the same patient with lung cancer. Their papers initiated interest in the possibility that neurological syndromes in patients with malignant tumors might not be explained by metastatic disease. The term *paraneoplastic neuropathy* was introduced. Cerebellar degeneration and limbic encephalitis joined the list. Progressive multifocal leukoencephalopathy seemed to be similar but was proven to be caused by a virus. Autoimmunity was adduced by finding antineuronal antibodies.

Brain, Croft, and Wilkinson[219] noted an excessive number of patients with MND among patients with lung and other cancers, an idea supported by W. King Engel and Forbes Norris. In 1965, Brain and Norris[220] organized a symposium on paraneoplastic syndromes. Norris and Engel[221] stated that 11 of 140 patients with ALS had had a malignancy; almost 8 percent seemed unduly high. However, Raymond Adams[222] said that this was not his experience, and there had been only one carcinoma among 80 autopsy-proven cases of ALS at the Montefiore Hospital in New York.[223]

For the next 2 decades, not much was heard of cancer and ALS. In 1989, Rosenfield and Posner[224] analyzed all reported series and concluded that there was no increase in the frequency of neoplasms with MNDs, merely the chance concurrence of two age-related diseases. The excessive numbers in Bethesda and at London Hospital could have been due to ascertainment bias—that is, investigators attracting patients with disorders of their special interest.

However, the controversy persisted for several reasons. First, Gubbay et al[225] avoided ascertainment bias in a population study in Israel, presumably missing no patients with MND; 10 percent had a malignant tumor. Second, the signs of MND sometimes disappeared after a tumor had been treated successfully.[226–230] Third, an association of MND with lymphoma became evident in 1963[231] and has become increasingly recognized.

Most reports of paraneoplastic syndromes described either mixed UMN and LMN disorders (ALS) or those confined to LMNs or PSMA. However, Forsyth et al[232] described three patients with elements of ALS among other CNS findings, as seen in paraneoplastic encephalomyelitis; all three had anti-Hu antibodies. The antibodies elevated this syndrome to the top of a small list of documented autoimmune MNDs. These antibodies have been found in sensory neuropathy and mixed CNS syndromes,[233] but in only one patient with an uncomplicated MND that included both LMN and UMN signs.[234] Patients with ALS and no tumor do not show these antibodies.[235]

The same authors described five women with carcinoma of the breast and PLS. However, some women have had breast cancer and typical ALS. One had an immunoglobulin A monoclonal gammopathy with antineuronal antibodies that reacted with neurofilaments[236] or other neuronal antigens,[237,238] but most lacked those antibodies. Among patients with presumed PLS, two autopsy-proven cases were associated with malignant neoplasms, one myeloma[11] and one lung cancer.[97] Because PLS may turn into ALS after months or years, it was little surprise to learn that three of the five cases of Forsyth et al ultimately developed LMN signs, meeting criteria for ALS, but one other patient had signs of PLS for 6 years before breast cancer was discovered.[239] It has not been proven that this association occurs more often than by chance; a case-control or population study would be necessary. Nevertheless it is now necessary to evaluate the possibility of breast cancer in any woman with PLS.

Motor neuron disorders may improve after a tumor is treated. Buchanan and Malamud[226] described a man with renal carcinoma and both UMN and LMN signs that improved after removal of the tumor; he was "nearly normal" neurologically for 4 years and then died of metastases. Autopsy showed loss of motor neurons and gliosis without change in the corticospinal tracts or peripheral nerves. Evans et al[240] described a similar case. We encountered a man with ALS, immunoglobulin M (IgM) monoclonal paraproteinemia and renal cancer. Removal of the tumor, however, did not reverse progression of the neurological disease, and he died of metastatic disease.[13]

In a study of 14 patients with ALS and different kinds of cancer, it was the ALS, not the tumor, that was responsible for the 8 deaths.[241] No antineuronal antibodies were found, and no patient improved with surgery or other treatment for the tumor. Whether malignant tumors are risk factors for ALS is still not known.

Amyotrophic Lateral Sclerosis and Lymphoma

In contrast to the uncertainty about the association of MNDs with cancers, there is growing interest in the link to lymphoproliferative diseases.[242–244] There has been no case-control study to prove that the association is more than a chance relationship, but there are now at least 65 reported cases.[245–247]

Although it was once thought that the neurological disorder is primarily one affecting the LMN (a neuronopathy[244]), more than half of reported cases have UMN signs in life and the corticospinal tracts have been affected in more than half of the autopsy cases.[242] Either the lymphomatous disease or the MND can appear first, or the two may occur together. When the lymphoma is first, the tumor may have been excised with an interval of as long as 25 years before neurological symptoms commence. That interval makes it unlikely that the lymphoma is producing an antineuronal antibody to cause the MND. In fewer than 10 percent of treated cases, immunosuppressive drugs improve the neurological disorder. The nature of the relationship is not known, but a spontaneous retroviral infection of wild mice results in a similar combination of lymphoma and an MND. If there is such a human viral infection, it has eluded detection and identification.

Clinically, the neurological syndromes do not differ from uncomplicated PSMA or ALS, and in most cases, it was the MND that was responsible for disability or death. Among the more esoteric lymphomatous conditions were Kikuchi disease, angiotropic lymphoma, and POEMS (polyneuropathy, organomegaly, endocrinopathy, monoclonal gammopathy, and skin changes) (Table 5.4). The diversity of disorders might be linked by a propensity for autoimmune neurological disorders.

The neurological disorder is usually responsible for disability or death, but the outcome in not easily predicted. Oppenshaw and Slatkin[248] noted that one patient died neurologically in 3 years, and another saw all neurological

Table 5.4 Lymphoproliferative diseases and motor neuron diseases: 65 patients

Lymphoproliferative disorder	No. of patients	%
Hodgkin lymphoma	24	36.9
Non-Hodgkin lymphoma	28	43.1
Macroglobulinemia	5	7.7
Myeloma	4	6.1
Angiotropic lymphoma	2	3.1
POEMS	1	1.5
Kikuchi necrotizing lymphadenitis	1	1.5
Lymphomatoid granulomatosis	1	1.5
Cutaneous T-cell lymphoma (mycosis fungoides)	1	1.5
Lymphoplasmacytic lymphoma	1	1.5
Monoclonal paraproteinemia	18/36	50.0

Data from Gordon PH, Rowland LP, Younger DS, et al. Lymphoproliferative disorders and motor neuron disease. Neurology 1997;48:1671–1678; and Chad D. Case records of the Massachusetts General Hospital case 16-1999. Lymphoplasmacytic lymphoma with motor neuronopathy and Waldenström macroglobulinemia. N Engl J Med 1999;340:1661–1669.

POEMS = polyneuropathy, organomegaly, endocrinopathy, monoclonal gammopathy, and skin changes.

symptoms disappear in 1 year. In another study, 23 patients were treated with immunosuppressive drugs, but only 3 responded in any way.[242]

Monoclonal Gammopathy (Plasma Cell Dyscrasia) and Amyotrophic Lateral Sclerosis/Motor Neuron Disease

Although cases had been recorded earlier, experience with one patient set us off on a decade of observations about monoclonal proteins in patients with ALS/MND. The patient[249] was a 48-year-old man with weakness, atrophy, and fasciculation and no UMN signs. Nerve conduction studies and autopsy provided evidence of a demyelinating neuropathy. Anterior horn cells showed chromatolysis but no reduction in numbers. Michael Shy et al[250] then found that 5 percent of patients with ALS and 1 percent of controls had a monoclonal protein. Immunofixation gave a higher figure, and in subsequent analyses, 5 to 10 percent of patients showed a monoclonal paraprotein, usually an IgM (in contrast to the immunoglobulin G monoclonal proteins found in asymptomatic elderly people). In Scotland, however, Willison et al[251] found no difference between patients with ALS and controls, which could result from geographical variations. However, the M protein does not always have antibody activity, and if it does, the reactive antigens have included G_{M1}, G_{D1b}, chondroitin sulfate, and neurofilament protein. At one time, some investigators thought there were anti-G_{M1} antibodies in most patients with ALS but that soon faded to a number less than 10 percent.[252] Currently, it seems that this antibody is found in patients with MMN but only rarely in patients with UMN signs. No animal model with MND and gammopathy has been produced. Injections of an M protein with anti-G_{M1} activity led to conduction block and demyelination.

Immunosuppressive treatment of patients with ALS and monoclonal gammopathy, with or without antibody activity, has not ameliorated the ALS/MND. Although patients with monoclonal paraproteinemia have been excluded from many therapeutic trials for ALS, the clinical pattern is no different than that of "ordinary" ALS.

Amyotrophic Lateral Sclerosis and Autoimmune Diseases

Except for Graves disease and lymphoproliferative diseases, ALS is only rarely associated with autoimmune diseases but has been recorded with multiple sclerosis,[253] rheumatoid arthritis,[254,255] systemic lupus erythematosus, pemphigus,[256] and scleroderma.[257,258] One woman had a combination of rheumatoid arthritis, pemphigus, myasthenia, Hashimoto thyroiditis, and MND.[259] Collectively, however, these cases are so few that it is difficult to make a case for autoimmunity.

Nevertheless, it is an idea that will not go away. Appel et al[260] and Drachman[261] have presented detailed and convincing arguments for and against an autoimmune etiology of sporadic ALS. In the most practical terms, there have been many trials of immunosuppressive trials, all failures. That may seem crushing, but a negative study does not rule out the possibility. It does mean that other therapies should be sought.

Amyotrophic Lateral Sclerosis with Thyrotoxicosis

One of our patients, a 40-year-old woman, had difficulty rising after kneeling to pray in church. She showed clinical signs of thyrotoxicosis and had proximal limb weakness, with no fasciculation. Her tendon jerks were overactive and there was clonus. The signs disappeared with treatment of the hyperthyroidism.[13]

Nineteen patients have been reported to have Graves disease and signs of ALS.[262–273] Four had limb weakness with fasciculations and normal or increased tendon reflexes with no definite UMN signs. All four improved with return of the euthyroid state, as did 11 of 14 with both LMN and UMN signs. One had solely UMN signs and also improved. All in all, 16 (84%) of the 19 reported cases improved with antithyroid medication. We were therefore profoundly disappointed to encounter a 43-year-old physician with carcinoma of the thyroid and thyrotoxicosis that was difficult to control as the ALS became worse and was ultimately fatal.[13]

The nature of the usually reversible syndrome, which includes both UMN and LMN signs, is not clear, but it affects the CNS and is therefore not merely a form of thyrotoxic myopathy. It reproduces the signs of ALS but is tied to the thyrotoxicosis and is reversed with return to a euthyroid state. The irreversible cases, which progress in the manner typical of ALS, are few and could be coincidental, but the number suggests some relationship to thyroid overactivity.

Motor Neuron Disorders in Multisystem Diseases

The elements of ALS may be seen in other hereditary diseases. For instance, G_{M2} gangliosidosis may be manifest as juvenile-onset SMA.[274,275] The clue to late-onset cases is sometimes a history of Tay-Sachs disease in a relative, but SMA is not the only manifestation; ataxia, areflexia, and proprioceptive sensory loss may resemble Friedreich's ataxia,[276] and the patient of Johnson et al[274] later suffered a disabling chronic depression. The neuronal pathology of these syndromes is that of a lysosomal storage disease, not the atrophic cell death found in ALS or related condition, and to that extent, the storage disease should be mentioned in a chapter on differential diagnosis, but not one describing the clinical manifestations of ALS. However, gangliosidosis was the first heritable MNDs in which the genetic fault was identified. Now LMN signs are encountered in some of the spinocerebellar atrophies.

AN OVERALL VIEW

ALS/MND is an age-related neurodegenerative disease with malignant clinical characteristics. Sporadic ALS may comprise several different syndromes, as suggested by variation in the symptoms and signs of upper and LMN dysfunction and by extreme variation in rapidity of course and duration of symptoms, as well as diverse possible etiologies. The cruel clinical manifestations give the disease a central position in discussions of physician-assisted death and patient autonomy. Although symptomatic therapy has become more effective, the greatest hope we can offer patients is the accelerating and increasingly molecular research of the past decade—since the discovery of the SOD1 mutation in FALS. If we could understand the pathogenesis of sporadic ALS, we could hope for a truly effective treatment.

REFERENCES

1. Rowland LP. Natural History and Clinical Features of Amyotrophic Lateral Sclerosis and Related Motor Neuron Diseases. In DN Calne (ed), Neurodegenerative Diseases (3rd ed). Philadelphia: WB Saunders, 1993;507–521.
2. Rowland LP. Diverse Forms of Motor Neuron Diseases. In LP Rowland (ed), Human Motor Neuron Diseases. New York: Raven Press, 1982;1–13.
3. Rowland LP. Motor Neuron Diseases: The Clinical Syndromes. In DW Mulder (ed), The Diagnosis and Treatment of Amyotrophic Lateral Sclerosis. Boston: Houghton Mifflin, 1980;7–27.
4. Swash M, Desai J. Motor neuron disease: classification and nomenclature. Amyotroph Lateral Scler Other Motor Neuron Disord 2000;1:105–112.
5. Wharton S, Ince PG. Pathology of Motor Neuron Disorders. In PJ Shaw, M Strong (eds), Blue Books of Practical Neurology: Motor Neuron Disorders. London: Butterworth-Heinemann, 2003.
6. Strong MJ. Progress in clinical neurosciences: the evidence for ALS as a multisystem disorder of limited phenotypic expression. Can J Neurol Sci 2001;28(4):283–298.
7. Machida Y, Tsuchiya K, Anno M, et al. Sporadic amyotrophic lateral sclerosis with multiple system degeneration: a report of an autopsy case without respirator administration. Acta Neuropathol (Berl) 1999;98(5):512–515.

8. Ellis CM, Suckling J, Amaro E Jr, et al. Volumetric analysis reveals corticospinal tract degeneration and extramotor involvement in ALS. Neurology 2001;57:1571–1578.

9. Wakabayashi K, Horikawa Y, Oyake M, et al. Sporadic motor neuron disease with severe sensory neuronopathy. Acta Neuropathol (Berl) 1998;95(4):426–430.

10. Cudkowicz ME, McKenna-Yasek D, Chen C, et al. Limited corticospinal tract involvement in amyotrophic lateral sclerosis subjects with the A4V mutation in the copper/zinc superoxide dismutase gene. Ann Neurol 1998;43(6):703–710.

11. Brownell B, Oppenheimer DR, Hughes JT. Central nervous system in motor neuron disease. J Neurol Neurosurg Psychiatry 1970;33:338–357.

12. Lawyer M, Netsky MG. Amyotrophic lateral sclerosis. Clinico-anatomic study of 53 cases. Arch Neurol Psychiatry 1953;69:171–192.

13. Rowland LP. Diagnosis of ALS. J Neurol Sci 1998;160:S6–S24.

14. Rowland LP, Leung D, Hays AP. A Clinically Pure Lower Motor Neuron Syndrome. In AHV Schapira, LP Rowland (eds), Clinical Cases in Neurology. Oxford: Butterworth-Heinemann, 2001;47–54.

15. Tsuchiya K, Shintani S, Kikuchi M, et al. Sporadic amyotrophic lateral sclerosis of long duration mimicking spinal progressive muscular atrophy: a clinicopathological study. J Neurol Sci 1999;162(2):174–178.

16. Ince PG, Evans J, Knopp M, et al. Corticospinal tract degeneration in the progressive muscular atrophy variant of ALS. Neurology 2003;60:1252–1258.

17. Younger DS, Rowland LP, Latov N, et al. Motor neuron disease and amyotrophic lateral sclerosis: relation of high CSF protein content to paraproteinemia and clinical syndromes. Neurology 1990;40:595–599.

18. Chan S, Shungu DC, Douglas-Akinwande AC, et al. Motor neuron diseases: comparison of single-voxel, proton MR spectroscopy of the motor cortex with MR imaging of the brain in motor neuron diseases. Radiology 1999;212:763–769.

19. Leung DK, Hays AP, Karlikaya G, et al. ALS: clinicopathologic analysis of 76 autopsies, Neurology 1999;52:A164.

20. Kuwabara S, Nakata M, Sung JY, et al. Hyperreflexia in axonal Guillain-Barré syndrome subsequent to *Campylobacter jejuni* enteritis. J Neurol Sci 2002;199(1–2):89–92.

21. Visser J, van den Berg-Vos RM, Franssen H, et al. Mimic syndromes in sporadic cases of progressive spinal muscular atrophy. Neurology 2002;58:1593–1596.

22. Van den Berg-Vos RM, Franssen H, Wokke JHJ, Van den Berg. Multifocal motor neuropathy: long-term clinical and electrophysiological assessment of intravenous immunoglobulin maintenance treatment. Brain 2002;125:1875–1886.

23. McCullagh S, Moore M, Gawel M, Feinstein A. Pathological laughing and crying in amyotrophic lateral sclerosis: an association with prefrontal cognitive dysfunction. J Neurol Sci 1999; 169(1–2):43–48.

24. Abrahams S, Goldstein LH, Al-Chalabi A, et al. Relation between cognitive dysfunction and pseudobulbar palsy in amyotrophic lateral sclerosis. J Neurol Neurosurg Psychiatry 1997; 62(5):464–472.

25. Rowland LP. Peripheral Neuropathy, Motor Neuron Disease, or Neuronopathy? In L Battistin, GA Hashim, A Lajtha (eds), Clinical and Biological Aspects of Peripheral Nerve Diseases. New York: Alan R. Liss, 1983:27–41.

26. Subcommittee on Motor Neuron Diseases of World Federation of Neurology Research Group on Neuromuscular Diseases. El Escorial "Clinical limits of ALS" workshop contributors. El Escorial World Federation of Neurology criteria for the diagnosis of amyotrophic lateral sclerosis. J Neurol Sci 1994;124:96–107.

27. Belsh JM. ALS diagnostic criteria of El Escorial revisited: Do they meet the needs of clinicians as well as researchers? Amyotroph Lateral Scler Other Motor Neuron Disord 2000;1(suppl 1): S57–S60.

28. Traynor BJ, Codd MB, Corr B, et al. Clinical features of amyotrophic lateral sclerosis according to the El Escorial and Airlie House diagnostic criteria. A population based study. Arch Neurol 2000;57:1171–1176.

29. Miller RG, Munsat TL, Swash M, Brooks BR, for the World Federation of Neurology Committee on Research. Consensus guidelines for the design and implementation of clinical trials in ALS. J Neurol Sci 1999;169:2–12.

30. Brooks BR, Miller RG, Swash M, Munsat TL, and the World Federation of Neurology Research Group on Motor Neuron Diseases. El Escorial revisited; revised criteria for the diagnosis of amyotrophic lateral sclerosis. Amyotroph Lateral Scler Other Motor Neuron Disord 2000;1:293–299.

31. Eisen A, Krieger C. Amyotrophic Lateral Sclerosis. A Synthesis of Research and Clinical Practice. New York: Cambridge University Press, 1998.
32. Finsterer J. Amyotrophic lateral sclerosis with very slow progression. Neuromusc Disord 2002;12:694–695.
33. Borasio GD, Grohme K, Maravic MV. Amyotrophic lateral sclerosis with very slow progression [response to comments by J. Finsterer]. Neuromusc Disord 2002;12:695–696.
34. Garcia-Redondo A, Bustos F, Seva BY, et al. Molecular analysis of the superoxide dismutase 1 gene in Spanish patients with sporadic or familial amyotrophic lateral sclerosis. Muscle Nerve 2002;26:274–278.
35. Andersen P. Genetic Aspects of Amyotrophic Lateral Sclerosis/Motor Neuron Disease. In PJ Shaw, M Strong (eds), Blue Books of Practical Neurology: Motor Neuron Disorders. Philadelphia: Butterworth-Heinemann, 2003.
36. Corcia P, Mayeux-Portas V, Khoris J, et al. Abnormal SMN1 gene copy number is susceptibility factor for amyotrophic lateral sclerosis. Ann Neurol 2002;51:243–246.
37. Parboosingh JS, Meininger V, McKenna-Yassek D, et al. Deletions causing spinal muscular atrophy do not predispose to amyotrophic lateral sclerosis. Arch Neurol 1999;56:710–712.
38. Veldink JH, van den Berg LH, Cobben JM, et al. Homozygous deletion of the survival motor neuron 2 gene is a prognostic factor in sporadic ALS. Neurology 2001;56(6):749–752.
39. Giess R, Holtmann B, Braga M, et al. Early onset of severe familial amyotrophic lateral sclerosis with a SOD-1 mutation: potential impact of CNTF as a candidate modifier gene. Am J Hum Genet 2002;70:1277–1286.
40. Mui S, Rebeck GW, McKenna-Yasek D, et al. Apolipoprotein E epsilon 4 allele is not associated with earlier age at onset in amyotrophic lateral sclerosis. Ann Neurol 1995;38(3):460–463.
41. Scarmeas N, Shih T, Stern Y, et al. Premorbid weight, body mass, and athletics in ALS and related syndromes. Neurology 2002;59:773–775.
42. Critchley M. Discussion on motor neurone disease. Proc Roy Soc Med 1962;55:1066.
43. Felmus MT, Patten BM, Swanke L. Antecedent events in amyotrophic lateral sclerosis. Neurology 1976;26:167–172.
44. Longstreth WT, Nelson LM, Koepsell TD, Van Belle G. Hypotheses to explain the association between vigorous physical activity and amyotrophic lateral sclerosis. Med Hypoth 1991; 34:144–148.
45. Wilbourn AJ, Mitsumoto H. Why are patients with amyotrophic lateral sclerosis so nice? Proceedings of the ninth International Symposium on ALS/MND; Munich; 1998.
46. Armon C. Epidemiology of Amyotrophic Lateral Sclerosis/Motor Neuron Disease. In PJ Shaw, M Strong (eds), Blue Books of Practical Neurology: Motor Neuron Disorders. Philadelphia: Butterworth-Heinemann, 2003.
47. Boothby J, deJesus PV, Rowland LP. Reversible forms of motor neuron disease: lead "neuritis." Arch Neurol 1974;31:18–23.
48. Galasko D, Salmon DP, Craig UK, et al. Clinical features and changing patterns of neurodegenerative disorders on Guam. Neurology 2002;58:90–97.
49. Plato SS, Galasko D, Garruto RM, et al. ALS and PDC of Guam; forty year follow-up. Neurology 2002;58:765–773.
50. Sacks O. The Island of the Colorblind. New York: Random House, 1998;97–177.
51. Cox PA, Sacks OW. Cycad neurotoxins, consumption of flying foxes, and ALS-PDC disease in Guam. Neurology 2002;58:956–959.
52. Chiò A, Mora G, Leone M, et al. Early symptom progression rate is related to ALS outcome. A prospective population-based study. Neurology 2002;59:99–103.
53. del Aguila MA, Longstreth WT Jr, McGuire V, et al. Prognosis in amyotrophic lateral sclerosis: a population-based study. Neurology 2003;60:813–819.
54. Munsat TL, Andres PL, Finison L, et al. The natural history of motoneuron loss in amyotrophic lateral sclerosis. Neurology 1988;38:409–413.
55. Sasaki S, Iwata M. Atypical form of amyotrophic lateral sclerosis. J Neurol Neurosurg Psychiatry 1999;66:581–585.
56. Katz JS, Wolfe F, Andersson PB, et al. Brachial amyotrophic diplegia. A slowly progressive motor neuron disorder. Neurology 1999;53:1071–1076.
57. Rosenfield H, Chang SW, Jackson CE, et al. Lower extremity amyotrophic diplegia (LAD): a new clinical entity in the spectrum of motor neuron disease. Neurology 2002;58(suppl 3):A411.
58. Gamez J, Cervera C, Codina A. Atypical form of amyotrophic lateral sclerosis: a new term to define a previously well known form of ALS. J Neurol Neurosurg Psychiatry 2000;68:118–119.

59. Hu MTM, Ellis CM, Al-Chalabi, et al. Flail arm syndrome: a distinctive variant of amyotrophic lateral sclerosis. J Neurol Neurosurg Psychiatry 1998;65:950–951.
60. Chancellor AM, Slattery JM, Fraser H, et al. The prognosis of adult-onset motor neuron disease: a prospective study based on the Scottish Motor Neuron Disease Register. J Neurol 1993; 240:339–346.
61. Mulder DW, Howard FM. Patient resistance and prognosis in amyotrophic lateral sclerosis. Mayo Clin Proc 1976;51:537–541.
62. Juergens SM, Kurland LT, Okazaki H, Mulder DW. ALS in Rochester, Minnesota, 1925–1977. Neurology 1980;30:463–470.
63. Tysnes OB, Vollset SE, Larsen JP, Aarli JA. Prognostic factors and survival in amyotrophic lateral sclerosis. Neuroepidemiology 1994;13:226–235.
64. Stambler N, Charatan M, Cedarbaum J, et al. Prognostic indicators of survival in ALS. ALS CNTF Treatment Study Group. Neurology 1998;50:66–72.
65. Norris F. Adult progressive muscular atrophy and the spinal muscular atrophies. In de Jong J.M.B.V. (ed): Handbook of Clinical Neurology: Diseases of the Motor System, vol 59, Amsterdam, 1992, Elsevier Science Publishers.
66. Norris F, Shepherd R, Denys E, et al. Onset, natural history and outcome in idiopathic adult motor neuron disease. J Neurol Sci 1993;118:48–55.
67. Wokke JHJ, Van den Berg-Vos M, Visser J, et al. Classification of sporadic adult onset lower motor neuron syndromes. Neurology 2002;58(suppl 3):A411.
68. Van den Berg-Vos RM, Visser J, Franssen J, et al. Sporadic lower motor neuron disease with adult onset: classification of subsets. Neurology (in press).
69. Mortara P, Chiò A, Rosso MD, et al. Motor neuron disease in the province of Turin, Italy, 1966–1980. J Neurol Sci 1984;66:165–173.
70. Ohi T, Saita K, Takechi S, et al. Familial ALS with a His46Arg mutation in SOD1. J Neurol Sci 2002;197(1–2):73–78.
71. McLeod JG, Prineas JW. Distal type of chronic spinal muscular atrophy. Clinical, electrophysiological and pathological studies. Brain 1971;94:703–714.
72. Petiot P, Gonon V, Froment JC, et al. Slowly progressive spinal muscular atrophy of the hands (O'Sullivan-McLeod syndrome): clinical and magnetic resonance imaging presentation. J Neurol 2000;247:654–655.
73. Van den Berg-Vos RM, Van den Berg LH, Jansen GH, et al. Hereditary pure lower motor neuron disease with adult onset and rapid progression. J Neurol 2001;248(4):290–296.
74. Swash M. Clinical Features and Diagnosis of Amyotrophic Lateral Sclerosis. In RH Brown Jr, V Meininger, M Swash (eds), Amyotrophic Lateral Sclerosis. London: Martin Dunitz, 2000;3–30.
75. Okamoto K, Hirai S, Amari M, et al. Oculomotor nuclear pathology in amyotrophic lateral sclerosis. Acta Neuropathol 1993;85:458–462.
76. Kushner MJ, Parrish M, Burke A, et al. Nystagmus in motor neuron disease: clinicopathological study of two cases. Ann Neurol 1984;16:71–77.
77. Shaunak S, Orrell RW, O'Sullivan E, et al. Oculomotor function in amyotrophic lateral sclerosis. Ann Neurol 1995;38:38–44.
78. Mizutami T, Sakamaki S, Tsuchiya N, et al. Amyotrophic lateral sclerosis with ophthalmoplegia and multisystem degeneration in patients on long-term use of respirators. Acta Neuropathol 1992;84:372–377.
79. Oey PL, Vos PE, Wieneke GH, et al. Subtle involvement of the sympathetic nervous system in amyotrophic lateral sclerosis. Muscle Nerve 2002;25:402–408.
80. Ono S. The skin in amyotrophic lateral sclerosis. Amyotroph Lateral Scler Other Motor Neuron Disord 2000;1(3):191–199.
81. Bradley MD, Orrell RW, Clarke J, et al. Outcome of ventilatory support for acute respiratory failure in motor neurone disease. J Neurol Neurosurg Psychiatry 2002;72:752–756.
82. Benditt JO, Smith TS, Tonelli MR. Empowering the individual with ALS at the end-of-life: disease-specific advance care planning. Muscle Nerve 2001;24:1706–1709.
83. Gelanis DF. Respiratory failure or impairment in amyotrophic lateral sclerosis. Curr Treat Options Neurol 2001;3:133–138.
84. Lyall RA, Donaldson N, Polkey MI, et al. Respiratory muscle strength and ventilatory failure in amyotrophic lateral sclerosis. Brain 2001;124:2000–2013.
85. Bach JR. Amyotrophic lateral sclerosis: prolongation of life by noninvasive respiratory aids. Chest 2002;122(1):92–98.
86. Ganzini L, Johnston WS, Silveira MJ. The final month of life in patients with ALS. Neurology 2002;59(3):428–431.

87. Mandler RN, Anderson FA Jr, Miller RG, et al, and the ALS CARE Study Group. The ALS patient care database: insights into end-of-life care in ALS. Amyotroph Lateral Scler Other Motor Neuron Disord 2001;2:203–208.
88. Rapkin JG, Wagner GJ, Del Bene M. Resilience and distress among amyotrophic lateral sclerosis patients and caregivers. Psychosom Med 2000;62:271–279.
89. Ganzini L, Johnston W, McFarlland B, et al. Attitudes of patients with amyotrophic lateral sclerosis and their caregivers toward assisted suicide. N Engl J Med 1998;339:967–973.
90. Moore MJ, Moore PB, Shaw P. Mood disturbances in motor neurone disease. J Neurol Sci 1998;160(suppl 1):S53–S54.
91. Veldink JH, Wokke JH, van der Wal G, et al. Euthanasia and physician-assisted suicide among patients with amyotrophic lateral sclerosis in the Netherlands. N Engl J Med 2002;346(21):1638–1644.
92. Rowland LP. Assisted suicide and alternatives in amyotrophic lateral sclerosis. N Engl J Med 1998;339:987–989.
93. Ganzini L, Block S. Physician-assisted death—a last resort? N Engl J Med 2002;346(21):1638–1644.
94. Murphy PL, Albert SM, Weber CM, et al. Impact of spirituality and religiousness on outcomes in patients with ALS. Neurology 2000;55:1581–1584.
95. Doyal L. The Case for Physician-Assisted Suicide and Active Euthanasia in Amyotrophic Lateral Sclerosis. In RH Brown Jr, V Meininger, M Swash (eds), Amyotrophic Lateral Sclerosis. London: Dunitz, 2000;423–440.
96. Bruyn RP, Koelman JH, Troost D, de Jong JM. Motor neuron disease (amyotrophic lateral sclerosis) arising from longstanding primary lateral sclerosis. J Neurol Neurosurg Psychiatry 1995;58:742–744.
97. Younger DS, Chou S, Hays AP, et al. Primary lateral sclerosis. A clinical diagnosis reemerges. Arch Neurol 1988;45:1304–1307.
98. Rowland LP. Primary lateral sclerosis: disease, syndrome, both or neither? J Neurol Sci 1999;170:1–4.
99. Konagaya M, Sakai M, Matsuoka Y, et al. Upper motor neuron predominant degeneration with frontal and temporal lobe atrophy. Acta Neuropathol 1998;96:532–536.
100. Watanabe R, Iino M, Honda M, et al. Primary lateral sclerosis. Neuropathology 1997;17:220–224.
101. Swash M, Desai J, Misra VP. What is primary lateral sclerosis? J Neurol Sci 1999;170:5–10.
102. Pringle CE, Hudson AJ, Munoz DG, et al. Primary lateral sclerosis. Clinical features, neuropathology and diagnostic criteria. Brain 1992;115:495–520.
103. Serratrice G. Primary lateral sclerosis. Myology 2002;21:31–32.
104. Gastaut JL, Michel B, Figarella-Branger D, Somma-Mauvais H. Chronic progressive spinobulbar spasticity; a rare form of primary lateral sclerosis. Arch Neurol 1988;45:509–513.
105. De Koning I, van Doorn PA, van Dongen HR. Slowly progressive isolated dysarthria: longitudinal course, speech features, and neuropsychological deficits. J Neurol 1997;244:664–667.
106. Weller M, Poremba M, Dichgans J. Opercular syndrome without opercular lesions; Foix-Cavany-Marie syndrome in progressive supranuclear motor system degeneration. Eur Arch Psychiatry Clin Neurosci 1990;239:370–372.
107. Smith CD. Serial MRI findings in a case of primary lateral sclerosis. Neurology 2002;58:647–649.
108. Hecht MJ, Fellner F, Fellner C, et al. Hyperintense and hypointense MRI signals of the precentral gyrus and corticospinal tract in ALS: A follow-up examination including FLAIR images. J Neurol Sci 2002;1999:59–65.
109. Waragai M, Shinotoh H, Hayashi M, Hattori T. High signal intensity on T1 weighted MRI of the anterolateral column of the spinal cord in amyotrophic lateral sclerosis. J Neurol Neurosurg Psychiatry 1997;62:88–91.
110. Le Forestier N, Maisonobe T, Piquard A, et al. Does primary lateral sclerosis exist? A study of 20 patients and a review of the literature. Brain 2002;124:1989–1999.
111. Le Forestier N, Maisonobe T, Spelle L, et al. Primary lateral sclerosis: further clarification. J Neurol Sci 2001;185:95–100.
112. Kuippers-Upmeijer J, de Jager AEJ, Hew JM, et al. Primary lateral sclerosis: clinical, neurophysiological and magnetic resonance findings. J Neurol Neurosurg Psychiatry 2001;71:615–620.
113. Williams TL, Shaw PJ, Lowe J, Bates D. Parkinsonism in motor neuron disease: case report and literature review. Acta Neuropathol 1995;89:275–283.
114. Qureshi AI, Wilmot G, Dihenia B, et al. Motor neuron disease with parkinsonism. Arch Neurol 1996;53:987–991.

115. Brait K, Fahn S, Schwarz GA. Sporadic and familial parkinsonism and motor neuron disease. Neurology 1973;23:990–1002.
116. Majoor-Krakauer D, Ottman R, Johnson WG, Rowland LP. Familial aggregation of amyotrophic lateral sclerosis, dementia, and Parkinson's disease: evidence of shared genetic susceptibility. Neurology 1994;44:1872–1877.
117. Cruz DC, Nelson LM, McGuire V, Longstreth WT Jr. Physical trauma and family history of neurodegenerative diseases in amyotrophic lateral sclerosis: a population-based case-control study. Neuroepidemiology 1999;18(2):101–110.
118. Al-Sarraj S, Makekawa S, Kibble M, et al. Ubiquitin-only intraneuronal inclusion in the substantia nigra is a characteristic feature of motor neurone disease with dementia. Neuropathol Appl Neurobiol 2002;28:120–128.
119. Lynch T, Vu TH, Pech RS, et al. Amyotrophic lateral sclerosis and dementia: a retrospective review of autopsy cases [abstract]. Ann Neurol 1994;36:321.
120. Drachman DA, Newell KL. Case Records of the Massachusetts General Hospital case 12-1999: A 67-year-old man with three years of dementia. N Engl J Med 1999;340:1269–1276.
121. Gustafson L. Frontal lobe degeneration of non-Alzheimer type, II: clinical picture and differential diagnosis. Arch Gerontol Geriatr 1987;6:209–223.
122. Brun A. Frontal lobe degeneration of non-Alzheimer type, I: neuropathology. Arch Gerontol Geriatr 1987;6:193–207.
123. Lowe J, Aldridge F, Lennox G, et al. A filamentous inclusion body within anterior horn neurones in motor neurone disease defined by immunocytochemical localization of ubiquitin. Neurosci Lett 1989;105(1–2):7–13.
124. Leigh PN, Anderton BH, Dodson A, et al. Ubiquitin deposits in anterior horn cells in motor neuron disease. Neurosci Lett 1988;93:197–203.
125. Neary D, Snowden JS, Northern B, Goulding PJ. Dementia of frontal lobe type. J Neurol Neurosurg Psychiatry 1988;51:353–361.
126. Brun A, Englund B, Gustafson L, et al. Consensus statement. Clinical and neuropathological criteria for frontotemporal dementia. J Neurol Neurosurg Psychiatry 1994;4:416–418.
127. Lynch T, Sano M, Marder KS, et al. Clinical characteristics of a family with chromosome 17-linked disinhibition-dementia-parkinsonism-amyotrophy-complex. Neurology 1994;44:1878–1884.
128. Hong M, Zhukareva V, Vogelsberg-Regaglia V. Mutation-specific functional impairments in distinct tau isoforms of hereditary FTDP-17. Science 1998;282:1914–1917.
129. Hutton M, Lendon CL, Rizzu P, et al. Association of missense and 5N-splice-site mutations in tau with the inherited dementia FTDPB17. Nature 1998;393:702–705.
130. Goedert M, Crowther RA, Spillantini MG. Tau mutations cause frontotemporal dementias. Neuron 1998;21:955–958.
131. Rosso SM, Van Swieten JC. New developments in frontotemporal dementia and parkinsonism linked to chromosome 17. Curr Opin Neurol 2002;15(4):423–428.
132. Orrell RW, King AW, Hilton DA, et al. Familial amyotrophic lateral sclerosis with a point mutation of SOD-1: intrafamilial heterogeneity of disease duration associated with neurofibrillary tangles. J Neurol Neurosurg Psychiatry 1995;59:266–270.
133. Al-Shahi R, Lynch T, Murphy PL, et al. Heterogeneity in amyotrophic lateral sclerosis dementia: autopsy data in 14 cases [abstract]. Ann Neurol 1997;42:397.
134. Ratnavalli E, Brayne C, Dawson K, Hodges JR. The prevalence of frontotemporal dementia. Neurology 2002;58:1608–1615.
135. Greicius MD, Geschwind MD, Miller BL. Presenile dementia syndromes: an update on taxonomy and diagnosis. J Neurol Neurosurg Psychiatry 2002;72:691–700.
136. Lomen-Hoerth C, Anderson T, Miller B. The overlap of amyotrophic lateral sclerosis and frontotemporal dementia. Neurology 2002;59:1077–1079.
137. Lomen-Hoerth C, Murphy J, Langmore S, et al. Are amyotrophic lateral sclerosis patients cognitively normal? Neurology (submitted).
138. Lomen-Hoerth C, Murphy J, Henry R, et al. The frequency of frontotemporal lobar dementia (FLTD) is an ALS population. Is neuropsychological testing or neuroimaging more sensitive? Ann Neurol (in press).
139. Evdokimidis I, Constdnatinidis TS, Gourtzelidis P, et al. Frontal lobe dysfunction in amyotrophic lateral sclerosis. J Neurol Sci 2002;195:25–33.
140. Hudson A. Amyotrophic lateral sclerosis and its association with dementia. Brain 1991;194:217–247.
141. Strong MJ, Grace GM, Orange JB, et al. A prospective study of cognitive impairment in ALS. Neurology 1999;53(8):1665–1670.

142. Strong MJ, Grace GM, Orange JB, Leeper HA. Cognition, language, and speech in amyotrophic lateral sclerosis: a review. J Clin Exp Neuropsychol 1996;18(2):291–303.
143. Massman PJ, Sims J, Cooke N, et al. Prevalence and correlates of neuropsychological deficits in amyotrophic lateral sclerosis. J Neurol Neurosurg Psychiatry 1996;61:450–455.
144. Newsom-Davis IC, Lyall RA, Leigh PN, et al. The effect of non-invasive positive pressure ventilation (NIPPV) on cognitive function in amyotrophic lateral sclerosis (ALS): a prospective study. J Neurol Neurosurg Psychiatry 2001;71(4):482–487.
145. Galasko D, Marder K. Picking away at frontotemporal dementia. Neurology 2002;58:1585–1586.
146. Neary D, Snowden JS, Gustafson L, et al. Frontotemporal lobar dementia: a consensus on clinical diagnostic criteria. Neurology 1998;51:1546–1554.
147. Vercelletto M, Ronin M, Huvet M, et al. Frontal type dementia preceding amyotrophic lateral sclerosis: a neuropsychological and SPECT study of five clinical cases. Eur J Neurol 1999;6:295–299.
148. Chow TW, Miller BW, Hayashi VN, Geschwind DH. Inheritance of frontotemporal dementia. Arch Neurol 1999;56:817–822.
149. Neary D, Snowden JS, Mann DM. Cognitive change in motor neurone disease/amyotrophic lateral sclerosis (MND/ALS). J Neurol Sci 2000;180(1–2):15–20.
150. Wilson CM, Grace GM, Munoz DG, et al. Cognitive impairment in sporadic ALS: a pathologic continuum underlying a multisystem disorder. Neurology 2001;57(4):651–657.
151. Jackson M, Lennox G, Lowe J. Motor neurone disease-inclusion dementia. Neurodegeneration 1996;5:339–350.
152. Abe K. Cognitive function in amyotrophic lateral sclerosis. Amyotroph Lateral Scler Other Motor Neuron Disord 2000;1:343–347.
153. Tomik B, Adamek D, Lechwacka A, et al. ALS-Plus syndrome. A clinical and neuropathological case study. Pol J Pathol 2000;51(4):191–196.
154. Kawashima T, Doh-ura K, Kikuchi H, Iwaki T. Cognitive dysfunction in patients with amyotrophic lateral sclerosis is associated with spherical or crescent-shaped ubiquitinated intraneuronal inclusions in the parahippocampal gyrus and amygdala, but not in the neostriatum. Acta Neuropathol 2001;102:467–472.
155. Houlden H, Baker M, Adamson J, et al. Frequency of tau mutations in three series of non-Alzheimer's degenerative dementia. Ann Neurol 1999;46(2):243–248.
156. Poorkaj P, Grossman M, Steinhart E, et al. Frequency of tau gene mutations in familial and sporadic cases of non-Alzheimer dementia. Arch Neurol 2001;58:383–387.
157. Miller BL. Tau mutations—center tent or sideshow? Arch Neurol 2001;58:351–352.
158. Rizzu P, Van Swieten JC, Joose M, et al. High prevalence of mutations in microtubule-associated protein tau in a population study of frontotemporal dementia in the Netherlands. Am J Hum Genet 1999;64:414–421.
159. Rosso SM, van Swieten JC. New developments in frontotemporal dementia and parkinsonism linked to chromosome 17. Curr Opin Neurol 2002;15(4):423–428.
160. Salazar AM, Masters CL, Gajdusek DC, Gibbs CJ Jr. Syndromes of amyotrophic lateral sclerosis and dementia: relation to transmissible Creutzfeldt-Jakob disease. Ann Neurol 1983;14(1):17–26.
161. Worrall BB, Rowland LP, Chin SS, Mastrianni JA. Amyotrophy in prion diseases. Arch Neurol 2000;57:33–38.
162. Gomez Esteban JC, Atarés B, Zarranz JJ, et al. Dementia, amyotrophy, and periodic complexes on the electroencephalogram. Arch Neurol 2001;58:1669–1672.
163. Niewiadomska M, Kulczycki J, Wochnik-Dyjas D, et al. Impairment of the peripheral nervous system in Creutzfeldt-Jakob disease. Arch Neurol 2002;59:1430–1436.
164. Robberecht W, Aguirre T, van den Bosch L, et al. Familial juvenile focal amyotrophy of the upper extremity (Hirayama disease). Superoxide dismutase 1 genotype and activity. Arch Neurol 1997;54(1):46–50.
165. Hirayama K, Tokumaru Y. Cervical dural sac and spinal cord in juvenile muscular atrophy of distal upper extremity. Neurology 2000;54(10):1922–1926.
166. Toma S, Shiozawa Z. Amyotrophic cervical myelopathy in adolescence. J Neurol Neurosurg Psychiatry 1995;58:56–64.
167. Chen CJ, Chen CM, Wu CL, et al. Hirayama disease: MR diagnosis. AJNR Am J Neuroradiol 1998;19(2):365–368.
168. Poewe W. Juvenile asymmetric segmental spinal muscular atrophy (Hirayama's disease): three cases without evidence of flexion myelopathy. Acta Neurol Scand 2001;104(5):320–322.
169. Schroder R, Keller E, Flacke S, et al. MRI findings in Hirayama's disease: flexion-induced cervical myelopathy or intrinsic motor neuron disease? J Neurol 1999;246(11):1069–1074.

170. Imai T, Shizukawa H, Nakanishi K, et al. Hyperexcitability of cervical motor neurons during neck flexion in patients with Hirayama disease. Electromyogr Clin Neurophysiol 2000;40(1):11–15.

171. Hirayama K, Tomonaga M, Kitano K, et al. Focal cervical poliopathy causing juvenile muscular atrophy of distal upper extremity: a pathological study. J Neurol Neurosurg Psychiatry 1987; 50(3):285–290.

172. Takemitsu M, Murayama K, Saga T, et al. Monomelic muscle atrophy. Neuromusc Disord 1993;3:311–317.

173. Di Muzio A, Pizzi CD, Lugaresi A, et al. Benign monomelic amyotrophy of lower limb; a rare entity with a characteristic muscular CT. J Neurol Sci 1994;126:153–161.

174. Tucker T, Layzer RB, Miller RG, Chad D. Subacute, reversible motor neuron disease. Neurology 1991;41(10):1541–1544.

175. Tsai CP, Ho HH, Yen DJ, et al. Reversible motor neuron disease. Eur Neurol 1993;33(5):387–389.

176. Miyoshi K, Ohyagi Y, Amano T, et al. A patient with motor neuron syndrome clinically similar to amyotrophic lateral sclerosis, presenting spontaneous recovery [in Japanese]. Rinsho Shinkeigaku 2000;40(11):1090–1095.

177. Sànchez-Juan P, Garcia-Penco C, Calleja J, et al. Reversible diffuse motor neuron syndrome related to Bacille Calmette-Guérin (BCG) for local bladder cancer. Muscle Nerve (submitted 2002).

178. Fetell MR, Smallberg G, Lewis LD, et al. A benign motor neuron disorder: delayed cramps and fasciculation after poliomyelitis or myelitis. Ann Neurol 1982;11:423–427.

179. Chad DA, Hammer K, Sargent J. Slow resolution of multifocal weakness and fasciculation: a reversible motor neuron syndrome. Neurology 1986;36(9):1260–1263.

180. Denny-Brown D, Foley JM. Myokymia and benign fasciculation of muscle. Trans Assoc Am Physicians 1948;61:88–96.

181. Eisen A, Stewart H. Not-so-benign fasciculation. Ann Neurol 1994;35:375.

182. Fleet WS, Watson RT. From benign fasciculation and cramps to motor neuron disease. Neurology 1986;36:997–998.

183. Reed DM, Kurland LT. Muscle fasciculations in a healthy population. Arch Neruol 1963; 9:363–367.

184. Mitsikostas DD, Karandreas N, Coutsopetras P, et al. Fasciculation potentials in healthy people. Muscle Nerve 1998;21(4):533–535.

185. Blexrud MD, Windebank AJ, Daube JR. Long-term follow-up of 121 patients with benign fasciculation. Ann Neurol 1993;334:622–625.

186. Okuda B, Kodama N, Tachibana H, Sugita M. Motor neuron disease following generalized fasciculation and cramps. J Neurol Sci 1997;150:129–131.

187. McShane MA, Boyd S, Harding B, et al. Progressive bulbar paralysis of childhood. A reappraisal of Fazio-Londe disease. Brain 1992;115(pt 6):1889–1900.

188. Tsuchiya K, Shintani S, Nakabayashi H, et al. Familial amyotrophic lateral sclerosis with onset in bulbar sign, benign clinical course, and Bunina bodies: a clinical, genetic, and pathological study of a Japanese family. Acta Neuropathol (Berl) 2000;100(6):603–607.

189. Gouri Devi M, Suresh TG. Madras pattern of motor neuron disease in south India. J Neurol Neurosurg Psychiatry 1988;51:773–777.

190. Santoro M, Thomas FP, Fink ME, et al. IgM deposits at nodes of Ranvier in a patient with amyotrophic lateral sclerosis, anti-G_{M1} antibodies, and multifocal conduction block. Ann Neurol 1990;28:373–377.

191. Roberts M, Willison HJ, Paterson G, et al. Human monoclonal anti-G_{M1} ganglioside antibodies derived from multifocal motor neuropathy patients block distal motor nerve conduction. Ann Neurol 1995;38:111–118.

192. Van den Beg-Vos RM, Franssen H, Wokke JH, Van den Berg LH. Multifocal motor neuropathy: long-term clinical and electrophysiological assessment of intravenous immunoglobulin maintenance treatment. Brain 2002;125:1875–1886.

193. Nobile-Orazio E, Cappellari A, Meucci N, et al. Multifocal motor neuropathy: clinical and immunological features and response to IVIg in relation to the presence and degree of motor conduction block. J Neurol Neurosurg Psychiatry 2002;72(6):761–766.

194. Pakiam A, Parry G. Multifocal motor neuropathy without evidence of conduction block. Neurology 1996;46;A234.

195. Wolfe GI, Katz JS, Bryan WW, et al. Is conduction block a necessary finding in patients with multifocal motor neuropathy? Neurology 1996;46:A234.

196. Katz JS, Wolfe GI, Bryan WW, et al. Electro-physiologic findings in multifocal motor neuropathy. Neurology 1997;47:700–707.

197. Adams D, Kuntzer T, Steck AJ, et al. Motor conduction block and high titres of anti-G_{M1} ganglioside antibodies; pathological evidence of a motor neuropathy in a patient with lower motor neuron syndrome. J Neurol Neurosurg Psychiatry 1993;56:982–987.

198. Oh SJ, Claussen GC, Odabasi Z, Palmer CP. Multifocal demyelinating motor neuropathy: pathologic evidence of "inflammatory demyelinating polyradiculoneuropathy." Neurology 1995;45: 1828–1832.

199. Veugelers B, Theys P, Lammends M, et al. Pathological findings in a patient with amyotrophic lateral sclerosis and multifocal motor neuropathy with conduction block. J Neurol Sci 1996; 136:64–70.

200. Molinuevo JL, Cruz-Martinez A, Graus F, et al. Central motor conduction time in patients with multifocal motor conduction block. Muscle Nerve 1999;22(7):926–932.

201. Rowland LP, Defendini R, Sherman W, et al. Macroglobulinemia with peripheral neuropathy simulating motor neuron disease. Ann Neurol 1982;11:532–536.

202. Gorson KC, Ropper AH, Adelman LS, et al. Chronic motor axonal neuropathy: pathological evidence of inflammatory polyradiculopathy. Muscle Nerve 1999;22:266–270.

203. Matsuzaki T, Nakagawa M, Nagai M, et al. HTLV-I–associated myelopathy (IHAM)/tropical spastic paraparesis (TSP) with amyotrophic lateral sclerosis–like manifestations. J Neurovirol 2000;6:544–548.

204. MacGowan DJ, Scelsa SN, Waldron M. An ALS-like syndrome with new HIV infection and complete response to antiretroviral therapy. Neurology 2001;57(6):1094–1097.

205. Moulignier A, Moulonguet A, Pialoux G, Rozenbaum W. Reversible ALS-like disorder in HIV infection. Neurology 2001;57(6):995–1001.

206. Nishio M, Koizumi K, Moriwaka F, et al. Reversal of HIV-associated motor neuron syndrome after highly active antiretroviral therapy. J Neurol 2000;248:233–234.

207. Zoccolella S, Carbonara S, Minerva D, et al. A case of concomitant amyotrophic lateral sclerosis and HIV infection. Eur J Neurol 2002;9(2):180–182.

208. Sastre-Garriga J, Tintoré M, Raguer N, et al. Lower motor neuron disease in an HIV-2 infected woman. J Neurol 2000;247:718–719.

209. Galassi G, Gentilini M, Ferrari S, et al. Motor neuron disease and HIV-1 infection in a 30-year-old HIV-positive heroin abuser: a causal relationship? Clin Neuropathol 1998;17(3):131–135.

210. Simpson DM, Morgello S, Citak K, et al. Motor neuron disease associated with HIV and anti-sialo G_{M1} antibody [abstract]. Muscle Nerve 1994;17:1091.

211. Behar R, Wiley C, McCutchan JA. Cytomegalovirus polyradiculoneuropathy AIDS. Neurology 1987;37:557–561.

212. Verma A, Berger JR, Snodgrass S, Petito C. Motor neuron disease: a paraneoplastic process associated with anti-Hu antibody and small-cell lung carcinoma. Ann Neurol 1996;40:112–116.

213. Sher J, Wzolek M, Shmuter Z. Motor neuron disease associated with AIDS [abstract]. J Neuropathol Exp Neurol 1999;47:303.

214. Goudreau G, Carpenter S, Beaulieu N, Jolicoeur P. Vacuolar myelopathy in transgenic mice expressing human immunodeficiency virus type 1 proteins under the regulation of the myelin basic protein gene promoter. Nat Med 1996;2(6):655–661.

215. Thomas FP, Chalk C, Lalonde R, et al. Expression of human immunodeficiency virus type 1 in the nervous system of transgenic mice leads to neurological disease. J Virol 1994;68(11):7099–7107.

216. Andrews WD, Tuke PW, Al-Chalabi A, et al. Detection of reverse transcriptase activity in the serum of patients with motor neuron disease. J Med Virol 2000;61(4):527–532.

217. Denny-Brown DE. Primary sensory neuropathy with muscular changes associated with carcinoma. J Neurol Neurosurg Psychiatry 1948;11:73–87.

218. Wyburn-Mason R. Bronchial carcinoma presenting as polyneuritis. Lancet 1948;1:203–206.

219. Brain WR, Croft PB, Wilkinson M. Motor neurone disease as a manifestation of neoplasm (with a note on the course of classical motor neurone disease). Brain 1965;88:479–500.

220. Lord Brain, Norris FH Jr, eds. The Remote Effects of Cancer on the Nervous System. New York: Grune and Stratton, 1965.

221. Norris FH Jr, Engel WK. Carcinomatous Amyotrophic Lateral Sclerosis. In Lord Brain, Norris FH Jr (eds), The Remote Effects of Cancer on the Nervous System. New York: Grune and Stratton, 1965;24–34.

222. Adams RD. Discussion of ref 221, Lord Brain, Norris FH Jr (eds), The Remote Effects of Cancer on the Nervous System. New York: Grune and Stratton, 1965;39.

223. Rowland LP. Discussion of ref 221, Lord Brain, Norris FH Jr (eds), The Remote Effects of Cancer on the Nervous System. New York: Grune and Stratton, 1965;40.

224. Rosenfield D, Posner JB. Motor Neuron Disease and Malignant Tumors. In LP Rowland (ed), Amyotrophic Lateral Sclerosis and Other Motor Neuron Diseases. New York: Raven Press, 1991;445–462.
225. Gubbay SS, Kahana E, Zilber N, et al. Amyotrophic lateral sclerosis. A study of its presentation and prognosis. J Neurol 1985;232:295–300.
226. Buchanan DS, Malamud N. Motor neuron disease with renal cell carcinoma and postoperative neurological remission. Neurology 1973;28:891–894.
227. Evans BS, Fagan C, Arnold T, et al. Paraneoplastic motor neuron disease and renal cell carcinoma; improvement after nephrectomy. Neurology 1990;40:960–963.
228. Gerling GM, Woolsey RM. Paraneoplastic motor neuron disease. Mo Med 1967;64:503–506.
229. Mitchell DM, Olczak SA. Remission of a syndrome indistinguishable from motor neuron disease after resection of bronchial carcinoma. BMJ 1979;2:176–177.
230. Stephens TW, Rougas A, Ghose MK. Pure motor neuropathy complicating carcinoma of the bronchus recovered after surgery. Br J Dis Chest 1966;60:107–109.
231. Rowland LP, Schneck S. Neuromuscular disorders associated with malignant neoplastic disease. J Chron Dis 1963;16:777–795.
232. Forsyth PA, Dalmau J, Graus F, et al. Motor neuron syndromes in cancer patients. Ann Neurol 1997;41:722–730.
233. Dalmau J, Graus F, Rosenblum MK, Posner JB. Anti-Hu–associated paraneoplastic encephalomyelitis/sensory neuropathy. Medicine 1992;71:59–72.
234. Verma A, Berger JR, Snodgrass S, Petito C. Motor neuron disease: a paraneoplastic process associated with anti-Hu antibody and small cell lung carcinoma. Ann Neurol 1996;40:112–116.
235. Kiernan JA, Hudson AJ. Anti-neurone antibodies are not characteristic of amyotrophic lateral sclerosis. Neuroreport 1993;4:427–430.
236. Hays AP, Roxas A, Sadiq SA, et al. A monoclonal IgA in a patient with amyotrophic lateral sclerosis reacts with neurofilaments and surface antigen on neuroblastoma cells. J Neuropathol Exp Neurol 1990;49:383–398.
237. Ferracci F, Fassetta G, Butler MH, et al. A novel antineuronal antibody in a motor neuron syndrome associated with breast cancer. Neurology 1999;53(4):852–855.
238. Khwaja S, Sripathi N, Ahmad BK, Lennon VA. Paraneoplastic motor neuron disease with type 1 Purkinje cell antibodies. Muscle Nerve 1998;21:943–945.
239. Corcia P, Honnorat J, Geunnoc AM, et al. Sclérose latérale primitive et cancer du sein: syndrome neologique paranéoplasique ou association fortuite? Rev Neurol (Paris) 2000;156:1020–1022.
240. Evans BK, Fagan C, Arnold T, et al. Paraneoplastic motor neuron disease and renal cell carcinoma; improvement after nephrectomy. Neurology 1990;40:960–962.
241. Vigliani MC, Polo P, Chiò A, et al. Patients with amyotrophic lateral sclerosis and cancer do not differ clinically from patients with sporadic amyotrophic lateral sclerosis. J Neurol 2000;247: 778–782.
242. Gordon PH, Rowland LP, Younger DS, et al. Lymphoproliferative disorders and motor neuron disease. Neurology 1997;48:1671–1678.
243. Rowland LP, Gordon PH, Younger DS, et al. Lymphoproliferative disorders and motor neuron disease [letter to the editor]. Neurology 1997;48:1671–1678.
244. Schold SC, Cho ES, Sonasundaram M, Posner JP. Subacute motor neuronopathy; a remote effect of lymphoma. Ann Neurol 1979;5:271–287.
245. Leone KV, Phillips LH. Lymphoproliferative disorders and motor neuron disease [letter]. Neurology 1998;50:576.
246. Rowland LP, Gordon PH, Younger DS, et al. Lymphoproliferative disorders and motor neuron disease [letter]. Neurology 1998;50:576.
247. Chad D. Case records of the Massachusetts General Hospital case 16-1999. Lymphoplasmacytic lymphoma with motor neuronopathy and Waldenström macroglobulinemia. N Engl J Med 1999; 340:1661–1669.
248. Oppenshaw H, Slatkin E. Motor neuron disease in Hodgkin's lymphoma. Neurology 1998;50:A31.
249. Rowland LP, Defendini R, Sherman WH, et al. Macroglobulinemia with peripheral neuropathy simulating motor neuron disease. Ann Neurol 1981;11:532–536.
250. Shy M, Rowland LP, Smith T, et al. Motor neuron disease and plasma cell dyscrasia. Neurology 1986;36:1429–1436.
251. Willison HJ, Chancellor AM, Patterson G, et al. Antiglycolipid antibodies, immunoglobulins and paraproteins in motor neuron disease: population-based case control study. J Neurol Sci 1993;114:209–215.

252. Rowland LP. Amyotrophic Lateral Sclerosis with Paraproteins and Autoantibodies. In G Serratrice, TL Munsat (eds), Pathogenesis and Therapy of Amyotrophic Lateral Sclerosis. Philadelphia: Lippincott-Raven Publishers, 1995:93–105.

253. Dynes GJ, Schwimer CJ, Staugatis SM, et al. Amyotrophic lateral sclerosis with multiple sclerosis: a clinical and pathological report. Amyotroph Lateral Scler Other Motor Neuron Disord 2000;1:349–353.

254. M'Bappe P, Moguilevski A, Arnal C, et al. Concomitant rheumatoid arthritis and amyotrophic lateral sclerosis. A puzzle illustrated by a new case. Joint Bone Spine 2000;67:242–244.

255. Sostarko M, Brzovic Z, Vranjes D. Motor neurone disease associated with several immunological disorders. J Neuro Sci 1994;124(suppl):70–71.

256. Chosidow O, Doppler V, Bensimon G, et al. Bullous pemphigoid and amyotrophic lateral sclerosis. Arch Dermatol 2000;136:521–524.

257. Ouhabi H, Bourazza A, Wouimi A, et al. Association of amyotrophic lateral sclerosis with scleroderma. Study of 2 cases [in French]. Rev Neurol (Paris) 1997;153:790–791.

258. Katz JS, Horoupian D, Ross MA. Multisystem neuronal involvement and sicca complex: broadening the spectrum of complications. Muscle Nerve 1999;22:404–407.

259. Priori R, Buoopane A, Francia A, Valesini G. Scleroderma and motor neuron disease: an unusual association. Clin Rheumatol 1993;12:428–429.

260. Appel SH, Alexianu M, Engelhardt JI, et al. Involvement of Immune Factors in Motor Neuron Cell Injury in Amyotrophic Lateral Sclerosis. In RH Brown Jr, V Meininger, M Swash (eds), Amyotrophic Lateral Sclerosis. London: Martin Dunitz Ltd, 2000;309–326.

261. Drachman DB. Does Autoimmunity Play a Role in Amyotrophic Lateral Sclerosis? In RH Brown Jr, V Meininger, M Swash (eds), Amyotrophic Lateral Sclerosis. London: Martin Dunitz Ltd, 2000;327–340.

262. Bulens C. Neurologic complications of hyperthyroidism. Remission of spastic paraplegia, dementia, and optic atrophy. Arch Neurol 1981;38:669–670.

263. Cashman N, Antel J, Wissman G, Bader P. Hyperthyroidism and familial ALS [abstract]. Ann Neurol 1983;14:118.

264. Cervino JM, Mussio-Fournier JC, Muxi F, et al. Pyramidal tract symptoms in Basedow's disease. Med Klin 1959;54:1692–1693.

265. Feibel JH, Campa JR. Thyrotoxic neuropathy (Basedow's paraplegia). J Neurol Neurosurg Psychiatry 1976;39:491–497.

266. Fisher M, Mateer JE, Ullrich I, Gutrecht JA. Pyramidal tract deficits and polyneuropathy in hyperthyroidism. Combination clinically mimicking ALS. Am J Med 1985;78:1041–1044.

267. Garcia CA, Fleming RH. Reversible corticospinal tract disease due to hyperthyroidism. Arch Neurol 1977;34:647–648.

268. Harman JB, Richardson AT. Generalized myokymia in thyrotoxicosis. Lancet 1954;2:473–474.

269. McMenanim J, Croxon M. Motor neurone disease and hyperthyroid Graves disease; a chance association? J Neurol Neurosurg Psychiatry 1980;43:46–49.

270. Melamed E, Berman M, Levy S. Posterolateral myelopathy associated with thyrotoxicosis [letter]. N Engl J Med 1975;295:778–779.

271. Ravera JJ, Cervina JM, Fernandez G, et al. Two cases of Graves disease with signs of a pyramidal lesion. Improvement in neurological signs during treatment with antithyroid drugs. J Clin Endocrinol Metab 1960;20:876–880.

272. Rosati G, Aiello I, Tola R, Granieri E. ALS associated with thyrotoxicosis. Arch Neurol 1980;37:530–531.

273. Rothberg MP, Shebert RT, Levey GS, Daroff RB. Propranolol and hyperthyroidism. Reversal of upper motor neuron signs. JAMA 1974;230(7):1017.

274. Johnson WG, Wigger HJ, Karp HR, et al. Juvenile spinal muscular atrophy: a new hexosaminidase deficiency phenotype. Ann Neurol 1982;11(1):11–16.

275. Navon R, Khosravi R, Melki J, et al. Juvenile-onset spinal muscular atrophy caused by compound heterozygosity for mutations in the HEXA gene. Ann Neurol 1997;41(5):631–638.

276. Willner JP, Grabowski GA, Gordon RE, et al. Chronic G_{M2} gangliosidosis masquerading as atypical Friedreich ataxia: clinical, morphologic, and biochemical studies of nine cases. Neurology 1981;31(7):787–798.

6
Cognitive Impairment in the Motor Neuron Disorders

Michael J. Strong, Catherine Lomen-Hoerth, and Wenchang Yang

The classic descriptions of amyotrophic lateral sclerosis (ALS) have focused largely on the degeneration of the motor neurons yielding a motor neuron–selective disorder.[1–3] The contemporary view, however, includes a more widespread neurodegenerative process in which the motor system degeneration is the core feature, but not the sole system affected.[4] Though historically there have been scattered reports of cognitive impairment occurring among individuals afflicted with ALS, leading Hudson[5] in 1981 to conclude that cognitively impaired patients with ALS formed a unique subset of patients with ALS, it has become increasingly evident that cognitive impairment may also form a key component of the degenerative process of ALS. There is, however, little consensus on the prevalence of cognitive dysfunction in ALS, with opinions ranging from rare[6–8] to much more common than traditionally thought.[5,9–11] Massman et al[12] observed a clinically significant cognitive impairment in 35.6 percent of individuals with ALS, whereas Lomen-Hoerth et al[13] observed that cognitive impairment manifested by deficits in frontal executive function occurred in more than 50 percent of a cohort of randomly selected patients with ALS.

SYNDROME OF FRONTOTEMPORAL DEMENTIA

In part, the discrepancy regarding the prevalence of cognitive impairment in ALS may reflect the fundamental nature of the neuropsychological deficits in ALS and the inability of classically used tools in dementia assessment (i.e., the Mini-Mental State Examination [MMSE]) to detect such deficits. To understand this, we must comprehend the nature of the frontotemporal dementias (FTDs). Though seemingly an intuitive observation, only in the past decade has the tremendous neuropathological breadth underlying the age-dependent dementias

145

become clear. Although Alzheimer's disease still accounts for the majority of dementia within the European and U.S. populations, increasingly non–Alzheimer-type dementias play a greater role.[14,15] These include vascular dementia (more common in China, Japan, and Russia), dementia with Lewy bodies, FTDs, and progressive nonfluent aphasia. Within the FTDs are a number of specific disease entities that include semantic dementia, dementia of the frontal type, dementia lacking distinct histopathology, progressive supranuclear palsy, and corticobasal degeneration. These latter illnesses share, as the basis of cognitive dysfunction, impairments in frontotemporal functioning in which the primary deficits arise from disturbances in attention and executive functioning with relatively intact memory.

The early detection of an FTD and then differentiation of FTD from Alzheimer's disease (AD) can be difficult. Among the FTDs, neuropsychiatric manifestations are more prominent and can include alterations in mood (e.g., euphoria, anxiety, suicidal ideation, apathy), behavior (e.g., inappropriate, disinhibition, agitation, hyperorality, eating disorders, perseveration, or hypersexuality), or psychotic features.[14] In a prospective analysis of 50 patients with FTD and 30 matched patients with AD, noncognitive deficits were more evident in the FTD group and included a loss of insight (90%), apathy and speech abnormalities (in more than two thirds), and overactivity (50%).[16] Of interest given the male predominance of ALS in the premenopausal years, almost all men studied in the FTD population suffered from a lack of insight, whereas this was preserved among women. Although both AD and FTD patients performed poorly on the Boston Naming Test and tests of verbal fluency (e.g., animals in 1 minute), no difference was observed between the two groups. Patients with AD performed more poorly on word list learning, delayed recall, and visuoconstruction. Subtle differences between the two groups in performance on the Boston Naming Test have been postulated to result because patients with AD possess greater difficulties with semantic affect, compared with patients with FTD who have greater impairments caused by general adynamia and impoverishment of motor responses. The MMSE was incapable of differentiating among early AD and FTD patients and indeed is unlikely to detect early cognitive changes characteristic of FTD. There is thus a need to use testing of attention and executive functioning as early markers of the disease process.

An example of such a testing paradigm and its utility in differentiating FTD from AD is the Addenbrooke cognitive examination (ACE).[17] The ACE incorporates aspects of the MMSE with additional emphasis on memory, language, and visuospatial components, as well as verbal fluency. In an analysis of 56 patients with AD and 24 patients with FTD using the ACE, Mathuranath et al[17] found that measures of *v*erbal fluency, *o*rientation, *l*anguage, and *m*emory (when used in a composite score, termed the VOLM ratio) could differentiate AD from FTD. Patients with AD performed more poorly on tests of orientation, attention, and memory, whereas patients with FTD performed more poorly on tests of letter fluency, language, and naming. These findings were mirrored in an analysis of autopsy-proven cases of FTD and AD, in which patients with FTD performed more poorly on word generation tasks and patients with AD performed more poorly on tests of visuospatial and constructional abilities.[18]

It is not particularly surprising therefore that the presence of cognitive impairment in ALS has been and continues to be largely overlooked if such an alteration in cognition is based on subtle deficits reflective of a frontotemporal degenerative process. Routine use of the MMSE is insensitive to this process, and the rather laborious application of detailed neuropsychological testing to the ALS population has been felt to be inappropriate in a population of patients in whom the mind has been considered to be free of the ravages of the disease process. As will become clear, however, the latter can no longer be held axiomatic, and ALS can be properly considered to be among the spectrum of diseases in which an FTD can exist and in which motor dysfunction is a cardinal clinical aspect (Table 6.1).

Accurate diagnosis of FTD may be significantly improved using a combination of neurobehavioral evaluation and neuroimaging.[19,20] The Neuropsychiatric Inventory (NPI) is a scale that measures the frequency and severity of ten dysfunctional areas, including aberrant motor behaviors, agitation, anxiety, apathy, delusions, depression, disinhibition, euphoria, hallucinations, and irritability. The NPI separates Alzheimer's disease from FTD and is administered to the caregiver, decreasing patient burden with testing. Patients with FTD have higher scores because they have more apathy, disinhibition, euphoria, and aberrant motor behavior.[21,22] These NPI scales alone accurately assigned 77 percent of patients with FTD and 77 percent of patients with AD to the correct diagnostic group. When combined with neuroimaging, these two dementias can be distinguished with greater certainty.

NATURE OF AMYOTROPHIC LATERAL SCLEROSIS WITH COGNITIVE IMPAIRMENT

Although cognitive impairment in ALS can antedate the appearance of motor neuron degeneration, more commonly it is reported as a subtle neurological presentation marked by deficits primarily in frontal and temporal functions.[23–26] The exception to this mode of presentation, in which alterations in cognition precede the motor system manifestations, has been termed "ALS plus dementia" (ALS + D).[27] These cases seem to differ somewhat from the more typical cases of ALS with cognitive impairment (ALSci) in which the impairments include alterations in mental flexibility, verbal and nonverbal fluency, abstract reasoning, and memory for both verbal and visual material.[11,12,28–33] Individuals with bulbar-onset disease appear to be at a greater risk of developing cognitive impairment manifested primarily as deficits in classic "frontal" functions such as mental flexibility, working memory, and word fluency, as well as in some aspects of memory and visual perception; however, these deficits may also be found in limb-onset patients but to a lesser degree.[13,33] Significant memory dysfunction[29,30,32,34] and impaired performance on verbal and nonverbal fluency tasks[11] have also been observed. In 1993 using an extensive neuropsychological test battery, Kew et al[28] found significantly poorer performance in their group of "nondemented" patients with ALS compared with age-matched controls on verbal fluency and picture recall tasks. In 1996 in a study investigating a large cohort of patients with ALS, Massman et al[12] found that the most common deficits included problem-solving, attention and mental control, continuous visual recognition memory, word fluency, and verbal recall. In addition,

Table 6.1   The spectrum of motor neuron disease and frontotemporal dementia

	ALS[a]	ALSci[b]	ALS[a] + D[c]	MNDID[d]	FTD[e]	Inherited variants of FTD		
						Chromosome 3 linked[f]	Chromosome 9 linked[g]	Chromosome 17 linked[h]
Clinical phenomenology								
Average age at onset	Age-dependent, peak in sixth and seventh decade	Age-dependent peak in sixth and seventh decade	61.5yr	61.8yr	57.8yr	57 yes	53.8yr	50yr
Neurogenic muscular atrophy	Yes	Yes	Yes	No	Rare	No	Yes	Rare
Pyramidal signs (hyperreflexia, Babinski signs, spasticity)	Yes	Yes	Rare	No	No	Late	Yes	No
Neuropsychiatric/behavioral signs at presentation	No	Rare	No	Yes	Yes	—	No	Yes
Cognitive deficit at initial presentation	No	Uncommon	—	Yes	50%	Yes	Yes	Yes
Progressive dementia	No	Yes	Yes	Yes	Yes	Yes	Yes	Yes
Urinary incontinence	No	No	No	No	No	Yes	No	No
Inherited variants	<10%	Uncommon	Uncommon	Uncommon	<50% First-degree relative affected	AD, high penetrance	AD	AD
Neuroimaging								
Cerebral atrophy	—	—	—	Global	Frontal	Yes	Frontal	—
Frontal lobar atrophy	—	—	Yes	Yes	Yes	—	Yes	—
Frontal predominant rCBF reduction	Variable	Yes	Yes	Yes	Yes	Global	Yes	—
Neuropathology								
Macroscopic frontal (lobar atrophy)	No	Yes	Yes	Yes	Yes	Global with frontal predominant	Yes	Yes

Motor system degeneration							
Betz cell loss	Yes	Yes	Yes	No	No	Unknown	—	No
Pyramidal tract degeneration	Yes	Yes	Uncommon	No	No	No	—	No
Loss of anterior horn cells	Yes	Yes	Yes	Yes	Yes	No	—	Rare (mutation specific)
Superficial linear spongiosis	Rare	Yes	Yes	Yes	Yes	Variable	Yes	Yes
Neuronal loss							
Frontotemporal cortex	No	Yes	Yes	Yes	Yes	Variable	—	Yes
Parahippocampal gyrus, amygdala	No	Yes	Yes	Yes	Yes	No	—	Yes
Substantia nigra	No	No	Yes	Rare	—	—	—	Yes
Astrocytosis							
Frontotemporal cortex	No	Yes	Yes	Yes	Yes	Variable	Yes	Yes
Parahippocampal gyrus, amygdalae	No	—	Yes	—	—	No	—	—
Substantia nigra	No	No	No	No	Uncommon	No	—	No
Spinal anterior horn	Yes	Yes	Yes	—	No	No	—	No
Ubiquitinated inclusions							
Hippocampal dentate granular cells	Rare	Yes	Yes	Yes	No	No	—	Yes
Frontotemporal cortex	No	Yes	Yes	Yes	Yes	No	—	No
Brain stem motor neurons	Yes	Yes	Yes	No	No	No	—	No

Table 6.1 (continued)

	ALS[a]	ALSci[b]	ALS[a] + D[c]	MNDID[d]	FTD[e]	Inherited variants of FTD		
						Chromosome 3 linked[f]	Chromosome 9 linked[g]	Chromosome 17 linked[h]
Spinal motor neurons	Yes	Yes	Yes	No	No	—	—	No
Inclusion								
Bunina bodies	Yes	Yes	Yes	No	No	—	—	No
Pick bodies	No	No	No	No	No	No	Rare	Rare (mutation specific)
Neurochemistry								
Neurofibrillary changes[i]								
Gallyas positive	No	Yes	Yes	No	No	No	—	—
Tau positive	No	Yes	Yes	No	No	Age related	Rare	—

AD = autosomal dominant; ALS = amyotrophic lateral sclerosis; ALSci = ALS with cognitive impairment; ALS + D = ALS with dementia; FTD = frontotemporal dementia; MNDID = motor neuron disease–inclusion dementia; rCBF = regional cerebral blood flow.
[a]Data taken from references 4, 45, 77.
[b]Data taken from references 72, 77, 132–135.
[c]Data taken from references 27, 36, 37, 39, 60, 119, 136, 137.
[d]Data taken from references 59, 138–140.
[e]Data taken from references 15, 16, 35, 141–144.
[f]Data taken from reference 145.
[g]Data taken from reference 146.
[h]Chromosome 17–linked FTD is a phenotypical and molecular group of disorders caused by mutations in the tau gene, with frontotemporal dementia and parkinsonism as the primary clinical features, but with certain mutations associated with motor neuron degeneration. Data taken from references 125, 147.
[i]Includes neurofibrillary tangle–like pathology and neuropil threads.

impairments in written verbal fluency, planning, problem solving, selective attention, and recognition memory for words have been described. Of the published studies reviewed, only one failed to find evidence of cognitive deficits.[8] However, tests sensitive to frontal lobe dysfunction were not administered in this latter study. Until recently, there was also lack of consensus as to what criteria defined the different subtypes of FTD, making it difficult to categorize patients.[31]

Despite these reported links between cognitive dysfunction and ALS, the prevalence of FTD and associated cognitive changes in ALS has not been determined. A recent study evaluated 36 patients with FTD with no known diagnosis of ALS with clinical and electrophysiological measures. Of the 36 patients studied, 5 met criteria for a definite diagnosis of ALS and an additional 13 patients met criteria for possible ALS. One of the patients with possible ALS developed definite ALS over the next year. This result suggested that ALS may be more common in FTD than had previously been reported.[35] A subsequent study administered word generation tests to 100 consecutive patients with ALS in an ALS multidisciplinary clinic. Any patient with a prior dementia diagnosis was excluded from the study. A subset of 44 patients agreed to undergo further neuropsychological testing and clinical interview to confirm or deny a diagnosis of dementia. Diminished word generation was found in one third. Of the patients with abnormal word generation who agreed to further evaluation, nearly all were shown to meet research criteria for FTD. In addition, one quarter of the patients with normal word generation who agreed to further evaluation met research criteria for FTD; these patients had new-onset personality changes. This study suggests that frontal executive deficits are present in half of patients with ALS, many of whom meet strict research criteria for FTD.[13]

As mentioned earlier and in seeming distinction to ALSci, there have been a number of reports among the Japanese ALS population of dementia followed by the manifestations of the motor system degeneration (see Table 6.1). This process, ALS + D or the "Mitsuyama variant of ALS," tends to affect a younger population (mean ages of men and women are 52.4 and 54.1 years, respectively) with a relatively short disease duration (mean, 2.5 years).[27] In the majority, the first manifestation is a progressive impairment of memory (observed in 100%), with mild to slight personality changes (85%) and emotional dysfunction (euphoria, indifference, and lability in 85%). Neurogenic muscle atrophy and motor symptoms become evident within a year with bulbar symptoms predominating. Only rarely were signs of pyramidal tract dysfunction observed, either clinically or neuropathologically in these initial reports. Subsequent reports were consistent with these observations,[36] although a recent analysis of eight cases with clinicopathological confirmation of ALS + D found clinical signs of pyramidal dysfunction and neuropathological evidence of corticospinal tract degeneration with loss of Betz cells.[37] Hence, it is not yet clear that ALSci and ALS + D can be justifiably considered as distinct entities.

Perhaps not surprisingly given the nature of language deficits that can be observed in the FTDs, the language characteristics of the ALS-dementia complex include word finding difficulty, lexical disorganization as manifested by problems on tests of word fluency, and reliance of stereotypic sentences.[9–11,34] Anterior-based language functions (e.g., fluency, syntax, and grammar) are more compromised than those associated with temporal-parietal lobe regions (e.g., auditory and reading comprehension, naming).[7,38,39] Such language deficits are differentiated from the speech characteristics of individuals with ALS that are directly attributable to the neuromuscular and physical difficulties of the disease processes. The mixed dysarthria (e.g., spastic, flaccid) demonstrated by patients with ALS is typically characterized by imprecise consonant production, hypernasality, harsh voice quality, and slow speaking rate.[40] In contrast, the language disorder presents either as a fluent aphasia with significant loss of word meaning, characteristic of semantic dementia, or as a nonfluent aphasia, characteristic of primary progressive aphasia.[31]

Neuroimaging in Amyotrophic Lateral Sclerosis with Cognitive Impairment

The recognition of cognitive dysfunction in ALS can be aided by the use of both static and dynamic neuroimaging. Computed tomographic (CT) scanning is of some value in visualizing frontal and temporal lobe cortical atrophy and may demonstrate involvement of the precentral and the postcentral gyrus, the anterior cingulate gyrus, the corpus callosum, and the brain stem tegmentum. With magnetic resonance imaging (MRI), an increase in the T2-weighted signal in the precentral and adjacent gyri, the frontal and temporal white matter, the pyramidal tracts, the globus pallidus, and the thalamus can be observed.[41] However, static imaging alone can be insensitive to the earliest manifestations of frontotemporal dysfunction in ALS.[8] For example, in 1989, Gallassi et al[9] observed cognitive impairments consisting of impaired associative functions (e.g., word fluency, phrase construction, temporal rule induction, and analogies) in 22 of 35 patients with ALS in the absence of overt dementia but found no evidence of CT changes.

New methods for assessing atrophy have been recently developed both with and without the use of standard templates for comparing patients. Voxel-based morphometry studies have been used to identify regions associated with pathology in various neurodisorders but have not been previously applied to patients with ALS. This method uses spatial transformation of all subjects' volumetric MRI brain scans to the Montreal Neurological Institute (MNI) 152 standard template and then represents each voxel with a value reflecting the local tissue volume. Statistical comparisons between groups are then performed on a voxel-by-voxel basis, and those voxels that are significantly different between the groups are noted. A recent comparison between patients with FTD and patients with AD and normal controls was useful in identification of regions specific to neurodegeneration.[42] In a recent study of 23 patients with ALS, Lomen-Hoerth assessed lobar atrophy by comparing volumes on MRI with normal age- and sex-matched controls (unpublished data). Thirteen had abnormal frontal and/or temporal atrophy, which correlated well with their poor performance on neuropsychological testing ($p < 0.05$) (Figure 6.1).

Functional neuroimaging techniques have proven to be a very sensitive marker of frontotemporal dysfunction in ALSci, including [123]I-*N*-isopropyl-*p*-iodoamphetamine[38,43] and [^{99m}Tc]-D,L-hexamethylpropyleneamine oxime (HMPAO)[44,45] in single photon emission computed tomography (SPECT) studies. Either isotope will demonstrate reduced frontal and temporal cortical

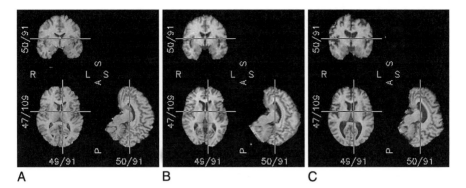

Figure 6.1 Coronal, axial, and sagittal views of T1-weighted extracted brain images that have been transformed into the normal space (Montreal Neurological Institute standard) using FSL subroutines. The subjects are **(A)** a 61-year-old normal, **(B)** a 57-year-old cognitively intact patient with amyotrophic lateral sclerosis (ALS), and **(C)** a 54-year-old cognitively impaired patient with ALS. Note the appearance of marked frontal atrophy in the cognitively impaired patient with ALS.

blood flow in ALSci. Similarly, positron emission tomography (PET) may be used to document frontotemporal hypometabolism and is a sensitive, though less readily available, marker.[46] Assays of regional cerebral blood flow (rCBF), though more readily available, have not been studied yet prospectively in ALSci. Their potential utility has however been highlighted in several studies.[28,47] The latter observations have been extended to include functional neuroimaging using PET in which reduced metabolism in the right dorsolateral prefrontal cortex (areas 46 and 9) and the left middle and superior temporal gyrus (areas 39 and 22) ($p < 0.001$) during a verbal fluency/word generation task with a PET activation program was observed only in ALSci.[48,49] In a prospective study of cognitive impairment in ALS using proton magnetic resonance spectroscopy (^{1}H-MRS) of the left anterior cingulate gyrus, a significant reduction was observed in the NAA/Cr ratio (consistent with neuronal loss) at the earliest time interval studied in those patients developing cognitive impairment.[33]

Neuropathology of Amyotrophic Lateral Sclerosis with Cognitive Impairment

As reviewed by Ince et al in Chapter 2, the diagnosis of ALS is established by the finding of degeneration of selective populations of motor neurons, including the descending supraspinal motor pathways and their neurons of origin, and of brain stem and spinal motor neurons.[1-3] These findings remain at the core of the disease and are accompanied by a wealth of intracellular inclusions in degenerating motor neurons in ALS involving both the cell body and neuritic processes.[50-52] These include intraneuronal aggregates immunoreactive to antibodies recognizing key cytoskeletal intermediate filament proteins such as phosphorylated neurofilament (NF), peripherin, and α-internexin.[53–55] Unique to ALS is the presence of Bunina bodies, eosinophilic intracellular aggregates of dense granular proteinaceous material that are immunoreactive for the lysosomal cysteine proteinase inhibitor cystatin C, but not NF, tau protein, or ubiquitin.[56] Distinct from these inclusions, ubiquitin immunoreactivity may be observed either as discrete skeins or homogenous aggregates of material or co-localizing to neurofilamentous aggregates.[57,58] The latter observation is important because the presence of ubiquitin-immunoreactive structures within spinal motor neurons, in the presence of the pathological features of an FTD but in the absence of overt clinical features of motor neuron disease (MND), has led to the concept of a unique FTD termed "MND-inclusion dementia" (MNDID)[59] (see Table 6.1). Whether this forms a crossover disease between true FTD and ALSci remains to be determined.

These features remain at the core of the neuropathology of ALSci. In addition, the most consistent feature of ALSci is the presence of spongiform degeneration in frontal and precentral gyrus cortical layers 2 and 3[23,27,60–67] (Figure 6.2). Given the clinical characterization of ALSci as an FTD, this is not unexpected given the prominence of superficial linear spongiosis among the FTD population.[65,66,68–70] Neuronal density is reduced in the anterior cingulate gyrus.[71] Superficial linear spongiosis is also evident in cognitively intact patients with ALS, though considerably less extensive than observed in ALSci.[72] In concert with previous studies, this suggests that ALS and ALSci may form a disease continuum.[73–77]

Although ubiquitin immunoreactive intraneuronal inclusions are often observed within the dentate granule cells, the superficial frontal and temporal

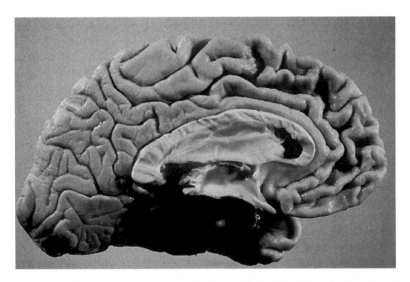

Figure 6.2 Cortical atrophy in amyotrophic lateral sclerosis with cognitive impairment (ALSci). Consistent with the findings from neuroimaging, marked frontal atrophy is evident in ALSci with prominent involvement of the precentral and cingulate gyrus. (Reprinted with permission from Strong MJ. The evidence for ALS as a multisystems disorder of limited phenotypic expression. Can J Neurol Sci 2001;28:283–298.)

cortical layers, and in the entorhinal cortex, these are not specific to ALSci and are observed in other forms of neurodegeneration.[70,77–82] By immunoelectron microscopy, these ubiquitin immunoreactive inclusions are composed of loosely arranged 10- to 15-nm linear filaments, the exact identity of which remains uncertain.[79,83] Although these ubiquitin immunoreactive inclusions are observed in other degenerative processes, those observed in ALSci are unique in lacking immunoreactivity to either microtubule-associated protein tau or α-synuclein.[27,70,79,80,83–87] This is not to say that tau immunoreactive structures are absent in ALS or ALSci. In 1999, Noda et al[60] first described three cases of late adult-onset ALS in which tau immunoreactive threadlike structures were observed in the neuropil and in glial cells (as coiled bodies) in the hippocampus, parahippocampal gyrus, and amygdala. In one case, neurofibrillary tangles (NFTs) were observed, rendering differentiation from early AD difficult. In the remaining two cases, the neuropil and glial tau immunoreactive structures occurred in the absence of pathology typical of AD.

In 2002, Yang and Strong[72] reported that in both ALSci and ALS patients the presence of neuronal, extraneuronal, and glial tau aggregates are readily observed using either Gallyas silver staining[88] or immunostaining with monoclonal antibodies directed against tau (tau-1 following dephosphorylation or AT8) (Figure 6.3). In this latter study, the immunostaining of tau-1 neuronal–positive inclusions was not restricted to ALSci but was also observed in cognitively intact patients with ALS. However, in ALSci, tau immunostaining was more intense and more likely to replace the cytoplasm. It was also considerably more frequent than observed in ALS in the absence of cognitive impairment, with dense tau-1 distribution in layer 2 and layer 3 being characteristic of ALSci. This latter finding was reminiscent of the distribution of NFTs in Guamanian ALS/parkinsonism-dementia.[89] Astrocytic tau immunoreactive inclusions were also observed in cortical layer 1, deep cortical layers, and subcortical white matter in ALS and ALSci patients, but not in control cases. Astrocytic proliferation in these layers was consistent with that observed by others in ALSci.[90–92] In addition to these neuronal and glial intracellular aggregates, extraneuronal tau aggregates were also evident and appeared uniquely in ALSci. These were most evident using Gallyas staining and assumed a number of morphologies, including curvilinear neuropil threads, rare argyrophilic granules, and dense rounded aggregates with irregular fibrillary margins that were easily distinguished from corpora amylacea by their indistinct margins and inhomogenous core.

These observations raise the intriguing possibility that ALSci has, as the basis of the pathogenic process, a fundamental abnormality in tau protein metabolism. In this sense, there may be a greater homology between ALSci, ALS (if ALSci is in fact one end of a spectrum of ALS pathology), and the neurodegenerative tauopathies than anticipated.

COGNITIVE DYSFUNCTION IN OTHER DEGENERATIVE MOTOR NEURON DISEASES

The preceding discussion has focused largely on the occurrence of cognitive dysfunction or dementia among a population of patients with classic ALS in

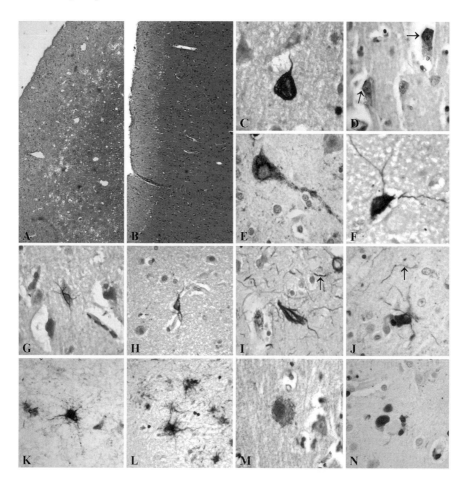

which both upper and lower motor neuron signs are evident, both clinically and neuropathologically. However, a number of neurodegenerative diseases exist in which motor neuron dysfunction is prominent. The intriguing question remains about whether these processes are unique disease entities or participants in a spectrum of motor neuron system neurodegenerations with a single underlying pathogenesis.

A variant of ALS known as the ALS/parkinsonism-dementia complex of Guam remains the only known hyperendemic variant of ALS and the best example to date of ALS among a population in which both genetic and environmental factors can be incriminated etiologically.[93–96] Although a tendency toward familial clustering had been observed, no single genetic defects have been associated with this population (including alterations in the copper/zinc superoxide dismutase gene (SOD1; the most common gene defect among autosomal dominantly inherited ALS), the high-molecular-weight neurofilament protein (NFH)[97] or to the microtubule-associated protein tau.[98] In this variant, affecting three geographically and genetically unique populations in the

Figure 6.3 Neuropathology of amyotrophic lateral sclerosis with cognitive impairment (ALSci). The features of pathology in ALSci are present in superficial linear spongiosis, tau neuronal, and glial aggregates and extraneuronal inclusions. As observed in a number of the frontotemporal dementias, (**A**) vacuolar changes within the second and third cortical layers (superficial linear spongiosis) is characteristic of patients with ALSci. A similar vacuolization can be observed in cognitively-intact patients with ALS (**B**), though less often and to a lesser extent. A variety of tau-immunoreactive neuronal, glial, and extraneuronal aggregates are also characteristic of ALSci. Neuronal aggregates are the core feature of ALSci; however, the morphology and immunoreactivity characteristics vary among the varying cortical layers. Gallyas positive filamentous neuronal aggregates are more typically dense, filamentous structures filling the cytoplasm in neurons of the fourth through sixth cortical layers (**C**), whereas fine, filamentous cellular threads are more typical of the neurons in the immediate subcortical white matter (**G**). Following dephosphorylation (*Escherichia coli* alkaline phosphatase), (**D**) dense and tufted tau-1 immunoreactive neuronal aggregates are readily observed in layers two through six *(arrows)*. Neurons with immunoreactivity to the monoclonal antibody AT8 (recognizing a tau epitope observed in Alzheimer's disease) were observed in layer two through subcortical white matter (**E, H**). Rarely, and only in ALSci, tau aggregates immunoreactive to a monoclonal antibody recognizing C-terminus tau hyperphosphorylation (Ser^{396}) were observed (**F**). Neuritic threads were often observed in the frontal cortex of both ALS and ALSci (Gallyas and AT8 staining, *arrow,* **I** and **J**, respectively). Tau immunoreactive astrocytic aggregates were also characteristic of ALSci (Gallyas and AT8 immunoreactive staining, **K** and **L**, respectively). These were most commonly observed in layers one and six and less often observed in the subcortical white matter. Extraneuronal tau-immunoreactive aggregates are another features of ALSci. Most commonly, these are dense, tau-1 immunoreactive aggregates with poorly defined margins (distinct from corpora amylacea) (**M**) or discrete tau immunoreactive globules (**N**). See color insert. (**A, B**, ×10; all other photomicrographs, ×40 before reproduction.)

Western Pacific including the Chamorros of the Mariana Islands, the Auyu and Jakai of West New Guinea, and residents of the Kii peninsula of southern Japan, the clinical manifestations of ALS are indistinguishable from those observed in the sporadic variant of ALS. Although parkinsonism/dementia can also exist as a separate entity, both ALS and parkinsonism/dementia can coexist in the same individual, leading to the diagnosis of the ALS/parkinsonism-dementia complex.[99–101] Close to 50 percent of the siblings of these patients developed parkinsonism and dementia, 25 percent developed ALS, and 5 percent of siblings had parkinsonism, dementia, and ALS.[102]

An intriguing aspect of the Western Pacific variant of ALS is the co-occurrence of the neurofilamentous pathology of ALS, with NFTs morphologically identical to those observed in Alzheimer's disease.[103–107] Severe cortical atrophy and widespread NFT formation are hallmarks of this disorder, with the NFTs bearing the immunohistochemical and ultrastructural characteristics of Alzheimer's disease NFTs.[103,104,108–110] In contrast to Alzheimer's disease, and as is discussed later in this chapter, the hyperphosphorylated, highly insoluble tau triplet protein (the fundamental constituent of the NFT) is more widely distributed in both cortical and subcortical structures in the Western Pacific variant of ALS.[111] Lewy-like bodies, containing accumulations of α-synuclein and typical of those observed in Parkinson's disease, are also observed predominantly with neurons of the amygdala.[112,113]

Familial ALS, parkinsonism, and dementia also occurs outside of the Western Pacific variant of ALS and is typified in "Family Mo".[114] In this family, personality and behavioral changes were the first symptoms in 12 of 13 affected patients. Onset was around age 45 on average and mean duration to death was 13 years. There was early memory loss, anomia, and poor construction with later involvement of orientation, speech, and calculations. All affected members had rigidity, bradykinesia, and postural instability. On neuropathologic examination, there was atrophy and spongiform change in the frontotemporal cortex, and neuronal loss and gliosis in the substantia nigra and amygdala. Two individuals had anterior horn cell loss and one subject had fasciculations and muscle wasting. There were no Lewy bodies, NFTs, or amyloid plaques. The genetic locus was linked to chromosome 17q21-q22 and a mutation was found in the intron adjacent to exon 10 (E10) in the tau gene.

More than 13 kindreds of families with FTD and linkage to chromosome 17 have been described.[115] Corticospinal disturbances, muscle wasting, and fasciculations were found in 4 or these 13 families, and there were occasional patients with dysphagia and dysarthria. Mutations in the tau gene, location on chromosome 17, were found in many of these families, particularly those with extrapyramidal disturbances; however, few FTD-ALS cases are caused by known tau mutations.[116–118] Subsequently 25 different mutations have been identified in the tau gene that are presumed to cause FTD symptoms. Although findings of ALS have been reported in only a few of the familial FTD cases, individuals with neuromuscular expertise have examined few of the patients.

In 1996, Jackson, Lennox, and Lowe[59] highlighted the existence of a disorder termed *MNDID* in an initial cohort of nine patients identified from a larger pool of patients with FTD and in whom no clinical evidence of either upper or lower motor neuron dysfunction was evident. Neuropathologically, there was microvacuolization in cortical layer 2 of the frontotemporal lobes, subcortical gliosis, and ubiquitin immunoreactive inclusion in the hippocampal dentate granule cells and remaining neurons of layer 2 of the frontotemporal cortex. Although this initial report did not have spinal cord tissue available, brain stem motor nuclei were normal. Subsequent reports have highlighted the loss of anterior horn cells in the absence of pyramidal tract degeneration or ubiquitinated motor neuronal inclusions.[119]

The appearance of progressive spasticity alone, in the absence of either clinical or laboratory evidence of lower motor neuron dysfunction, is a rare variant of MND termed primary lateral sclerosis (PLS).[120,121] In an analysis of nine patients with PLS, Caselli, Smith, and Osborne[122] observed mild cognitive dysfunction consistent with frontal lobe dysfunction in eight patients. Six patients underwent HMPAO-SPECT studies of rCBF with evidence of bilateral posterior hypoperfusion.

RELATIONSHIP BETWEEN AMYOTROPHIC LATERAL SCLEROSIS WITH COGNITIVE IMPAIRMENT AND FRONTOTEMPORAL DEMENTIA

As discussed earlier, among the FTDs are a clinically heterogeneous group of diseases manifesting as dementia with parkinsonism due to mutations in chromosome 17 at the tau gene.[123] Some are associated with motor dysfunction. It is likely that these latter cases are similar to a case described by Gilbert et al[124] in 1988 termed the "dementia-parkinsonism-motor neuron disease" syndrome complex. At the core of the chromosome 17–linked FTD with parkinsonism (FTDP-17) syndrome are behavioral changes, psychosis, loss of executive functioning, and for the majority of variants, a lack of motor phenomenon with the exception of a progressive loss of speech output. The neuropathological features consist of prominent frontotemporal atrophy, with or without degeneration of the basal ganglia, substantia nigra, or amygdala. Superficial linear spongiosis is evident in frontotemporal cortical layer 2. Tau immunoreactive neuropil threads are prominent, as are glial tangles and dense intracellular deposits of tau.

The primary function of tau proteins is to bind to microtubules and to both promote their assembly and enhance their stability in a polymerized state. Hyperphosphorylated tau, as observed in a number of the tauopathies, is a highly insoluble protein that will polymerize in the somatodendritic neuronal compartment and form NFTs. Six alternatively spliced tau isoforms exist in the adult human nervous system, containing either three (3R) or four (4R) microtubule binding domains, with the additional microtubule binding domain encoded by E10 (Figure 6.4). Mutations in the tau gene appear to cause tau protein accumulations by at least two broad mechanisms.[125] In one group, intronic mutations adjacent to the 3′ end of the E10 can lead to an increased expression of the E10-encoded domain, producing a predominance of the 4R tau isoform and thus a greater predominance of the four microtubule binding domain tau isoforms (for an excellent detailed review of the tau protein chemistry, see Lee et al[123]). An example of such a mutation is the N279K mutation, which strengthens the expression of an exon-splicing enhancer, leading to increased E10 expression. In contrast, the Δ280K mutation results in a loss of the exon-splicing enhancer and a loss of E10 expression, leading to a predominance of the 3R tau isoform (with less avid microtubule binding). Within E10 is another regulatory element, the "exon-splicing silencer," which is abolished with the L284L mutation and thus leads to increased E10 expression. Intronic mutations immediately 5′ adjacent to E10 also appear to result in increased E10 expression. In the second group of tau mutations, the mutations are associated with abnormalities of tau protein function leading to a reduction in tau affinity and binding to microtubules (e.g., G272V, V337M, and R406W mutations).

CONCLUSION

Although the original clinicopathological descriptions of ALS focused on a disorder in which the neuropathological process was restricted to degeneration of both the upper and the lower motor neuron, our understanding of the neuropathological basis of ALS has rapidly extended beyond this.[126–128] Shortly after these descriptions, reports (though rare) began to appear within the literature describing the occurrence of "mental" symptoms among the ALS population; symptoms that we now consider to be reflective of the behavioral deficits of frontotemporal dysfunction.[5,129–131] The involvement of nonmotor neuronal systems can no longer be questioned, and indeed cognitive dysfunction should

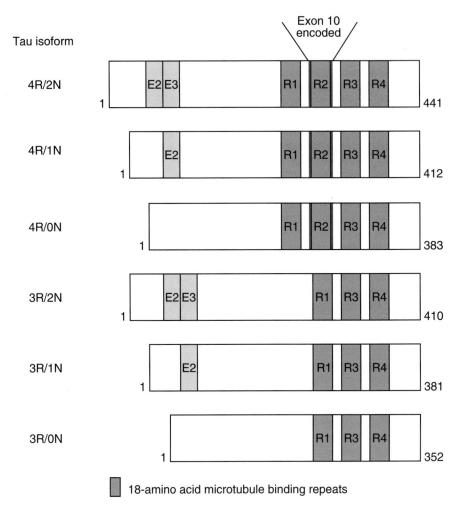

Figure 6.4 Tau isoforms. Six human tau isoforms are generated by alternative splicing of the tau gene, which includes 16 exons. Alternative splicing of the E2, E3 and E10 exons produce the six isoforms, with E10 encoding an 18–amino acid microtubule binding repeat. The isoforms range from 352 to 441 amino acids in length.

justifiably be considered an integral component of the disease process of ALS. However, questions remain about the exact prevalence of cognitive dysfunction in ALS and the extent to which such deficits progress to a florid dementia. Moreover, the relationship among the various subgroups of motor neuron degenerative diseases in association with dementia (ALSci, ALS + D, the Western Pacific variant of ALS, and MNDID) needs clarification but likely awaits a greater molecular understanding. Ultimately, the key question remains about the relationship between alterations in tau protein metabolism and the appearance of tau immunoreactive neuronal, glial, and neuropil pathology in ALS and whether ALSci represents yet another manifestation of the neurodegenerative tauopathies.

REFERENCES

1. Lawyer T, Netsky MG. Amyotrophic lateral sclerosis. Arch Neurol 1963;8:117–127.
2. Brownell B, Oppenheimer DR, Hughes JT. The central nervous system in motor neurone disease. J Neurol Neurosurg Psychiatry 1970;33:338–357.
3. Hirano A. Cytopathology of Amyotrophic Lateral Sclerosis. In LP Rowland (ed), Amyotrophic Lateral Sclerosis and Other Motor Neuron Disorders. New York: Raven Press, 1991;91–101.
4. Strong MJ. The evidence for ALS as a multisystems disorder of limited phenotypic expression. Can J Neurol Sci 2001;28:283–298.
5. Hudson A. Amyotrophic lateral sclerosis and its association with dementia, parkinsonism and other neurological disorders: a review. Brain 1981;194:217–247.
6. Lishman WA. Organic Psychiatry (2nd ed). Oxford: Blackwell Scientific Publications, 1987.
7. Montgomery GK, Erickson LM. Neuropsychological perspectives in amyotrophic lateral sclerosis. Neurol Clin 1987;5:61–81.
8. Poloni M, Capitani E, Mazzini L, Ceroni M. Neuropsychological measures in amyotrophic lateral sclerosis and their relationship with CT scan–assessed cerebral atrophy. Acta Neurol Scand 1986;74:257–260.
9. Gallassi R, Montagna P, Morreale A, et al. Neuropsychological, electroencephalogram and brain computed tomography findings in motor neuron disease. Eur Neurol 1989;29:115–120.
10. Gallassi R, Montagna P, Ciardulli C, et al. Cognitive impairment in motor neuron disease. Acta Neurol Scand 1985;71:480–484.
11. Ludolph AC, Langen KJ, Regard M, et al. Frontal lobe function in amyotrophic lateral sclerosis: a neuropsychological and positron emission tomography study. Acta Neurol Scand 1992;85:81–89.
12. Massman PJ, Sims J, Cooke N, et al. Prevalence and correlates of neuropsychological deficits in amyotrophic lateral sclerosis. J Neurol Neurosurg Psychiatry 1996;61:450–455.
13. Lomen-Hoerth C, Murphy J, Langmore S, et al. Are amyotrophic lateral sclerosis patients cognitively normal? Neurology 2003 (in press).
14. Ritchie K, Lovestone S. The dementias. Lancet 2002;360:1759–1766.
15. Bozeat S, Gregory CA, Ralph MAL, Hodges JR. Which neuropsychiatric and behavioral features distinguish frontal and temporal variants of frontotemporal dementia from Alzheimer's disease? J Neurol Neurosurg Psychiatry 2000;69:178–186.
16. Diehl J, Kurz A. Frontotemporal dementia: patient characteristics, cognition, and behavior. Int J Geriatr Psychiatry 2002;17:914–918.
17. Mathuranath PS, Nestor PJ, Berrios GE, et al. A brief cognitive test battery to differentiate Alzheimer's disease and frontotemporal dementia. Neurology 2000;55:1613–1620.
18. Rascovsky K, Salmon DP, Ho GJ, et al. Cognitive profiles differ in autopsy-confirmed frontotemporal dementia and AD. Neurology 2002;58:1801–1808.
19. Miller BL, Ikonte C, Ponton M A, et al. A study of the Lund-Manchester research criteria for frontotemporal dementia: clinical and single-photon emission CT correlations. Neurology 1997;48:937–942.
20. Read SL, Miller BL, Mena I, et al. SPECT in dementia: clinical and pathological correlation. J Am Geriatr Soc 1995;43:1243–1247.
21. Levy ML, Miller BL, Cummings JL, et al. Alzheimer disease and frontotemporal dementias. Arch Neurol 1996;53:687–690.
22. Cummings JL, Mega M, Gray K, et al. The neuropsychiatric inventory: comprehensive assessment of psychopathology in dementia. Neurology 1994;44:2308–2314.
23. Caselli RJ, Windebank AJ, Petersen RC, et al. Rapidly progressing aphasic dementia and motor neuron disease. Ann Neurol 1993;33:200–207.
24. Devinsky O, Morrell MJ, Vogt BA. Contributions of anterior cingulate cortex to behavior. Brain 1995;118:279–306.
25. Strong MJ, Grace GM, Orange JB, Leeper HA. Cognition, language and speech in amyotrophic lateral sclerosis: a review. J Clin Exp Neuropsychol 1996;18:291–303.

26. Vercelletto M, Ronin M, Huvet M, et al. Frontal type dementia preceding amyotrophic lateral sclerosis: a neuropsychological and SPECT study of five clinical cases. Eur J Neurol 1999;6:295–299.
27. Mitsuyama Y. Presenile dementia with motor neuron disease in Japan: clinico-pathological review of 26 cases. J Neurol Neurosurg Psychiatry 1984;47:953–959.
28. Kew JJM, Goldstein LH, Leigh PN, et al. The relationship between abnormalities of cognitive function and cerebral activation in amyotrophic lateral sclerosis. Brain 1993;116:1399–1423.
29. David AS, Gillham RA. Neuropsychological study of motor neuron disease. Psychosomatics 1986;27:441–445.
30. Iwasaki Y, Kinoshita M, Ikeda K, et al. Neuropsychological dysfunctions in amyotrophic lateral sclerosis: relation to motor disabilities. Int J Neurosci 1990;54:191–195.
31. Neary D, Snowden JS, Gustafson L, et al. Frontotemporal lobar degeneration. A consensus on clinical diagnostic criteria. Neurology 1998;51:1546–1554.
32. Peterson RC, Ivnik RJ, Litchy WJ, et al. Cognitive function in amyotrophic lateral sclerosis. Neurology 1990;40:315.
33. Strong MJ, Grace GM, Orange JB, et al. A prospective study of cognitive impairment in ALS. Neurology 1999;53:1665–1670.
34. Iwasaki Y, Kinoshita M, Ikeda K, et al. Cognitive impairment in amyotrophic lateral sclerosis and its relation to motor disabilities. Acta Neurol Scand 1990;81:141–143.
35. Lomen-Hoerth C, Anderson T, Miller B. The overlap of amyotrophic lateral sclerosis and frontotemporal dementia. Neurology 2002;59:1077–1079.
36. Morita K, Kaiya H, Ikeda T, Namba M. Presenile dementia combined with amyotrophy: a review of 34 Japanese cases. Arch Gerontol Geriatr 1987;6:263–277.
37. Tsuchiya K. Constant involvement of the Betz cells and pyramidal tract in amyotrophic lateral sclerosis with dementia: a clinicopathological study of eight autopsy cases. Acta Neuropathol 2002;104:249–259.
38. Ludolph AC, Elger CE, Böttger IW, et al. *N*-Isopropyl-*p*-^{123}I-amphetamine single photon emission computer tomography in motor neuron disease. Eur Neurol 1989;29:255–260.
39. Neary D, Snowden JS, Mann DMA, et al. Frontal lobe dementia and motor neuron disease. J Neurol Neurosurg Psychiatry 1990;53:23–32.
40. Darley FL, Aronson AE, Brown JR. Differential diagnostic patterns of dysarthria. J Speech Hear Res 1969;12:246–269.
41. Kato S, Hayashi H, Yagishita A. Involvement of the frontotemporal lobe and limbic system in amyotrophic lateral sclerosis: as assessed by serial computed tomography and magnetic resonance imaging. J Neurol Sci 1993;116:52–58.
42. Rosen HJ, Gorno-Tempini ML, Goldman WP, et al. Patterns of brain atrophy in frontotemporal dementia and semantic dementia. Neurology 2002;58:198–208.
43. Ohnishi T, Hoshi H, Nagamachi S, et al. Regional cerebral blood flow study with ^{123}I-IMP in patients with degenerative dementia. Am J Neuroradiol 1991;12:513–520.
44. Waldemar G, Varstrup S, Jensen TS, et al. Focal reductions in cerebral blood flow in amyotrophic lateral sclerosis: A [99mTc]-D,L-HMPAO SPECT study. J Neurol Sci 1992;107:19–28.
45. Talbot PR, Goulding PJ, Lloyd JJ, et al. Inter-relation between "classic" motor neuron disease and frontotemporal dementia: neuropsychological and single photon emission computed tomography study. J Neurol Neurosurg Psychiatry 1995;58:541–547.
46. Dalakas MC, Hatazawa J, Brooks RA, Di Chiro G. Lowered cerebral glucose utilization in amyotrophic lateral sclerosis. Ann Neurol 1987;22:580–586.
47. Tanaka M, Kondo S, Hirai S, et al. Cerebral blood flow and oxygen metabolism in progressive dementia associated with amyotrophic laterals sclerosis. J Neurol Sci 1993;120:22–28.
48. Abrahams S, Leigh PN, Kew JJM, et al. A positron emission tomography study of frontal lobe function (verbal fluency) in amyotrophic lateral sclerosis. J Neurol Sci 1995;129:44–46.
49. Abrahams S, Goldstein LH, Lloyd CM, et al. Cognitive deficits in non-demented amyotrophic lateral sclerosis patients: a neuropsychological investigation. J Neurol Sci 1995;129:54–55.
50. Carpenter S. Proximal axonal enlargement in motor neuron disease. Neurology 1968;18:841–851.
51. Delisle MB, Carpenter S. Neurofibrillary axonal swellings and amyotrophic lateral sclerosis. J Neurol Sci 1984;63:241–250.
52. Averback P. Unusual particles in motor neuron disease. Arch Pathol Lab Med 1981;105:490–493.
53. Migheli A, Pezzulo T, Attanasio A, Schiffer D. Peripherin immunoreactive structures in amyotrophic lateral sclerosis. Lab Invest 1993;68:185–191.
54. Wong N, He BP, Strong MJ. Characterization of neuronal intermediate filament protein expression in cervical spinal motor neurons in sporadic amyotrophic lateral sclerosis (ALS). J Neuropathol Exp Neurol 2000;59:972–982.

55. Strong MJ. Neurofilament metabolism in sporadic amyotrophic lateral sclerosis. J Neurol Sci 1999;169:170–177.
56. Wada M, Uchihara T, Nakamura A, Oyanagi K. Bunina bodies in amyotrophic lateral sclerosis on Guam: a histochemical, immunohistochemical and ultrastructural investigation. Acta Neuropathol 1999;98:150–156.
57. Murayama S, Mori H, Ihara Y, et al. Immunocytochemical and ultrastructural studies of lower motor neurons in amyotrophic lateral sclerosis. Ann Neurol 1990;27:137–148.
58. Leigh PN, Dodson A, Swash M, et al. Cytoskeletal abnormalities in motor neuron disease. An immunohistochemical study. Brain 1989;112:521–535.
59. Jackson M, Lennox G, Lowe J. Motor neuron disease-inclusion dementia. Neurodegeneration 1996;5:339–350.
60. Noda K, Katayama S, Watanabe C, et al. Gallyas- and tau-positive glial structures in motor neuron disease with dementia. Clin Neuropathol 1999;18:218–225.
61. Morris HR, Khan MN, Janssen JC, et al. The genetic and pathological classification of familial frontotemporal dementia. Arch Neurol 2001;58:1813–1816.
62. Ferrer I, Roig C, Espino A, et al. Dementia of frontal lobe type and motor neuron disease. A Golgi study of the frontal cortex. J Neurol Neurosurg Psychiatry 1991;54:932–934.
63. Kato S, Oda M, Hayashi H, et al. Participation of the limbic system and its associated areas in the dementia of amyotrophic lateral sclerosis. J Neurol Sci 1994;126:62–69.
64. Kawashima T, Kikuchi H, Takita M, et al. Skein-like inclusions in the neostriatum from a case of amyotrophic lateral sclerosis with dementia. Acta Neuropathol 1998;96:541–545.
65. Munoz DG. The Pathology of Pick Complex. In A Kertesz, DG Munoz (eds), Pick's Disease and Pick Complex. New York: John Wiley & Sons, 1998;211–239.
66. Neary D, Snowden J. Fronto-temporal dementia: nosology, neuropsychology, and neuropathology. Neurology 1998;51:1546–1554.
67. Horoupian DS, Katzman R, Terry RD, et al. Dementia and motor neuron disease: morphometric, biochemical and Golgi studies. Ann Neurol 1984;16:305–313.
68. Brun A, Passant U. Frontal lobe degeneration of non-Alzheimer type. Acta Neurol Scand 1996;168:28–30.
69. Giannakopoulos P, Hof PR, Bouras C. Dementia lacking distinctive histopathology: clinicopathological evaluation of 32 cases. Acta Neuropathol (Berl) 1995;89:346–355.
70. Jackson M, Lowe J. The new neuropathology of degenerative frontotemporal dementias. Acta Neuropathol 1996;91:127–134.
71. Soni W, Luthert PJ, Leigh PN, Mann DMA. A morphometric study of the neuropathological substrate of dementia in patients with motor neuron disease. Neuropathol Appl Neurobiol 1993; 19:203.
72. Yang WC, Strong MJ. Is the frontotemporal dementia of ALS a tauopathy? ALS and other motor neuron disorders 2002;3(suppl 2):50.
73. Hayashi H, Kato S. Total manifestations of amyotrophic lateral sclerosis. J Neurol Sci 1989;93:19–35.
74. Hayashi H, Kato S, Kawada A. Amyotrophic lateral sclerosis patients living beyond respiratory failure. J Neurol Sci 1991;105:73–78.
75. Kishikawa M, Nakamura T, Iseki M, et al. A long surviving case of amyotrophic lateral sclerosis with atrophy of the frontal lobe: a comparison with the Mitsuyama type. Acta Neuropathol 1995;89:189–193.
76. Mizutani T, Aki A, Shiozawa R, et al. Development of ophthalmoplegia in amyotrophic lateral sclerosis during long-term use of respirators. J Neurol Sci 1990;99:311–319.
77. Wilson CM, Grace GM, Munoz DG, et al. Cognitive impairment in sporadic ALS. A pathological continuum underlying a multisystem disorder. Neurology 2001;57:651–657.
78. Cooper PN, Jackson M, Lennox G, et al. τ, ubiquitin, and αB-crystallin immunohistochemistry define the principal causes of degenerative frontotemporal dementia. Arch Neurol 1995;52:1011–1015.
79. Okamoto K, Hirai S, Yamazaki T, et al. New ubiquitin-positive intraneuronal inclusions in the extra-motor cortices in patients with amyotrophic lateral sclerosis. Neurosci Lett 1991;129:233–236.
80. Wightman G, Anderson VER, Martin J, et al. Hippocampal and neocortical ubiquitin-immunoreactive inclusions in amyotrophic lateral sclerosis with dementia. Neurosci Lett 1992;139:269–274.
81. Lowe J, Blanchard A, Morrell K, et al. Ubiquitin is a common factor in intermediate filament inclusion bodies of diverse type in man, including those of Parkinson's disease, Pick's disease, and

Alzheimer's disease, as well as Rosenthal fibers in cerebellar astrocytomas, cytoplasmic bodies in muscle, and Mallory bodies in alcoholic liver disease. J Pathol 1988;155:9–15.

82. Lowe J, Mayer RJ, Landon M. Ubiquitin in neurodegenerative diseases. Brain Pathol 1993;3:55–65.

83. Okamoto K, Murakami N, Kusaka H, et al. Ubiquitin-positive intraneuronal inclusions in the motor cortices of presenile dementia patients with motor neuron disease. J Neurol 1992;239:426–430.

84. Anderson VER, Cairns NJ, Leigh PN. Involvement of the amygdala, dentate and hippocampus in motor neuron disease. J Neurol Sci 1995;129:75–78.

85. Ikemoto A, Hirano A, Akiguchi I, Kimura J. Comparative study of ubiquitin immunoreactivity of hippocampal granular cells in amyotrophic lateral sclerosis with dementia, Guamanian amyotrophic lateral sclerosis and Guamanian parkinsonism-dementia complex. Acta Neuropathol 1997;93:265–270.

86. Leigh PN. Pathogenic Mechanisms in Amyotrophic Lateral Sclerosis and Other Motor Neuron Disorders. In DB Calne (ed), Neurodegenerative Diseases. Philadelphia: WB Saunders, 1994;474–477.

87. Lowe J. New pathological findings in amyotrophic lateral sclerosis. J Neurol Sci 1994;124:38–51.

88. Munoz DG. Stains for the differential diagnosis of degenerative dementias. Biotech Histochem 1999;74:311–320.

89. Buée-Scherrer V, Buée L, Hof PR, et al. Neurofibrillary degeneration in amyotrophic lateral sclerosis/parkinsonism-dementia complex of Guam. Immunochemical characterization of tau proteins. Am J Pathol 1995;146:924–932.

90. Berry RW, Quinn B, Johnson N, et al. Pathological glial tau accumulations in neurodegenerative disease: review and case report. Neurochem Int 2001;39:469–479.

91. Cruz-Sanchez FF, Moral A, Tolosa E, et al. Evaluation of neuronal loss, astrocytosis and abnormalities of cytoskeletal components of large motor neurons in the human anterior horn in aging. J Neural Trans 1998;105:689–701.

92. Ikeda K, Akiyama H, Arai T, Nishimura T. Glial tau pathology in neurodegenerative diseases: their nature and comparison with neuronal tangles. Neurobiol Aging 1998;19:S85–S91.

93. Reed DM, Brody JA. Amyotrophic lateral sclerosis and parkinsonism-dementia on Guam, 1945–1972, I: descriptive epidemiology. Am J Epidemiol 1975;101:287–301.

94. Garruto RM, Gajdusek DC, Chen KM. Amyotrophic lateral sclerosis among Chamorro migrants from Guam. Ann Neurol 1980;8:612–619.

95. Torres J, Iriarte LLG, Kurland LT. Amyotrophic lateral sclerosis among Guamanians in California. Calif Med 1957;86:385–388.

96. Yanagihara RT, Garruto RM, Gajdusek DC. Epidemiological surveillance of amyotrophic lateral sclerosis and parkinsonism-dementia in the Commonwealth of the Northern Mariana Islands. Ann Neurol 1983;13:79–86.

97. Figlewicz DA, Garruto RM, Krizus A, et al. The Cu/Zn superoxide dismutase gene in ALS and parkinsonism-dementia of Guam. Neuroreport 1994;5:557–560.

98. Poorkaj P, Tsuang D, Wijsman E, et al. TAU as a susceptibility gene for amyotrophic lateral sclerosis-parkinsonism dementia complex of Guam. Arch Neurol 2001;58:1871–1878.

99. Garruto RM. Amyotrophic lateral sclerosis and parkinsonism-dementia of Guam: clinical, epidemiological and genetic patterns. Am J Hum Biol 1989;1:367–382.

100. Garruto RM. Cellular and molecular mechanisms of neuronal degeneration: amyotrophic lateral sclerosis, parkinsonism-dementia, and Alzheimer disease. Am J Human Biol 1989;1:529–543.

101. Trojanowski JQ, Ishihara T, Higuchi M, et al. Amyotrophic lateral sclerosis/parkinsonism dementia complex: transgenic mice provide insights into mechanisms underlying a common tauopathy in an ethnic minority on Guam. Exp Neurol 2002;176:1–11.

102. McGeer PL, Schwab C, McGeer EG, et al. Familial nature and continuing morbidity of the amyotrophic lateral sclerosis-parkinsonism dementia complex of Guam. Neurology 1997;47:400–409.

103. Hirano A, Arumugasamy N, Zimmerman HM. Amyotrophic lateral sclerosis. A comparison of Guam and classical cases. Arch Neurol 1967;16:357–363.

104. Hirano A. Neuropathology of Amyotrophic Lateral Sclerosis and Parkinsonism-Dementia Complex on Guam. In L Luthy, A Bischoff (eds), Proceedings of the Fifth International Congress of Neuropathology. Amsterdam: Excerpta Medica, 1966;190–194.

105. Malamud N, Hirano A, Kurland LT. Pathoanatomic changes in amyotrophic lateral sclerosis on Guam. Arch Neurol 1961;5:401–415.

106. Oyanagi K, Makifuchi T, Ohtoh T, et al. Amyotrophic lateral sclerosis of Guam: the nature of the neuropathological findings. Acta Neuropathol 1994;88:405–412.

107. Kuzuhara S, Kokubo Y, Sasaki R, et al. Familial amyotrophic lateral sclerosis and parkinsonism-dementia complex of the Kii Peninsula of Japan: clinical and neuropathological study and tau analysis. Ann Neurol 2001;49:501–511.

108. Rodgers-Johnson P, Garruto RM, Yanigahara R, et al. Amyotrophic lateral sclerosis and parkinsonism-dementia on Guam: a 30-year evaluation of clinical and neuropathological trends. Neurology 1986;36:7–13.

109. Shankar SK, Yanagihara R, Garruto RM, et al. Immunocytochemical characterization of neurofibrillary tangles in amyotrophic lateral sclerosis and parkinsonism-dementia of Guam. Ann Neurol 1989;25:146–151.

110. Hirano A, Dembitzer HM, Kurland LT, Zimmerman HM. The fine structure of some intraganglionic alterations: neurofibrillary tangles, granulovacuolar bodies, and "rod-like" structures in Guam amyotrophic lateral sclerosis and parkinsonism-dementia complex. J Neuropathol Exp Neurol 1968;27:167–182.

111. Buée-Scherrer V, Buée L, Hof PR, et al. Neurofibrillary degeneration in amyotrophic lateral sclerosis/parkinsonism-dementia complex of Guam. Am J Pathol 1995;68:924–932.

112. Yamazaki M, Arai Y, Baba M, et al. Alpha-synuclein inclusions in amygdala in the brains of patients with the parkinsonism-dementia complex of Guam. J Neuropathol Exp Neurol 2000;59:585–591.

113. Forman MS, Schmidt ML, Kasturi S, et al. Tau and a-synuclein pathology in amygdala of parkinsonism-dementia complex patients of Guam. Am J Pathol 2002;160:1725–1731.

114. Lynch T, Sano M, Marder KS, et al. Clinical characteristics of a family with chromosome 17-linked disinhibition-dementia-parkinsonism-amyotrophy complex. Neurology 1994;44:1878–1884.

115. Foster NL, Wilhelmsen K, Sima AAF, et al. Frontotemporal dementia and parkinsonism linked to chromosome 17: a consensus conference. Ann Neurol 1997;41:706–715.

116. Clark LN, Poorkaj P, Wszolek Z, et al. Pathogenic implications of mutations in the tau gene in pallido-ponto-nigral degeneration and related neurodegenerative disorders linked to chromosome 17. Proc Natl Acad Sci USA 1998;95:13103–13107.

117. Hutton M, Lendon CL, Rizzu P, et al. Association of missense and 5′-splice-site mutations in tau with the inherited dementia FTDP-17. Nature 1998;393:702–705.

118. Spillantini MG, Goedert M. Tau protein pathology in neurodegenerative diseases. Trends Neurosci 1998;21:428–433.

119. Bergmann M, Kuchelmeister K, Schmid KW, et al. Different variants of frontotemporal dementia: a neuropathological and immunohistochemical study. Acta Neuropathol 1996;92:170–179.

120. Pringle CE, Hudson AJ, Munoz DG, et al. Primary lateral sclerosis. Clinical features, neuropathology and diagnostic criteria. Brain 1992;115:495–520.

121. Hudson AJ, Keirnan JA, Munoz DA, et al. Clinicopathological features of primary lateral sclerosis are different from amyotrophic lateral sclerosis. Brain Res Bull 1993;30:359–364.

122. Caselli RJ, Smith BE, Osborne D. Primary lateral sclerosis: a neuropsychological study. Neurology 1995;45:2005–2009.

123. Lee VMY, Goedert M, Trojanowski JQ. Neurodegenerative tauopathies. Annu Rev Neurosci 2001;24:1121–1159.

124. Gilbert JJ, Kish SJ, Chang L-J, et al. Dementia, parkinsonism and motor neuron disease: neurochemical and neuropathological correlates. Ann Neurol 1988;24:688–691.

125. D'Souza I, Poorkaj P, Hong M, et al. Missense and silent tau gene mutations cause frontotemporal dementia with parkinsonism-chromosome 17 type, by affecting multiple alternative RNA splicing regulatory elements. Proc Natl Acad Sci USA 1999;96:5598–5603.

126. Aran FA. Recherches sur une maladie non encore décrite du système musculaire (atrophie musculaire progressive). Arch Gén Méd 1850;24:5–35.

127. Aran FA. Recherches sur une maladie non encore décrite du système musculaire (atrophie musculaire progressive) (2ᵉ article-suite et fin). Arch Gén Méd 1850;24:172–214.

128. Charcot JM, Joffroy A. Deux cas d'atrophie musculaire progressive avec lésions de la substance grise et des faisceaux antérolatéraux de la moelle épinière. Arch Physiol Norm Pathol 1869;2: 354–744.

129. Ziegler LH. Psychotic and emotional phenomena associated with amyotrophic lateral sclerosis. Arch Neurol Psychiatry 1930;24:930–936.

130. Lawyer T, Netsky MG. Amyotrophic lateral sclerosis, a clinicoanatomic study of fifty-three cases. Arch Neurol Psychiatry 1953;69:171–192.

131. Wechsler IS, Davison C. Amyotrophic lateral sclerosis with mental symptoms. Arch Neurol Psychiatry 1932;27:857–880.

132. Ince PG, Lowe J, Shaw PJ. Amyotrophic lateral sclerosis: current issues in classification, pathogenesis and molecular pathology. Neuropathol Appl Neurobiol 1998;24:104–117.

133. Kawashima T, Doh-ura K, Kikuchi H, Iwaki T. Cognitive dysfunction in patients with amyotrophic lateral sclerosis is associated with spherical or crescent-shaped ubiquitinated intraneuronal inclusions in the parahippocampal gyrus and amygdala, but not in the neostriatum. Acta Neuropathol 2001;102:467–472.

134. Abrahams S, Goldstein LH, Kew JJM, et al. Frontal lobe dysfunction in amyotrophic lateral sclerosis. A PET study. Brain 1996;119:2105–2120.

135. Gunnarsson L-G, Dahlbom K, Strandman E. Motor neuron disease and dementia reported among 13 members of a single family. Acta Neurol Scand 1991;84:429–433.

136. Uematsu S. Amyotrophic lateral sclerosis and its mental symptoms. Shindan To Chiryo 1935;22:838–844.

137. Furukawa T. Clinical and epidemiological studies on amyotrophic lateral sclerosis. Osaka Daigaku Igaku Zasshi 1959;11:4087–4099.

138. Jackson M, Lennox G, Ward L, Lowe J. Frontal dementia with MND inclusions without clinical ALS: report of eleven cases. Neuropathol Appl Neurobiol 1995;21:148–145.

139. Mann DM. Dementia of frontal type and dementia with subcortical gliosis. Brain Pathol 1998;8:325–338.

140. Mann DMA, South PW, Snowden JS, Neary D. Dementia of frontal lobe type: neuropathology and immunohistochemistry. J Neurol Neurosurg Psychiatry 1993;56:605–614.

141. Tolnay M, Probst A. Frontal lobe degeneration: novel ubiquitin-immunoreactive neurites within frontotemporal cortex. Neuropathol Appl Neurobiol 1995;21:492–497.

142. Martin JA, Craft DK, Su JH, et al. Astrocytes degenerate in frontotemporal dementia: possible relation to hypoperfusion. Neurobiol Aging 2001;22:195–207.

143. Chow TW, Miller BL, Hayashi VN, Geschwind DH. Inheritance of frontotemporal dementia. Arch Neurol 1999;56:817–822.

144. Curcio SAM, Kawarai T, Paterson DA, et al. A large Calabrian kindred segregating frontotemporal dementia. J Neurol 2002;249:911–922.

145. Gydesen S, Brown JM, Brun A, et al. Chromosome 3 linked frontotemporal dementia (FTD-3). Neurology 2002;59:1585–1594.

146. Hosler BA, Siddique T, Sapp PC, et al. Linkage of familial amyotrophic lateral sclerosis with frontotemporal dementia to chromosome 9q21-q22. JAMA 2000;284:1664–1669.

147. Janssen JC, Warrington EK, Morris HR, et al. Clinical features of frontotemporal dementia due to the intronic *tau* 10^{+16} mutation. Neurology 2002;58:1161–1168.

7

Epidemiology of Amyotrophic Lateral Sclerosis/Motor Neuron Disease

Carmel Armon

DEFINITION AND CLASSIFICATIONS

Amyotrophic lateral sclerosis (ALS), or motor neuron disease (MND) is the most common neurodegenerative disorder of motor neurons. It is a multilevel neurodegenerative disease. It results from progressive loss of upper motor neuron (UMN) and lower motor neuron (LMN) at two or three levels of the neuraxis. Loss of pyramidal, spinal and bulbar motor neurons affecting multiple regions of the body leads to progressive motor dysfunction, disability, and death. Loss of prefrontal motor neurons, when it occurs, results in a unique pattern of cognitive impairment that affects mainly executive functions, akin to that seen in frontotemporal dementia, but usually milder, and not the limiting factor in patients' disability.

Case Definitions

Two consensus meetings convened under the auspices of the World Federation of Neurology (WFN) Subcommittee on MND/ALS resulted in definitions for ALS/MND for research purposes that are accepted widely.[1,2] Although it would not have been possible to apply criteria adopted in the 1990s to classifying ALS/MND in earlier years, the distinctions between ALS/MND and other motor neuron disorders have long been appreciated. Currently, the application of WFN criteria to making the diagnosis of ALS/MND in nonresearch settings is constrained by the practical need for a binary approach to the diagnosis of ALS/MND ("yes" or "no") in the clinical setting. However, with rare exceptions, patients with progressive motor dysfunction who are classified initially as "suspected" or "possible" ALS and for whom an alternative diagnosis is not found will progress to "probable" or "definite" ALS. In contrast to the "splitting" approach of neuromuscular specialists, most epidemiological data derived

167

from public health registries rely on the *International Classification of Diseases,* ninth edition (ICD-9), classification that lumps all chronic progressive motor neuron disorders together under one code: 335.20. This code captures, in all likelihood, not only forms of degenerative MNDs that are not ALS/MND (see below), but also the immune-mediated multifocal motor neuropathy, late seque-lae of poliomyelitis, and ALS/MND look-alikes that went unrecognized. Pre-vious chapters have discussed the differentiation of ALS/MND from other degenerative MNDs (pure UMN [primary lateral sclerosis] or pure LMN [the spinal muscular atrophies and progressive muscular atrophy]) and nondegener-ative motor neuron disorders. These conditions represent less than 10 percent of all motor neuron disorders. Consequently, they introduce only a minor error when making inferences about ALS/MND from data based on the ICD-9 clas-sification using code 335.20. In contrast, underascertainment of patients with ALS/MND in passively acquired national registries introduces a greater uncer-tainty in the numbers derived from these sources, the magnitude of which cannot be estimated readily. More recently, actively ascertained, population-based data from the service areas of specialized ALS/MND clinics have com-bined the precision of diagnosis based on WFN criteria with completeness of ascertainment. These data are excellent, are useful for comparisons with data, present or future, ascertained similarly, but cannot be used to draw inferences based on comparisons with data, mainly past data, based on passive ascertain-ment. In summary, although there has been an evolution of the case definition of ALS/MND for the purpose of research in the past decade, its impact on the generation of epidemiological data has been limited. Future reliance on WFN criteria to report actively ascertained patients will increase the confidence in their diagnosis and in the soundness of the epidemiological data thus derived.

Epidemiological Classification of Amyotrophic Lateral Sclerosis

Epidemiological and genetic factors permit classifying ALS into three classes or forms[3]:

1. Sporadic
2. Familial
3. Western Pacific

The latter was first described among the indigenous population (Chamorros) of Guam, often in association with another progressive and fatal disorder, a parkinsonism-dementia complex (PDC).[4,5] It was recognized subsequently in two villages in the Kii Peninsula of Japan[6,7] and among the Auyu and Jakai people of Irian Jaya (western New Guinea),[8] resulting in a total of three Western Pacific foci for ALS.

ETIOLOGICAL CONSIDERATIONS

The causes of ALS/MND are not known, although genetic risk factors have been identified. There are abundant data at the clinical, histological, ultrastructural, and molecular levels regarding its consequences. A currently favored working hypothesis for the initiation of ALS/MND postulates genetic–environmental interactions. Even though specifics are lacking, this hypothesis is useful by providing a framework for conceptualizing about causation in ALS/MND and for planning research. As I have considered ALS/MND, I have found one of its most salient clinical features to be that it usually starts in one place and spreads. One mode of spread within the central nervous system is by direct contiguity. Weakness first spreads within the initially affected limb, then frequently crosses to the contralateral limb at the same spinal level, and then proceeds to affect spinal levels contiguous to those in which it began. A second mode of spread is the dissemination of the pathology of ALS/MND up and down the motor neuron system of the neuraxis. This behavior is conceptually similar to that of a malignancy that has metastasized by the time of clinical diagnosis, except that subcellular components, rather than entire cells, are involved in the spread of the malignancy. Two specific *hypothetical* examples based on known processes may be considered. First, a conformational change in a protein, such as the one that occurs in the spongiform encephalopathies, except that instead of affecting a structural protein, a protein involved in cellular function, or intercellular communication undergoes this conformational change. Second, a post-translational mutation: a change in DNA, except that instead of causing uninhibited cellular proliferation (as is the case in the usual malignancies) an abnormal protein results, which interferes with normal cell function or with intercellular communication. Under all these hypothetical scenarios, the abnormal protein, or the abnormally conformed protein, may be merely a non-functional analogue of the native protein, which is not recognized by the body's immune system. Conceptually, the change need not be a big one, if a critical function is incapacitated.

The biochemical trigger that sets off the processes that lead to motor neuron loss can be conceptualized as a malignant biochemical transformation (Figure 7.1). This is a hypothetical concept, because the nature of this biochemical trigger has remained elusive. There is probably more than one trigger and more than one possible malignant biochemical transformation. Similarly, there is no basis to determine whether the transformation is triggered as a single random event, as a nonrandom cumulative result of a sequence of events that lead to a threshold being crossed inevitably, or as a result of nonrandom cumulative events that increase the likelihood that a threshold will be crossed, triggering disease onset. It is likely that all these options play a part in some instances of ALS/MND. What is certain is that once the process is detectable clinically, it is inexorably progressive. This framework, even though hypothetical, is useful because it permits us to think of processes that precede this transformation ("upstream") and of processes that are consequences of this transformation ("downstream"). It is worthwhile to distinguish between upstream factors that make the occurrence of the transformation more likely to happen and those that actually mediate the transformation. Factors that increase the likelihood of the transformation happening are best termed "risk factors" for the disease. The best example for these is carrying a gene for familial ALS. Not all carriers will develop the disease. The "causes" of ALS/MND are the biochemical processes

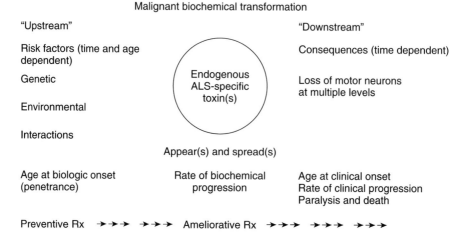

Figure 7.1 Malignant biochemical transformation hypothesis. Risk factors operate "upstream" to a malignant biochemical transformation, which causes the appearance of "endogenous amyotrophic lateral sclerosis (ALS)–specific toxins." These putative toxins spread, behaving like a metastasizing biochemical malignancy, and cause the "downstream" biochemical, histological, and clinical consequences of ALS. (Adapted with permission from Armon C. ALS: Clinical and Epidemiologic Clues to Pathogenesis. In Neurobiology of ALS. Course Syllabus, 51st Annual Meeting. American Academy of Neurology, 1999.)

upstream to the transformation that mediate between risk factors and disease by taking normally functioning cells and converting them into abnormally functioning cells. Once a point of no return has been crossed, the malignant biochemical transformation has occurred and all the processes may be considered downstream, consequences, or modes of execution of ALS/MND. It remains to be seen to what extent the analogy to carcinogenesis will be found to be relevant to some of the forms of ALS/MND.

The continuum between risk factors and biochemical causes and consequences of ALS has yet to be elucidated even for the best-defined forms of ALS/MND—the familial forms. However, study of the nonrandom patterns of occurrence of the disease,[9] that is, the epidemiology of ALS/MND, has been and remains the only way of identifying risk factors in sporadic ALS/MND. Furthermore, the past few years have seen an evolution in our understanding of the methods needed to search for environmental risk factors for sporadic ALS/MND. This chapter provides first the descriptive epidemiology of ALS/MND, scrutinizing it for etiological clues, and then proceeds to examine the results of studies designed with the specific goal of identifying risk factors for ALS/MND ("analytical epidemiology"). This emphasis reflects the hope that the identification of risk factors will permit plausible efforts to be directed to identify the biochemical processes that cause ALS/MND. Further, avoidance of modifiable risk factors may provide the best hope for preventing, if only in part, the occurrence of ALS/MND.

DESCRIPTIVE EPIDEMIOLOGY

Methodological Considerations

There are several methodological factors to consider in studying the epidemiology of ALS/MND.[3] Of these, the most important relate to case definition, case ascertainment, competing causes of mortality in a susceptible population, referral bias in data that are not population based, and the impacts of earlier diagnosis and proactive supportive treatment on survival. Those related to case definition have been discussed earlier in this chapter. Improved ascertainment wherever special effort is made to identify cases will result in the appearance of increased incidence, compared to a reference population (in which such an effort was not made), without a true increase in incidence. The impact of increased survival of a population at risk, due to the loss of competing causes of mortality, needs to be factored into any consideration of time-dependent trends in the incidence of ALS/MND in the developed countries. The nonrepresentative aspects of referral-based case series are well recognized. Specifically, case series of referral patients with ALS/MND consistently report a mean age at onset that is 10 years younger and survival that is longer than those of patients in well-ascertained population-based series. Other differences may not be as easy to recognize. Earlier diagnosis and proactive supportive treatment[10] will result in longer survival from diagnosis, without a true change in the biology of the disease. Variability in how the date of diagnosis is defined may confound data regarding survival from onset or regarding onset-to-diagnosis latency. Is the date of diagnosis considered the date the diagnosis was first considered (by whom?), the date the patient was first told of the possibility, or the date a firm diagnosis was made?[11] Hence, survival from disease onset is a better measure. However, I have found that focused questioning of patients often results in the establishment of a date of clinical disease onset that is earlier than the one obtained through routine questioning, particularly if patients are given a chance to think back on the period leading to what they initially considered disease onset. If neurologists who are experienced in early diagnosis of ALS/MND establish concurrently an earlier date of disease onset, the average onset-to-diagnosis latency might remain unchanged and an apparent increase in patient survival from onset and from diagnosis will appear to have occurred, without any change in the biology of the disease or the actual longevity of affected patients. These considerations limit the ability to draw conclusions about changes in the natural history of the disease or to establish the efficacy of current interventions by making comparisons to historical controls.

Incidence and Mortality Data

Where ascertainment is complete, excluding the Western Pacific foci, the incidence of sporadic ALS is geographically fairly constant, ranging from 0.86 to 2.5 per 100,000 per year.[4,12–16] The more recent studies provide an approximate crude rate of 2 per 100,000 per year. With an average duration of 3 years, the prevalence rate may be estimated at three times the incidence rate, or about 6 per 100,000 on any given date.

It should be recognized that the denominator for incidence rates is usually based on the total general population. If only a subset of the population is considered in the denominator, for example, those aged 20 years or older, then the annual incidence rate might range from 3.0 to 4.0 per (100,000 individuals aged 20 years or older) per year. This point is illustrated by Example 1. The proportions of individuals in each age bracket approximate the data from the 2000 United States population census. The age-specific incidence rates are approximations based on the Rochester, Minnesota data.[16]

Example 1

Calculation A: All the population is considered when calculating the total incidence rate.

Age (yr)	No. of people	Incidence rate (cases/100,000/yr)	Incident cases
0–19	3,000,000	0	0
20–49	4,300,000	1	43
50–59	1,100,000	5	55
60–69	750,000	15	113
70 and older	850,000	5	43
Total	10,000,000	2.54	254

Calculation B: Only persons aged 20 years and older are considered when calculating the total incidence rate.

Age (yr)	No. of people	Incidence rate (cases/100,000/yr)	Incident cases
20–49	4,300,000	1	43
50–59	1,100,000	5	55
60–69	750,000	15	113
70 and older	850,000	5	43
Total	7,000,000	3.63	254

It may be shown similarly that national incidence rates (using the total population as the denominator) also will be influenced by the age composition of the population, even if age-specific incidence rates do not vary from one population to the other, and cases ascertainment is complete or equal across the populations. Example 2 derives the incidence rate expected in a population with a younger age composition than that of the United States population used in Example 1. The same age-specific incidence rates were used as in Example 1. The overall incidence rate is 1.5 per 100,000 per year in this second population.

Example 2

In a population with a younger age composition, all the population is considered when calculating the total incidence rate.

Age (yr)	No. of people	Incidence rate (cases/100,000/yr)	Incident cases
0–19	5,000,000	0	0
20–49	3,500,000	1	35
50–59	1,000,000	5	50
60–69	400,000	15	60
70 and older	100,000	5	5
Total	10,000,000	1.5	150

Comparison of the incidence rate derived in Example 2 (1.5/100,000/year) to the incidence rate in Calculation A of Example 1 (2.54/100,000/year) illustrates also the expected rise in total incidence rates over time that might result from aging of the population.

Mortality would be expected to track incidence fairly closely, as almost all patients with ALS/MND die of their disease. The reported mortality rate in the United States during the 1980s was less than 1.5 per 100,000 per year for all ages combined. This was considered to be due, in part, to under-reporting on death certificates. It was projected to increase in the 1990s and subsequently.[17] Indeed, most ALS/MND morbidity and mortality data demonstrate higher rates in recent years than previously.[14–16,18–20] This increase may be accounted for by the aging of the population, improved ascertainment, better reporting, and loss of competing causes of mortality in a susceptible cohort.[21–25] The putative susceptible cohort may be a true subset of the population or may be a conceptualization of the maximal risk of the entire population. Peaking in age-specific incidence rates is cited in support of there being a true subpopulation at risk. However, age-specific incidence rates have been shown to increase into older age-groups in population-based series,[13,15,19,26] rather than peaking at 55 to 60 years, as shown in referral-based case series.[27,28] More recent population-based series have shown the peaks at older ages. However, even there, if ascertainment is less complete in patients older than 80 years in Italy[15] or 85 years in Norway,[19] the peak (caused by the following drop-off) may be artefactual and probably may not be used to support the inference that the population is at risk for ALS/MND, is a subset of the entire population, or that there is a finite period of susceptibility to putative exogenous risk factors for developing ALS/MND.

Case Series Variability

In population-based series, mean and median ages at onset are approximately 65 years, and mean and median disease duration from clinical onset to death are approximately 3 years,[13,26] where use of ventilatory support and invasive nutritional support are limited. Recent mortality data from Norway[19] provide a similar indication: The median age at death for the 1989 to 1994 period was 70 years. Assuming mean survival of 3 years, this suggests a mean age at onset of 67 years. In referral series, including most reported clinical trials, mean age at onset has been approximately 10 years younger, that is, 55 years. Median survival from disease onset in referral series has varied and usually has been more than 3 years. The relationship between age at onset and incidence rates in several studies[29–32] illustrates the potential effect of referral bias and ascertainment bias: A higher incidence rate was associated with a higher mean age at onset and with a shorter survival. This observation suggests that improved diagnosis and ascertainment may identify more patients with a course shorter than the previously considered median of 3 years and with an older age at onset. This is consistent with observations that older age at onset is associated with a shorter course.[13,33–35]

Individual Variability: "Endogenous" Risk Factors for Disease Occurrence or Shorter Survival

Increasing age is the principal individual risk factor for the occurrence of sporadic ALS. Age-specific incidence rates increase in men and women. In addition, the overall incidence and age-specific incidence rates of sporadic ALS/MND in men are more than those in women (1.6 : 1 to 1.3 : 1 overall).[3] In this context, it is worth considering that Kennedy's disease, a lower MND caused by a trinucleotide repeat expansion on chromosome X, affects men only, but not the female carriers,[36,37] and that a gene for familial ALS/MND has been identified on chromosome X. This suggests that there may a susceptibility gene also for sporadic ALS/MND on the X chromosome, which may be the same or adjacent to the genes for Kennedy's disease or for X-linked familial ALS, but with lesser penetrance. More recent reports suggest a decline in the gender ratio for sporadic ALS/MND.[16,19] This may reflect greater improvement of ascertainment in women, greater decrease of mortality from competing causes in women, with more living to ages where their risk to develop ALS/MND may be realized, or equalization of opportunities to be exposed to exogenous risk factors.

There are some indications that a family history of neurodegenerative disease may be a risk factor for the occurrence of sporadic ALS,[38,39] although others have not found this to be the case.[40] Similarly, reports regarding the role of apolipoprotein E-4 (ApoE-4) as a risk factor for disease occurrence, earlier age at onset, or shorter survival have been conflicting.[41–45]

Racial differences in death rates from ALS/MND in the United States were noted in 1959 to 1961 mortality data studies: The rates for whites exceeded those for non-whites by 1.7 : 1.[28,46] Subsequent studies of the rates for 1971 and 1973 to 1978 and 1962 to 1984 continued to show lower rates among non-whites, particularly those older than 60 years, especially women. These differences may represent continued underascertainment in this population. Given the potential confounding effect of underascertainment, it is difficult to make any statement regarding the effect of race on the true incidence of ALS. Although this point has been illustrated with data from the United States, it may apply also to international comparisons.

Assessment of risk factors for shorter survival requires recognition of the potential role of supportive care, including ventilatory support, on survival. To date, use of tracheostomy-free survival as an endpoint has been the chief concession given to the impact of ventilatory support on survival. Other than reporting on the percentage of individuals using other interventions, it had been difficult to control for their impact on survival data. Consequently, with some exceptions,[47] interpretation of the data is constrained by lack of control for level of supportive care.

Traditional risk factors for shorter survival have been older age and non-limb onset (worst if involves respiratory tract muscles).[3,35,44,47,48] There is one mention that patients with predominant spasticity have longer survival,[49] and this conforms with our own observations. Features in patients' status at the time of assessment that predict worse survival *from that point in time* are lower forced vital capacity (expressed as percent of predicted value), subnormal body mass index, greater recent weight loss, and lower serum chloride.[44,50,51] All of these are late consequences of advanced stages of the disease, foretelling patients' imminent demise.

Attention has also focused on how rate of disease progression, determined relatively early in its course, may be used to predict survival. This is the most direct way to capture the variability among individual patients early and use it for prognosis.[52] An indirect measure is the interval from symptom onset to diagnosis: A shorter interval has been shown to predict shorter survival.[35,44,49,50] A second indirect measure of the speed with which ALS progresses is the extent of clinical involvement at the time of initial diagnosis. The WFN classification[1] is based on the number of body levels in which UMN and LMN findings are present. Patients who at the time of initial diagnosis can be classified as "definite" ALS have a worse prognosis than those classified as "probable" or "possible" ALS.[47] Direct calculations of rates of disease progression also predict survival from onset or from the date of the calculations. In addition to calculations of rate of disease progression based on serial measures of muscle strength, ventilatory function, bulbar function, or global function,[47,53–55] it is possible to obtain linear estimates of disease progression (LEP) based on strength or ventilatory function measurements at one time and the interval from disease onset.[56,57] All these measures are excellent predictors of tracheostomy-free survival: Patients with a faster rate of disease progression die or require tracheostomy sooner. LEP based on motor unit number estimates (MUNEs) have been shown, in a small series, to be better predictors of survival than those based on regionally concordant muscle strength.[58] We speculated that this might be the case because MUNEs reflect the primary process, loss of motor neurons, whereas all other measures reflect also the effects of reinnervation, and further, that the rate of loss of motor neuron dominates patients' course, and thus is the best determinant of survival.

Specific treatments that extend survival include feeding gastrostomy,[59–61] noninvasive ventilatory support,[62,63] and riluzole.[64] All other things being equal, personality traits or psychological states that would result in declining these interventions may be considered risk factors for reduced survival. Of these, depression is genetically mediated[65] and thus is an endogenous risk factor for reduced survival. Cultural factors that might impact the acceptability of these treatments and lack of social support for their implementation also are risk factors for reduced survival.

Epidemiological Implications for Clinical Trials

Median survival in clinical trials depends strongly on the specific patient sample enrolled, based on the inclusion/exclusion criteria. Patients in studies with more recently diagnosed patients will have a shorter survival than those in studies with patients with longer disease duration. Due to the numerous factors that may impact survival, data should be provided to permit comparisons of clinical trial cohorts: within treatment arms of individual trials, among clinical trials, and between clinical trial populations and other patient cohorts. This requires providing all individual factors that might influence the rate of disease progression or mortality, as listed earlier, and data that will permit deriving measures of the rate of disease progression—the most important prognostic factor. Consideration should be given to performing stratified randomization to ensure arms balanced for the most important factors, and nonexperimental therapeutic interventions should be standardized and accounted for. Although homogeneity of the study participants increases the likelihood of detecting a treatment effect, it is their heterogeneity that makes them more representative of the general patient population.

An imbalance in prognostic factors favoring the placebo arm may mask the efficacy of an effective treatment. This can be corrected, if there is enough faith in the efficacy of the intervention, by performing another trial, with more attention to balancing the treatment arms. Conversely, if the placebo arm has a higher mortality because of an imbalance in risk factors among the arms, the treatment may appear effective even if survival was no better than in the placebo arms of other studies. Such a conclusion may or may not be corrected by a subsequent study. This is thought to have occurred in the first trial on brain-derived neurotrophic factor (BDNF), where treatment appeared effective because of a poorly performing placebo arm, only to be shown ineffective in the second trial on BDNF.[66] In contrast, it is noteworthy that the second pivotal trial for riluzole[64] included the fastest declining placebo cohort in recent clinical trial experience—the French and Belgian subgroup. The entire demonstration of benefit of riluzole in the second riluzole trial[64] was driven by showing efficacy in the French and Belgian subgroup. Moreover, this subgroup was drawn from the same population base as the first cohort that demonstrated efficacy of riluzole, also in a rapidly declining (bulbar-onset) subgroup.[67] An alternative interpretation of these data is that both treatments (BDNF and riluzole) are effective only in patients declining at faster than average rates. From the epidemiological perspective, the unique characteristics of the study populations in whom efficacy was demonstrated, with a worse than average prognosis for the placebo arms, raise questions regarding the possible role of an imbalance of risk factors among treatment arms in producing the apparent efficacy. It also raises questions about the generalizability of the data to other populations, decisions of regulatory agencies notwithstanding.

ANALYTICAL EPIDEMIOLOGY

Trends in Focus

The past 10 years have seen a significant shift in the focus of analytical studies in ALS/MND.[68] First, there has been a shift away from looking for risk factors in the form of isolated events and toward looking for them in the form of chronic, lifelong exposures. This shift has been driven chiefly by considerations of biological plausibility and the need to ensure that risk factors precede disease onset. Second is the expansion of exposures to include not only environmental or exogenous factors but also endogenous factors, such as diet or smoking. Third is the increased emphasis on the genetic–environmental interaction model, with time or age as a modifier.

Trends in Methodology

Over the past 10 years, significant advances have occurred both in the methodology of ALS/MND epidemiological research and the methodology of analyzing the published literature. Recognizing the limitations of earlier epidemiological research, more recent studies have been designed more rigorously. Particular strength has resulted from the population-based case-control study design, with meticulous attention to case definition, completeness of ascertainment, and standardized quantification of exposures, with great effort to avoid or minimize recall bias. Research adhering to these higher standards costs more and requires expertise and infrastructure in place that is more complex than in years past and that typically cannot be maintained just for the study of risk factors for ALS/MND. Research adhering to these higher standards will typically require external funding and will necessitate collaborations between the people with the questions and the people with the expertise to answer them. This expertise will need to come from the fields of epidemiology and genetics, if the genetic–environmental model of disease etiology is to be advanced. Clinicians highly competent in diagnosing ALS/MND will need to be involved as full partners to ensure complete and accurate case ascertainment and diagnosis. Individual investigators or individual centers will find it difficult to advance the field.

A second shift in methodology that has taken place over the past 10 years relates to the way that data in the literature are analyzed and summarized. Readers of epidemiological reviews and chapters 15 and 20 years ago may have encountered what today might be considered relatively uncritical summaries of the published literature. Between 15 and 20 years ago, the idea of a critical review of the literature began to have an impact on the way data were summarized and presented: Not all reports were accorded equal weight. Approximately 10 years ago, the idea was introduced that meta-analysis might be a method to summarize and condense the results of many studies that individually might be ambiguous or conflicting. However, limitations of this method when the ingredients were less than perfect have not permitted its proper application to the epidemiology of ALS/MND.

The past 10 years have also seen "evidence-based medicine" (EBM) introduced into the way we think about drawing conclusions from the published literature. The application of these concepts has not been done uniformly. It varies among professional organizations and has undergone changes and refinements over time within individual organizations, including, for example, the American Academy of Neurology. There are advantages to applying this method to the analytical epidemiology of ALS/MND,[68] of which three are discussed here. First, it makes explicit the expectation that review of data in the literature is done for the purpose of drawing conclusions. Where that is not possible, the purpose of the review is to determine what additional data would need to be generated to be able to draw conclusions in the future. This would counteract the potential for "circular epidemiology."[69] Second, it establishes the rule that all data are not equal, as far as the ability to draw conclusions from them. Third, it makes explicit the discussion regarding how data should be classified, and how firm a conclusion can be drawn from data that cross a threshold of conclusion worthiness. As a result, if agreement is established regarding the way the method is to be applied, the results of its application tend to be highly reproducible. However, EBM has limitations, of which three are discussed. First, the choice of the way it is applied is based on individual opinion or a consensus of opinions, rather than on evidence. This may result in data being excluded from impacting conclusions under one set of criteria, but being included under another set, changing the conclusions in specific cases. A second limitation is that the choice of how the method is to be applied is made with some knowledge of the data to which it is to be applied. This differs from what happens in a research setting, where the experiment is done and the results become known only after the methods have been established. Finally, EBM is prone to type II errors (avoiding making a recommendation or drawing a conclusion when one is warranted) even as it tries to decrease the likelihood of type I errors (making a recommendation or drawing a conclusion with insufficient basis). In contrast to other research efforts and, in particular, clinical trials, it is usually impossible to estimate the magnitude of the likelihood of a type II error when applying EBM methods, whereas the likelihood of a type I error is usually explicit, and kept low. Thus the magnitude of impact of this particular limitation is difficult to assess prospectively. A type II error in the application of EBM is discovered only in retrospect. Consequently, it is important to keep in mind that absence of evidence should not be construed as evidence of absence. EBM may be applied to take advantage of its strengths, but with due recognition of its limitations.

New Challenges: How to Classify the Results, and When Do they Matter?

In applying the EBM approach to classifying the evidence in the analytical epidemiology of ALS, a first step is to develop a classification method, including (1) the method of rating articles and (2) the method of translating the evidence into conclusions. A preliminary attempt is presented in Tables 7.1 and 7.2.[68]

This effort draws on examples of rating systems for classification of evidence developed over the past few years by the American Academy of Neurology[71,72] and similar organizations but has not gone through a comparable process to establish a prepublication consensus in support of it. A second challenge of thinking of the analytical epidemiology of ALS/MND in terms of EBM is that it may be necessary to deal with results that cross various thresholds of conclusion worthiness and decide how to rank their potential important to the general public. Some considerations regarding the strength of the conclusions and their impact, as they might influence their importance to the general public, are summarized in Table 7.3.[68] This approach may be subjected to critique

Text continued on p. 183

Table 7.1 Proposed system for classification of evidence of risk factors in amyotrophic lateral sclerosis

Rating of analytic epidemiological articles
Class I: One of the following:
1. Prospective or retrospective cohort study with parallel controls.
   a. Exposure and hence assignment to the "exposed" cohort, established before knowledge of diagnostic status, or without knowledge of diagnostic status, or confirmable independently of the knowledge of diagnostic status. Consideration of and accounting for possible misclassification.
   b. Unexposed cohort is appropriate to the risk factor in question, is well matched to the exposed cohort on factors other than the exposure, and is otherwise representative of the general population.
   c. Diagnosis of amyotrophic lateral sclerosis (ALS) made applying uniform efforts and criteria to exposed and unexposed cohorts.
   d. Loss to follow-up low and comparable in exposed and unexposed cohorts. Possible roles of competing causes of mortality accounted for—preferably, all mortality data available for both cohorts.
   e. Exposure quantified, where possible, to permit assessment of dose-response relationships.
   f. Sources of biases and confounding identified and accounted for.
   g. Conclusion based on large numbers. Appropriate statistical analysis.
2. Population-based case-control studies.
   a. Putative risk factor or exposure occurred before probable biological onset of disease.
   b. Demonstration that ascertainment of patients is complete in the given population.
   c. Appropriate choice of controls, to ensure they are matched to the patients and are representative of the general population. (Ensure adequate matching, avoid "overmatching.")
   d. High response rates from patients and controls.
   e. Uniform effort to gather information equally from affected and unaffected individuals.
   f. Blinding of information-gathering method to individuals' disease status ideal; if not done, adequate justification about why this does not affect the assessment of the risk factor in question.
   g. Blinding of subjects and individuals gathering the data about the hypotheses being tested. If not done, adequate justification about why this does not affect the assessment of the risk factor in question.
   h. Meticulous attention to avoiding recall bias or if not possible to evaluating its impact, estimating the magnitude of its impact and controlling for it.
   i. Diagnosis of ALS made by applying established criteria.
   j. Exposure quantified, where possible, to permit assessment of dose-response relationships.
   k. Sources of biases and confounding identified and accounted for.
   l. Conclusions based on large numbers. Appropriate statistical analysis.
      Methods state if hypotheses were selected a priori for confirmatory analysis. If more than one exposure considered in exploratory analysis, statistical significance is established with correction for multiple comparisons.
Class II
1. Cohort studies with parallel controls meeting most of criteria (b) through (g), where the findings may be considered valid for the risk factor in question. This requires justification. (Criterion [a] is mandatory.)
2. Population-based case-control studies meeting most of criteria (c) through (l), where the findings may be considered valid for the risk factor in question. This requires justification. (Criteria [a] and [b] are mandatory.)
3. Well-designed case-control studies that are not population-based, meeting most of criteria (c) through (l). Criterion (a) is mandatory. Justification is necessary, why the findings may be considered valid for the risk factor in question, with initial attention to referral bias.

Table 7.1 (continued)

Class III
1. Cohort studies with parallel controls where not all of the criteria (b) through (g) have been met, and consequently bias or confounding may account for the findings with regards to the risk factor in question, but not to an extent that would invalidate the findings completely.
2. Case-control studies where not all the criteria (b) through (l) have been met, and consequently bias and confounding may account for the findings with regards to the risk factor in question, but not to an extent that would invalidate the findings completely.

    Findings that result from otherwise unbiased exploratory analysis or encountered through the performance of multiple comparisons may belong in this class, provided no sources of bias or other material limitations are present. If there are additional limitations, then the evidence is class IV or V. Assignment to level III requires justification.

Class IV: All other studies with controls, where the risk factor occurred before biological disease onset. Results that do not attain statistical significance. Results of post hoc analyses, uncorrected for implicit multiple comparisons.

Class V:
1. Studies with controls where the risk factor studied most likely occurred after biological disease onset. Assignment to this class is specific to that risk factor.
2. Uncontrolled data (case series, case reports, chance observations, and expert opinions that are not based on verifiable data).

    Comment: Epidemiological studies are designed to look for presence and magnitudes of associations. Findings of absence of association require special consideration. *Absence* of *evidence* (of association) is not equivalent to *evidence* of *absence*. In general, power calculations are needed to provide an estimate of the type II error (the likelihood of missing a true association where one is present). This information is needed to know how likely it is that absence of association is due to chance or to a sample size too small to detect a true effect of a predetermined magnitude. If power calculations are available, failure to find an association may be construed as class I or class II evidence in support of a conclusion that there is no association if the power is sufficiently large, typically more than 80%. In the absence of power calculations, failure to find an association might be considered at most as class III evidence in support of a conclusion that there is no association. However, power calculations are usually not performed when designing epidemiological studies, and do not guide sample size. In fact, sample size is usually determined by practical constraints of resources (time and budget). Power calculations are not provided in published reports and may be difficult to derive in retrospect.

    Therefore I am proposing an additional criterion that might permit considering failure to find an association as (at most) class II evidence for lack of association. It has two elements: (1) The finding is based on a large sample of patients and a large proportion of patients in the sample and (2) the 95% confidence interval (CI) around the odds ratio of 1.0 is "tight." There are no universally accepted definitions of "large number of patients" or of "tight 95% CI." I propose that the number of patients may be considered "large" if the actual number of patients in the sample is more than 50 and the proportion of patients be considered "large" if all, or close to all, of the patients in the sample inform the conclusion. A 95% CI of round 1.0 may be considered "tight" if its upper limit (UL) is less than 2.0 (to conclude "no increased risk") or if its lower limit (LL) is more than 0.5 (to conclude "no protective effect"). If this criterion is to be applied, then the number and proportion of patients on whom this conclusion is based should be provided, as well as the actual 95% CI, so that readers may decide how robust they consider the conclusion.

Table 7.2 Translating evidence implicating an alleged risk factor for amyotrophic lateral sclerosis into conclusions

Level A rating: This is an established risk factor ("overwhelming evidence")
> Two class I studies, or one class I and two class II studies, or three class II studies, with no contradictory evidence of equal or higher quality ranking, and which lend themselves to the application of the criteria for inferring causation from association.[70]

Level B rating: This is a probable risk factor ("more likely than not")
1. One class I study or two class II studies, with no contradictory evidence of equal or higher quality ranking, and which lend themselves to the application of the criteria for inferring causation from association.[70]
2. Two class I studies, or one class I and two class II studies, or three class II studies, with some contradictory evidence of equal quality ranking. The evidence in favor of inferring risk factor status preponderates, through the application of the criteria for inferring causation from association.[70]

Level C rating: This is a possible risk factor (does not attain a "more likely than not" status). Better designed studies may be warranted regarding this risk factor.
> One class II study or several class III studies, with or without contradictory evidence of equal or lesser quality. If there is contradictory evidence of equal quality ranking, there must be less such evidence than there is evidence favoring risk factor status. The inconsistencies in the evidence do not permit consideration of inferences about causation.
> Biological plausibility is not necessary for assignment to this category.

Level U rating: It is unknown whether this is a risk factor.
> Evidence regarding this risk factor is from conflicting or an insufficient number of class I through class III studies, without a preponderance of evidence one way or another, or is from class IV or V studies, or there is no evidence.
> If evidence that this is not a risk factor outweighs the evidence in support of this being a risk factor, assignment should be to a level A or B rating, as outlined in the following comments.

Comments:
1. This table is designed to permit moving from the default position—that it is not known if a putative risk factor is a risk factor (level U)—to a position that a risk factor has been identified. Consistent evidence in the form of class I through III studies that permit inferring lack of association from failure to find an association (see comment for Table 7.1) should also result in a shift away from level U. However, assignment to level C ("possibly not a risk factor") is meaningless in this setting. Hence, to translate evidence that there is a no association, a simpler system is proposed, whereby a level B rating ("probably not a risk factor") is assigned if there is stronger quality of evidence that there is no association than that there is an association, and a level A rating ("definitely not a risk factor") is assigned if there is a preponderance of evidence for lack of association. Further, it should be recognized that realistically, there will be very little impetus for the scientific and funding communities to replicate even one class II study that establishes that there is no association for a particular presumptive risk factor; hence, one class II study unopposed by equal or higher class evidence is a realistic minimal requirement for assignment of a level B rating for absence of association. This is a small relaxation of the requirements to establish level B rating in support of presence of association.
2. Biological onset of ALS precedes clinical onset, but it is not known by how many years. In all likelihood, the slower the disease progression, the longer it is reasonable to assume its preclinical course has been. Exposures or events that happened within the 1 to 3 years before clinical onset of ALS most likely happened after its biological onset, thus cannot have caused the disease, and constitute class V evidence for risk factor status. Studies may choose to exclude from consideration exposures or events within 5 or even 10 years of clinical onset, to avoid this limitation.

Table 7.2 (continued)

3. Invoking Hill's criteria of inferring causation from association[70] to the process of assignment of risk factor level is done intentionally, recognizing that "risk factor" and "cause" are not synonymous. The purpose is that those risk factors that are assigned higher levels will be further along the road toward potential causal status than if they were mere associations.
4. Biological plausibility. In general, a critical link between a well-established risk factor and causation is biological plausibility. Biological plausibility is proved either by producing the disease in excess in an appropriate animal model exposed to the risk factor or by knowing with certainty how the risk factor would interact with the established biological mechanism of disease causation. In the case of ALS, the biological mechanisms underlying disease causation are not known, animal models of sporadic ALS are lacking, and the animal models of familial ALS may or may not be relevant to the pathogenesis of sporadic ALS. Thus biological plausibility cannot be proven for most risk factors for ALS under consideration. However, biological plausibility may be considered within the framework of existing hypotheses regarding the pathogenesis of ALS, recognizing the speculative or hypothetical nature of this process, for the time being. This is required for levels A and B.

Table 7.3 Considerations in ranking the importance of risk factors in amyotrophic lateral sclerosis

1. Level of establishment of the risk factor status
   a. Greater weight given to a higher level ("established" and "probable")
   b. Some weight given to "possible," with appropriate caveats
   c. No weight given to "unknown"
2. What is the public health impact of the risk factor?
   a. Greater weight given if a large percentage of the population is impacted
   b. Some weight given even if only a small percentage of the population is affected
3. Is the risk factor modifiable?
   a. Greater weight given to modifiable risk factors
   b. Some weight given to non-modifiable risk factors
4. Does the risk factor have co-morbidities unrelated to amyotrophic lateral sclerosis (ALS), or does it have "redeeming features?"
   a. Greater weight given to risk factor with known co-morbidities unrelated to ALS or no "redeeming features"
   b. Lesser weight given if risk factor for ALS may be protective for other more prevalent conditions that might cause earlier morbidity and mortality

resulting in future refinements. Finally, when results point in a particular direction, but do not quite reach the level of drawing conclusions, it is necessary to state what additional data would make a conclusion possible, to make the research cycle regarding a particular question finite. This may influence funding priorities.

The Role of Clusters in Risk Factor Identification

Clusters arising from community reports of patients with ALS/MND have so far yielded no epidemiologically useful information.[73] The most likely cause for that is failure to consider the role of implicit multiple comparisons, which lead to the generation of community-identified clusters resulting from chance alone.[73] Several approaches have been suggested to compensate for the effect of chance in assessing the potential significance of clusters arising from the community.[28,73,74] To conserve clinical and public health resources, we have proposed[73] that the lowest value for the ratio of observed to expected cases that may be considered of potential epidemiological significance should be increased. Case ascertainment and field investigations would be reserved only for those reports that, if confirmed, would represent a cluster not due to chance alone.[73] The likelihood of small clusters to yield epidemiologically meaningful information is small.

Classification of Analytical Studies

Three major types of analytical studies may identify potential risk factors for disease: cross-sectional or prevalence studies, cohort (prospective or retrospective) studies, and case-control studies. Because of the relatively low incidence of ALS, cross-sectional studies and prospective cohort studies have so far been considered impractical as a means of identifying risk factors. This has left the case-control study as the most efficient method for generating or confirming hypotheses regarding possible causal agents. A retrospective cohort study might be used to follow up on hypotheses generated by a case-control study with regards to specific risk factors but cannot be used to identify risk factors. To my knowledge, only two retrospective cohort studies have been done in ALS/MND[75,76]; both showed no increased incidence in the cohorts studied. The chief disadvantages of case-control studies are the multiple sources of biases to which they are subjected[77] and the concern that by testing multiple hypotheses (a "fishing expedition") some may attain significance by chance alone. Unfortunately, most case-control studies to date have not been rigorously designed. Furthermore, there is concern that publication bias, whereby a positive finding is more likely to be published than the lack of such a finding, may favor the identification of spurious risk factors.[78,79] The six major considerations in designing and assessing the significance of published case-control studies are patient homogeneity, choice of controls, recall bias, quantification of activities or exposures, testing of multiple hypotheses, and power of study.[80] Insufficient power[81] may be the most common cause for associations that do not meet clinical significance within case-control studies. The diversity of patient selection criteria and study methodologies in case-control studies of ALS/MND precludes using meta-analysis to overcome this shortcoming.

Retrospective Cohort Studies

A retrospective cohort study[75] showed no increased incidence of ALS/MND in patients who had sustained head trauma. However, because of the fairly low lifetime cumulative risk of ALS/MND (1/1000), even a large cohort, such as that reviewed by Williams et al,[75] which included 821 patients, might not show a modest increase in risk. Conversely, a chance occurrence of ALS/MND in one or two extra people might result in a statistically significant elevation in the attributed risk. A recent mortality study[76] that resulted from an epidemiological investigation of a large number of patients with ALS associated with former work at Kelly Air Force Base in San Antonio, Texas, showed that for now, there is no evidence for excess mortality from ALS there. The recognized limitations of a mortality study done when most of the affected population is alive do not detract from its strengths, in providing a scientifically sound platform for the identification of any large, early excess of cases, if such an excess had been evident. Going forward, it will be necessary to take into consideration the effects of active ascertainment of ALS in this population, when comparing their rates to those of reference populations in which case ascertainment has been passive. This is discussed in more detail elsewhere.[68] These cohort studies did not apply parallel controls but compared observed rates to rates expected from the same or appropriate comparison populations. Hence, they may be considered class II evidence. There are no sources of bias that may affect the validity of their conclusions (which would require assignment to class III or lower). Power calculations are absent, but there was no a priori hypothesis regarding the magnitude of effect (increased incidence of or mortality from ALS/MND) that they set out to detect, and no increase was found.

Case-Control Studies Reported Before 1990

Case-control studies have pointed to numerous potential risk factors including previous mechanical, chemical, and electrical trauma, exposure to heavy metals, occupations dealing with leather, physical labor, and physical activity.[82–111] The results at times are conflicting. Even when they are not, methodological limitations, highlighted by reference to Table 7.1, make it inappropriate to draw inferences from the results of these studies. Most would be considered class IV evidence; those in which biological disease onset likely preceded the occurrence of the risk factor would be considered class V evidence. None are class II evidence, which could provide a basis for a level B "more likely than not" rating. Examining whether any might be class III evidence, which may give rise to a level C "possible" rating is not a fruitful exercise at this time. Of the putative risk factors for ALS, one of the most controversial—recent trauma—was the subject of much discussion that centered around the inadequacies of the data purporting to show such an association; other data showed no association.[3,28,112,113] A later population-based case-control study of risk factors for ALS/MND that showed no association of ALS/MND with antecedent trauma[40] provided additional direct confirmation for the lack of association of excess trauma, before disease onset, with ALS.

Case-Control Studies Reported Since 1990

As a result of the recognized limitations in many of the case-control studies reported before 1990, a higher level of scientific rigor has been reflected in most studies reported in the last decade. Those that may be considered class I through III evidence are discussed here.[68]

Population-Based Case-Control Study in Western Washington State from 1990 to 1994

This was a rigorously designed population-based case-control study that followed on an incidence study[114] and resulted in five articles.[40,115–118] Such a study would be expected to provide class I evidence (see Table 7.1). However, the published methods state that interviewers were not blinded to disease status of respondents, do not state whether interviewers were aware of any of the hypotheses being tested, do not state the total number of hypotheses tested, and do not state if any hypotheses were designated a priori as confirmatory (versus exploratory). Furthermore, approximately one third of eligible controls refused to participate. This resulted in 64.4 percent of controls who had more than high school education, compared with 52.3 percent of cases. Even though education was used as a covariate in the analysis to adjust for this difference, it would increase the likelihood to find exposures associated with jobs requiring less education in patients. Thus in general, the highest level of evidence should be a conservative class II and may be warranted for positive findings (presence of association) where there are strong elements to support an association not due to chance or bias, such as a particularly low p value and a robust dose–response effect (rather than the minimal threshold for statistical significance $p < 0.05$ or a 95% confidence interval [CI] that excludes 1.0). Class III or IV assignment is warranted for all other positive associations because of lack of control for the multiple hypotheses tested and the risk of recall bias by patients. In cases in which it is clear that the exposure was assessed after biological disease onset, a class V assignment is appropriate. Findings of absence of association require separate consideration (see Table 7.1, "Comments"). This discussion depends on absence of other sources of bias that should result in assignment to a lower class of evidence. Using this approach, the study showed the following:

1. An association with exposure to agricultural chemicals in men only[115] (class III). The authors also state that this finding should be considered exploratory. No associations were found for exposures to metals and solvents when relying on assessment by a panel of industrial hygienists evaluating job histories, blinded to participant status (class III evidence, due to upper limit [UL] 95% CI usually >2.0, and small numbers of patients and controls), although such associations were found when relying on self-report (class IV evidence, due to risk of recall bias).
2. Overall no difference in physical activity between patients and controls[116] (class II evidence). This classification is assigned because the absence of statistically significant association is based on findings derived from a study

that was designed to be confirmatory, as reflected by the meticulous methods, even though this is not stated explicitly. Data were quantified from all 174 patients in the sample. In addition to the authors' own analyses, direct inspection shows that in multiple analyses, the proportions of patients grouped based on levels of activity are similar in patients and controls.

3. Slightly more patients reporting participating in organized high school sports (class III evidence), and some indication (in exploratory analysis) of increased risk with greater levels of leisure physical activity approximately 40 years before disease onset (class IV evidence).[116] These are interdependent data.

4. No associations with a family history of neurodegenerative diseases other than ALS (class III evidence: small numbers, concern for underascertainment); an association with a positive family history of ALS was found, as expected.[40]

5. No associations with other factors, including history of physical trauma (fractures [class II], electric shocks [class II for "no injury" shocks, class III for shocks associated with unconsciousness of burns], or surgeries [class II]), residence in rural areas (class II), and (all class III) travel to Western Pacific foci, history of polio, polio immunization, or tetanus immunization.[40] Class II level was assigned if UL 95% CI was <1.5 and more than 50 of the 174 patients informed the result.

6. An association with lifetime cigarette smoking[117] (class II, because of a significant dose–response effect and little chance of these data being influenced by bias).

7. No association with alcohol consumption[117] (class II, UL 95% CI < 1.4 after adjustment for education and smoking, approximately 54% of 161 patients and 59% of 321 controls reported alcohol consumption).

8. Putative dietary risk factors (high glutamate or fat intake increases risk, dietary fiber intake decreases risk).[118] This is class V evidence, because the dietary history was obtained for the year before clinical onset, when the disease was biologically active; hence, the dietary survey cannot be construed as risk factors assessment. The findings may even reflect dietary adjustments made in response to preclinical disease. The multiple comparisons further limit the ability to make any inferences from these findings.

New England 1993 to 1996 Case-Control Study

This was a well-designed study that compared recently diagnosed patients recruited at two referral clinics to population controls identified by random-digit dialing. The findings were reported in three publications.[119–121] Such a study might yield class I evidence with regards to risk factors unlikely to be influenced by referral, self-selection, and recall biases. However, there are limitations similar to that of the Washington county study. For example, only 71 percent of eligible cases and 76 percent of eligible controls participated in the study. Of the controls, 78 percent had a level of education above high school, compared to 67 percent of cases ($p = 0.005$); however, cases tended to have a higher income 5 years before the interview date than controls ($p = 0.082$). It cannot be stated whether these differences in the samples reflect truly differences between the general patient and control populations. However, odds ratio (OR) calculations were adjusted for education (and other factors). These limitations suggest that at best, a lower assignment of class of evidence (class II) is warranted even in cases in which these biases are unlikely to have influenced the findings. If the likelihood of the impact of biases is high, then class IV assignment is appropriate. Dietary exposures were assessed for 5 years before the interview, and patients were enrolled within 2 years of initial diagnosis, which is equivalent, on average, to within 3 years of clinical onset. Thus dietary exposures were assessed, on average, 2 years before clinical onset; however, the disease was probably biologically active at the time, at least in some patients (class V evidence). Other risk factors were assessed for periods that extended earlier, but also included periods of active disease, and the authors were careful to point out when they may have been detecting consequences of disease rather than its causes. An exception to these general rules is the evaluation of lead exposure, where the authors' intent to perform "confirmatory" analysis is clear: The authors state that this was the primary intent of the study and they invested special effort to collect biological samples from patients and controls.[121] The issues in the lead exposure component of the study are not whether multiple comparisons may have resulted in positive findings due to chance alone, but the extent to which biases may have affected the findings, and how biological samples in patients who are already ill should be interpreted: Do they reflect the cause of the disease or its consequence. Applying these criteria, the New England study showed the following:

1. An association with cigarette smoking[119] (class II evidence). A dose–response trend was demonstrated, but the level of statistical significance varied: It was 0.046 using "cigarettes per day" as the measure and 0.084 when using "pack-years" as the measure. Statistical significance was not attained when using "years smoked" as the measure; however, 12 percent of patients, compared to 4 percent of controls, had stopped smoking within the 5 years before the interview date. This likely reflects a case in which the consequences of the disease interfered with continued exposure to the risk factor. The authors considered whether potential population controls who declined to participate may have had an impact on these findings and reported that compared to participants, refusers were less educated and less likely to have ever smoked. This increases the confidence in the findings that cases had greater frequency and quantity of smoking than controls.
2. No association with alcohol use, marijuana use, or family history of neurological disease other than ALS[119] (class III evidence). An association with family history of ALS was found, as expected.
3. Inconclusive data regarding dietary intake. Dietary intake of calcium and antioxidants was not strongly related to risk of ALS (authors' wording)[120] (class V evidence).
4. An association of ALS with self-reported occupational exposure to lead and with elevated blood and bone lead levels, but no association with residential or recreational exposures. Adjusting for occupational exposures had little effect on the association of blood and patella levels, but weakened the association of tibia levels with ALS.[121] The latter observation suggests that blood and patella levels may not be good biological markers for lifetime lead

exposure or that exposure estimates based on the self-reported occupational histories are unreliable. The half-life for lead is 1 month in blood, 3 to 5 years in patella, and 15 to 25 years in tibia.[121] Tibia lead levels would thus be better markers for lifetime exposure, and adjusting for lifetime exposure would thus tend to decrease their association with ALS, as was found to be the case. The self-report results were driven by a small number of cases who provided the margin of excess occupational exposure: approximately 12 of 102. Considering that 154 patients were eligible and 110 are listed as having participated, it is possible that this study of lead as a risk factor for ALS was enriched by patients with such an exposure, who may have been more willing to participate than those who did not have such an exposure. If the denominator had been 154, rather than 102, then the apparent excess would no longer be evident (35/154 = 22.7%, a proportion similar to 54 of 247 controls [21.8%] who reported exposure to lead fumes, dust or particles 10 or more times). Such a self-selection bias would also have enriched the proportion of patients with ALS with elevated blood and bone lead levels, if these were related to lifetime exposure. If the levels are a consequence of the disease, rather than markers of its cause, this discussion is moot. Thus the strength of evidence provided by this study for the association of exposure to lead with ALS is best assigned as class III. The authors conclude that "the hypothesis that lead exposure plays a role in the etiology of ALS deserves further consideration," a conclusion that is consistent with class III evidence.

Scottish Motor Neuron Disease Register 1990/1991 Case-Control Study

A case-control study was performed of 103 of 147 patients with sporadic ALS diagnosed between May 1, 1990, and October 31, 1991, identified from the Scottish MND Register.[122] A structured interview was used to gather data. General practitioners' medical records for patients and controls were reviewed to supplement and corroborate the data from the interviews. The results may be summarized as follows:

1. Results regarding an association of a history of fractures with ALS are inconclusive. A matched case-control analysis for lifetime history of fractures results in an OR of 1.3, with a 95% CI of 0.7 to 2.5. This does not attain statistical significance. The OR for men alone is 0.7 (a putative protective effect) and for women 2.8. Matched analysis for fractures within 5 years of symptom onset shows a highly significant excess in cases. However, in all likelihood, disease was biologically active at the time, and subclinical disease may have caused the fractures.[113] Interestingly, if all 16 fractures within 5 years of clinical onset are excluded, there are 13 case-only couplets, compared to 20 control-only couplets, which might lead to a speculation that remote fractures reduce the likelihood of ALS. Thus the entire association is based on class V evidence (risk factor likely occurred after biological disease onset). There was no correlation between site of fracture and the anatomical area in which the disease began.

2. There was no significant difference between patients and controls in the number of nonbony traumatic events requiring medical attention, total number of operations, or electric shocks (class IV evidence for lack of association, due to lack of actual numbers and CIs).

3. An occupational history that included manual work was more common in patients with MND (OR = 2.6, 95% CI, 1.1 to 6.3). This was based on a detailed lifetime employment history classified according to the Office of Population and Censuses and Surveys (class III evidence, due to low likelihood of bias, but obtained in the context of many comparisons).

4. Regular exposure for a period over 12 months for lead, chemicals/solvents, pesticides, and minerals/ores was reported by patients more frequently than controls. The 95% CI excluded 1.0 for lead and chemicals/solvents (class IV evidence, due to risk of recall bias, difficulties quantifying the exposure, and risk of confounders).

5. No statistically significant associations with environment in childhood, social class, common childhood infections, contact with poliomyelitis, vascular disease, or tobacco use (class IV evidence for lack of association, due to limited data provided).

Epidemiological Correlates of Sporadic Amyotrophic Lateral Sclerosis Case-Control Study

A case-control study was conducted in 1988/1989 using a referral population at the Mayo Clinic, in Rochester, Minnesota.[38] It was designed to be a state-of-the-art case-control study and indeed tried to avoid many of the shortcomings of previous studies. A total of 74 patients were compared to 201 matched controls using a sequential questionnaire/interview technique to gather quantitative data regarding risk factors, with five hypotheses designated a priori as those for which the study would be considered confirmatory. After the classification of evidence system (see Table 7.1), the results of such a study might be considered class II evidence. However, because I am evaluating my own work, and because of methodological limitations of the study, particularly when judged by today's standards, it may be more appropriate to represent the results as class III evidence. The study showed an association with greater exposure to lead and no associations of ALS with hard physical labor, trauma or major surgery, or years lived in a rural community. There was also no statistically significant association of ALS with a family history of neurodegenerative diseases: 68.5 percent of patients reported at least one affected family member, compared to 56.8 percent of controls (OR = 1.65, 95% CI, 0.70 to 2.62, $p = 0.085$). The median percentage of relatives older than 60 years with neurodegenerative diseases was 12.5 percent for patients, compared to 8.3 percent for controls ($p = 0.128$). However, performing the analysis using time to failure or survival methods, as done in another study,[39] may have shown the result to be statistically significant.

Medical Conditions as Risk Factors for Amyotrophic Lateral Sclerosis

In a population-based case-control study,[123] no association was shown between antecedent medical conditions and ALS/MND, based on review of lifetime medical records maintained equally for patients and controls, from before disease onset (class I evidence; no sources of bias evident).

Inferring Causation from Associations: Rules of Evidence

Even if robust associations were provided by epidemiologically sound studies, it is necessary to remember that association does not prove causation. The initial criteria used to establish a causal relationship between agent and disease were Koch's postulates, which were developed to identify infectious agents.[124] These criteria, though rigorous and specific, are not appropriate for settings in which the causal agents may not be infective or may not be present at the time of diagnosis of the illness. For such causes, a different set of rules was developed and proposed concurrently by the Surgeon General's Advisory Committee on Smoking and Health[125] and by Hill.[70] These rules contain seven cardinal requirements for consideration:

1. Chronological relationship
2. Specificity of association
3. Strength of association
4. "Dose-response effect"
5. Consistency of the findings
6. Replicability of the findings
7. Biological plausibility

They are discussed in detail elsewhere.[3,70,126] A special consideration with regards to the requirement of chronological relationship arises when trying to apply these rules to ALS: Cause must precede effect. The risk of ignoring this requirement, particularly in past studies, is recognized better currently, because it is now well established that the biological onset of ALS/MND probably precedes its clinical manifestation by years, in most cases. On average, about 12 months elapses between the onset of the first clinical symptom of ALS/MND and its diagnosis.[13,16,27,38,95] However, the first clinical symptoms occur after the disease has been biologically active, probably for several years, because emergence of weakness requires cumulative loss of motor neurons to have occurred at a rate that is greater than can be compensated for by the rate of reinnervation of muscle by surviving motor neurons. Assuming that progression from clinical onset to death averages 3 years (when approximately 90% of the anterior horn cells at affected levels have degenerated) and that clinical disease can be recognized when half the motor neurons are affected, we have estimated that biological onset might predate clinical onset by at least 3 years. However, motor neuron death is not the first biochemical manifestation of ALS/MND. Hence, the true lower limit for average duration of biological activity of disease before its clinical onset is likely greater than 3 years and perhaps as much as a decade.[112] A longer preclinical course should be postulated in individuals with slowly progressive disease. Data from human studies in partial support of these estimates may be found in a recent, prospective, longitudinal study of asymptomatic individuals with SOD1 mutations for familial ALS with serial MUNE evaluations.[127] It showed that a precipitous drop in motor units occurred, in two carriers of the Val148Gly mutation, several months before symptom onset. In these patients, detectable weakness was present at the time of a 37- to 51-percent reduction in regionally concordant[128] MUNEs, but not when regionally concordant MUNEs were reduced by 12 to 23 percent from baseline. Patient survival from clinical onset was not available in this report.[127]

Conclusions from Analytical Studies

Five recent reviews of the epidemiology of ALS,[113,129–132] as well as several book chapters,[3,80,133] have considered environmental risk factors for ALS. They did not apply a formal EBM approach, and most were broader in the number of factors and studies considered than presented here. However, if evaluated by contemporary standards, the studies that I elected not to consider here would mostly rank as class IV and V evidence. The front-running hypotheses raised by the pre-1990 studies were the focus of the studies reviewed earlier. All the previous reviews came to similar conclusions: No association of an exogenous environmental risk factor with ALS has been demonstrated consistently and convincingly. Causation has not been an issue, given the uncertain and often conflicting nature of most associations shown.

However, I will attempt at this point to apply the criteria presented in Tables 7.2 and 7.3 to place in perspective the data from the evidence classified earlier, which I consider the best available data. The results are summarized in Table 7.4.

Smoking is the only risk factor that merits a level B rating for a probable positive association. There are two studies providing class II evidence to support this level.[117,119] Of note, reference to Table 7.3 shows this risk factor to warrant a high ranking of importance according to all four criteria listed: It is considered "probable," it is modifiable, it has no redeeming features, and it affects a relatively large segment of the population. It is intriguing to speculate that some of the reduction of the male-to-female preponderance of ALS in more recent epidemiological studies is due to the rise in prevalence of smoking among women in the latter part of the last century. Smoking has not been thought of within the framework of "environmental" risk factors in the past, and thus the significance of the two recent studies implicating it may not have struck the scientific and patient community with the same force as would have even one study of equal quality implicating an exogenous, truly environmental, risk factor.

It is possible to assign a level B rating to the statement that the following are *not* risk factors for ALS (only supporting studies providing class I or II evidence listed):

1. Trauma[40,71]
2. Physical activity[116]
3. Residence in rural areas[40]

Table 7.4 Exogenous risk factors for amyotrophic lateral sclerosis/motor neuron disease and their public health implications

Status as risk factor	Modifiable?	Population affected (%)	Redeeming features
A. Probable risk factor			
Smoking[117,119]	Yes	Large	None
B. Probably not risk factor			
1. Trauma[40,71]			
2. Physical activity[116]			
3. Residence in rural areas[40]			
4. Alcohol consumption[117]			
5. Antecedent medical conditions[123]			
C. Selected unproven risk factors (illustrative examples)			
1. Lead	Yes	Small	None
2. Agricultural chemicals	Yes	Small	None
3. Physical prowess	Yes	Small	Yes
4. Dietary glutamate intake	Yes	Unknown	Unknown

4. Alcohol consumption[117]
5. Antecedent medical conditions[123]

Currently, there are no conflicting data of equal or higher evidence class. This rating may be revised if conflicting, high-quality data become available.

All other putative risk factors carry a level C rating or lower. Their potential public health impact is variable. For example, referring to the criteria in Table 7.3, exposure to lead or to agricultural chemicals is modifiable, that is, avoidable, exposures and have no redeeming features. Unfortunately, even if these are ultimately shown to be risk factors, they may play a role only in a minority of patients. The issue of "physical prowess," and, in particular, of excelling in athletics in high school remains of continued interest, but the level of evidence in support of considering it is class III or lower. This includes a recent referral-based case-control study[134] (class IV evidence). Even if physical prowess and slim physique are shown in the future to be robust risk factors for ALS, it will be necessary to control for the survival advantage of being fit, which puts individuals at risk of developing ALS, due to reduced competition from other causes of mortality (gompertzian consideration). The best current data are that physical activity is *not* a risk factor for developing ALS.[116] Dietary risk factors have aroused interest; however, the actual data (outside of Guam) are class V evidence. Although it is intriguing to speculate that high glutamate intake (mainly due to high protein intake) may expose motor neurons to a chronic excitotoxic stimulus, this hypothesis could be tested directly by checking whether different amounts of dietary glutamate change cerebrospinal fluid glutamate in a small number of healthy volunteers. This has not been shown to occur in healthy dogs.[135]

In summary, to date there is no convincing evidence for an exogenous environmental risk factor for developing sporadic ALS. There are two studies[117,119] providing class II evidence in support of the conclusion that smoking is a probable risk factor, with further evidence to support a causal role for it. Both show, to varying degrees, a dose–response effect. Because smoking does not confer a survival advantage, the association with ALS could not be due to lack of competition from other causes of mortality. There is some biological plausibility to consider a role for smoking, a known carcinogen, in producing a condition that acts like a biochemical malignancy. Reduction in the ability to detoxify smoking-related carcinogens by some postmenopausal women[136] may explain that the increased mortality from ALS in a recent report[19] occurred predominantly in women older than 65 years. This is a modifiable risk factor with no redeeming features.

EPIDEMIOLOGY OF FAMILIAL AMYOTROPHIC LATERAL SCLEROSIS

The epidemiological observations that some cases of ALS occurred in families were the basis for the search for causal genes. Identification of the SOD1 mutation underlying one form of familial ALS/MND[137] and of the trinucleotide repeat underlying X-linked spinobulbar muscular atrophy,[138,139] as well as subsequent advances in the genetics of ALS/MND, have transformed the field of familial ALS in the space of less than 10 years. It is now thought of in terms of its genetic classification, rather than its epidemiology. Six loci and two genes have been identified.[140–142] However, epidemiological observations continue to identify the families for genetic research, and the mode of inheritance predicts the effect expected of the abnormal genes. An autosomal dominant mode suggests gain of function; an autosomal recessive mode suggests loss of function. Phenotypic differences based on whether inheritance is maternal or paternal suggest interaction with, or involvement of, mitochondrial genes. Anticipation has been shown to occur in neurological diseases mediated by trinucleotide repeats. Other mechanisms, such as genomic imprinting and germline mosaicism,[143] may also be sought in the future in some forms of familial ALS/MND.

This section provides a brief summary of some of the epidemiological observations in familial ALS/MND. In most series, familial cases make up 5 to 10 percent of patients with ALS/MND.[26,144–148] Familial ALS/MND may be inherited in either an autosomal dominant, an autosomal recessive, or an X-linked recessive pattern.[144,148–156] The most common form of inheritance is autosomal dominant, suggesting a toxic "gain of function."[157,158] Rarely, inheritance is autosomal recessive. In the autosomal dominant families, the male-to-female ratio is close to 1:1. A total of 15 percent of familial cases are due to mutations at the SOD1 gene on chromosome 21, with more than 100 alleles recognized. All result in an autosomal dominant pattern of inheritance, except for the D90A mutation, which is recessive in 20 families with a common founder but dominant in 8 other families without a shared founder.[159] Additional chromosomes implicated in autosomal recessive ALS/MND are chromosomes 15[160] and chromosome 2, on which the responsible gene ("ALS2") was isolated.[140,141] The deletions in the gene identified on chromosome 2 may cause either an autosomal recessive form of juvenile ALS or an autosomal recessive form of PLS. Kennedy's disease, X-linked spinobulbar muscular atrophy, is due to a CAG trinucleotide repeat.[138,139]

Although some forms of familial ALS are indistinguishable from sporadic ALS, other forms of familial ALS have special phenotypes. The mean age at onset for familial ALS is approximately 15 to 20 years earlier than the mean age at onset for the sporadic form. Variability within families is smaller than variability between families with regards to age at onset and duration of disease.[161] This has been shown also in transgenic mouse models of familial ALS. Autosomal dominant familial ALS has variable penetrance (approximately 80%), suggesting the interaction of the gene with other factors. Between 40 and 50 percent of the familial cases show initial involvement of the lower extremities and at least half will have, in addition to anterior horn cell degeneration, clinically silent involvement of spinocerebellar tracts, posterior columns, and the columns of Clarke. Some patients with familial ALS lack UMN signs or evidence of UMN involvement on autopsy.[162]

There has been evidence for phenotypic and genotypic variability of familial ALS.[163,164] Some of the distinguishing features of familial ALS may be the result of selective recognition of stronger familial aggregation among cases with a low mean age at onset.[146] A review of parental sex effect on familial ALS[165] showed that the proportion of maternally transmitted cases increased significantly with age and that the age of the affected parent at disease onset was significantly correlated with the offspring age at onset only when the affected parent was the mother. In addition, in late-onset ALS occurring at ages older than 50 years, the mean offspring age at onset was 9.6 years lower than that of the parent in maternally transmitted cases but was 15.1 years lower in paternally transmitted cases. Anticipation, namely development of ALS in the child at an age before the age at which it developed in the parent, was found in 13 of 15 patients with an affected father and 19 of 26 patients with an affected mother. Based on a similar parental sex effect in Huntington's disease and in autosomal dominant cerebellar ataxia, the speculation that some cases of familial ALS (other than Kennedy's disease) also may be due to excessive numbers on trinucleotide repeats is tantalizing. Alternatively, the effect could involve the existence of a mitochondrial, maternally transmitted protective factor or could be a consequence of either inherited DNA methylation or chromosomal imprinting.[165]

The genetic classification of familial ALS/MND is expected to consolidate its preeminence in the study of these disorders. Clinical and epidemiological observations will continue to be the means of identifying affected families, characterizing their patterns of inheritance and clinical findings, and documenting the phenotypic heterogeneity for patients with similar genetic abnormalities.

EPIDEMIOLOGY OF WESTERN PACIFIC AMYOTROPHIC LATERAL SCLEROSIS

The Western Pacific form of ALS has aroused interest over the past 50 years because its incidence, prevalence, and mortality rates when first identified were 50 to 100 times those of the sporadic form in the continental United States. The male-to-female ratio approximated 2 : 1, the median age at onset was 44 years, and ALS was often associated with a PDC. More recently, the frequency of ALS has declined, although it is still higher than on the continental United States, and the frequency of dementia has increased.[166] The tantalizing implication of a temporary exposure to an environmental risk factor, possibly in a genetically susceptible population, has fueled decades of search and speculation.[167] Three Western Pacific geographical isolates were identified[178]: in the southern Mariana Islands of Guam, in two villages of the Kii Peninsula of Japan, and among the Auyu and Jakai people in a small area of Irian Jaya (western New Guinea). Familial aggregation of ALS/PDC on Guam was recognized in the first published reports from Guam.[168–170] This pattern has persisted to date. However, the pattern of putative inheritance within "afflicted families" has not followed simple mendelian patterns. Genetic explanations of variations from simple mendelian patterns might be possible by postulating involvement of multiple genes, or mitochondrial inheritance of a predisposition to ALS/PDC or of protective factors preventing expression in carriers of a gene, or considering the possibility of false paternity. The prevalence of excessive neurofibrillary tangles in asymptomatic Chamorros, which may suggest a predisposition to neurodegenerative disorders, is also a possible clue. A more recent report suggests separate familial clustering of ALS and PDC on Guam.[171] However, a genetic etiology is not the only possible explanation of familial clustering of disease. Families may share common exposures to dietary or other environmental risk factors, resulting in the familial aggregation. For example, before bacille Calmette-Guérin, the infectious agent causing tuberculosis, was isolated, the tendency of tuberculosis to occur in more than one family member led to speculations that tuberculosis might be a hereditary condition.

Several observations support an environmental etiology for Western Pacific ALS/PDC: the involvement of three apparently different populations; the apparent excess of ALS or PDC among Filipinos who have settled in Guam as young adults[172]; and the trend of increasing age at onset of ALS and PDC in the southern villages of Guam over time.[166] Presence of an exogenous toxin common to the three foci and absence of essential minerals have been considered. A leading candidate as a source for an exogenous toxin has been the seed of the false sago palm, *Cycas circinalis*. Low levels of calcium and magnesium in the soil were also considered to support an environmental deficiency hypothesis.[173,174] However, subsequent studies on Guam have shown an adequate calcium and magnesium content of water and foods grown in the soil of areas such as Umatac, where ALS and PDC are particularly prevalent.[175] The persistence of a high prevalence of neurodegenerative disease in some villages on Guam suggests that the causal factors are still present. However, the changing spectrum suggests changes in the susceptibility of individuals, changes in the burden of environmental risk factors, or changes in the interaction of susceptible individuals with the environmental factors.

The leading hypothesis has postulated exposure to an environmental toxin that peaked during World War II and declined but did not disappear. According to this hypothesis, individuals exposed to higher doses of that toxin developed ALS at a relatively early age, with or without associated PDC, and individuals exposed to a lesser dose developed at a later date ALS with or without PDC, PDC alone, or dementia alone. The seed of the false sago palm, *Cycas circinalis,* and its products have been a focus of investigation in support of this hypothesis. It was identified as a potential cause in field studies by Margaret Whiting.[176] The most immediately active toxin of *Cycas circinalis* is cycasin, a glycoside component with hepatotoxic and carcinogenic effects, but only minimal neurotoxic effects. This toxin is usually removed by the soaking process used to prepare cycad for consumption. A single animal experiment by Dastur in 1964[177] described production of muscle weakness and degeneration of anterior horn cells in a young rhesus monkey fed washed cycad in which cycasin was not detected using the methods of assay available at the time. This finding appeared to be an isolated observation. The cycad hypothesis was kept alive by Kurland[178,179] and received new impetus from Spencer and et al.[180] They suspected that there might be parallels between the neurotoxicity of β-N-oxalyl-amino-L-alanine (BOAA), the compound responsible for lathyrism, and β-N-methylamino-L-alanine (BMAA), which is present in the cycad, both of which have structures similar to glutamic acid. Using a purified L-isomer of BMAA, Spencer was able to produce in monkeys an illness with features of human ALS and possible Parkinson's disease.[181,182] Spencer has further reported use of unwashed cycad as a medicinal in both other foci of Western Pacific ALS, namely, the Irian Jaya focus in western New Guinea (as a poultice) and the Kii Peninsula of Japan (as a "tonic" made from dried seeds of *Cycas revoluta*).[183,184] However, the results of Spencer's feeding experiment in monkeys have not been replicated.[185] The chief difference between the course of animals exposed to exogenous toxins and human disease is the lack of progression of the disease in those animals.[186,187] A pattern of continuous exposure to the toxin would be required to explain a progressive syndrome. Recognizing the limitations of the neurotoxicity hypothesis, Spencer currently favors methylazoxymethanol, a potent alkylating agent, the aglycone of cycasin, as the primary mechanism for the long-latency induction of Western Pacific ALS.[188,189] He postulates that methylazoxymethanol may produce postmitotic DNA damage and interfere with DNA repair, up-regulate the expression of tau messenger RNA by itself or in conjunction with an endogenous excitotoxic agent (neurotransmitter glutamate), and thus promote the accumulation of tau protein and neuronal degeneration in Western Pacific ALS/PDC. However, the primary neurotoxicity hypothesis remains alive, with current focus on a new group of non–water-soluble neurotoxic agents that may be found in washed cycad: three sterol β-D-glucosides.[190,191] They appear to have distinct effects on N-methyl-D-aspartate (NMDA) receptor activation, and NMDA antagonists can block their various actions in vitro. Their acute mode of action results in induction of release of glutamate and lactate dehydrogenase. It remains to be shown whether these neurotoxins can produce chronic, progressive neurodegenerative disease, possibly at a time remote from the time of their consumption, even though other neurotoxins affecting the motor and cognitive systems have not been shown to do so. A recent contribution to the discussion of how a toxic product originating in the cycad may be transmitted to humans, bypassing the detoxification process that usually precedes human consumption of cycad-derived products, has been a hypothesis that consumption of bats who feed on cycad may place humans at risk for ALS/PDC.[192] Further postulated is that biomagnification may occur, by concentrating the putative cycad-derived toxin in the body of the bat. This hypothesis has been debated.[193,194]

CONCLUSION

I find Spencer's proposal of an alkylating agent as causal for Western Pacific ALS/PDC appealing within the framework of my biochemical malignancy hypothesis.[195] In both Western Pacific and sporadic ALS, damaged DNA might result in the emergence of one or more members of a class of altered gene products that would mediate a malignant biochemical transformation. The simplest way for this to occur is if altered gene products belonging to this class had affinity for the target receptors of the natural products, had less biological activity or lacked it altogether, and possibly were less degradable than the natural products. They could interfere with the function of the natural gene products by means of competitive or noncompetitive inhibition. By destabilizing interneuronal feedback mechanisms, the presence of this class of molecules might lead to exhaustion of cells attempting to compensate for their effects, in addition to their primary deleterious actions. A mechanism for Western Pacific ALS/PDC, whereby a remote exposure may increase vulnerability to the effect of endogenous glutamate is consistent also with the role shown for glutamate in sporadic ALS. However, that role appears to be limited. Thus a chronic excitotoxic process may play a secondary role in the clinical course of ALS, possibly by determining (together with the individual's age) the size of the initial motor neuron pool and by serving as one of the factors that influence the rate of disease progression. The truth for Western Pacific ALS/PDC, as for sporadic ALS/MND, may contain elements of both postulated mechanisms of action and additional mechanisms, as yet unenvisioned.

It is gratifying to see clinical, epidemiological, genetic, biochemical, and molecular information derived from many sources converge in the quest to understand why ALS/MND happens, and how its course may be averted or modified. However, the major lesson of the past decades may be that the time frame for progress in unraveling the causes of this condition may need to be measured in decades, or even investigator lifetimes, rather than in 1 or several years or grant-funding cycles. If future epidemiological research is influenced by this assumption, then well-designed cohort studies may be initiated to enhance the armamentarium of epidemiological tools of investigators seeking to elucidate the causes of ALS/MND. Attaching an ALS/MND component to ongoing cohort studies may be the most efficient way to begin. It is hoped that combining more ambitious epidemiological study designs with the current capabilities of gathering, storing, and analyzing genetic material will result in even greater gains in insights into the etiology of ALS 10 years from now than have been attained over the past decade.[195,196]

Acknowledgments

I would like to acknowledge with gratitude the contribution of colleagues, not only through the published literature and interactions in open conferences, but also within recent conferences and meetings coordinated by the ALS Association, California, including a recent workshop on Environmental Factors and Genetic Susceptibility in Amyotrophic Lateral Sclerosis held May 29 through 31, 2002, in Keystone, Colorado.[196] Portions of the material in this chapter have been published previously.[3,68,80,131,133,195]

REFERENCES

1. Brooks BR. El Escorial World Federation of Neurology criteria for the diagnosis of amyotrophic lateral sclerosis. Subcommittee on Motor Neuron Diseases/Amyotrophic Lateral Sclerosis of the World Federation of Neurology Research Group on Neuromuscular Diseases and the El Escorial "Clinical limits of amyotrophic lateral sclerosis" workshop contributors. J Neurol Sci 1994;124: 96–107.
2. Miller RG, Munsat TL, Swash M, Brooks BR. Consensus guidelines for the design and implementation of clinical trials in ALS. World Federation of Neurology committee on research. J Neruol Sci 1999;169:2–12.
3. Armon C. Motor Neuron Disease. In PB Gorelick, M Alter (eds), Handbook of Neuroepidemiology. New York: Marcel Dekker, 1994;407–456.
4. Hirano A, Kurland LT, Krooth RS, Lessell S. Parkinsonism-dementia complex, an endemic disease on the island of Guam. I. Clinical features. Brain 1961;84:642–661.
5. Hirano A, Malamud N, Kurland LT. Parkinsonism-dementia complex, an endemic disease on the island of Guam. II. Pathological features. Brain 1961;84:662–679.
6. Kimula K, Yase Y, Higashi Y, et al. Epidemiological and geomedical studies on amyotrophic lateral sclerosis. Dis Nerv Syst 1963;24:155–159.
7. Shiraki H. The Neuropathology of Amyotrophic Lateral Sclerosis (ALS) in the Kii Peninsula and Other Areas of Japan. In FH Norris Jr, LT Kurland (eds), Motor Neuron Diseases: Research on Amyotrophic Lateral Sclerosis and Related Disorders. New York: Grune & Stratton, 1969;80–84.
8. Gajdusek DC, Salazar AM. Amyotrophic lateral sclerosis and parkinsonian syndromes in high incidence among the Auyu and Jakai people of West New Guinea. Neurology 1982;32:107–126.
9. Fox JP, Hall CE, Elveback LR. Epidemiology: Man and Disease. London: Macmillan, 1970.
10. Miller RG, Rosenberg JA, Gelinas DF, et al. Practice parameter: the care of the patient with amyotrophic lateral sclerosis (an evidence-based review): report of the Quality Standards Subcommittee of the American Academy of Neurology: ALS Practice Parameters Task Force. Neurology 1999; 52:1311–1323.
11. Iwasaki Y, Ikeda K, Ichikawa Y, et al. The diagnostic interval in amyotrophic lateral sclerosis. Clin Neurol Neurosurg 2002;104:87–89.
12. Kurtzke JF. Which "neurodegenerative diseases" are on the rise? Health Environ Digest 1989;3: 3–4, 8.
13. Christensen PB, Hojer-Pedersen E, Jensen NB. Survival of patients with amyotrophic lateral sclerosis in two Danish counties. Neurology 1990;40:600–604.
14. Traynor BJ, Codd MB, Corr B, et al. Incidence and prevalence of ALS in Ireland, 1995–1997: a population-based study. Neurology 1999;52:504–509.
15. Piemonte and Valle d'Aosta Register for Amyotrophic Lateral Sclerosis (PARALS). Incidence of ALS in Italy: evidence for a uniform frequency in Western countries. Neurology 2001;56:239–244.
16. Sorenson EJ, Stalker AP, Kurland LT, Windebank AJ. Amyotrophic lateral sclerosis in Olmsted County, Minnesota, 1925 to 1998. Neurology 2002;59:280–282.
17. Lilienfeld DE, Perl DP. Projected neurodegenerative disease mortality in the United States, 1990–2040. Neuroepidemiology 1993;12:219–228.
18. Ludolph AC, Langen KJ, Regard M, et al. Frontal lobe function in amyotrophic lateral sclerosis: a neuropsychologic and positron emission tomography study. Acta Neurol Scand 1992;85:81–89.

19. Seljeseth YM, Vollset SE, Tysnes OB. Increasing mortality from amyotrophic lateral sclerosis in Norway? Neurology 2000;55:1262–1266.
20. Maasilta P, Jokelainen M, Loytonen M, et al. Mortality from amyotrophic lateral sclerosis in Finland, 1986–1995. Acta Neurol Scand 2001;104:232–235.
21. Gompertz B. On the nature of the function expressive of the law of human mortality. Philos Trans R Soc London 1825;115:513–585.
22. Nielson S, Robinson I, Hunter M. Longitudinal gompertzian analysis of ALS mortality in England and Wales, 1963–1989: estimates of susceptibility in the general population. Mech Ageing Dev 1992;64:210–216.
23. Riggs JE. Longitudinal gompertzian analysis of amyotrophic lateral sclerosis mortality in the U.S., 1977–1986: evidence for an inherently susceptible population subset. Mech Ageing Dev 1990;55: 207–220.
24. Riggs JE, Schochet Jr S. Rising mortality due to Parkinson's disease and amyotrophic lateral sclerosis: a manifestation of the competitive nature of human mortality. J Clin Epidemiol 1992;45: 1007–1012.
25. Chio A, Magnani C, Schiffer D. Gompertzian analysis of amyotrophic lateral sclerosis mortality in Italy, 1957–1987; application to birth cohorts. Neuroepidemiology 1995;1496:269–277.
26. Yoshida S, Mulder DW, Kurland LT, et al. Follow-up study on amyotrophic lateral sclerosis in Rochester, Minnesota, 1925–1984. Neuroepidemiology 1986;5:61–70.
27. Gunnarsson L-G, Lindberg F, Soderfelt B, Axelson O. The mortality of motor neuron disease in Sweden. Arch Neurol 1990;47:42–46.
28. Kurtzke JF. Risk factors in amyotrophic lateral sclerosis. Adv in Neurol 1991;56:245–270.
29. DeDomenico P, Malara CE, Marabello L, et al. Amyotrophic lateral sclerosis: an epidemiologic study in the province of Messina, Italy, 1976–1985. Neuroepidemiology 1988;7:152–158.
30. Lopez-Vega JM, Calleja J, Combarros O, et al. Motor neuron disease in Cantabria. Acta Neurol Scand 1988;77:1–5.
31. Salemi G, Fierro B, Arcara A, et al. Amyotrophic lateral sclerosis in Palermo, Italy: an epidemiologic study. Ital J Neurol Sci 1989;10:505–509.
32. Scarpa M, Colombo A, Panzetti P, Sorgato P. Epidemiology of amyotrophic lateral sclerosis in the province of Modena, Italy. Influence of environmental exposure to lead. Acta Neurol Scand 1988; 77:456–460.
33. Brooks BR, Sufit RL, Depaul R, et al. Design of Clinical Therapeutic Trials in Amyotrophic Lateral Sclerosis. In LP Rowland (ed), Advances in Neurology (vol 56), Amyotrophic Lateral Sclerosis and Other Motor Neuron Diseases. New York: Raven Press, 1991;521–546.
34. Munsat TL, Hollander D, Andres P, Finison L. Clinical trials in ALS: measurement and natural history. Adv Neurol 1991;56:515–519.
35. Louwerse ES, Visser CE, Bossuyt PM, Weverling GJ. The Netherlands ALS Consortium. Amyotrophic lateral sclerosis: mortality risk during the course of the disease and prognostic factors. J Neurol Sci 1997;152(suppl 1):S10–S17.
36. Barkhaus PE, Kennedy WR, Stern LZ, Harrington RB. Hereditary proximal spinal and bulbar motor neuron disease of late onset. A report of six cases. Arch Neurol 1982;39:112–116.
37. Igarashi S, Tanno Y, Onodera O, et al. Strong correlation between the number of CAG repeats in androgen receptor genes and the clinical onset of features of spinal and bulbar muscular atrophy. Neurology 1992;42:2300–2302.
38. Armon C, Kurland LT, Daube JR, O'Brien PC. Epidemiologic correlates of sporadic amyotrophic lateral sclerosis. Neurology 1991;41:1077–1084.
39. Majoor-Krakauer D, Ottman R, Johnson WG, Rowland LP. Familial aggregation of amyotrophic lateral sclerosis, dementia, and Parkinson's disease: evidence of shared genetic susceptibility. Neurology 1994;44:1872–1877.
40. Cruz DC, Nelson LM, McGuire V, Longstreth WT Jr. Physical trauma and family history of neurodegenerative diseases in amyotrophic lateral sclerosis: a population-based case-control study. Neuroepidemiology 1999;18:101–110.
41. Mui S, Rebeck GW, McKenna-Yasek D, et al. Apolipoprotein E epsilon 4 allele is not associated with earlier age at onset in amyotrophic lateral sclerosis. Ann Neurol 1995;38:460–463.
42. Moulard B, Sefiani A, Laamri A, et al. Apolipoprotein E genotyping in sporadic amyotrophic lateral sclerosis: evidence for a major influence on the clinical presentation and prognosis. J Neurol Sci 1996;139(suppl):34–37.
43. Siddique T, Pericak-Vance MA, Caliendo J, et al. Lack of association between apolipoprotein E genotype and sporadic amyotrophic lateral sclerosis. Neurogenetics 1998;1:213–216.

44. Thijs V, Peeters E, Theys P, et al. Demographic characteristics and prognosis in a Flemish amyotrophic lateral sclerosis population. Acta Neurol Belg 2000;100:84–90.
45. Drory VE, Birnbaum M, Korczyn AD, Chapman J. Association of APOE epsilon4 allele with survival in amyotrophic lateral sclerosis. J Neurol Sci 2001;190:17–20.
46. Kurland LT, Kurtzke JF, Goldberg ID, Choi NW. Amyotrophic Lateral Sclerosis and Other Motor Neuron Disease. In LT Kurland, JF Kurtzke, ID Goldberg (eds), Epidemiology of Neurologic and Sense Organ Disorders [Vital and Health Statistics Monograph, American Public Health Association]. Cambridge, MA: Harvard University Press, 1973;108–127.
47. Chio A, Mora G, Leone M, et al. Piemonte and Valle d'Aosta Register for ALS (PARALS). Early symptom progression rate is related to ALS outcome: a prospective population-based study. Neurology 2002;59:99–103.
48. Preux PM, Couratier P, Boutros-Toni F, et al. Survival prediction in sporadic amyotrophic lateral sclerosis. Age and clinical form at onset are independent risk factors. Neuroepidemiology 1996;15:153–160.
49. Tysnes OB, Vollset SE, Larsen JP, Aarli JA. Prognostic factors and survival in amyotrophic lateral sclerosis. Neuroepidemiology 1994;13:226–235.
50. Stambler N, Charatan M, Cedarbaum JM. Prognostic indicators of survival in ALS. ALS CNTF Treatment Study Group. Neurology 1998;50:66–72.
51. Desport JC, Preux PM, Truong TC, et al. Nutritional status is a prognostic factor for survival in ALS patients. Neurology 1999;53:1059–1063.
52. Johnston SC. Prognostication matters. Muscle Nerve 2000;23:839–842.
53. Smith RA, Melmed S, Sherman B, et al. Recombinant growth hormone treatment of amyotrophic lateral sclerosis. Muscle Nerve 1993;16:624–633.
54. Ringel SP, Murphy JR, Alderson MK, et al. The natural history of amyotrophic lateral sclerosis. Neurology 1993;43:1316–1322.
55. Magnus T, Beck M, Giess R, et al. Disease progression in amyotrophic lateral sclerosis: predictors of survival. Muscle Nerve 2002;25:709–714.
56. Armon C, Moses D. Linear estimates of rates of disease progression as predictors of survival in patients with ALS entering clinical trials. J Neurol Sci 1998;160(suppl 1):S37–S41.
57. Armon C, Graves MC, Moses D, et al. Linear estimates of disease progression predict survival in patients with amyotrophic lateral sclerosis. Muscle Nerve 2000;23:874–882.
58. Armon C, Brandstater ME. Motor unit number estimate-based rates of progression of ALS predict patient survival. Muscle Nerve 1999;22:1571–1575.
59. Mazzini L, Corra T, Zaccala M, et al. Percutaneous endoscopic gastrostomy and enteral nutrition in amyotrophic lateral sclerosis. J Neurol 1995;242:695–698.
60. Strong MJ, Rowe A, Rankin RN. Percutaneous gastrojejunostomy in amyotrophic lateral sclerosis. J Neurol Sci 1999;169:128–132.
61. Hardiman O. Symptomatic treatment of respiratory and nutritional failure in amyotrophic lateral sclerosis. J Neurol 2000;247:245–251.
62. Kleopa KA, Sherman M, Neal B, et al. BiPAP improves survival and rate of pulmonary function decline in patients with ALS. J Neurol Sci 1999;164:82–88.
63. Aboussouan LS, Khan SU, Banerjee M, et al. Objective measures of the efficacy of noninvasive positive-pressure ventilation in amyotrophic lateral sclerosis. Muscle Nerve 2001;24:403–409.
64. Lacomblez L, Bensimon G, Leigh PN, et al. Dose-ranging study of riluzole in amyotrophic lateral sclerosis. Amyotrophic Lateral Sclerosis/Riluzole Study Group II. Lancet 1996;347:1425–1431.
65. Blackwood D, Muir W. Molecular genetics and the epidemiology of bipolar disorder. Ann Med 2001;33:242–247.
66. A controlled trial of recombinant methionyl human BDNF in ALS: the BDNF Study Group (Phase III). Neurology 1999;52:1427–1433.
67. Bensimon G, Lacomblez L, Meininger V. A controlled trial of riluzole in amyotrophic lateral sclerosis. ALS/Riluzole Study Group. N Engl J Med 1994;330:585–591.
68. Armon C. An evidence-based medicine approach to the evaluation of the role of exogenous risk factors in sporadic amyotrophic lateral sclerosis [editorial]. Neuroepidemiology 2003;22 (in press).
69. Kuller LH. Circular epidemiology. Am J Epidemiol 1999;150:897–903.
70. Hill AB. The environment and disease: association or causation? Proc R Soc Med 1965;56:295–300.
71. Hirtz D, Ashwal S, Berg A, et al. Practice parameter: evaluating a first nonfebrile seizure in children: report of the quality standards subcommittee of the American Academy of Neurology, The Child Neurology Society, and The American Epilepsy Society. Neurology 2000;55:616–623.

72. Lewis DW, Ashwal S, Dahl G, et al. Practice parameter: evaluation of children and adolescents with recurrent headaches: report of the Quality Standards Subcommittee of the American Academy of Neurology and the Practice Committee of the Child Neurology Society. Neurology 2002;59: 490–498.
73. Armon C, Daube JR, O'Brien PC, et al. When is an apparent excess of neurologic cases epidemiologically significant? Neurology 1991;41:1713–1718.
74. Kurtzke JF. On statistical testing of prevalence studies. J Chron Dis 1966;19:909–922.
75. Williams DB, Annegers JF, Kokmen E, et al. Brain injury and neurologic sequelae: a cohort study of dementia, parkinsonism, and amyotrophic lateral sclerosis. Neurology 1991;41:1554–1557.
76. Mundt DJ, Dell LD, Luippold RS, et al. Cause-specific mortality among Kelly Air Force Base civilian employees, 1981–2001. J Occup Environ Med 2002;44:989–996.
77. Schlesselman JJ. Case-Control Studies Design, Conduct, Analysis. Oxford, United Kingdom: Oxford University Press, Inc., 1982.
78. Koren G, Klein N. Bias against negative studies in newspaper reports of medical research. JAMA 1991;266:1824–1826.
79. Dickersin K, Min Y-I, Meinert CL. Factors influencing publication of research results. Follow-up of applications submitted to two institutional review boards. JAMA 1992;267:374–378.
80. Armon C, Kurland LT, Smith GE, Steele JC. Sporadic and Western Pacific ALS: Epidemiological Implications. In RA Smith (ed), Handbook of Amyotrophic Lateral Sclerosis. New York: Marcel Dekker, 1992;93–132.
81. Hennekens CH, Buring JE. Epidemiology in Medicine. Boston/Toronto: Little, Brown and Company, 1987.
82. Campbell AMG, Williams ER, Barltrop D. Motor neurone disease and exposure to lead. J Neurol Neurosurg Psychiatry 1970;33:877–885.
83. Felmus MT, Patten BM, Swanke L. Antecedent events in amyotrophic lateral sclerosis. Neurology 1976;26:167–172.
84. Hanish R, Divorsky RL, Henderson BE. A search for clues to the cause of amyotrophic lateral sclerosis. Arch Neurol 1976;33:456–457.
85. Palo J, Jokelainen M. Geographic and social distribution of patients with amyotrophic lateral sclerosis. Arch Neurol 1977;34:724.
86. Kondo K. Population Dynamics of Motor Neuron Disease. In T Tsubaki, Y Toyokura (eds), Amyotrophic Lateral Sclerosis. Baltimore: University Park Press, 1979;61–103. Japan Medical Research Foundation publication no. 8.
87. Kurtzke JF, Beebe GW. Epidemiology of amyotrophic lateral sclerosis; a case-control comparison based on ALS deaths. Neurology 1980;30:453–462.
88. Hawkes CH, Fox AJ. Motor neurone-disease in leather workers. Lancet 1981;1:507.
89. Kondo K, Tsubaki T. Case-control studies of motor neuron disease. Association with mechanical injuries. Arch Neurol 1981;38:220–226.
90. Pierce-Ruhland R, Patten BM. Repeat study of antecedent events in motor neuron disease. Ann Clin Res 1981;13:102–107.
91. Angelini C, Armani M, Bresolin N. Incidence and risk factors of motor neuron disease in the Venice and Padua districts of Italy. 1972–1979. Neuroepidemiology 1983;2:236–242.
92. Buckley J, Warlow C, Smith P, et al. Motor neuron disease in England and Wales, 1959–1979. J Neurol Neurosurg Psychiatry 1983;46:197–205.
93. Bharucha NE, Schoenberg BS, Raven RH, et al. Geographic distribution of motor neuron disease and correlation with possible etiologic factors. Neurology 1983;33:911–915.
94. Gawel M, Zaiwalla Z, Rose FC. Antecedent events in motor neuron disease. J Neurol Neurosurg Psychiatry 1983;46:1041–1043.
95. Granieri E, Murgia SB, Rosati G, et al. The frequency of amyotrophic lateral sclerosis among workers in Sardinia. IRCS Med Sci 1983;11:898.
96. Murros K, Fogelhom R. Amyotrophic lateral sclerosis in Middle-Finland: an epidemiological study. Acta Neurol Scand 1983;67:41–47.
97. Gunnarsson L-G, Palm R. Motor neuron disease and heavy manual labor: an epidemiologic survey of Varmland County, Sweden. Neuroepidemiology 1984;3:195–206.
98. Roelofs-Iverson RA, Mulder DW, Elveback LR, et al. ALS and heavy metals: a pilot case-control study. Neurology 1984;34:393–395.
99. Granieri E, Rosati G, Paolino E, et al. The risk of amyotrophic lateral sclerosis among laborers in Sardinia, Italy: a case-control study. J Neurol 1985;232(suppl):15.30.25(abstract).
100. Tarras S, Schenkman N, Boesch R, et al. ALS and pet exposure. Neurology 1985;35:717–720.

101. Tandan R, Bradley WG. Amyotrophic lateral sclerosis. Part I. Clinical features, pathology, and ethical issues in management. Ann Neurol 1985;18:271–280.
102. Gresham LS, Molgaard CA, Golbeck AL, Smith R. Amyotrophic lateral sclerosis and occupational heavy metal exposure: a case-control study. Neuroepidemiology 1986;5:29–38.
103. Holloway SM, Mitchell JD. Motor neurone disease in the Lothian Region of Scotland 1961–1981. J Epidemiol Commun Health 1986;40:344–350.
104. Imaizumi Y. Mortality rate of amyotrophic lateral sclerosis in Japan: effects of marital status and social class, and geographical variation. Jpn J Hum Genet 1986;31:101–111.
105. Plato CC, Garruto RM, Fox KM, Gajdusek DC. Amyotrophic lateral sclerosis and parkinsonism-dementia on Guam: a 25-year prospective case-control study. Am J Epidemiol 1986;124:643–656.
106. Gallagher JP, Sanders M. Trauma and amyotrophic lateral sclerosis: a report of 78 patients. Acta Neurol Scand 1987;75:145–150.
107. Buchman AS, Eisen AA, Hoirch M, et al. Epidemiology of ALS in British Columbia, Canada: evidence for prior environmental toxic exposure. Neurology 1988;38:(suppl 1):271(abstract).
108. Currier RD, Conwill DE. Is amyotrophic lateral sclerosis caused by influenza and physical activity? Results of a twin study. Ann Neurol 1988;24:148(abstract).
109. Granieri E, Carreras M, Tola R, et al. Motor neuron disease in the province of Ferrara, Italy in 1964–1982. Neurology 1988;38:1604–1608.
110. Hawkes CH, Fox AJ. Motor neurone-disease in leather workers. Lancet 1981;1:507.
111. Martyn CN. Motoneuron disease and exposure to solvents. Lancet 1989;1:394.
112. Kurland LT, Radhakrishnan K, Smith GE, et al. Mechanical trauma as a risk factor in classic amyotrophic lateral sclerosis: lack of epidemiologic evidence. J Neurol Sci 1992;113:133–143.
113. Nelson LM. Epidemiology of ALS. Clin Neurosci 1995–96;3:327–331.
114. McGuire V, Longstreth WT Jr, Koepsell TD, van Belle G. Incidence of amyotrophic lateral sclerosis in three counties in western Washington State. Neurology 1996;47:571–573.
115. McGuire V, Longstreth WT Jr, Nelson LM, et al. Occupational exposures and amyotrophic lateral sclerosis. A population-based case-control study. Am J Epidemiol 1997;145:1076–1088.
116. Longstreth WT, McGuire V, Koepsell TD, et al. Risk of amyotrophic lateral sclerosis and history of physical activity: a population-based case-control study. Arch Neurol 1998;55:201–206.
117. Nelson LM, McGuire V, Longstreth WT Jr, Matkin C. Population-based case-control study of amyotrophic lateral sclerosis in western Washington State. I. Cigarette smoking and alcohol consumption. Am J Epidemiol 2000;151:156–163.
118. Nelson LM, Matkin C, Longstreth WT Jr, McGuire V. Population-based case-control study of amyotrophic lateral sclerosis in western Washington State. II. Diet. Am J Epidemiol 2000;151:164–173.
119. Kamel F, Umbach DM, Munsat TL, et al. Association of cigarette smoking with amyotrophic lateral sclerosis. Neuroepidemiology 1999;18:194–202.
120. Longnecker MP, Kamel F, Umbach DM, et al. Dietary intake of calcium, magnesium and antioxidants in relation to risk of amyotrophic lateral sclerosis. Neuroepidemiology 2000;19:210–216.
121. Kamel F, Umbach DM, Munsat TL, et al. Lead exposure and amyotrophic lateral sclerosis. Epidemiology 2002;13:311–319.
122. Chancellor AM, Slattery JM, Fraser H, Warlow CP. Risk factors for motor neuron disease: a case-control study based on patients from the Scottish Motor Neuron Disease Register. J Neurol Neurosurg Psychiatry 1993;56:1200–1206.
123. Armon C, Kurland LT, O'Brien PC, Mulder DW. Antecedent medical diseases in patients with amyotrophic lateral sclerosis. A population-based case-controlled study in Rochester, Minn, 1925 through 1987. Arch Neurol 1991;48:283–286.
124. Tyler CW Jr, Last JM. Epidemiology. In JM Last, RB Wallace (eds), Maxcy-Rosenau-Last Public Health and Preventive Medicine. Norwalk, CT: Appleton & Lange, 1991;11–39.
125. US Department of Health, Education and Welfare. Smoking and Health: A Report of the Surgeon General. Washington, DC: US Government Printing Office, 1964.
126. Ibrahim ME. Rules of Evidence. In ME Ibrahim (ed), Epidemiology and Health Policy. Rockville, MD: Aspen, 1985;39–49.
127. Aggarwal A, Nicholson G. Detection of preclinical motor neurone loss in SOD1 mutation carriers using motor unit number estimation. J Neurol Neurosurg Psychiatry 2002;73:199–201.
128. Armon C, Brandstater ME, Peterson GW. Motor unit number estimates and quantitative muscle strength measurements of distal muscles in patients with amyotrophic lateral sclerosis. Muscle Nerve 1997;20:499–501.
129. Roman GC. Neuroepidemiology of amyotrophic lateral sclerosis: clues to aetiology and pathogenesis. J Neurol Neurosurg Psychiatry 1996;61:131–137.

130. Mitchell JD. Amyotrophic lateral sclerosis: toxins and environment. Amyotroph Lateral Scler Other Motor Neuron Disord 2000;1:235–250.
131. Armon C. Environmental risk factors for amyotrophic lateral sclerosis. Neuroepidemiology 2001; 20:2–6.
132. Noonan CW, Sykes L, Hilsdon R. Motor Neuron Disease/Amyotrophic Lateral Sclerosis: Preliminary Review of Environmental Risk Factors and Mortality in Bexar County, Texas. Agency for Toxic Substances and Disease Registry. March 5, 2002. Available at *www.atsdr.cdc.gov/NEWS/als_032002.html*.
133. Armon C, Kurland LT. Classic and Western Pacific Amyotrophic Lateral Sclerosis: Epidemiologic Comparisons. In AJ Hudson (ed), Amyotrophic Lateral Sclerosis: Concepts in Pathogenesis and Etiology. Toronto: University of Toronto Press, 1989;144–165.
134. Scarmeas N, Shih T, Stern Y, et al. Premorbid weight, body mass, and varsity athletics in ALS. Neurology 2002;59:773–775.
135. Schaeffer MC, Rogers QR, Leung PM, et al. Changes in cerebrospinal fluid and plasma amino acid concentrations with elevated dietary protein concentration in dogs with portacaval shunts. Life Sci 1991;48:2215–2223.
136. Ambrosone CB, Freudenheim JL, Graham S, et al. Cigarette smoking, *N*-acetyltransferase 2 genetic polymorphisms, and breast cancer risk. JAMA 1996;276:1494–1501.
137. Rosen DR, Bowling AC, Patterson D, et al. A frequent ala 4 to val superoxide dismutase-1 mutation is associated with a rapidly progressive familial amyotrophic lateral sclerosis. Hum Mol Genet 1994;3:981–987.
138. Amato AA, Prior TW, Barohn RJ, et al. Kennedy's disease: a clinicopathologic correlation with mutations in the androgen receptor gene. Neurology 1993;43:791–794.
139. Nakamura M, Mita S, Murakami T, et al. Exonic trinucleotide repeats and expression of androgen receptor gene in spinal cord from X-linked spinal and bulbar muscular atrophy. J Neurol Sci 1994; 122:74–79.
140. Yang Y, Hentati A, Deng HX, et al. The gene encoding alsin, a protein with three guanine-nucleotide exchange factor domains, is mutated in a form of recessive amyotrophic lateral sclerosis. Nat Genet 2001;29:160–165.
141. Hadano S, Hand CK, Osuga H, et al. A gene encoding a putative GTPase regulator is mutated in familial amyotrophic lateral sclerosis. Nat Genet 2001;29:166–173.
142. Hand CK, Rouleau GA. Familial amyotrophic lateral sclerosis. Muscle Nerve 2002;25:135–159.
143. Cunniff C. Molecular mechanisms in neurologic disorders. Semin Pediatr Neurol 2001;8:128–134.
144. Mulder DW, Kurland LT, Offord KP, Beard CM. Familial adult motor neuron disease: amyotrophic lateral sclerosis. Neurology 1986;36:511–517.
145. Li T-M, Alberman E, Swash M. Comparison of sporadic and familial disease amongst 580 cases of motor neuron disease. J Neurol Neurosurg Psychiatry 1988;51:778–784.
146. Williams DB, Floate DA, Leicester J. Familial motor neuron disease: differing penetrance in large pedigrees. J Neurol Sci 1988;86:215–230.
147. Williams DB, Windebank AJ. Motor neuron disease (amyotrophic lateral sclerosis). Mayo Clin Proc 1991;66:54–82.
148. Swash M, Leigh N. Criteria for diagnosis of familial amyotrophic lateral sclerosis. Neuromusc Disord 1992;2:7–9.
149. Kurland LT, Mulder DW. Epidemiologic investigations of amyotrophic lateral sclerosis. 2. Familial aggregations indicative of dominant inheritance. Neurology 1955;5:182–258.
150. Hirano A, Kurland LT, Sayre GP. Familial amyotrophic lateral sclerosis: a subgroup characterized by posterior and spinocerebellar tract involvement and hyaline inclusions in the anterior horn cells. Arch Neurol 1967;16:232–243
151. Husquinet H, Franck G. Hereditary ALS transmitted for five generations. Clin Genet 1980;18: 109–115.
152. Emery AE, Holloway S. Familial motor neuron diseases. Adv Neurol 1982;36:139–147.
153. Sobue G, Hashizume Y, Mukai E, et al. X-linked recessive bulbospinal neuronopathy. A clinico-pathological study. Brain 1989;112(pt 1):209–232.
154. Ben Hamida M, Hentati F, Ben Hamida C. Hereditary motor system diseases (chronic juvenile amyotrophic lateral sclerosis). Conditions combining a bilateral pyramidal syndrome with limb and bulbar amyotrophy. Brain 1990;113(pt 2):347–363.
155. Veltema AN, Roos RA, Bruyn GW. Autosomal dominant adult amyotrophic lateral sclerosis. A six generation Dutch family. J Neurol Sci 1990;97:93–115.
156. Appelbaum JS, Roos RP, Salazar-Grueso EG, et al. Intrafamilial heterogeneity in hereditary motor neuron disease. Neurology 1992;42:1488–1492.

157. Siddique T, Figlewicz DA, Pericak-Vance MA, et al. Linkage of a gene causing familial amyotrophic lateral sclerosis to chromosome 21 and evidence of genetic-locus heterogeneity. N Engl J Med 1991;324:1381–1384.
158. Siddique T, Nijhawan D, Hentati A. Familial amyotrophic lateral sclerosis. J Neuroal Transm Suppl 1997;49:219–233.
159. Al-Chalabi A, Anderson PM, Chioza B, et al. Recessive amyotrophic lateral sclerosis families with the D90A SOD1 mutation share a common founder: evidence for a linked protective factor. Hum Mol Genet 1998;7:2045–2050.
160. Hentati A, Oahchi K, Pericak-Vance MA, et al. Linkage of a commoner form of recessive amyotrophic lateral sclerosis to chromosome 15q15-122 markers. Neurogenetics 1998;2:55–60.
161. Juneja T, Pericak-Vance MA, Laing NG, et al. Prognosis in familial amyotrophic lateral sclerosis: progression and survival in patients with glu100gly and ala4val mutations in Cu,Zn superoxide dismutase. Neurology 1997;48:55–57.
162. Cudkowicz ME, McKenna-Yasek D, Chen C, et al. Limited corticospinal tract involvement in sclerosis subjects with the A4V mutation in the copper/zinc superoxide dismutase gene. Ann Neurol 1998;43:703–710.
163. Chio' A, Brignolio F, Meineri P, Schiffer D. Phenotypic and genotypic heterogeneity of dominantly inherited amyotrophic lateral sclerosis. Acta Neurol Scand 1987;75:277–282.
164. Horton WA, Eldridge R, Brody JA. Familial motor neuron disease. Neurology 1976;26:460–465.
165. Leone M. Parental sex effect in familial amyotrophic lateral sclerosis. Neurology 1991;41:1292–1294.
166. Lavine L, Steele JC, Wolf N, et al. Amyotrophic Lateral Sclerosis/Parkinsonism Dementia Complex in Southern Guam. Is It Disappearing? In LP Rowland (ed), Advances in Neurology. New York: Raven Press, 1991;271–285.
167. Kurland LT. Geographic isolates: their role in neuroepidemiology. Adv Neurol 1978;19:69–82.
168. Kurland LT, Mulder DW. Epidemiologic investigations of amyotrophic lateral sclerosis: 1. preliminary report on geographic distribution, with special reference to the Mariana Islands, including clinical and pathologic observations. Neurology 1954;4:355–378.
169. Koerner DR. Amyotrophic lateral sclerosis on Guam: a clinical study and review of the literature. Ann Intern Med 1952;37:1204–1220.
170. Arnold A, Edgren DC, Palladino VS. Amyotrophic lateral sclerosis: fifty cases observed on Guam. J Nerv Ment Dis 1953;117:135–139.
171. McGeer PL, Schwab C, McGeer EG, et al. Familial nature and continuing morbidity of the amyotrophic lateral sclerosis–parkinsonism dementia complex of Guam. Neurology 1997;49:400–409.
172. Garruto RM, Gajdusek DC, Chen K-M. Amyotrophic lateral sclerosis and parkinsonism-dementia among Filipino migrants of Guam. Ann Neurol 1981;10:341–350.
173. Gajdusek DC, Garruto RM, Salazar AM. Ecology of High Incidence Foci of Motor Neuron Disease in Eastern Asia and Western Pacific and the Frequent Occurrence of Other Chronic Degenerative Neurological Diseases in These Foci. Proceedings of the Tenth International Congress on Tropical Medicine and Malaria; Manila, Philippines; Nov. 9–15, 1980;382.
174. Yase Y. The basic process of amyotrophic lateral sclerosis as reflected in Kii Peninsula and Guam. Excerp Med Int Cong Ser 1977;434:413–427.
175. Zolon WJ, Ellis-Neill L. Concentrations of aluminum, manganese, iron, and calcium in four southern Guam rivers. University of Guam Technical Report Water and Energy Research Institute of the Western Pacific, No. 64, 1986.
176. Whiting MG. Toxicity of cycads. Econ Bot 1963;17:271–302.
177. Dastur DK. Cycad toxicity in monkeys: clinical, pathological, and biochemical aspects. Fed Proc 1964;23:1368–1369.
178. Kurland LT, Molgaard CA. Guamaniam ALS: Hereditary or Acquired? In LP Rowland (ed), Human Motor Neuron Diseases. New York: Raven Press, 1982;165–171.
179. Kurland LT, Mulder DW. Overview of Motor Neurone Disease. In M Gourie-Devi (ed), Motor Neurone Disease: Global Clinical Patterns and International Research. New Delhi: Oxford and IBH, 1987;31–44.
180. Spencer PS, Schaumburg HH. Lathyrism: a neurotoxic disease. Neurobehav Toxical Teratol 1983;5:625–629.
181. Spencer PS. Guam ALS/parkinsonism-dementia: a long-latency neurotoxic disorder caused by "slow toxin(s)" in food? Can J Neurol Sci 1987;14:347–357.
182. Spencer PS, Nunn PB, Hugon J, et al. Motor neuron disease on Guam: possible role of a food toxin. Lancet 1986;1:965.

183. Spencer PS, Palmer VS, Herman A, Asmedi A. Cycad use and motor neurone disease in Irian Jaya. Lancet 1987;2:1273–1274.
184. Spencer PS, Ohta M, Palmer VS. Cycad use and motor neurone disease in the Kii Peninsula of Japan. Lancet 1987;2:1462–1463.
185. Garruto RM, Yanagihara R, Gajdusek DC. Cycads and amyotrophic lateral sclerosis/parkinsonism dementia. Lancet 1988;2:1079.
186. Spencer PS, Allen CN, Kisby GE, et al. Lathyrism and Western Pacific Amyotrophic Lateral Sclerosis: Etiology of Short and Long Latency Motor System Disorders. In LP Rowland (ed), Advances in Neurology. New York: Raven Press, 1991;287–299.
187. Duncan MW. Role of the Cycad Neurotoxin BMAA in the Amyotrophic Lateral Sclerosis-Parkinsonism Dementia Complex of the Western Pacific. In LP Rowland (ed), Advances in Neurology. New York: Raven Press, 1991;301–310.
188. Esclaire F, Kisby G, Spencer P, et al. The Guam cycad toxin methylazoxymethanol damages neuronal DNA and modulates tau mRNA expression and excitotoxicity. Exp Neurol 1999;155:11–21.
189. Kisby GE, Kabel H, Hugon J, Spencer P. Damage and repair of nerve cell DNA in toxic stress. Drug Metab Rev 1999;31(3):589–618.
190. Khabazian I, Bains JS, Williams DE, et al. Isolation of various forms of sterol beta-D-glucoside from the seed of *Cycas circinalis:* neurotoxicity and implications for ALS-parkinsonism dementia complex. J Neurochem 2002;82:516–528.
191. Wilson JM, Khabazian I, Wong MC, et al. Behavioral and neurological correlates of ALS-parkinsonism dementia complex in adult mice fed washed cycad flour. Neuromolecular Med 2002;1:207–221.
192. Cox PA, Sacks OW. Cycad neurotoxins, consumption of flying foxes, and ALS-PDC disease in Guam. Neurology 2002;58:956–959.
193. Chen KM, Craig UK, Lee CT, Haddock R. Cycad neurotoxin, consumption of flying foxes, and ALS/PDC disease in Guam. Neurology 2002;59:1664.
194. Cox PA, Sacks OW. Cycad neurotoxin, consumption of flying foxes, and ALS/PDC disease in Guam. Neurology 2002;59:1664–1665.
195. Armon C. ALS: Clinical and Epidemiologic Clues to Pathogenesis. In Neurobiology of ALS. Course Syllabus, 51st Annual Meeting. American Academy of Neurology, 1999.
196. Workshop on Environmental Factors and Genetic Susceptibility in Amyotrophic Lateral Sclerosis; May 29–31, 2002; Keystone, Colorado. Available at *www.alsa.org/research/workshops1.cfm.*

8

Genetic Aspects of Amyotrophic Lateral Sclerosis/Motor Neuron Disease

Peter M. Andersen

A HISTORICAL PERSPECTIVE

Some 20 years before J.-M. Charcot and Joffroy coined the term *amyotrophic lateral sclerosis* (ALS) (1869, 1873), another French doctor, Aran, had presented and published 11 cases of what was then called *progressive muscular atrophy* (PMA).[1–3] Case number 7 is particularly interesting: A 43-year-old sea captain presented with cramps in the muscles of the upper extremities followed by the later development of wasting and paresis. The disease became generalized, affecting also the lower limbs and the patient died 2 years after onset. Aran reports that one of the patient's three sisters and two maternal uncles had died from a similar disease. Charcot apparently ignored Aran's familial case and though his own original description of ALS was based on only 20 cases, claimed that ALS was never hereditary (1873).[2] This belief has unfortunately persisted in many textbooks of neurology up to the present day. The description by Aran was so detailed that later investigators have diagnosed case number 7 as most likely a case of familial ALS (FALS).

EPIDEMIOLOGY OF FAMILIAL AMYOTROPHIC LATERAL SCLEROSIS

Epidemiological studies (Table 8.1) find 0.8 to 13.5 percent of ALS cases to have a family history of the disease (FALS). The tenfold differences in frequency of FALS in these studies can be explained in a number of ways (Table 8.2).

Doctors' inattention and failure to record pertinent family history, as well as incomplete disease penetrance, is probably the most important: In a study of mutations in the copper/zinc superoxide dismutase (SOD1) gene among patients with ALS in the Scandinavian countries, the referring neurologists were

Table 8.1   Frequency of familial amyotrophic lateral sclerosis in some epidemiological studies

Study area	FALS (%)	n	Year	Reference
Germany	13.5	251	1959	4
Central Finland	11.6	36	1983	5
United States	9.5	1200	1995	6
Nova Scotia, Canada	5.8	52	1974	7
Värmland, Sweden	5.6	89	1984	8
England	5.0	580	1988	9
United States	4.9	668	1978	10
Northern Sweden	4.7	128	1983	11
Sardinia	4.4	182	1983	12
Jutland, Denmark	2.7	186	1989	13
Hong Kong	1.2	84	1996	14
Finland	0.8	255	1977	15

FALS = familial amyotrophic lateral sclerosis.

Table 8.2   Factors that may lead to underrepresentation of familial amyotrophic lateral sclerosis cases

1. Different diagnostic criteria have been used
2. Inadequate recording of pertinent family history in the patients charts
3. The ALS disease expresses itself with different subtypes of ALS in different members of the family and are therefore not recognized as being one disease entity
4. Reluctance of the patient to report a hereditary disease
5. Loss of contact between different members of a family
6. Early death to other causes of individuals in the family who transmit the gene defect
7. The child develops ALS before the parent who transmitted the gene defect
8. Incomplete disease penetrance
9. Family members with ALS were misdiagnosed
10. Illegitimacy

ALS = amyotrophic lateral sclerosis.

specifically asked whether the patient had a family history of ALS. About 72 (17%) of the 427 patients included in this study reportedly had a family history of ALS.[16]

Another caveat of the epidemiological studies listed in Table 8.1 are their retrospective nature and lack of medical genealogical studies of the cause of deaths of the ALS patients' relatives. In an unpublished study of the medical genealogy of 153 randomly selected patients with ALS in northern Sweden in the period from 1983 to 1993, 26 (17.4%) were found to have a blood relative with ALS. In more than half the cases, this relative's disease was unknown to the index patient. A traditionally performed epidemiological study in the same geographical area had reported the frequency of FALS to be 4.7 percent.[11]

Table 8.3 Characteristics of familial amyotrophic lateral sclerosis compared with sporadic amyotrophic lateral sclerosis

1. Earlier age at presentation[9,20,21]
2. Relative female preponderance (near unity)[9,20,21]
3. More frequent onset in the lower limbs[20,21]
4. Earlier and persistent absence of ankle reflexes[20]
5. Shorter survival time[9,20,21]
6. More frequent occurrence of sensory features at presentation[9]
7. Normally distributed age at onset in FALS compared with age-dependent incidence in SALS[22]
8. Finding of degeneration of the posterior columns, dorsal spinocerebellar tracts, and nucleus dorsalis of Clarke in 70 percent of patients with FALS[23]

FALS = familial amyotrophic lateral sclerosis; SALS = sporadic amyotrophic lateral sclerosis.

ARE FAMILIAL AND SPORADIC CASES OF AMYOTROPHIC LATERAL SCLEROSIS IDENTICAL?

The poor recording of FALS has made it difficult to delineate any possible differences between FALS and sporadic ALS (SALS). Frequently, SALS and FALS are claimed to be clinically indistinguishable in individual cases,[9,17–20] but some group differences have been noted (Table 8.3).

FALS with posterior column involvement is found in about 70 percent of autopsied FALS cases, although this has rarely been detected clinically ante-mortem.[23] Based on genetic, pathoanatomical and clinical features, FALS has been divided into three major types:[23]

Type I Rapid, progressive loss of motor function with predominantly lower motor neuron (LMN) features and a duration of less than 5 years. Neuropathological changes are limited to the ventral horns and pyramidal tracts

Type II Clinically identical to type I, but at autopsy additional changes are found in the posterior columns, Clarke's column, and the spinocerebellar tracts

Type III Clinically distinguished by survival of more than 10 years but with the same pathological features as found in type II

Supporting the clinical observation that *most* cases of SALS are similar to *most* cases of FALS is a recent discovery of similar neurotoxicity of cerebrospinal fluid (CSF) from 5 patients with ALS with the D90A SOD1 mutation, 5 patients with FALS, and 16 patients with SALS (all tested negative for SOD1 mutation) to rat spinal cord neurons cultured in vitro. This finding tentatively suggests a common pathological pathway in SALS and FALS with or without SOD1 mutation.[24]

There is general agreement that intrafamilial variation in site of onset (bulbar/upper limbs/trunk/lower limbs/diffuse) is common in FALS pedigrees and that within the same family cases with PMA, Charcot-classic type of ALS, progressive bulbar palsy (PBP), flail arm syndrome (Vulpian-Bernhardt form of ALS), and even primary lateral sclerosis (PLS) may be found.[9,17–20] Rare cases with frontotemporal dementia (sometimes preceding the onset of motor symptoms) and ALS have been reported in pedigrees in which other affected cases have not had obvious cognitive dysfunction, whereas in some rare pedigrees, all affected members develop both severe cognitive dysfunction and ALS.[25]

It is important to observe the variable age at onset of symptoms among members of the same family, an intrafamilial variation of 15 to 25 years is a common finding.[9] Also, the disease progression rate may differ markedly among different members of the same family,[26] although in certain pedigrees, the disease progression rate appears to be identical in all affected members.[17]

It has been claimed that female patients may have longer survival than affected males,[27] but this statement is based on small pedigrees with few affected members and has not been substantiated in larger studies.[22,28] A review of the world literature on FALS (84 families with 249 affected cases in 1999) found that in contrast to the age-dependent incidence of SALS, the age at onset of FALS was normally distributed about a mean of 45.7 years (SD ± 11.3 years). Survival curves for FALS demonstrated a markedly skewed distribution with 74 percent surviving at 1 year, 48 percent at 2 years, and 23 percent at 5 years. Age at onset, gender, and site of onset were unrelated variables, and age at onset was the only predictor of survival. It was found that the older the age at onset of FALS, the shorter the survival.[22]

INHERITANCE OF FAMILIAL AMYOTROPHIC LATERAL SCLEROSIS

ALS is not a rare disease and with a lifetime risk of approximately 1 : 1000 in the Western World,[29] the possibility exists that two family members could develop ALS from different causes, including environmental influences. In this context, the very rare occurrence of conjugal ALS should be mentioned to illustrate that the existence of ALS in more than one member of a family does not necessarily imply a common genetic cause for a familial clustering of the disease.

Many FALS pedigrees contain only two affected, sometimes distantly related, blood relatives and it may be difficult to determine whether this reflects common genetic or environmental influences.

In this book, FALS is defined as ALS existing in at least two blood-related individuals separated by not more than four generations. I have investigated a Finnish FALS pedigree in which three siblings in one part of the pedigree had ALS caused by a SOD1 mutation, and two affected second-degree cousins once removed tested negative for a SOD1 mutation. In a Swedish FALS pedigree, ALS was reported to exist in both the paternal and the maternal line of the propositus. DNA analysis revealed the patient to carry a mutation in the SOD1 gene, which was also found in a young paternal cousin, the son of a deceased patient with ALS. Surprisingly, the propositus was also found to have a maternally inherited CAG trinucleotide expansion of the androgen receptor gene on the X chromosome. Investigation and DNA analysis of the reported "ALS cases" in the mother's family showed them to be four cases of spinobulbar muscular atrophy (SBMA). Third, in a large U.S. FALS pedigree, one of the affected was found to be homozygous for the D90A SOD1 mutation, and other affected members of the same family tested negative for a mutation in the SOD1 gene.[30]

Albeit probably rare, the possibility of different etiological causes for ALS among affected members of a family should not be forgotten. This rare possibility complicates research into the cause of the disease and the evaluation of the effect of treatment among different members of the family, raises ethical questions, and makes genetic counseling difficult.

Three mendelian patterns of inheritance have been recognized in adult-onset FALS: By far the most commonly reported is dominant inheritance with high, if not complete, penetrance (all carriers of the single gene defect will eventually develop ALS in an age-dependent manner specific for that gene defect in that particular family).[9,17,18,20,21,25–28] Dominant inheritance with incomplete penetrance (some carriers of the single gene defect will—even though they live to advanced age—not develop ALS but may, with 50% risk, pass the gene defect on to their children) and recessive inheritance (the patient has inherited two identical gene defects: one from the mother and the other from the father who remain unaffected because they have only one defect gene each) have only rarely been reported.[31]

No formal study of the frequency of the three different modes of inheritance exists, but it is my experience from studying FALS pedigrees both in Europe and in North America that families with dominant inheritance with incomplete penetrance (from biological causes or for reasons listed in Table 8.2) are not infrequent and are often diagnosed as SALS cases. Few articles deal with this important issue, which may illuminate the causes of many ALS cases and suggest possible prevention of the disease in genetically predisposed individuals. Many SOD1 mutations have been found in apparently SALS cases or in FALS pedigrees with obvious reduced disease penetrance (see Table 8.8). In fact it may be that many SALS cases are FALS cases with very low disease penetrance. Supporting this notion, Williams et al[31] reported the mean age at onset in eight Australian families with low penetrance to be 60.8 years (i.e., comparable to what is reported for SALS in epidemiological studies) contrasting with 47.8 years in a family with high penetrance.

It has proved to be difficult to find the genes predisposing to ALS. The age-dependent onset in adults (sometimes in individuals with advanced age), short disease duration, genetic heterogeneity, incomplete disease penetrance, misdiagnosis, and other factors have hampered the availability of large pedigrees with multiple affected members in multiple generations, from whom DNA is available for genetic linkage analysis. Linkage analysis is a powerful method to find disease genes: The distribution of genetic markers (traits) in the DNA from affected individuals is compared with DNA from unaffected relatives to find a common set of adjacent markers (a so-called haplotype) that is carried by all the affected individuals and very few if any of the unaffected relatives. The defective gene will, with a certain probability, be in the DNA sequence where the patients but not the unaffected relatives share a common haplotype.

Genetic studies in ALS have been restricted to the few available large pedigrees with mendelian dominant or recessive inheritance with high penetrance, and at present only two genes have been identified. Seven additional gene loci have been identified (Figure 8.1). As an alternative to linkage analysis, based

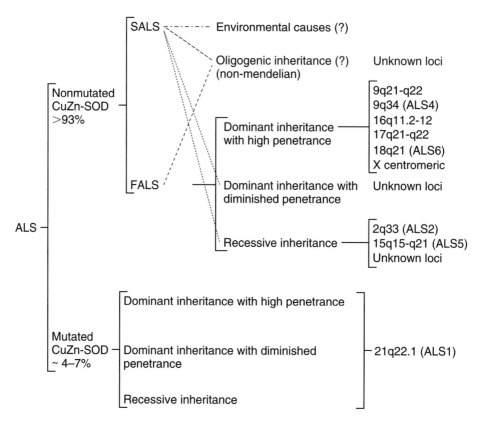

Figure 8.1   The different patterns of inheritance and genetic loci found in ALS. It cannot be excluded that there within the ALS syndrome exist types of ALS that have purely non-genetic causes.

on neuroanatomical findings in ALS and other degenerative diseases, and hypotheses of how the motor system degenerates in ALS, a number of candidate genes have been studied for possible involvement in both FALS and SALS, alas with meager results to date.

GENES KNOWN TO CAUSE AMYOTROPHIC LATERAL SCLEROSIS

Copper/Zinc Superoxide Dismutase

In 1993 an international consortium reported the finding of 11 missense mutations in the gene encoding the enzyme SOD1 (EC 1.15.1.1, superoxide:superoxide oxidoreductase) in 13 of 18 FALS pedigrees.[32] The human SOD1 gene spans 12 kilobases on the long arm of chromosome 21, with five exons and four introns. The five exons code for 153 highly conserved amino acids that, together with a catalytic copper ion and a stabilizing zinc ion, form a subunit. The subunit is further stabilized by an important disulfide bridge C57 to C146, making the subunit extremely stable. Two identical subunits combine through non-covalent binding to form the homodimeric SOD1 enzyme. The known function of SOD1 is to catalyze the reduction of superoxide anion (O_2^-) to molecular oxygen O_2 and hydrogen peroxide (H_2O_2), which is then reduced to H_2O by glutathione peroxidases and catalase. It is ubiquitously expressed in the cytosol of all cells in all organisms above the bacteria and constitutes about 1 percent of the soluble protein in the human brain.

The discovery of mutations in SOD1 in FALS sparked a worldwide search for mutations in the SOD1 gene. The small size of the exons and the absence of repetitive sequences facilitate mutational analysis. Since 1993 some 105 disease-associated mutations in the SOD1 gene have been found, 89 of which are listed in Table 8.4 (an additional 16 are in the process of being published). An earlier reported mutation D109N (GAC to AAC) was later recalled.

Also, six silent mutations and four intronic variants have been reported. Of the 105 disease-associated mutations, 94 are missense mutations causing a change of one amino acid to another but keeping the polypeptide length of 153 amino acids. The 94 missense mutations are in 63 different codons throughout the five exons, including six in exon 3, which codes for the catalytic site. The remaining eleven mutations are nonsense and deletion mutations that either introduce new nucleotides or remove nucleotides in the DNA sequence in exon 4 or exon 5. The result is a change in the length of the final polypeptide. The shortest of these polypeptides is 121 and the longest 156 amino acids long.[70,80] Although most missense mutations are in exon 4 and the nonsense mostly in the beginning of exon 5, there is no obvious correlation of the mutated sites and conserved residues through evolution, enzymic stability, or enzymatic function.[16,85] Some mutants (e.g., H46R and D90A) are as stable as the native SOD1 molecule, whereas others (e.g., L126X and G127X) are highly unstable.[16] Whereas most mutations have been found to cause a reduction in dismutation, four (L37R, A89V, D90A, G93A) have been found to possess essentially normal or only slightly reduced erythrocyte SOD activity (Table 8.5).[57,85,86] These studies were done in different cell systems using various assays in different laboratories, and the results are not directly comparable.

The finding of essentially normal SOD activity for some mutants, combined with the discovery of a murine motor neuron disease (MND) in transgenic mice overexpressing human G93A SOD and absence of motor degeneration in mice genetically engineered to lack expression of SOD1, led to the conclusion that the mutant SOD1 protein causes neurodegeneration by an acquired novel cytotoxic function.[87,88] (The proteotoxicity of mutant SOD1 is further discussed in Chapter 9.)

Unfortunately, only few clinical data have been published for most mutants. An earlier 1996 review concluded that with few exceptions, there are no clinical correlates between a specific mutation and phenotype.[85] Now more data are available and some of the mutants can be grouped according to survival time (Table 8.6), variability in site of onset (Table 8.7), complete or incomplete disease penetrance (Table 8.8), with reservations for small numbers for some mutants. Inexplicably some mutants (i.e. A4V, C6F, G10V, G41S, G93A) are

Text continued on p. 219

Table 8.4 Summary of copper/zinc superoxide dismutase mutations associated with amyotrophic lateral sclerosis

Exon	Pub#	Codon	Genotype	Sequence change	Amino acid change	Location found	Principal reference
Missense and Nonsense Mutations							
I	1	4	A4V	GCC to GTC	Ala-Val	Italy, Sweden, U.S.A.	33
1–23	2		A4S	GCC to TCC	Ala-Ser	Japan	34
	3	4	A4T	GCC to ACC	Ala-Thr	Cyprus, Japan, U.S.A.	35
	4	6	C6F	TGC to TTT	Cys-Phe	Japan	36
	5	6	C6G	TGC to GGC	Cys-Gly	Japan	37
	6	7	V7E	GTG to GAG	Val-Glu	Japan	38
	7	8	L8Q	CTG to CAG	Leu-Gln	Austria	39
	8	8	L8V	CTG to GTG	Leu-Val	U.K., U.S.A.	81
	9	10	G10V	GGC to GGT	Gly-Val	Korea	81
	10	12	G12R	GGC to CGC	Gly-Arg	Italy	40
	11	14	V14M	GTG to ATG	Val-Met	U.S.A.	41
	12	14	V14G	GTG to GGG	Val-Gly	Sweden	16
	13	16	G16A	GGC to GCC	Gly-Ala	U.S.A.	42
	14	16	G16S	GGC to AGC	Gly-Ser	Japan	43
	15	21	E21K	GAG to AAG	Glu-Lys	Scotland	44
	16	21	E21G	GAG to GGG	Glu-Gly	France	45
II	17	37	G37R	GGA to AGA	Gly-Arg	Spain, Turkey, U.S.A.	32
24–55	18	38	L38V	CTG to GTG	Leu-Val	Australia, Belgium, U.S.A.	32
	19	38	L38R	CTG to CGG	Leu-Arg	France	45
	20	41	G41S	GGC to AGC	Gly-Ser	Italy, U.S.A.	32
	21	41	G41D	GGC to GAC	Gly-Asp	U.S.A.	32
	22	43	H43R	CAT to CGT	His-Arg	Australia	32
	23	45	F45C	TTC to TGC	Phe-Cys	Italy	46
	24	46	H46R	CAT to CGT	His-Arg	France, Japan, U.S.A.	47
	25	47	V47F	GTT to TTT	Val-Phe	Italy	46

			Mutation	Codon change	Amino acid	Country	
	26	48	H48Q	CAT to CAG	His-Gln	United Kingdom	48
	27	49	E49K	GAG to AAG	Glu-Lys	France	45
III 56–79	28	65	N65S	AAT to AGT	Asn-Ser	Spain, U.S.A.	49
	29	67	L67R	CTA to CGA	Leu-Arg	France	45
	30	72	G72S	GGT to AGT	Gly-Ser	England	50
	31	76	D76Y	GAT to TAT	Asp-Tyr	Canada, Denmark, New Zealand, U.K.	16
	32	76	D76V	GAT to GTT	Asp-Val	Spain	51
IV 80–118	33	80	H80R	CAT to CGT	His-Arg	Ireland	52
	34	84	L84F	TTG to TTC	Leu-Phe	France, Italy, United Kingdom, U.S.A.	53
	35	84	L84V	TTG to GTG	Leu-Val	Japan, U.S.A.	54
	36	85	G85R	GGC to CGC	Gly-Arg	U.S.A.	32
	37	86	N86S	AAT to AGT	Asn-Ser	Japan, Scotland (Pakistan), Norway	55
	38	89	A89V	GCT to GTT	Ala-Val	Sweden (Finland), U.S.A.	56
	39	90	D90A	GAC to GCC	Asp-Ala	Australia, Belgium, Canada, Estonia, Finland, France, Germany, Italy, Norway, Russia, Sweden, U.K., U.S.A.	57
	40	90	D90V	GAC to GTC	Asp-Val	Japan	58
	41	93	G93A	GGT to GCT	Gly-Ala	U.S.A.	32
	42	93	G93C	GGT to TGT	Gly-Cys	U.S.A.	32
	43	93	G93R	GGT to CGT	Gly-Arg	United Kingdom	59
	44	93	G93D	GGT to GAT	Gly-Asp	U.S.A., Italy	60
	45	93	G93S	GGT to AGT	Gly-Ser	Iceland, Japan, U.S.A.	61
	46	93	G93V	GGT to GTT	Gly-Val	U.S.A., U.K.	62
	47	95	A95V	GCC to GTC	Ala-Val	Ireland	52
	48	95	A95T	GCC to ACC	Ala-Thr	Italy	46

Table 8.4 (continued)

Exon	Pub#	Codon	Genotype	Sequence change	Amino acid change	Location found	Principal reference
	49	96	D96N	GAT to AAT	Asp-Asn	France	63
	50	97	V97M	GTG to ATG	Val-Met	U.S.A.?	42
	51	100	E100G	GAA to GGA	Glu-Gly	New Zealand, U.K., U.S.A.	32
	52	100	E100K	GAA to AAA	Glu-Lys	Afro-American, Germany	64
	53	101	D101N	GAT to AAT	Asp-Asn	Asia/U.K.	65
	54	101	D101G	GAT to GGT	Asp-Gly	United Kingdom	66
	55	104	I104F	ATC to TTC	Iso-Phe	Japan	67
	56	105	S105L	TCA to TTA	Ser-Leu	Sweden	56
	57	106	L106V	CTC to GTC	Leu-Val	Japan, U.S.A.	32
	58	108	G108V	GGA to GTA	Gly-Val	United Kingdom	68
	59	112	I112M	ATC to ATG	Ile-Met	Spain	49
	60	112	I112T	ATC to ACC	Ile-Thr	U.S.A.	60
	61	113	I113F	ATT to TTT	Ile-Phe	Finland	56
	62	113	I113T	ATT to ACT	Ile-Thr	Australia, Canada, France, Italy, Japan, Norway, U.K., U.S.A.	32
	63	114	G114A	GGC to GCC	Gly-Ala	Sweden	56
	64	115	R115G	CGC to GGC	Arg-Gly	Germany	69
	65	118	V118KTGPX	delGinsAAAAC	Val-LysÉstop	United Kingdom	70
	66	118	V118L	GTG to TTG?	Val-Leu	Japan	71
V	67	124	D124V	GAT to GTT	Asp-Val	Australia, U.S.A.	62
119–153	68	125	D125H	GAC to CAC	Asp-His	United Kingdom	48
	69	126	L126GQRWK X	TTG to **G	Leu-...	Japan	72
	70	126	L126X	TTG to TAG	Leu-stop	U.S.A.	73
	71	126	L126S	TTG to TCG	Leu-Ser	Japan	74

72	127	G127GGQRWKX	insTGGG after bp 1450	Gly-...Éstop	Denmark	75
73	132	E132DX	insTT	Glu-Aspstop	United Kingdom	76
74	133	E133deltaE	delGAA	Glu–	U.S.A.	62
75	134	S134N	AGT to AAT	Ser-Asn	Japan	77
76	139	N139K	AAC to AAA	Asn-Lys	U.S.A.	78
77	139	N139D	AAC to GAC	Asn-Asp	France	79
78	144	L144F	TTG to TTC	Leu-Phe	Croatia, Italy, Serbia, U.S.A.	33
79	144	L144S	TTG to TCG	Leu-Ser	U.S.A.	80
80	145	A145T	GCT to ACT	Ala-Thr	U.S.A.	80
81	145	A145G	GCT to GGT	Ala-Gly	Yugoslavia	81
82	146	C146R	TGT to CGT	Cys-Arg	Japan	64
83	147	G147D	GGT to GAT	Gly-Asp	France	79
84	148	V148G	GTA to GGA	Val-Gly	U.S.A., Germany	33
85	148	V148I	GTA to ATA	Val-Ile	Japan	82
86	149	I149T	ATT to ACT	Ile-Thr	U.K., U.S.A.	78
87	151	I151T	ATC to ACC	Ile-Thr	Germany	83
88	intron 4		T to G 10 bp before exon 5		U.S.A.	80
89	intron 4		A to G 11 bp before exon 5		U.S.A.	73

Silent Mutations

1	10	G10G	GGC to GGT	Gly	United Kingdom	70
2	59	S59S	AGT to AGC	Ser	U.S.A.	62
3	116	T116T	ACA to ACG	Thr	New Zealand	84
4	139	N139N	AAC to AAT	Asn	Sweden	16
5	140	A140A	GCT to GCA	Ala	Sweden, U.S.A.	62
6	153	Q153Q	CAA to CAG	Gln	Norway	16

Table 8.5   Copper/zinc superoxide dismutase activity in amyotrophic lateral sclerosis with different mutations

Essentially preserved compared to native protein: G37R, A89V, D90A, G93A
Reduced activity: A4V, C6F, V7E, L38V, H43R, H46R, D76Y, L84V, G85R (inactive), N86S, G93C, G93R, G93V, E100G, I104F, I112T, I113T, D125H, L126X, G127X, E132DX, N139K, V148G, V148I, I149T

Table 8.6   Disease survival time in amyotrophic lateral sclerosis associated with copper/zinc superoxide dismutase mutations (without artificial ventilation)

Fast (<3 yr)	Medium (3–10 yr)	Slow (>10 yr)	Variable
A4T	G93R	G41D	E21G
A4V	G93V	D90A hom	L38V
C6G	D101G	G93D	L84V
L8Q	D101N	E100K	N86S
G10V	—	—	—
G41S	G108V	—	D90A het
H43R	—	—	G93R
H48Q	—	—	I104F
L84V	—	—	I113T
D90V	—	—	L144F
G93A	—	—	—
L106V	—	—	—
I112T	—	—	—
L126X	—	—	—
V148G	—	—	—
V148I	—	—	—

het = heterozygous; hom = homozygous.

Table 8.7   Site of onset in amyotrophic lateral sclerosis associated with a copper/zinc superoxide dismutase mutation

Uniform	Variable	Bulbar onset
H46R	A4V	A4V
D76V	C6G	C6G
L84V	G41S	L8Q
D90A hom	N86S	D76Y
E100K	D90A het	D90A
—	I113T	V148I
—	L144F	I51T
—	V148I	—

het = heterozygous; hom = homozygous.

Table 8.8 Disease penetrance in amyotrophic lateral sclerosis associated with a copper/zinc superoxide dismutase mutation

Complete	Incomplete
A4V	A4T
G41S	L8Q
H46R	D76Y
D76V	N86S
L84V	D90A het
D90A hom	A95T
G108V	I104F
G114A	I113T
L144F	—
V148I	—

het = heterozygous; hom = homozygous.

consistently associated with a very rapid disease independently of site of onset, and other mutants (G41D, H46R, homozygosity for D90A) are always associated with onset in the lower limbs and very slowly ascending paresis. In a third group of mutants, some individuals have very short survival and others in the same family survive for a decade or more. This is best illustrated by the G37R (survival range 2 to 36 years), I104F (3 to 38 years), and I113T mutations (2 to 20 years).[89,90]

Without any obvious correlation to survival time, some mutants consistently have onset in the lower limbs (H46R, D76V, D90A homozygous, E100K) or upper limbs (L84V).[47,51] Variable site of onset is the rule for most mutations (see Table 8.7). For most mutants, there appears to be both intrafamilial and interfamilial variation in sites of onset, with somewhat more frequent onset in the lower limbs than in ALS not associated with SOD1 mutations. Bulbar onset has been claimed to be rare among patients with SOD1 mutations[76,85] but has been reported in some patients (see Table 8.7).

The pedigrees used to find linkage to the SOD1 gene were pedigrees with high penetrance. Unfortunately, only few detailed pedigrees have been published, and at present it is only safe to state that ten mutations are associated with high if not complete penetrance (see Table 8.8). Likewise, some mutations appear to regularly be inherited with reduced penetrance, sometimes obscuring the heredity of the disease. This is particularly the case for the widespread I113T mutation, which interestingly is also associated with a higher mean age at onset (58 years) than that most commonly reported for SOD1 mutations (47 years).[28,91] It is well documented that I113T can pass asymptomatic from a patient down to the grandchildren or even great grandchildren before becoming manifest again.[92,93] Surprisingly, in a U.S. study of the epidemiology of the ALS and SOD1, it was found that I113T shows 100 percent penetrance.[28] This was a retrospective database analysis, with all the limitations of such a study. The author had the opportunity in 1999 to meet both patients and old unaffected members of one of these I113T families. Reduced disease penetrance was clearly evident in at least two branches of the pedigree (but had not been recorded in the charts).

The grouping listed in Tables 8.6 and 8.8 is based on available published data and may change as more patients are diagnosed and data are published. For many mutants, no clinical data are available or the mutation has been found only in single patients, making characterization impossible at present.

The mean age at onset of first symptom is 47 years for patients with an SOD1 mutation, 50.5 years for FALS, and 56 to 58 years for SALS, both without an SOD1 mutation.[28,67,85,91,94] The youngest age at onset of ALS in a patient with an SOD1 mutation was 6 years (I104F)[89] and the oldest 84 years (A4V; I113T)[28] and 94 years (D90A homozygous).[94] The shortest survival time was 14 weeks (N86S homozygous),[95] and the longest 36 years (G37R)[28] and 38 years (I104F).[89] There is surprisingly little variability in the mean age at onset for nearly all mutants, with the exception of G10V, G37R, and L38V, which have a somewhat lower mean age at onset (perhaps biased by small numbers)[28] and I113T with a somewhat older age at onset, as mentioned earlier. That the mutants have the same mean age at onset but very different disease progression rates, uniformity in site of onset or disease penetrance implies that onset of the disease and expression may be two different processes.

Although many patients with SOD1 mutations reportedly are clinically identical to patients without SOD1 mutations (patients with G108V, D125H, and G127X can present with a phenotype complete in accordance with J.-M. Charcot's depictions of 1873),[16,68] a predominantly LMN pattern is the rule for patients with an SOD1 mutation.[16,28,67,76,82,85] No case with predominantly upper motor neuron (UMN) features has been reported. Some mutants may show features of involvement of other parts of the nervous system. Autonomic failure has been reported in cases with G93S and V118L mutations.[61,71] Sensory symptoms, paraesthesia, lancinating pain in the back, localized neuralgic pain in the buttocks, hips or knees, or bladder disturbance have been reported for some mutants.[16,61,84,89,94] In many instances (V14G, E21G, H46R, D90A, E100G), these atypical features have preceded the onset of motor symptoms and have caused difficulties and delay in establishing the ALS diagnosis.[84,94] In H46R and in D90A homozygous patients, this preparetic phase may last for a few months to several years.[94] Autopsy studies have shown that in patients with ALS with SOD1 mutations, the disease process is not confined to the motor system and are type II or III according to the Horton classification.[23]

The most common SOD1 mutation globally is the D90A, followed by the A4V (accounting for about half of all cases in the United States) and the I113T. The D90A is also the only one of the 105 mutations to show recessive inheritance and has as such been found in many SALS cases. Homozygosity for the D90A mutation gives rise to an easily identifiable phenotype with initially a preparetic phase, followed months to years later by slowly ascending creeping paresis and wasting always beginning asymmetrically in the lower limbs.[94] After a mean of some 4 years from onset in the legs, paresis appears in the upper limbs, and 1.5 years later, bulbar symptoms appear. With time, bulbar symptoms have progressed to anarthria and aphagia, and some patients have shown slight pseudobulbar palsy. A few patients have also shown ataxia in the earlier stages of the disease, but it disappears later. At end stage, the patient is completely tetraplegic, with generalized wasting, cachectic, and in some cases with bladder incontinence. Dementia has not been seen in even very long surviving D90A cases but was recently reported for a single case with L144F.[96]

The background for the frequent finding of D90A homozygous ALS cases in Scandinavia is the occurrence of the D90A allele in heterozygous form in a substantial proportion of the population; 5 percent of the population in the Torney Valley in northern Sweden are heterozygous carriers of D90A. In Finland alone, it is estimated that there are 99,000 heterozygous carriers of the D90A allele.[94] A few D90A homozygous ALS patients with the same characteristic phenotype have also been found in Germany, southern France, Italy, Canada, Norway, Russia, and the United States.[97] A haplotype study has shown that all D90A homozygous cases have a common ancestor.[98] Surprisingly, a few D90A *heterozygous* ALS patients have been found in Belgium, Great Britain, northern France, the United States, and Belorussia.[97] Most of these patients have presented a phenotype very different from the D90A homozygous cases with variable sites of onset, disease progression rates, and disease penetrance, showing that the D90A allele can act in a dominant fashion as all other mutations. To explain the uniform phenotype and very slow progression in the D90A homozygous cases, it has been suggested that these patients, in addition to the disease-causing two D90A alleles, also carry a protective or modifying gene that is co-inherited with the D90A SOD1 alleles.[16,94,97] Studies are in progress to identify this modifying gene.

Presently, only the D90A mutation has been proven to show recessive inheritance, but homozygosity for three other mutations (L84F,[45] N86S,[95] L126S[99]) has been found in single individuals in heavily inbred families. In these families, heterozygous individuals also develop ALS and the inheritance is therefore not recessive. Interestingly, the phenotype in at least two of these homozygous cases appears to be far more aggressive than in the heterozygous cases, suggesting a dose effect.[95]

Recently, two siblings with ALS were found to be carriers of both a D90A and a D96N SOD1 allele and the phenotype was rather similar to the D90A homozygous cases.[100] This is the only instance of compound heterozygosity in ALS, but the published pedigree is also consistent with dominant inheritance of D96N with incomplete penetrance, as has been shown for many other SOD1 mutations (see Table 8.8). Presently, this is the only known family with D96N, and until the mutation has been found in more individuals, it is not possible to state with certainty its mode of inheritance.

The prevalence of patients with SOD1 mutations varies greatly from country to country and may partly explain the varying frequencies of FALS reported in different countries (see Table 8.1 and Table 8.9). No patient with an SOD1 mutation has been found in the Netherlands or in Switzerland, and only four mutations in a few patients in Germany, contrasting with four mutations in Scotland and six in Sweden. In Scotland, the I113T has been found in several FALS and apparently SALS cases (all shown to have the same common ancestor),[93] and in Scandinavia, the D90A mutation is very common, particularly in SALS cases.[94] Other mutations found in patients with apparent sporadic disease include V14G, G16S, N19S, E21K, G72S, D76Y, H80R, L84F, N86S, D90A, A95T, D101N, I113T, V118L, V118KTGPX, and E133ΔE. For only one of these, the H80R, has it been possible, through paternity studies, to show that it is a de novo mutation not occurring in the patients' parents.[52] The others are

Table 8.9 Frequency of copper/zinc superoxide dismutase
mutations

In apparently SALS	In FALS
7% (4/56) in Scotland[101]	23.5% in Scandinavia[16]
4% (14/355) in Scandinavia[16]	23.4% in the United States[28]
3% (5/155) in England[70]	21% in the United Kingdom[53]
	20% in the United Kingdom[76]
	14.3% in France[45]

FALS = familial amyotrophic lateral sclerosis; SALS = sporadic amyotrophic
lateral sclerosis.

likely to be FALS with low penetrance, although this has been proven only for
D76Y, D90A, and I113T.

The high prevalence of the A4V in the white population in North America
has, in a haplotype study, been shown to be unrelated to the three small
A4V families found in Italy and Sweden. The widespread occurrence of A4V
in both the United States and Canada implies that it must have been introduced
with some of the first immigrants to North America, or alternatively, that it
already existed in the Indian populations and was introduced into the white
population.[16]

Screening for SOD1 mutations has revealed that SOD1 mutations are not
found in diseases other than ALS,[85] that the only SOD1 polymorphism is the
D90A, and that about one fifth of all diagnosed FALS cases and a small percentage of apparently SALS cases carry an SOD1 mutation (see Table 8.9). The
differences in the prevalence of SOD1 mutations in different countries can be
explained by the different ethnic backgrounds, whether only FALS cases were
studied, the number of studied cases, and the laboratory technique used to
analyze for mutation. Most laboratories have used single-stranded conformational polymorphism (SSCP) as the screening method admitting that its sensitivity is only 85 to 90 percent, depending on the polymerase chain reaction
(PCR) conditions and primers used. Some laboratories have experienced difficulties detecting some mutations[66,72]: Using SSCP and the original published
primer sequences, one laboratory failed to find the D76Y in an apparently SALS
case. Using a different primer set for exon 3, the aberrant banding pattern caused
by the mutation was easily seen on SSCP, and DNA sequencing revealed the
D76Y alteration.[16]

Another example is the V14G, which is very hard to see under different PCR-
SSCP conditions. However, this mutation causes a severe reduction in erythrocyte SOD1 activity, which encouraged the sequencing of the entire gene to find
the V14G mutation.[16] To obtain high sensitivity, we screen for SOD1 mutations
by analyzing SOD activity in erythrocytes (because almost all known mutants
cause a reduction in activity; see Table 8.5) coupled with SSCP denaturing high-
performance liquid chromatography of all five exons. Other laboratories have
opted to do double SSCP under different conditions, and others use automated
DNA sequencing.[66,78]

The 105 mutations that cause a change in the SOD1 polypeptide are probably all disease causing and though for only a small part statistical analysis have shown linkage to ALS or have been shown to cause an MND when expressed in transgenic mice (G37R, G85R, G93A, G93D, D90A, G127X) or transgenic rats (H46R, G93A). The possibility that some mutants found in single patients (i.e., V14G, G16S, S134N) are coincidental findings cannot be excluded until further studies have been done.

In this context, the finding of six silent mutations (mutations that causes a DNA nucleotide change but not a change in the resulting amino acid sequence, because some amino acids are coded for by more than one trinucleotide sequence) should be mentioned. Silent mutations are usually considered to "innocent bystanders" unrelated to the disease. One of the silent mutations A140A deserves special attention because it has now been found in affected cases in a Swedish FALS pedigree with reduced disease penetrance,[16] in a Swedish SALS case, and in two U.S. SALS cases,[62] but never in any controls. A140A could be a coincidental finding, a marker for another disease gene, or—because the protein sequence is unaffected—the mutated messenger RNA (mRNA) sequence may be cytotoxic. Cytotoxic mutated SOD1 mRNA as the gained novel cytotoxic function in ALS could explain the finding of A140A in several ALS cases and not in controls.

ALS2

Recently a second gene was shown to cause a rare juvenile form of ALS called ALS2 by some and RFALS type 3 by others. In 1990, Tunisian researchers described three different forms of juvenile-onset ALS (mean 12 years, range 3 to 15 years) with slow progression and very long survival, in 17 highly inbred families, suggesting recessive inheritance.[102]

Genetic linkage analysis of the single family with type 3 juvenile ALS linked the disease to chromosome 2q33 and recently a mutation in a new gene, ALS2, was shown to co-segregated with the disease.[103] ALS2 is a very large gene of 34 exons coding for a new protein (by some termed ALSIN[104]) of 184 kilodaltons and 1657 amino acids in its long variant and—by alternate splicing after exon 4—of 396 amino acids in a short variant. The short and long variants appear to be expressed in most tissues, including neurons throughout the central nervous system, except in liver where the shorter transcript is predominantly expressed. The protein contains multiple domains that have homology to RanGEF and RhoGEF, suggesting that it is involved in membrane-proximity activities of small guanosine triphosphatases (GTPases) involved in vesicle transport.

In the Tunisian pedigree, a homozygous deletion of nucleotide 261A in codon 46 in exon 3 was found.[103] The mutation causes a frameshift, the introduction of three novel amino acids, and a premature stop codon in codon 50, dramatically truncating the polypeptide at 49 amino acids.

Since then, six more mutations have been reported in ALS2: In an inbred Kuwaiti family with juvenile PLS, a homozygous deletion of nucleotides 1548AG in codon 475 in exon 5 was found. This mutation causes a frameshift and the introduction of 70 novel amino acids followed by a stop codon.[103] In a

consanguineous Saudi Arabian family with juvenile PLS, a homozygous deletion of two nucleotides in exon 9, causing a frameshift and truncation at 645
amino acids, was reported.[104] A further four mutations in the ALS2 gene have
recently been reported in infantile-onset slowly ascending hereditary spastic
paralysis. The mutations all cause premature truncation of the polypeptide, and
because the patients are homozygous for the mutations, loss of protein function
can be predicted. The phenotype of the patients is that of juvenile onset of
slowly evolving spastic tetraparesis, in some individuals with pronounced
pseudobulbar disturbances of affect. Cognitive functioning is not affected. Only
the Tunisian patients also show a peripheral involvement with loss of LMN
function.

Mutations in ALS2 have not so far been reported in patients with typical ALS.
The prevalence of ALS2 in different subtypes of MND is unknown but is probably rare.

Other Genetic Loci Being Investigated

The finding that mutations in SOD1 only accounts for one fifth of all FALS
cases is a disappointment. A hunt to find other genes predisposing to ALS is
being hampered by the lack of suitable pedigrees. A number of loci have been
proposed to be linked to FALS (see Figure 8.1):

9q21-q22 has been associated with ALS with frontal lobe–type dementia.[105]

9q34 has been found in a single large Anglo-American pedigree with dominantly inherited juvenile ALS (mean age at onset, 17 years) with complete
penetrance and very long survival time over many decades.[106] Apparently,
some patients in this family do not die of the disease but do become
severely debilitated. This extends the phenotypical range of ALS.

17q21-q22 maps the gene encoding tau protein. Three affected members
in a family with an exon-10 tau mutation showed ALS-like features with
frontotemporal dementia, and other members developed frontotemporal
dementia with parkinsonism. Age at onset was between 30 and 56 years
and complete penetrance was found in three generations.[107]

18q linkage has been found in a single large European FALS pedigree with
dominant inheritance and complete penetrance. The phenotype is typical
adult-onset ALS.[108]

X-centromeric–linked dominant inheritance has been briefly reported in a
U.S. family with typical adult-onset ALS. Male patients were reported to
have much earlier onset (>20 years) than females in this one family.[109]

15q15-q21 linkage has been found in Tunisian pedigrees with juvenile ALS
and recessive inheritance pattern (juvenile ALS type 1).[110] A third type of
juvenile FALS in Tunisia has failed to show linkage to this locus or to
2q33, showing that there must be at least one more gene or genes involved
in recessively inherited juvenile ALS.

Mutations in the SOD1 gene were originally found in FALS pedigrees with
typical ALS and dominant inheritance over several generations. The finding of
patients with ALS with SOD1 mutations with atypical features, short, medium,
long, or variable survival times with different patterns of inheritance and in

apparently SALS cases, makes it plausible that similar variabilities may be the case for other FALS genes. All studies on the genetics of ALS have focused on monogenic mendelian inheritance. However, the possibility of oligogenic inheritance in both FALS and SALS should not be discounted.

Non-mendelian Inheritance of Amyotrophic Lateral Sclerosis: Risk Factors and Predisposing Genes

A number of observations suggest that genetic factors play a role in SALS. There is a significant male preponderance in SALS, in particular among patients younger than 60 years.[6,11,13,15] Also, certain phenotypical subtypes show a gender preference: Bulbar onset is far more common among women than men,[6,13] and flail arm syndrome or the Vulpian-Bernhardt form of ALS is nine times more frequent among men than women.[111] Interestingly, the Vulpian-Bernhardt form of ALS can be seen both in patients with and in patients without an SOD1 mutation, suggesting that the factor causing this phenotypical expression is not the primary cause of the disease. Longitudinal epidemiological analysis of ALS mortality in Norway,[112] Sweden,[113] and the United States[114] found that ALS affects an inherently susceptible population subset. Table 8.10 lists a number of genes proposed to be risk factor genes, or genes that modify the phenotypical expression of the disease.

Kinesins are microtubule-anchored motor proteins involved in intracellular trafficking. Accumulation of kinesins in spheroids in the spinal cord have been reported in five patients with ALS who have undergone autopsy, and mutation in the neuron-specific kinesin heavy-chain gene in *Drosophila melanogaster* cause progressive distal paralysis.[115] However, at present no study has linked ALS to the loci for neuron-specific kinesins.[115]

Allelic variants of the twin SMNt and SMNc genes and the neighboring NAIP gene are associated with spinal muscular atrophy (SMA) types I through III

Table 8.10 Summary of proposed modifying genes and risk factor genes in amyotrophic lateral sclerosis

Locus	Protein	Principal reference
2, 19q13	Neuron-specific kinesins	115
5q13	SMN and/or NAIP	116, 117
6p21.3	VEGF	118
6q25	Mn-SOD (SOD2)	119
9p13	CNTF receptor α	120
11p12	CNTF	121
11q13	EAAT2	122
14q11.2-q12	APEX nuclease	123
17q21	Tau	107
19q13	Apolipoprotein E	124, 125
22q12	NF-H	126
X	Androgen receptor	127
Mitochondrial DNA	Cytochrome *c* oxidase	128

(described in Chapter 16). Several groups have investigated these genes for possible involvement in adult-onset ALS. In a British study of 130 patients with SALS, 17 patients with FALS, and 5 patients with SBMA, the only finding was a homozygous exon 5 NAIP deletion in a single SALS case.[116] In a French study of SMNt and SMNc in 177 patients with SALS, 66 patients with FALS, and 14 patients with LMN-only MND (PMA type IV), the only finding was homozygous SMNt deletion in 2 and SMNc deletion in 5 of the patients with PMA type IV. None of the 243 patients with ALS had an SMN mutation.[117] NAIP was not studied in this study. A large U.S. study of 194 SALS and 69 FALS (without SOD1 mutations) patients revealed no SMN or NAIP mutations.[129]

Vascular endothelial growth factor (VEGF) is a potent angiogenic factor both in vivo and in vitro, and it is possible that VEGF has neurotrophic functions. The most important regulator of VEGF expression is hypoxia. VEGF is rapidly upregulated in neural tissues and in particular in motor neurons and interneurons upon hypoxia.[130] The regulation is incompletely understood, but a major regulator appears to be the hypoxia-responsive element (HRE). Surprisingly, targeted deletion of the HRE in the VEGF promoter in mice causes an adult-onset MND phenotype with progressive degeneration confined to the LMN in the spinal cord and brain stem.[118] No obvious pathology was found in the UMN in these mice, but it should be remembered that the UMN system is very difficult to study in mice because of the low number of UMNs in mice. The human VEGF gene spans 14 kilobases and consists of seven introns and eight exons. Alternative RNA splicing gives rises to three gene products termed VEGF-121, VEGF-165, and VEGF-189, depending on the length of the final polypeptide. VEGF-165 is the most prevalent form and is a heparin-binding homodimeric glycoprotein of 45 kilodaltons with domains similar to those of platelet-derived growth factor. The role of VEGF in ALS is presently being investigated.

Manganese-containing SOD (SOD2) is a mitochondrial isoenzyme of the cytosolic SOD1, earlier described in ALS. This made SOD2 an obvious candidate gene, but the initial study of exons 3 through 5 of the SOD2 gene in 73 ALS cases was negative.[131] SOD2 is synthesized in the cytosol and through a regulatory polypeptide sequence transported into the mitochondrial matrix, where the regulatory sequence is removed. Three groups have studied whether a known dimorphism A-9V in this regulatory sequence is associated with SALS. A small U.S. study of 20 SALS cases was compared with 10 controls, and homozygosity for the V9 allele was found among the patients with SALS.[132] The opposite result was found in a Swedish study of 72 patients with SALS and 132 controls; homozygosity for A9 was a significant risk factor for ALS, particularly among elderly women.[119] The opposite results of these two studies can be explained by the very small numbers of individuals and the lack of Hardy-Weinberg equilibrium in the U.S. study. However, a third study from the United Kingdom failed to detect any mutations or polymorphisms in SOD2 associated with disease in 77 cases of ALS.[133]

Ciliary neurotrophic factor (CNTF) has a survival-promoting effect on motor neurons. Inactivation of the CNTF gene causes mild progressive motor neuron loss in adult mice but does not result in an MND phenotype. A splice site acceptor mutation in the CNTF gene causes a null mutant allele lacking biological activity. Homozygosity for this null allele has been found in 1 to 2.3 percent of the normal human population. Three studies have failed to find an association with CNTF genotype or the CNTF-α receptor and SALS or any phenotypical subtype of ALS.[120,121]

Variant mRNA transcripts of the astroglial glutamate transporter excitatory amino acid transporter type 2 (EAAT2) have been proposed to play a major role in glutamate excitotoxicity in ALS, although this has not been found in all studies.[134] Two large studies, one American and the other German, searched for genomic mutations in the EAAT2 gene. The only finding was a single missense mutation N206S in an American patient with SALS. The mutation alters a glycosylation site, but the functional significance of this is uncertain.[122]

The levels of apurinic-apyrimidinic endonuclease, or APEX nuclease, have been found to be reduced in the frontal cortex of 11 patients with SALS compared with 6 controls. A reported finding of missense mutations in 8 of 11 U.S. patients with ALS, but not in 5 controls, has not been reproduced by others.[135] A Scottish group examined 117 SALS and 36 FALS cases and found only a four-nucleotide deletion in a SALS case and a silent mutation in 3 patients with SALS. Interestingly, in this study the D148E dimorphism was significantly overrepresented in the SALS group.[123]

Four studies have addressed the issue of whether there is an association between the three apolipoprotein E (ApoE) alleles and ALS. A British study of 124 ALS cases found an association with bulbar onset and the ApoE ε4 allele,[136] and a French study of 130 SALS cases found an even stronger association with bulbar onset, as well as earlier onset of disease in carriers of ApoE ε4. In the French study only, possession of the ApoE ε2 allele was associated with both longer survival and limb onset.[124] In contrast to these two European studies, two large North American studies have failed to find an association between ApoE ε4 genotype and ALS.[125,137]

Neurofilament accumulation is a hallmark of ALS pathology both in ALS with and in ALS without SOD1 mutations and occurs early in the disease in the proximal axons and cell bodies of LMNs. The neurofilament structure is a heteropolymer of three subunits of light, medium, and heavy molecular weights (NF-L, NF-M, NF-H). The genes encoding these subunits are complex and difficult to analyze. In particular, the NF-H gene contains a repeat X-lysine-serine-proline-Y motif. Two polymorphic variants of this motif have been identified with 44 and 43 KSP-repeat motifs, respectively. Five studies of neurofilament mutations in ALS have been published. In the pooled subjects of these studies, 10 of 1047 SALS cases and one of 295 FALS cases were found to have one of seven different mutations in the KSP domain in the NF-H gene. The deletions all occurred within a small region of the NF-H tail. Interestingly, clinical examination of the older brother of the single FALS case with a KSP deletion revealed that he had suffered from focal amyotrophy of the lower limbs for more than 2 decades. No mutations have been found in NF-L and NF-M in humans. NF-H mutations are probably very rare, and their pathological significance is unknown.[126,138–141]

Dynamic, unstable expansion in the CAG trinucleotide tandem sequence is the cause of the ALS-mimic disease SBMA. SBMA is an X-linked recessive disorder, usually with adult onset of very slowly progressive LMN signs, occasionally combined with slight sensory symptoms, tremor, gynecomastia, testicular atrophy, and oligospermia. SBMA can be misdiagnosed as ALS.[127,142] It is my experience that the asymmetrical facial fasciculations with low frequency and high amplitude are distinctive for SBMA and never seen in ALS. A study of CAG repeats in the androgen receptor gene in ALS did not find an association.

Early mitochondrial pathology has been found in transgenic mice with human SOD1 mutations. A single case of SALS with predominantly UMN features has been found to carry a heteroplasmic five-nucleotide deletion in the mitochondrial DNA-encoded cytochrome *c* oxidase.[128]

These studies exclude neuron-specific kinesins, SMNt, SMNc, NAIP, CNTF, CNTF-α, EAAT2, and tau as major disease modifiers in ALS. Further studies are needed to clarify the roles of VEGF, SOD2, APEX nuclease, and NF-H in ALS.

GENETIC TESTING IN AMYOTROPHIC LATERAL SCLEROSIS

At present, only two genes SOD1 and ALS2 have been shown to cause ALS. Whereas the SOD1 gene is small and simple to analyze for mutations, the ALS2 gene is very large and it will be prohibitively expensive to routinely screen ALS cases for mutations in this gene. Testing for mutations in the SOD1 gene has now become part of the clinical investigation of ALS, although it should be remembered that only a small group of patients carry such a mutation. Often not only FALS but also SALS patients request to be tested for an SOD1 mutation. A positive test result for an SOD1 mutation can expedite the diagnostic process, making it possible to start the patient earlier on neuroprotective drugs like riluzole, which may be most effective when administered early in the disease process. Many patients with an SOD1 mutation have predominantly LMN features (e.g., cases with A4V), and because of no or few UMN signs, these patients have earlier been excluded from participating in drug trials. The new revised diagnostic ALS criteria now couple the finding of progressive LMN lesions with an SOD1 mutation as sufficient to establish the diagnosis of ALS, and these patients can now be included in clinical trials. In addition, some patients with ALS with an SOD1 mutation present with a preparetic phase and atypical features. Many of these patients undergo very extensive and expensive investigations before the ALS diagnosis is established. Furthermore, some SOD1 mutations are associated with a specific phenotype, allowing some prognostic estimations (see Table 8.6) and genetic counseling to the family.

Genetic testing in a suspected ALS case should only be performed with the full consent of the patient. Likewise, genetic testing of the patient's relatives should only be done if the patient has been found to carry a specific SOD1 mutation. Screening for SOD1 mutations among unaffected relatives of deceased ALS patients with unknown SOD1 genotype or living patients who do not want to be DNA tested should not be done. Like the presenting individual, the patient with ALS has the right to decide whether or not genetic testing should be performed. Also, presymptomatic testing should be performed only with the full consent of all involved individuals. The test result should not reveal the genotype of an unaffected individual who has declined to be tested. As an example, the grandchild of a patient with ALS with a known SOD1 mutation should not be tested if the child's father or mother has declined testing. Finding a mutation in the grandchild would reveal the parent also to be a gene carrier. If the parent is deceased from other causes, the grandchild can be tested.

Presymptomatic genetic testing in ALS should follow the internationally accepted guidelines for presymptomatic testing in Huntington's disease and hereditary breast cancer.[143] Guidelines for presymptomatic genetic testing in ALS are listed in Table 8.11. The guidelines should be modified to suit the cultural, religious, and legal conditions in the community in which the test subject resides.

We and others have performed presymptomatic genetic testing in individuals belonging to families with the following SOD1 mutations: A4V, H43R, D90A homozygous, E100G, S105L, I113T, G114A, and V148G. If the test subject is a child of a D90A homozygous patient, it is recommended first to test the patient's spouse. The child will at a minimum be obligatorily D90A heterozygous. The spouse genotype will decide whether the child will become

Table 8.11 Proposed guidelines for presymptomatic genetic testing in amyotrophic lateral sclerosis

---

1. The test subject should belong to a family with a known copper/zinc superoxide dismutase mutation.
2. The test subject should be a first-degree relative of an affected blood relative, or second-degree relative of an affected patient if the first-degree relative is deceased from other causes.
3. The test subject should be 18 years or older.
4. The test subject should be mentally and physically healthy.
5. The test subject should not be under emotional stress (e.g., recently married or divorced, have become unemployed, pregnant, etc.).
6. The test subject should participate as a volunteer without influence from a third party.
7. The test subject can at any time demand that the blood sample and test records be destroyed.
8. The test subject should receive a minimum of two genetic counseling sessions before the blood is drawn.
9. The test subject can request more than two genetic counseling sessions.
10. Genetic counseling should be given by professionals with a specific knowledge about amyotrophic lateral sclerosis and genetics.
11. After the blood sample has been drawn, the mutation analysis should be performed as fast as possible to minimize the emotional discomfort of the procedure.
12. The test subject should be informed of the test result at a personal meeting with a genetic counselor. The test result should never be given by letter or electronic communication.
13. The test subject should be accompanied by a close friend at the genetic counseling sessions and when the test result is announced.
14. The test subject can at any time and without explanation withdraw from the test procedure and can choose not to be informed of the test result.
15. Professional and community resources should be available to deal with the impact of test results in the test subject and relatives.
16. The test result is private and should be kept in a separate file in the medical chart.
17. The test result is private and no third party can request taking part in the result.

---

homozygous for D90A. In an anonymous study of the spouses of 18 D90A homozygous ALS patients in Finland and Sweden, two were found to be heterozygous for the D90A mutation and had passed the defective gene on to some of their children, giving rise to D90A homozygosity and ALS in multiple generations.[16,57]

In my experience it is difficult to perform presymptomatic genetic testing in FALS pedigrees with reduced disease penetrance (see Table 8.8). Unless there are very special reasons, presymptomatic testing in these families should be avoided. Relatives of patients with the D90A mutation in heterozygous form or the I113T SOD1 mutation who request genetic counseling should receive particular attention. The unpredictable disease penetrance and the very variable survival time in pedigrees with the I113T mutation make it, in my opinion, virtually impossible to provide good counseling. The uncertainty about the future is most often the main reason for wanting to receive presymptomatic testing in Sweden. A positive test result in a subject from an ALS family with high disease penetrance gives predictable implications, allowing the individual to plan for the future, compared with the test subject from a family with reduced disease penetrance. In the latter case, the uncertainty is not relieved by the positive test result and can cause much emotional discomfort.

Antenatal testing for the SOD1 mutation has to my knowledge not been done in ALS. Before any genetic testing in ALS is done, considerate and careful genetic counseling should be provided.

REFERENCES

1. Charcot J-M, Joffroy A. Deux cas d'atrophie musculaire progressive avec lésions de la substance grise et des faisceaux antéro-latéraux de la moelle épinière. Arch Physiol Neurol Pathol 1869;2:744–760.
2. Charcot J-M. Lecons sur les maladies du système nerveux. Second series, collected by Bourneville 1873. In G Sigerson (translator and ed). Charcot J-M. Lectures on the Diseases of the Nervous System (vol 2, series 2). London: New Sydenham Society, 1881;163–204.
3. Aran FA. Researches sur une maladie non encore décrite du système musculaire (atrophie musculaire progressive). Arch Gen Med 1850;24:5–35, 172–214.
4. Haberlandt WF. Genetic aspects of amyotrophic lateral sclerosis and progressive bulbar paralysis. Acta Genet Med Gemell 1959;8:369–373.
5. Murros K, Fogelholm R. Amyotrophic lateral sclerosis in middle-Finland: an epidemiological study. Acta Neurol Scand 1983;67:41–47.
6. Haverkamp LJ, Appel V, Appel SH. Natural history of amyotrophic lateral sclerosis in a database population. Brain 1995;118:707–719.
7. Murray TJ, Pride S, Haley G. Motor neuron disease in Nova Scotia. CMA J 1974;110:814–817.
8. Gunnarsson L-G, Palm R. Motor neuron disease and heavy labour: an epidemiological survey of Värmland county, Sweden. Neuroepidemiology 1984;3:195–206.
9. Li T-M, Alberman E, Swash M. Comparison of sporadic and familial disease amongst 580 cases of motor neuron disease. J Neurol Neurosurg Psychiatry 1988;51:778–784.
10. Rosen AD. Amyotrophic lateral sclerosis. Clinical features and prognosis. Arch Neurol 1978;35:638–642.
11. Forsgren L, Almay BGL, Holmgren G, Wall S. Epidemiology of motor neuron disease in northern Sweden. Acta Neurol Scand 1983;68:20–29.
12. Giagheddu M, Puggioni G, Masala C, et al. Epidemiologic study of amyotrophic lateral sclerosis in Sardinia, Italy. Acta Neurol Scand 1983;68:394–404.

13. Højer-Pedersen E, Christensen PB, Jensen NB. Incidence and prevalence of motor neuron disease in two Danish counties. Neuroepidemiology 1989;8:151–159.
14. Fong KY, Yu YL, Chan YW, et al. Motor neuron disease in Hong Kong Chinese: epidemiology and clinical picture. Neuroepidemiology 1996;15:239–245.
15. Jokelainen M. Amyotrophic lateral sclerosis in Finland, II: clinical characteristics. Acta Neurol Scand 1977;56:194–204.
16. Andersen PM, Nilsson P, Keränen M-L, et al. Phenotypic heterogeneity in MND—patients with CuZn-superoxide dismutase mutations in Scandinavia. Brain 1997;10:1723–1737.
17. Kurland KT, Mulder DW. Epidemiological investigations of amyotrophic lateral sclerosis. Familial aggregations indicative of dominant inheritance. Part I & II. Neurology 1955;5:182–267.
18. Emery AEH, Holloway S. Familial Motor Neuron Diseases. In LP Rowland (ed), Human Motor Neuron Diseases. New York: Raven Press, 1982;139–145.
19. Tandan R, Bradley WG. Amyotrophic lateral sclerosis. Part 1 & 2. Ann Neurol 1985;18:271–280, 419–431.
20. Mulder DW, Kurland LT, Offord KP, Beard CM. Familial adult motor neuron disease: amyotrophic lateral sclerosis. Neurology 1986;36:511–517.
21. Veltema AN, Ross RAC, Bruyn GW. Autosomal dominant adult amyotrophic lateral sclerosis: a six-generation Dutch family. J Neurol 1990;97:93–115.
22. Strong MJ, Hudson AJ, Alvord WG. Familial amyotrophic lateral sclerosis, 1850–1989: a statistical analysis of the world literature. Can J Neurol Sci 1991;18:45–58.
23. Horton WA, Eldridge R, Brody JA. Familial motor neuron disease. Evidence for at least three different types. Neurology 1976;26:460–465.
24. Tikka TM, Vartiainen NE, Goldsteins G, et al. Minocycline prevents neurotoxicity induced by cerebrospinal fluid from patients with motor neurone disease. Brain 2002;125:722–731.
25. Gunnarsson L-G, Dahlbom K, Strandman E. Motor neuron disease and dementia reported among 13 members of a single family. Acta Neurol Scand 1991;84:429–433.
26. Giménez-Roldán S, Esteban A. Prognosis in hereditary amyotrophic lateral sclerosis. Arch Neurol 1977;34:706–708.
27. Espinosa RE, Okihiro MM, Mulder DW, Sayre GP. Hereditary amyotrophic lateral sclerosis. A clinical and pathologic report with comments on classification. Neurology 1962;12:1–7.
28. Cudkowicz ME, McKenna-Vasek D, Sapp PE, et al. Epidemiology of mutations in superoxide dismutase in amyotrophic lateral sclerosis. Ann Neurol 1997;2:210–221.
29. Bobowick AR, Brody JA. Epidemiology of motor-neuron diseases. N Engl J Med 1973;288: 1047–1055.
30. Siddique T, *personal communication,* 2002.
31. Williams DB, Floate DA, Leicester J. Familial motor neuron disease: differing penetrance in large pedigrees. J Neurol Sci 1988;86:215–230.
32. Rosen DR, Siddique T, Patterson D, et al. Mutations in CuZn superoxide dismutase gene are associated with familial amyotrophic lateral sclerosis. Nature 1993;362:59–62.
33. Deng H-X, Hentati A, Tainer JA, et al. Amyotrophic lateral sclerosis and structural defects in CuZn superoxide dismutase. Science 1993;261:1047–1051.
34. Nakanishi T, Kishikawa M, Miyazaki A, et al. Simple and defined method to detect SOD-1 mutants from patients with familial amyotrophic lateral sclerosis by mass spectrometry. J Neurosci Methods 1998;81:41–44.
35. Nakano R, Sato S, Inuzuka T, et al. A novel mutation in Cu/Zn superoxide dismutase gene in Japanese familial amyotrophic lateral sclerosis. Bichem Biophys Res Commun 1994;200:695–703.
36. Morita M, Aoki M, Abe K, et al. A novel two-base mutation in the CuZn-superoxide dismutase gene associated with familial ALS in Japan. Neurosci Lett 1996;205:79–82.
37. Kohno S, Takahashi Y, Miyajima H, et al. A novel mutation (Cys6Gly) in the Cu/Zn superoxide dismutase gene associated with rapidly progressing familial amyotrophic lateral sclerosis. Neurosci Lett 1999;276:135–137.
38. Hirano M, Fujii J, Nagai Y, et al. A new variant CuZn superoxide dismutase (Val7'Glu) deduced from lymphocyte mRNA sequences from Japanese patients with familial amyotrophic lateral sclerosis. Biochem Biophys Res Commun 1994;204:572–577.
39. Bereznai B, Winkler A, Borasio GD, Gasser T. A novel SOD1 mutation in an Austrian family with amyotrophic lateral sclerosis. Neuromusc Disord 1997;7:113–116.
40. Penco S, Schjenone A, Bordo D, et al. A SOD1 gene mutation in a patient with slowly progressive familial ALS. Neurology 1999;53:404–406.
41. Deng H-X, Tainer JA, Mitsumoto H, et al. Two novel SOD1 mutations in patients with familial amyotrophic lateral sclerosis. Hum Mol Genet 1995;4:1113–1116.

42. Hung W-Y. American Society for Human Genetics Conference [abstract], Denver; 1998.
43. Kawamata J, Shimohama S, Takano S, et al. Novel G16S (GGC-AGC) mutation in the SOD-1 gene in a patient with apparently sporadic young-onset amyotrophic lateral sclerosis. Hum Mutat 1997;9:356–358.
44. Jones CT, Swingler RJ, Brock DJH. Identification of a novel SOD1 mutation in an apparently sporadic amyotrophic lateral sclerosis patient and the detection of Ile113Thr in three others. Hum Mol Genet 1994;3:649–650.
45. Boukaftane Y, Khoris J, Moulard B, et al. Identification of six novel SOD1 gene mutations in familial amyotrophic lateral sclerosis. Can J Neurol Sci 1998;25:192–196.
46. Gellera C, Castelotti B, Riggio MC, et al. Superoxide dismutase gene mutations in Italian patients with familial and sporadic amyotrophic lateral sclerosis: identification of three novel missense mutations. Neuromusc Disord 2001;11:404–410.
47. Aoki M, Ogasawara M, Matsubara Y, et al. Mild ALS in Japan associated with novel SOD mutation. Nat Genet 1993;5:323–324.
48. Enayat ZE, Orrell RW, Claus A, et al. Two novel mutations in the gene for copper zinc superoxide dismutase in UK families with amyotrophic lateral sclerosis. Hum Mol Genet 1995;4:1239–1240.
49. Esteban J, *personal communication,* 1999.
50. Orrell RW, Marklund SL, de Belleroche JS. Familial ALS is associated with mutations in all exons of SOD1: a novel mutation in exon 3 (Gly72Ser). J Neurol Sci 1997;153:46–49.
51. Segovia-Silvestre T, Andreu LA, Vives-Bauza C, et al. A novel exon 3 mutation (D76V) in the SOD1 gene associated with slowly progressive ALS. Amyotroph Lateral Scler Other Motor Neuron Disord (in press).
52. Hardiman O, *personal communication,* 2000.
53. Shaw CE, Enayat ZE, Chioza BA, et al. Mutations in all five exons of SOD-1 may cause ALS. Ann Neurol 1998;43:390–394.
54. Aoki M, Abe K, Houi K, et al. Variance of age at onset in a Japanese family with amyotrophic lateral sclerosis associated with a novel CuZn-superoxide dismutase mutation. Ann Neurol 1995;37:676–679.
55. Maeda T, Kurahashi K, Matsunaga M, et al. On intra-familial clinical diversities of a familial amyotrophic lateral sclerosis with a point mutation of Cu/Zn superoxide dismutase (Asn86-Ser). No To Shinkei 1997;49:847–851.
56. Jacobsson J, Jonsson PA, Andersen PM, et al. Superoxide dismutase in CSF from ALS patients with and without CuZn-superoxide dismutase mutations. Brain 2001;124:1461–1466.
57. Andersen PM, Nilsson P, Ala-Hurula V, et al. Amyotrophic lateral sclerosis associated with homozygosity for an Asp90Ala mutation in CuZn-superoxide dismutase. Nat Genet 1995;10:61–66.
58. Morita M, Abe K, Takahashi M, et al. A novel mutation Asp90Val in the SOD1 gene associated with Japanese familial ALS. Eur J Neurol 1998;5:389–392.
59. Elshafey A, Lanyon WG, Connor JM. Identification of a new missense mutation in exon 4 of the Cu/Zn superoxide dismutase (SOD-1) gene in a family with amyotrophic lateral sclerosis. Hum Mol Genet 1994;2:363–364.
60. Esteban J, Rosen DR, Bowling AC, et al. Identification of two mutations and a new polymorphism in the gene for CuZn-superoxide dismutase in patients with amyotrophic lateral sclerosis. Hum Mol Genet 1994;3:997–998.
61. Kawata A, Kato S, Hayashi H, Hirai S. Prominent sensory and autonomic disturbances in familial amyotrophic lateral sclerosis with a Gly93Ser mutation in the SOD1 gene. J Neurol Sci 1997;153:82–85.
62. Hosler BA, Nicholson GA, Sapp PC, et al. Three novel mutations and two variants in the gene for Cu/Zn superoxide dismutase in familial amyotrophic lateral sclerosis. Neuromusc Disord 1996;6:361–366.
63. Hand CK, Mayeux-Portas V, Khoris J, et al. Compound heterozygous D90A and D96N SOD1 mutations in a recessive amyotrophic lateral sclerosis family. Ann Neurol 2001;49:267–271.
64. Siddique T, Deng H-X. Genetics of amyotrophic lateral sclerosis. Hum Mol Genet 1996;5:1465–1470.
65. Jones CT, Shaw PJ, Chari G, Brock DJH. Identification of a novel exon 4 SOD1 mutation in a sporadic amyotrophic lateral sclerosis patient. Mol Cell Probes 1994;8:329–330.
66. Yulug IG, Katsanis N, de Belleroche J, et al. An improved protocol for the analysis of SOD1 mutations, and a new mutation in exon 4. Hum Mol Genet 1995;4:1101–1104.
67. Abe K, Aoki M, Ikeda M, et al. Clinical characteristics of familial amyotrophic lateral sclerosis with Cu/Zn superoxide dismutase gene mutations. J Neurol Sci 1996;136:108–116.

68. Orrell RW, Jabgood JJ, Shepherd DI, et al. A novel mutation of SOD1 (Gly108Val) in familial amyotrophic lateral sclerosis. Eur J Neurol 1997;4:48–51.
69. Kostrzewa M, Burck-Lehmann, Müller U. Autosomal dominant amyotrophic lateral sclerosis: a novel mutation in the CuZn superoxide dismutase-1 gene. Hum Mol Genet 1994;3:2261–2262.
70. Jackson M, Al-Chalabi A, Enayat ZE, et al. Copper/zinc superoxide dismutase 1 and sporadic amyotrophic lateral sclerosis: analysis of 155 cases and identification of a novel insertion mutation. Ann Neurol 1997;42:803–807.
71. Shimizu T, Kawata A, Kato S, et al. Autonomic failure in ALS with novel SOD1 gene mutation. Neurology 2000;54:1534–1537.
72. Pramatarova A, Goto J, Nanba E, et al. A two basepair deletion in the SOD1 gene causes familial amyotrophic lateral sclerosis. Hum Mol Genet 1994;3:2061–2062.
73. Zu JS, Deng H-X, Lo TP, et al. Exon 5 encoded domain is not required for the toxic function of mutant SOD1 but essential for the dismutase activity: identification and characterization of two new SOD1 mutations associated with familial amyotrophic lateral sclerosis. Neurogenetics 1997;1:65–71.
74. Murakami T, Warita H, Hayashi T, et al. A novel SOD1 gene mutation in familial ALS with low penetrance in females. J Neurol Sci 2001;189:45–47.
75. Hansen C, Gredal O, Werdelin L, et al. Novel 4-bp Insertion in the CuZn-Superoxide Dismutase (SOD1) gene associated with familial amyotrophic lateral sclerosis. Hum Mutat 1998;suppl 1:S327–S328.
76. Orrell RW, Habgood JJ, Gardiner I, et al. Clinical and functional investigation of 10 missense mutations and a novel frameshift insertion mutation of the gene for copper-zinc superoxide dismutase in UK families with amyotrophic lateral sclerosis. Neurology 1997;48:746–751.
77. Watanabe Y, Kuno N, Kono Y, et al. Absence of the mutant SOD1 in familial amyotrophic lateral sclerosis (FALS) with two base pair deletion in the SOD1 gene. Acta Neurol Scand 1997;95: 167–172.
78. Pramatarova A, Figlewicz DA, Krizus A, et al. Identification of new mutations in the CuZn superoxide dismutase gene of patients with familial amyotrophic lateral sclerosis. Am J Hum Genet 1995;56:592–596.
79. Jafari-Schluep HF, Khoris J, Mayeux-Portas V, et al. Les anomalies du gene superoxyde dismutase 1 dans la sclerose laterale amyotrophique familiale: correlations phenotype-genotype et implications pratiques. Rev Neurol 2003 (In press).
80. Sapp PC, Rosen DR, Hosler BA, et al. Identification of three novel mutations in the gene for CuZn superoxide dismutase in patients with familial amyotrophic lateral sclerosis. Neuromuscular Dis 1995;5:353–357.
81. Accessed May 19, 2003 from *www.alsod.org.*
82. Ikeda M, Abe K, Aoki M, et al. A novel point mutation in the CuZn superoxide dismutase gene in a patient with familial amyotrophic lateral sclerosis. Hum Mol Genet 1995;4:491–492.
83. Kostrzewa M, Damian MS, Müller U. Superoxide dismutase 1: identification of a novel mutation in a case of familial amyotrophic lateral sclerosis. Hum Genet 1996;98:48–50.
84. Calder VL, Domigan NM, George PM, et al. Superoxide dismutase (Glu100Gly) in a family with inherited motor neuron disease: detection of mutant superoxide dismutase activity and the presence of heterodimers. Neurosci Lett 1995;189:143–146.
85. Radunovic A, Leigh PN. CuZn superoxide dismutase gene mutations in ALS. Correlation between genotype and clinical features. J Neurol Neurosurg Psychiatry 1996;61:565–572.
86. Marklund SL, Andersen PM, Forsgren L, et al. Normal binding and reactivity of copper in mutant superoxide dismutase isolated from amyotrophic lateral sclerosis patients. J Neurochem 1997;69:675–681.
87. Gurney ME, Pu H, Chiu AY, et al. Motor neuron degeneration in mice expressing a human CuZn superoxide dismutase mutation. Science 1994;264:1772–1775.
88. Reaume AG, Elliott JL, Hoffman EK, et al. Motor neurons in Cu/Zn superoxide dismutase-deficient mice develop normally but exhibit enhanced cell death after axonal injury. Nat Genet 1996;13:43–47.
89. Ikeda M, Abe K, Aoki M, et al. Variable clinical symptoms in familial amyotrophic lateral sclerosis with a novel point mutation in the CuZn-superoxide dismutase gene. Neurology 1995; 45:2038–2042.
90. Shaw CE, Enayat ZE, Powell JF, et al. Familial amyotrophic lateral sclerosis. Molecular pathology of a patient with a SOD1 mutation. Neurology 1997;49:1612–1616.
91. Juneja T, Pericak-Vance MA, Laing NG, et al. Prognosis in familial amyotrophic lateral sclerosis: progression and survival in patients with Glu100Gly and Ala4Val mutations in CuZn-superoxide dismutase. Neurology 1997;48:55–57.

92. Suthers G, Laing N, Wilton S, et al. "Sporadic" motoneuron disease due to familial SOD1 mutation with low penetrance. Lancet 1994;344:1773.
93. Jones CT, Swingler RJ, Simpson SA, Brock DJH. Superoxide dismutase mutations in an unselected cohort of Scottish amyotrophic lateral sclerosis patients. J Med Genet 1995;32:290–292.
94. Andersen PM, Forsgren L, Binzer M, et al. Autosomal recessive adult-onset ALS associated with homozygosity for Asp90Ala CuZn-superoxide dismutase mutation. A clinical and genealogical study of 36 patients. Brain 1996;119:1153–1172.
95. Hayward C, Minns RA, Swingler RJ, Brock DJH. Homozygosity of Asn86Ser mutation in the CuZn-superoxide dismutase gene produces a severe clinical phenotype in a juvenile onset case of familial amyotrophic lateral sclerosis. J Med Genet 1998;2:174.
96. Masé G, Ros S, Gemma A, et al. ALS with variable phenotypes in a six-generation family caused by Leu144Phe mutation in the SOD1 gene. J Neurol Sci 2001;191:11–18.
97. Skvortsova VI, Limborska SA, Slominsky PA, et al. Sporadic ALS associated with the D90A CuZn-superoxide dismutase mutation in Russia. Eur J Neurol 2001;8:167–172.
98. Al-Chalabi A, Andersen PM, Chioza B, et al. Recessive amyotrophic lateral sclerosis with the D90A SOD1 mutation shares a common founder: evidence for a linked protective factor. Hum Mol Genet 1998;13:2045–2050.
99. Kato M, Aoki M, Ohta M, et al. Marked reduction of the Cu/Zn superoxide dismutase polypeptide in a case of familial ALS with the homozygous mutation. Neurosci Lett 2001;312:165–168.
100. Hand CK, Mayeux-Portas V, Khoris J, et al. Compound heterozygous D90A and D96N SOD1 mutations in a recessive amyotrophic lateral sclerosis family. Ann Neurol 2001;49:267–271.
101. Jones CT, Swingler RJ, Simpson SA, Brock DJH. Superoxide dismutase mutations in an unselected cohort of Scottish amyotrophic lateral sclerosis patients. J Med Genet 1995;32:290–292.
102. Hamida MB, Hentati F, Hamida CB. Hereditary motor system diseases (chronic juvenile amyotrophic lateral sclerosis). Brain 1990;113:347–363.
103. Hadano S, Hand CK, Osuga H, et al. A gene encoding a putative GTPase regulator is mutated in familial amyotrophic lateral sclerosis. Nat Genet 2001;29:166–173.
104. Yang Y, Hentati A, Deng H-X, et al. The gene encoding alsin, a protein with three guanine-nucleotide exchange factor domains, is mutated in a form of recessive ALS. Nat Genet 2001;29:160–165.
105. Hosler BA, Siddique T, Sapp PC, et al. Linkage of familial amyotrophic lateral sclerosis with frontotemporal dementia to chromosome 9q21-q22. JAMA 2000;284:1664–1669.
106. Chance PF, Rabin PA, Ryan SG, et al. Linkage of the gene for an autosomal dominant form of juvenile amyotrophic lateral sclerosis to chromosome 9q34. Am J Hum Genet 1998;62:633–640.
107. Lynch T, Sano M, Marder KS, et al. Clinical characteristics of a family with chromosome 17-linked disinhibition-dementia-parkinsonism-amyotrophy complex. Neurology 1994;44:1878–1884.
108. Hand CK, Khoris J, Salachas F, et al. A novel locus for familial amyotrophic lateral sclerosis, on chromosome 18q. Am J Hum Genet 2002;70:251–256.
109. Hong S, Brooks SR, Hung WY, et al. X-linked dominant locus for late-onset familial amyotrophic lateral sclerosis. Soc Neurosci Abst 1998;24:478.
110. Hentati A, Bejaoui K, Pericak-Vance MA, et al. Linkage of a commoner form of recessive ALS to chromosome 15q15-q22 markers. Neurogenetics 1998;2:55–60.
111. Tomik B, Nicotra A, Ellis CM, et al. Phenotypic differences between African and white patients with motor neuron disease: a case-control study. J Neurol Neurosurg Psychiatry 2000;69:251–253.
112. Neilson S, Robinson I, Nymoen EH. Longitudinal analysis of amyotrophic lateral sclerosis mortality in Norway, 1966–1989: evidence for a susceptible subpopulation. J Neurol Sci 1994; 122:148–154.
113. Neilson S, Gunnarsson LG, Robinson I. Rising mortality from motor neurone disease in Sweden 1961–1990: the relative role of increased population life expectancy and environmental factors. Acta Neurol Scand 1994;3:150–159.
114. Riggs JE. Longitudinal Gompertzian analysis of amyotrophic lateral sclerosis mortality in the U.S., 1977–1986. Evidence for an inherently susceptible subset. Mech Ageing Dev 1990;55:207.
115. Toyoshima I, Sugawara M, Kato K, et al. Kinesin and cytoplasmic dynein in spinal spheroids with motor neuron disease. J Neurol Sci 1998;1:38–44.
116. Jackson M, Morrison KE, Al-Chalabi A, et al. Analysis of chromosome 5q13 genes in amyotrophic lateral sclerosis: homozygous NAIP deletion in a sporadic case. Ann Neurol 1996;39:796–800.
117. Moulard B, Salachas F, Chassande B, et al. Association between centromeric deletions of the SMN gene and sporadic adult-onset lower motor neuron disease. Ann Neurol 1998;5:640–644.
118. Oosthuyse B, Moons L, Storkebaum E, et al. Deletion of the hypoxia-response element in the vascular endothelial growth factor causes motor neuron degeneration. Nat Genet 2002;28:131–138.

119. Van Landeghem GF, Tabatabaie P, Beckman L, et al. Mn-SOD signal sequence polymorphism associated with sporadic motor neuron disease. Eur J Neurol 1999;6:639–644.

120. Imura T, Shimohama S, Kawamata J, Kimura J. Genetic variation in the ciliary neurotrophic factor receptor α gene and familial amyotrophic lateral sclerosis. Ann Neurol 1998;2:275.

121. Giess R, Goetz R, Schrank B, et al. Potential implications of a ciliary neurotrophic factor gene mutation in a German population of patients with motor neuron disease. Muscle Nerve 1998;21:236–238.

122. Aoki M, Lin Cl, Rothstein JD, et al. Mutations in the glutamate transporter EAAT2 gene do not cause abnormal EAAT2 transcripts in amyotrophic lateral sclerosis. Ann Neurol 1998;5:645–653.

123. Hayward C, Colville S, Swingler RJ, Brock DJH. Molecular genetic analysis of the APEX nuclease gene in amyotrophic lateral sclerosis. Neurology 1999;52:1899–1901.

124. Moulard B, Sefiani A, Laamri A, et al. Apolipoprotein E genotyping in sporadic amyotrophic lateral sclerosis: evidence for a major influence on the clinical presentation and prognosis. J Neurol Sci 1996;139(suppl):34–37.

125. Mui S, Rebeck GW, McKenna-Yasek D, et al. Apolipoprotein E ε4 allele is not associated with earlier age at onset in amyotrophic lateral sclerosis. Ann Neurol 1995;38:460–463.

126. Figlewicz DA, Krizus A, Martinoli MG, et al. Variants of the heavy neurofilament subunit are associated with the development of amyotrophic lateral sclerosis. Hum Mol Genet 1994;3:1757–1761.

127. Shaw PJ, Thagesen H, Tomkins J, et al. Kennedy's disease: unusual molecular pathologic and clinical features. Neurology 1998;1:252–255.

128. Comi GP, Bordoni A, Salani S, et al. Cytochrome c oxidase subunit I microdeletion in a patient with motor neuron disease. Ann Neurol 1998;43:110–116.

129. Parboosingh JS, Meininger V, McKenna-Yasek D, et al. Deletions causing spinal muscular atrophy do not predispose to amyotrophic lateral sclerosis. Arch Neurol 1999;56:710–712.

130. Hayashi T, Sakurai M, Abe K, et al. Expression of angiogenic factors in rabbit spinal cord after transient ischemia. Neuropathol Appl Neurobiol 1999;25:63–71.

131. Parboosingh JS, Rouleau GA, Meninger V, et al. Absence of mutations in the Mn superoxide dismutase or catalase genes in familial amyotrophic lateral sclerosis. Neuromusc Disord 1995;1:7–10.

132. Tomblyn M, Kasarskis EJ, Xu Y, St. Clair DK. Distribution of MnSOD polymorphisms in sporadic ALS patients. J Mol Neurosci 1998;1:65–66.

133. Tomkins J, Banner SJ, McDermott CJ, Shaw PJ. Mutation screening of manganese superoxide dismutase in amyotrophic lateral sclerosis. Neuroreport 2001;12:1–4.

134. Flowers JM, Powell JF, Leigh PN, et al. Intron-7 retention and exon-9 skipping EAAT2 mRNA variants are not associated with ALS. Ann Neurol 2001;49:643–649.

135. Olkowski ZL. Mutant AP endonuclease in patients with amyotrophic lateral sclerosis. Neuroreport 1998;9:239–242.

136. Al-Chalabi A, Enayat ZE, Bakker MC, et al. Association of apolipoprotein E ε4 allele with bulbar-onset motor neuron disease. Lancet 1996;347:159–160.

137. Smith RG, Haverkamp LJ, Case S, et al. Apolipoprotein E ε4 in bulbar-onset motor neuron disease. Lancet 1996;348:334–335.

138. Al-Chalabi A, Andersen PM, Nilsson P, et al. Deletions of the heavy neurofilament subunit tail in amyotrophic lateral sclerosis. Hum Mol Genet 1999;8:157–164.

139. Tomkins J, Usher P, Slade JY, et al. Novel NF-H insertion in ALS. Neuroreport 1998;9:3967–3970.

140. Vechio JD, Bruijn LI, Xu Z, et al. Sequence variants in human neurofilament proteins: absence of linkage to familial amyotrophic lateral sclerosis. Ann Neurol 1996;40:603–610.

141. Rooke K, Figlewicz DA, Han FY, Rouleau GA. Analysis of the KSP repeat of the neurofilament heavy subunit in familial amyotrophic lateral sclerosis. Neurology 1996;46:789–790.

142. Parboosingh JS, Figlewicz DA, Krizus A, et al. Spinobulbar muscular atrophy can mimic ALS: the importance of genetic testing in male patients with atypical ALS. Neurology 1997;49:568–572.

143. de Wert G. Ethics of predictive DNA-testing for hereditary breast and ovarian cancer. Patient Educ Couns 1998;1:43–52.

9
Cellular Biological Effects of Copper/Zinc Superoxide Dismutase Mutations

Andrew J. Grierson and Pamela J. Shaw

GENETICS OF SOD1

Mutations in copper/zinc superoxide dismutase (SOD1) are associated with 15 to 20 percent of cases of familial motor neuron disease (MND). This accounts for only 1 to 2 percent of all MND cases, but the clinical features of disease in SOD1 families are virtually indistinguishable from those seen in sporadic patients. By using appropriate molecular techniques, we are now able to make robust laboratory models of SOD1-mediated MND. Because of the clinical similarities between sporadic and familial MND, the cellular biological effects of mutant SOD1 in these model systems are likely to be relevant to many if not all forms of the disease. In particular, the availability of transgenic mice and motor neuron–like cellular models expressing mutant SOD1 permits the identification of neuroprotective agents that may be beneficial in patients with MND.

SOD1 MUTATIONS CAUSE A TOXIC GAIN OF FUNCTION

The discovery of mutations in the SOD1 gene in 1993 provided the first insight into the molecular basis of MND.[1] The fact that SOD1 is a widely expressed protein, representing approximately 1 percent of total cellular protein content in the central nervous system (CNS), was at odds with the development of selective motor neuron degeneration. Many laboratories have confirmed the presence of SOD1 mutations in familial MND, and there are at least 100 mutations characterized to date (a continuously updated list is available at *www.alsod.org*). SOD1 is known to convert superoxide radicals to hydrogen peroxide and water,

237

so the first studies carried out on mutant SOD1 addressed the impact of mutations on this function. It was proposed that the mutations might reduce SOD1
dimerization, producing disease by a loss of function mechanism.[2] Experiments
using postmortem brain samples and red blood cell lysates from patients with
MND, as well as transfected cells in culture, suggested a reduced superoxide-
scavenging function and a reduced half-life of some forms of mutant SOD1,[3–8]
but other mutations studied showed apparently normal SOD1 activity.[9] In addition, mutant SOD1 expression in cells did not appear to influence the function
or half-life of the endogenous wild type protein.[10] Taken together, these experiments suggested that alterations in superoxide-scavenging function of SOD1
are unlikely to cause MND, but that a novel function attributed to the mutant
protein may be involved. To test this hypothesis, mouse models that overexpressed mutant SOD1 or that carried deletions of the endogenous SOD1 gene
were generated.[11,12] SOD1 knockout mice did not develop MND-like symptoms,
but a careful study of motor unit physiology and a morphometric analysis
demonstrated subtle motor symptoms by 6 months.[13] In contrast, mice expressing a G93A mutant SOD1 minigene, a human genomic DNA clone containing
the SOD1 promoter, coding region, and introns, developed clinical signs of
MND at about 3 months of age, despite having much higher levels of SOD1
activity than control mice.[12] Three further lines of transgenic mice carrying
mutant SOD1 minigenes were made, each with normal or increased SOD1
activity. These mice all developed MND symptoms, demonstrating that loss of
SOD1 activity is not associated with the development of disease and supporting the gain of a novel toxic function by the mutant protein as the mechanism
of disease. These mouse models of MND have been extensively characterized
and have lead to insights into the cellular effects of mutant SOD1. These are
described in detail in the following sections.

INSIGHTS GAINED FROM STUDYING
SOD1 BIOCHEMISTRY

SOD1 is a free-radical–scavenging enzyme that catalyzes the conversion of
superoxide to hydrogen peroxide (Figure 9.1). There are three SOD enzymes
that are specifically localized to cytosol (SOD1), mitochondria (SOD2), and the
extracellular space (SOD3). SOD1 is a metalloenzyme with copper- and zinc-
binding sites, and it functions in cells as a homodimer. It accounts for 1 percent
of total brain protein[14] and is thought to be particularly abundant in motor
neurons, which may have consequences for the selective vulnerability of these
cells in MND (see Selective Vulnerability of Motor Neurons).

To investigate the toxic gain of function associated with mutant SOD1, many
groups have investigated its biochemical properties. As discussed earlier, the
mutations do not cause a loss-of-function phenotype; in fact many mutant SOD1
proteins show only a mild loss of enzymatic activity. An alternative mechanism
was suggested. In the presence of mutations that alter the structure of the SOD1
homodimer giving the active channel a more open configuration, mutant SOD1
is able to catalyze the production of toxic free radicals by reacting with

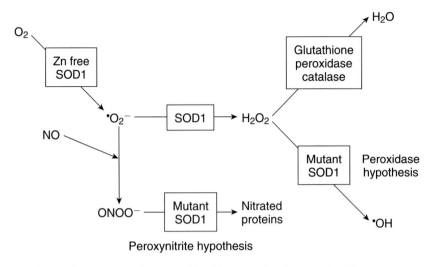

Figure 9.1 Biochemical pathways mediated by normal and mutant SOD1.

aberrant substrates. If the active copper site is more accessible in mutant homodimers, then the enzyme might be able to catalyze reactions with inappropriate substrates, or even release free copper, which could catalyze unwanted oxidative reactions. Two pathways were proposed:

1. *Peroxynitrite hypothesis:* The biochemical implications of this hypothetical pathway are shown in Figure 9.1. Two cellular free radicals, superoxide and nitric oxide (NO), may spontaneously form highly reactive peroxynitrite (‾ONOO). When this reacts with mutant SOD1, nitration of protein tyrosine residues is postulated to occur.[15] Indeed, there is some evidence for nitration of tyrosine components in MND (see later discussion). An alternative peroxynitrite hypothesis was suggested in 1999, when it was demonstrated that some mutant SOD1 proteins bind zinc less well in vitro. The reduction in bound zinc may allow reduced Cu^{1+} SOD1 to work backward and convert O_2 to superoxide, which then reacts with NO, as in the original peroxynitrite hypothesis.[16]
2. *Peroxidase hypothesis:* Mutant SOD1 may react with its normal reaction product, hydrogen peroxide, to yield the highly reactive hydroxyl free radical (see Figure 9.1).

The possible cellular effects of these hypothetical pathways are explained in further detail in the following sections.

CELLULAR EFFECTS OF MUTANT SOD1

Oxidative Stress

In postmitotic motor neurons, oxidative stress may result in a slowly progressing degeneration associated with a cumulative increase in oxidatively damaged cellular components. Alterations in the function of vital pathways due to oxidative damage may eventually lead to motor neuron cell death, and there is neurochemical evidence for oxidative disease mechanisms in sporadic and familial MND. In support of the peroxynitrite hypothesis, transgenic mice expressing mutant SOD1 have two- to three-fold increased levels of free, but not protein-bound, nitrotyrosine.[17,18] It was also suggested that there was no increase in protein-bound nitrotyrosine in postmortem human SOD1 patient spinal cord samples.[17] However, Beal et al[19] showed that nitrotyrosine immunoreactivity was increased in the motor neurons of SOD1 patients. Furthermore, some investigators have found evidence for lipid peroxidation by using immunohistochemical approaches in mutant SOD1-expressing transgenic mice.[18] These findings were not supported by biochemical studies in mutant SOD1 transgenic mice,[17] which raises methodological questions over the sensitivity and specificity of the tests used. The demonstration of increased protein oxidation in mutant SOD1 transgenic mice suggested the involvement of highly reactive hydroxyl radicals in the later stages of disease.[20] Indeed in this latter study, SOD1 itself was identified as a protein that was oxidatively damaged (Figure 9.2).

Using genetic approaches, the peroxynitrite hypothesis has been challenged. Overexpression or elimination of wild type SOD1 in transgenic mice that express mutant SOD1 would be expected to modulate the production of peroxynitrite from superoxide by either increased superoxide-scavenging activity by overexpression or by decreased scavenging on the knockout background.[21] In fact, in neither case did the crossbreeding of mutant SOD1 transgenic with wild type SOD1 transgenic or knockout mice alter the phenotype.[21] In a subsequent study, another group of investigators was able to exacerbate mutant SOD1 toxicity by co-overexpressing wild type and mutant SOD1.[22]

Cell culture models offer some advantages for studying the biochemistry of short-lived free radicals, and several groups have used these systems to address the role of oxidative stress in SOD1-mediated MND. Differentiated rat pheochromocytoma PC12 cells infected with adenoviruses expressing mutant but not wild type SOD1 showed slightly increased intracellular superoxide production as assayed by single-cell microfluorometry to measure ethidium fluorescence.[23] In transfected SK-N-MC neuroblastoma cells expressing mutant SOD1, several markers of increased oxidative stress have been reported, including increased lipid peroxidation, 3-nitrotyrosine and protein carbonyl levels.[24] Finally, in transfected NSC34 motor neuron–like cells, both wild type and mutant SOD1 decreased the release of superoxide from cells into the media; however, they showed divergent effects with respect to NO handling. Cells expressing wild type SOD1 showed increased NO release into the media, whereas mutant SOD1–expressing cells released less NO. Therefore it seems likely that mutant SOD1–expressing cells have alterations in free-radical handling compared with wild type cells.[25]

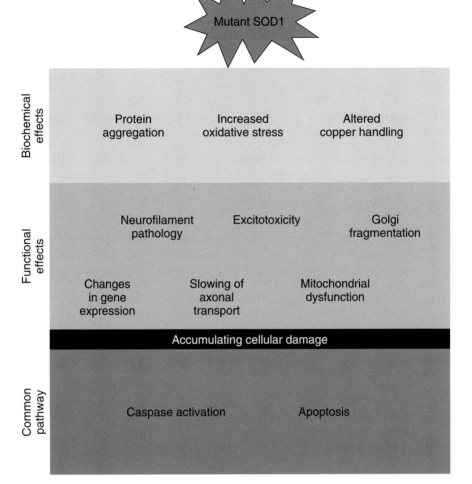

Figure 9.2 The cascade of cellular effects of mutant SOD1 includes biochemical and functional effects that probably lead to a common final pathway.

Thus evidence exists for oxidative and nitrative free-radical damage in SOD1-mediated MND, but the exact mechanisms responsible for the damage are not fully understood. It is quite likely that a combination of the mechanisms described here may be involved.

Alterations in Intracellular Copper and Zinc

The discovery in yeast that copper binding by SOD1 requires a specific copper chaperone for SOD1 (CCS), has allowed further insights into the role of copper binding in SOD1-mediated disease. Some SOD1 mutants maintain the ability to bind copper in vitro,[26] and by cloning the murine CCS gene, it was now possible to use genetic crossbreeding approaches to study the effect of reduced copper binding on mutant SOD1–mediated disease in mice. CCS knockout mice were generated and crossed with three lines of SOD1 transgenic mice.[27] In all cases, there was no effect on disease onset or progression mediated by the absence of CCS. One possible caveat of this approach is that tissue extracts from the CCS knockout/G37R and G93A transgenic mice show residual SOD1 activity of 10 to 20 percent. Whether this is an artefact of the in vitro assay, perhaps due to tissue homogenization, is not clear. Regardless of this, it is clear that the SOD1 in these mice bound no radioactive copper in vivo, suggesting that CCS-mediated delivery of copper to SOD1 in MND did not contribute to the toxicity of the mutant enzyme. Recently, an alternative strategy to deplete copper from mutant SOD1 has been tested.[28] There are four histidines in SOD1 that coordinate copper binding.[29] Using a genetic approach, one group has systematically mutated two of these histidine residues, H46R and H48Q, in a single SOD1 molecule to mimic two of the mutations found in human SOD1 patients.[30,31] These artificially engineered chimeras would be predicted to bind less copper in vivo and therefore could potentially block any in vivo copper binding that is mediated by chaperones other than CCS. Several lines of transgenic mice were generated that expressed these mutant SOD1 chimeras at a range of expression levels, and these mice developed symptoms of MND in a dose-dependent fashion. Therefore it seems likely that deficient copper binding is not a key factor in the development of mutant SOD1–mediated MND.

It has been suggested that mutant SOD1 does not bind copper tightly and may release free copper, which catalyzes unwanted reactions. Therefore sequestration of free copper in motor neurons may represent a clinical approach in MND. To test this, the copper-chelating agents diethyldithiocarbamate and neocuproin were used in an in vitro assay[32] of motor neuron viability and outgrowth. These experiments showed a dramatic 200-percent increase in survival and an increase in neurite outgrowth in cultures grown in the presence of copper-chelating compounds.

Aggregation of Mutant SOD1

A significant finding in SOD1-mediated disease is the presence of aggregates of the mutant protein observed in both human MND patients and transgenic models.[21,33–36] This is of potential interest because protein aggregation is found in other neurodegenerative diseases including Huntington's disease, Parkinson's disease, and Alzheimer's disease. One suggestion is that protein aggregation in these diseases may represent a common toxic mechanism or alternatively may reflect a common neuronal salvage pathway in response to protein misfolding. Because of the potential toxicity of SOD1 aggregates, several models of SOD1-mediated MND have been studied. First, in mutant SOD1 mice, aggregates immunoreactive with anti-SOD1 antibodies are observed in neurons and astrocytes.[21] A sensitive filter assay has been developed to quantify the amount of aggregated SOD1 in central nervous system (CNS) extracts prepared from transgenic mice expressing mutant SOD1.[37] This assay has revealed a dramatic temporal increase in aggregated SOD1 in these animals, and most mice with filterable SOD1 aggregates also showed hindlimb weakness.[37]

Cellular models of SOD1 aggregation have also been developed. The overexpression of mutant SOD1 protein in motor neurons, COS7 cells, HEK293, and PC12 cells leads to the formation of aggregates.[38–41] In a striking example of these studies, the formation of aggregates of mutant SOD1 in microinjected primary motor neurons preceded cell death that could be partially rescued by apoptosis inhibitors.[40] The study by Johnston et al[38] in HEK293 cells supported a role for proteasome inhibition in the development of SOD1 "aggresomes." When cells expressing mutant SOD1 were treated with inhibitors of the proteasome degradation pathway, insoluble aggregates of high-molecular-weight SOD1-immunoreactive material were generated. These experiments are consistent with different models of disease pathogenesis: Firstly, it is possible that SOD1 aggregation leads to inhibited proteasome activity. Alternatively, SOD1 aggregates may lead to a loss of function of important proteins that are sequestered into protein aggregates.

Evidence for a role for heat shock proteins (Hsp) in SOD1-mediated MND was suggested by Durham et al[40], who showed that aggregation of mutant SOD1 in microinjected motor neurons could be prevented by Hsp70.[40] In a subsequent study using transfected NIH3T3 cells and G93A mutant transgenic mouse spinal cords, the same group reported that Hsp40, Hsp70, and αB-crystallin were associated with mutant but not wild type SOD1.[42] Furthermore these complexes were found in a detergent-insoluble fraction that contained up to 10 percent of total mutant SOD1. The authors suggest that something other than SOD1 mutation is required to render mutant SOD1 insoluble, and that Hsp association with this modified SOD1 may be a protective response, possibly by preventing aberrant protein–protein interactions.[42] Recently a supporting study in transfected Neuro2α cells demonstrated that coexpression of either Hsp40 or Hsp70 suppressed aggregate formation by mutant SOD1.[43]

In conclusion, aggregation of mutant SOD1 is a common finding in cellular and mouse models of SOD1-mediated MND. The suggested links between aggregates of SOD1 and motor neuron cell death make this mechanism a potential neurotherapeutic target in MND.

SOD1 Slows Axonal Transport and Induces Aberrant Cytoskeletal Pathology

The pathology of sporadic and familial MND is characterized by the presence of abnormal accumulations of neurofilament proteins. These may be in the form of hyaline conglomerate inclusions in SOD-linked familial cases or axonal swellings in sporadic disease.[44] Neurofilaments are the major intermediate filaments found in neurons and are formed by the polymerization of three individual subunits: neurofilament light (NF-L), medium (NF-M), and heavy (NF-H). Several groups have reported that the levels of steady-state NF-L messenger RNA (mRNA) are reduced in spinal cord motor neurons in sporadic and SOD1-mediated MND.[45–47] These findings are replicated when mutant but not wild type SOD1 is expressed in a motor neuron–like cell line and in G93A mutant transgenic mice,[47] suggesting that the reduction in NF-L may be a primary consequence of mutant SOD1 expression, and not an end-stage epiphe-nomenon. To better understand neurofilament function in vivo, several trans-genic and knockout mouse models have been generated. Although the results of these studies are covered in more detail elsewhere in this volume, it is worth pointing out that overexpression of any one of the neurofilament proteins alone can give rise to perikaryal neurofilament inclusions. For instance, NF-H over-expression leads to severe motor dysfunction but not neuronal death, and the motor phenotype could be rescued by coexpression of NF-L.[47–49] These exper-iments emphasize the necessity for subunit stoichiometry for normal assembly and transport of neurofilaments, which may be relevant to the idea that loss of NF-L in spinal motor neurons leads to perikaryal neurofilament inclusions seen in MND.

To investigate the effects of mutant SOD1 on axonal transport and cytoskele-tal pathology, experiments were devised to radiolabel newly synthesized pro-teins in the ventral horn and then study their distribution in the axonal process 28 days later. Because cytoskeletal proteins are transported by "slow" axonal transport, at a rate of 0.1 to 3.0 mm per day, it is possible to measure transport of neurofilaments in this way. In an elegant study, Williamson and Cleveland[50] showed that neurofilament and tubulin transport is perturbed in transgenic mice expressing G37R and G85R mutant SOD1, and this occurs before the onset of symptoms in these mice. At present the mechanism responsible for this slowing is not known, although it seems logical that the primary cause may be damage to either neurofilament proteins, the motor proteins that transport them, or the microtubule tracks along which the motors move. In SOD1-mediated MND patients and transgenic mice, abnormal localization of phosphorylated neuro-filaments has been reported, which may be associated with these putative disease mechanisms.[44,51]

Because the neurofilament transgenic and knockout mice showed motor neu-ronal effects, several have been crossbred with mutant SOD1 mice to look for possible synergistic effects. Remarkably, it was shown that knockout of NF-L or overexpression of human NF-H, or mouse NF-L or NF-H, extended the life span of mutant SOD1 mice by up to 65 percent.[50,52,53] Although these results seem counterintuitive, one possible explanation is that the alteration in neuro-filament distribution between the cell body and the axon in motor neurons arising from abnormal subunit stoichiometry acts as a protective factor. This may be due to the increased perikaryal neurofilaments acting as a "sink" to reduce damaging biochemical perturbations such as increased intracellular calcium or by the reduction in axonal neurofilaments, which might otherwise contribute in some way to the toxicity of SOD1.[53–57]

Therefore mutant SOD1 expression in cells is responsible for functional and pathological alterations in the cytoskeleton of motor neurons. However, the precise significance of the perikaryal neurofilament accumulations, and the reduced expression of NF-L, seen in SOD1-mediated MND is still unclear.

Organelle Dysfunction

Studying the ultrastructural changes that are observed in MND has suggested that dysfunction of specific organelles may be part of the disease process. These organelles include mitochondria, the Golgi apparatus, and the cytoskeleton (discussed earlier). Although many of these experiments were performed before the identification of SOD1 mutations, the correlation between sporadic and SOD1-mediated disease may represent a common mechanism.

Studies on postmortem material from sporadic MND patients have shown that the Golgi apparatus is fragmented in motor neurons.[58,59] These studies used antisera against MG160, a conserved membrane sialoglycoprotein found in the medial cisternae of the Golgi apparatus.[60] When these antibodies were tested on spinal cord sections prepared from mutant SOD1 transgenic mice, it was shown that fragmentation of the Golgi apparatus is an early event in this model of disease.[61] Subsequent studies of the pathology of SOD1 patients have demonstrated similar fragmentation of the Golgi apparatus can be observed in the surviving motor neurons of these patients. Although it is not clear what may be responsible for these effects in SOD1-mediated disease, one hypothesis suggests that the retrograde pathways that normally regulate the distribution of the Golgi apparatus, and/or the rough endoplasmic reticulum-to-Golgi transport, may be disrupted.

Afifi et al[62] first reported mitochondrial pathology in atrophic muscle of sporadic MND patients in 1966. Subsequent studies have identified structurally abnormal mitochondria in intramuscular nerves, liver, spinal cord anterior horn cells, corticospinal tracts, and the synapses of degenerating motor neurons.[63–67] One of the key functions of mitochondria is to generate adenosine triphosphate (ATP) via the electrochemical gradient across their inner membrane. There are five subunits arranged in an electron transport chain, termed complex I through complex V. Supporting evidence for mitochondrial involvement in MND came from studies of the function of these complexes purified from MND CNS material. In the first study, increased complex I activity was observed in the frontal cortex of MND patients with SOD1 mutations.[8] The activities of complexes II, III, and IV showed no alterations in this study. In an extension of this work, the same group later studied three CNS regions: the motor cortex, parietal cortex, and cerebellum.[68] Increases in complexes I, II, and III were seen in the motor cortex of patients with an SOD1 mutation, but not in any sporadic MND patients. In the parietal cortex, complex I activity was increased, and in the cerebellum, the activity of complexes II and III was increased. It has been suggested that these increases in mitochondrial electron transport chain activities are a compensatory mechanism for the oxidative damage to mitochondria when damage to the inner membrane leads to proton leakage and the "uncoupling" of the electron transport chain. Other studies have not demonstrated an increase in complex I activity; however, decreased complex IV activity has been reported by several groups. Fujita et al[69] measured decreased complex IV activity in all areas of the spinal cord in sporadic MND patients, although the decrease was particularly marked in the ventral region. Borthwick et al[70] used a histochemical approach to demonstrate decreased complex IV activity in individual residual spinal motor neurons of sporadic MND cases. To further investigate the role of SOD1 in mitochondrial abnormalities in MND, model systems have been used. In mutant SOD1 transgenic mice, it was demonstrated that mitochondria undergo a degenerating phase associated with the formation of vacuoles in spinal motor neurons, and that this immediately precedes the onset of rapidly progressing clinical disease.[71,72] In a motor neuron–like cell culture model of

SOD1-mediated MND, Menzies et al[73] showed that expression of mutant SOD1 was able to reproduce some of the effects observed in patients with SOD1 mutations. Structurally abnormal mitochondria were commonly seen in cells expressing G93A mutant but not wild type SOD1, and there were significant reductions in the activity of complexes II and IV of the electron transport chain.[73] Previously, overexpression of mutant but not wild type SOD1 was shown to lead to a significant loss of mitochondrial membrane potential that was associated with increased intracellular calcium levels. Therefore there are several model systems, including transgenic mice and cell culture models of mutant SOD1–associated MND that recapitulate the clinical and pathological mitochondrial phenotype observed in patients. These models allow a unique opportunity to further investigate the pathways upstream and downstream of mitochondrial dysfunction in MND.

Recently, several groups of investigators have confirmed earlier experiments that showed that SOD1 is present in mitochondria and the cytosol. Two groups found SOD1 in the mitochondrial inter membrane space of yeast and in rat liver extracts.[74,75] It has now been shown that mutant SOD1 protein in SOD1 transgenic mice is localized to mitochondria, and that in this model of ALS, SOD1 may accumulate in vacuolated mitochondria.[76,77] A novel hypothesis for mutant SOD1–mediated MND has been suggested by Okado-Matsumoto and Fridovich.[78] They demonstrated that mitochondrial uptake of SOD1 requires demetallation, and that the chaperones Hsp70 and Hsp25 preferentially bind to mutant forms of SOD1. These experiments led them to conclude that the mode of action of mutant SOD1 may be to deplete the levels of available Hsp in motor neurons, making them unavailable for antiapoptotic defense mechanisms.[78]

Abnormalities of mitochondrial structure and function are thus widely reported in both SOD1-mediated and sporadic MND. Thus neurotherapeutic strategies targeting mitochondrial function may be beneficial in MND. Klivenyi et al[79] demonstrated that administration of creatine in the drinking water of G93A mutant SOD1 mice was able to increase their survival and motor function in a dose-dependent manner. Creatine buffers energy levels in the cell, maintaining ATP levels, and stabilizes mitochondrial creatine kinase, which inhibits the opening of the mitochondrial transition pore. This treatment also reduced oxidative damage in the mice, as measured by levels of 3-nitrotyrosine in the spinal cord.

Proapoptotic Effect of Mutant SOD1

As described earlier, microinjection of mutant but not wild type SOD1 into primary motor neurons results in apoptosis.[40] Furthermore, evidence for involvement of members of the Bcl-2 and caspase families in SOD1-mediated MND suggests that apoptosis may be the predominant cell death mechanism. Activation of caspase-1 and caspase-3 appears to occur sequentially in the spinal cords of mutant SOD1 transgenic mice.[80–82] In support of this, expression of a dominant-interfering form of caspase-1 or intraventricular administration of a caspase inhibitor both slowed disease progression in G93A mutant SOD1 mice.[80,83] Other caspases have also been linked to SOD1-mediated disease in transgenic mice. Caspase-9 and caspase-7 were also reported to be sequentially activated, with the caspase-9 activity occurring concomitantly with the translocation of Bax from the cytoplasm to the mitochondria, the cleavage of Bid, and the release of cytochrome *c* from the mitochondria.[84,85]

Bcl-2 family members have also been investigated in mutant SOD1 transgenic mice. In symptomatic mice, expression of Bcl-2 and Bcl-XL, which inhibit apoptosis, is reduced, whereas expression of Bad and Bax, which stimulate apoptosis, is increased.[86] In support of this as a mechanism underlying cell death, crossing mutant SOD1 mice with transgenic mice overexpressing Bcl-2 delays the onset of disease and mortality by 1 month.[87]

There is also evidence that mutant SOD1 might activate p53 in motor neurons, because p53 immunoreactivity has been reported in motor neuron nuclei in mutant SOD1 transgenic mice.[88] This may be associated with apoptotic cell death, but evidence from crossbreeding experiments with p53 knockout mice suggests that removal of p53 from motor neurons has no beneficial effects in this model of MND.[89]

Analysis of mRNA expression in mutant SOD1 transgenic mice spinal cords demonstrated that the X-linked inhibitor of apoptosis protein (XIAP) is downregulated in motor neurons in this model of MND.[90] This raises the possibility that decreased levels of XIAP may be causally related to the apoptotic pathways reported in SOD1-mediated MND. To further investigate this possibility, the investigators overexpressed XIAP in Neuro2α cells expressing mutant SOD1. They were able to demonstrate that this inhibited both caspase-3 activity and cell death in this cellular model.[91]

A recent survey of levels of mRNA from apoptosis-related genes in the spinal cords of G93A SOD1 mutant mice revealed that all caspases investigated (caspase-1, -2, -3, -6, -7, -8, -10, -11, and -12) were upregulated in 120-day-old mice.[92] In the same study, a number of cytokines, including tumor necrosis factor-α (TNF-α) and its receptor, were found to be upregulated at 80 days, leading these investigators to conclude that neuroinflammatory changes occur as a result of SOD1 expression and precede the upregulation of apoptotic genes in this model.[92]

Pulling together the work of several groups, there is increasing evidence for apoptosis in SOD1-mediated MND. The various transgenic mouse models of mutant SOD1 have been invaluable in these experiments. Further discussion of cell death pathways in SOD1-related and other forms of MND are discussed in Chapter 14.

Alterations in Gene and Protein Expression

It is conceivable that changes in the expression of some cellular genes and proteins are associated with the MND phenotype. By identifying these changes in expression, we are able to identify molecules that are potentially important in disease pathogenesis. New technologies are available, including complementary DNA (cDNA) microarrays and two-dimensional gel electrophoresis of proteins, followed by mass spectrometry (proteomics), which allow large-scale screening of disease models for alterations in gene and protein expression. These protocols have the advantage of offering a very high throughput approach that should in principle be fully quantitative.

Recently, several groups have used cDNA arrays to identify important changes in gene expression in MND. Malaspina et al[93] used pooled mRNA extracted from the lumbar spinal cord of sporadic MND cases and controls. They identified 13 upregulated and one downregulated transcript. These genes fell into several categories, including antioxidants, neuroinflammatory pathways and lipid metabolism. To specifically look at the role played by mutant SOD1 on levels of gene expression, Olsen et al[94] used spinal cord mRNA from transgenic mice expressing G93A mutant SOD1 at four key stages of disease, compared with non-transgenic litter mates and wild type SOD1 expressing mice. They showed that a number of transcripts consistent with glial cell activation, including glial fibrillary acidic protein (GFAP), CD63, vimentin, were increased at the onset of disease (3 months). This is consistent with a neuroinflammatory response in SOD1-mediated MND. Whether this response to dying motor neurons is likely to be beneficial or harmful is unclear, because glial cells can release factors that are both neurotrophic and neurotoxic to motor neurons. The same study also showed a dramatic fivefold increase in apolipoprotein E (ApoE) expression in mice aged 4 months. It was suggested that this is produced by macrophages to aid in the metabolism of lipid and cholesterol associated with degenerating myelinated axons. There was also evidence of upregulation of other "scavenging" pathways in the affected mice, which are likely to represent the mobilization of lipids and glycoproteins, for example, hexosaminidase B, fatty acid–binding protein, or the catabolism of proteins, such as cathepsin D and cathepsin S. Immediately before end-stage disease (4 months), mice showed increases in genes involved in metal ion regulation—for example, metallothionein I and III and ferritin H and L. These changes might represent an adaptive response to the stress caused by massive degeneration of motor neurons at this age.

A second study using the same G93A mutant line of mice, but different cDNA arrays, confirmed the findings relating to the neuroinflammatory response in SOD1-mediated MND.[90] They showed increases in vimentin, TNF-α, P selectin glycoprotein ligand-1, CD147, junD1, cathepsin D, CD68, proenkephalin-2, serine protease inhibitor 2 through 4, and cystatin C precursor. Therefore it appears that a dramatic neuroinflammatory response is a robust finding in the G93A transgenic mice. These authors also showed that the caspase-1 and Bcl-XL genes were upregulated, whereas XIAP was downregulated after the onset of disease. These changes in expression indicate that activation of neuronal apoptotic pathways may be involved in this mouse model of MND.

Although these studies have highlighted the nature of the immune response in SOD1-related MND, the dilution effect of non-neuronal cells present in the spinal cord has probably masked many changes in gene expression that occur selectively in motor neurons. To address this problem, Kirby et al[95] used cDNA microarrays to investigate changes in gene expression in motor neuron–like cell lines expressing wild type or mutant SOD1. This study identified 29 genes showing altered expression in each of three cell lines expressing three different SOD1 mutations (G37R, G93A, I113T), compared with cells expressing wild type SOD1. Of these genes, the authors concentrated on the seven genes that were significantly decreased in the presence of mutant SOD1. The levels of four mRNAs were confirmed to be decreased in the presence of mutant SOD1 in the motor neuron cell lines: KIF3B, a motor protein of the kinesin family[96]; c-Fes, which may play a role in the regulation of vesicle trafficking[97]; intracellular adhesion molecule-1 (ICAM-1), an adhesion molecule[98]; and Bag1, a protein involved in apoptosis.[99] These changes are currently being investigated in motor neurons from human SOD1 cases.

In summary, alterations in gene expression linked with inflammatory processes and neuronal degeneration have been reported using spinal cord mRNA from mutant SOD1 transgenic mice. To take this work further, it will be important to develop strategies that allow motor neuron–specific gene expression to be studied, and as a step toward this the use of motor neuron–like cells in culture may identify some of the relevant genes.

Selective Vulnerability of Motor Neurons

Global expression of the mutant protein in SOD1-associated MND patients results in a significant loss of motor neurons, but relative sparing of other cell types. This apparent paradox suggests that motor neurons may be especially vulnerable to the toxicity of mutant SOD1, compared with other cells including other types of neurons. Several hypotheses have been put forward to explain the selective vulnerability of motor neurons in MND: First, the unique size of motor neurons, with an axon up to 1 meter long in humans, demands efficient intracellular transport[100] and places a high demand on cellular energy production.[101] Second, motor neurons lack the calcium-buffering proteins parvalbumin and calbindin$_{D28k}$,[102] which may increase susceptibility to calcium-mediated neurodegeneration in MND. Third, motor neurons express low levels of the GluR2 subunit of the AMPA (α-amino-3-hydroxy-5-methyl-4-isoxazole propionic acid) receptor, which normally confers calcium impermeability on this glutamate receptor subtype.[103,104] This suggests that motor neurons might be more susceptible to AMPA receptor–mediated increases in intracellular calcium. In support of this, motor neurons microinjected with cDNA that encode mutant SOD1 display prominent aggregation of mutant SOD1, which can be prevented by blocking AMPA receptors with a selective receptor antagonist.[105]

Although motor neurons are the ultimate targets for SOD1 toxicity in MND, the increases in non-neuronal cells in the spinal cord of MND patients,[106–108] the occurrence of SOD1 aggregates in glial cells in G85R transgenic mice,[109] and the selective loss of excitatory amino acid transporter type 2 (EAAT2) in transgenic rats expressing mutant SOD1[110] all support the idea that glial cells may be mediators of SOD1 toxicity. A number of lines of transgenic mice have been generated to address this, by using both neuron-specific and astrocyte-specific promoters to drive the expression of the mutant SOD1 transgene.[111–113] Eighteen-month-old mice overexpressing G37R mutant SOD1 driven by the neuron-specific NF-L promoter did not develop disease,[111] and mice expressing the G85R mutant SOD1 gene under a Thy1 promoter also did not develop disease.[112] In the latter study, crossbreeding studies with G93A mutant mice under the control of the endogenous SOD1 promoter demonstrated no exacerbation of the disease phenotype by doubling the expression of mutant SOD1 in neurons.[112] The authors argue that this supports the idea that expression of SOD1 in neurons alone is not sufficient to cause disease.[112] The expression of mutant

SOD1 under the control of the astrocyte-specific GFAP promoter leads to a progressive astrocytosis in the spinal cord of mice, in the absence of any overt motor neuron loss.[113] This suggests that the astrocytosis observed in mutant SOD1 minigene mice may not arise purely in response to dying motor neurons, because the expression of mutant SOD1 in astrocytes alone causes a similar expansion in astrocyte cells within the spinal cord.[113] Thus it appears likely that mutant SOD1 expression in both neuronal and non-neuronal cells may be necessary to model mutant SOD1-mediated disease in transgenic mice.

Neuroprotection

The lack of an effective therapy for treatment of MND remains the most important issue in the field of MND research. The expression of mutant SOD1 in cell lines and transgenic mice mimics some of the major clinical and pathological features of both familial and sporadic MND. Therefore we are able to test novel therapies in these systems and look for any treatments that might be beneficial to patients with MND. Both cell and mouse systems have their advantages. Cell lines offer a relatively high throughput system, because they can be grown in high-density arrays, and very large numbers of therapeutic compounds can potentially be tested at the same time.[114] Mouse models of MND, though essentially low throughput, offer the unique opportunity to study the effects of new compounds and treatments on disease onset in vivo and allow us to study effects on motor neuron survival and pathology.[115]

Many investigations of this type have already been carried out using cells and mice expressing mutant SOD1. Most studies using potential therapeutic compounds have used G93A mutant SOD1 transgenic mice, because these develop MND in a relatively short period (onset approximately 100 days, paralysis by approximately 140 days). Therefore the costs involved in housing mice and administering therapeutic agents are minimized. It should be noted that in most studies, drugs are given to mice before the onset of clinical symptoms, a situation that is not usually possible in human patients. A summary of the results of these experiments is outlined in Table 9.1, and clinical trials of some of these agents in human MND are described in detail in Chapter 21.

Many agents tested had no effect or only a small effect (up to a 10% increase) on survival, but a few studies have shown an extension in life span of more than 20 percent. These include intrathecal delivery of the broad-spectrum caspase inhibitor zVAD-fmk[80] and the addition of creatine, a mitochondrial-buffering drug, to the drinking water.[80] It is likely that other effective compounds will be identified using the mutant SOD1 transgenic mice, and that future clinical trials in human MND patients with these compounds will be a natural progression of these experiments.

Table 9.1 Therapeutic agents that have been tested in experimental models of SOD1-related motor neuron disease

Type	Therapeutic agent	Reference
Antioxidants	Ascorbate/trientine	116
	Carboxyfullerenes	117
	Catalase	118
	Desmethylselegiline	119
	Ginkgo biloba	120
	Ginseng root	121
	Glutathione peroxidase	122
	Lipoic acid	119
	N-acetylcysteine	123
	NOS inhibition	124
	SOD1	21, 22, 125
	Vitamin E	126
	DMPO	127
Metal ion related	Trientine	116
	D-penicillamine	128
	CCS knockout	27
Anti-inflammatory	Cyclosporin	129
	Aspirin	130
	Minocycline	131
Apoptosis related	zVAD-fmk	80, 83
	p53	89, 132
	Bcl-2	87
	Caspase-1	83
	PARP	119
	Minocycline	133
Cytoskeleton	NF-H overexpression	53
	NF-L overexpression	52
	NF-L knockout	56
Glutamate	Riluzole	126
Mitochondria/energy	Creatine	79
Neurotrophic factors	GDNF	134–137
	HGF	138
	FGF	139
	LIF	140
	BMP	141
Others	JAK inhibitor	142
	Gabapentin	126
	Genistein	143

BMP = bone morphogenic protein; CCS = copper chaperone for SOD1; DMPO = 5′,5′-dimethylpyrroline-*N*-oxide; FGF = fibroblast growth factor; GDNF = glial cell–derived neurotrophic factor; HGF = hepatocyte growth factor; JAK = janus kinase; LIF = leukemia inhibitory factor; NF-H = neurofilament heavy; NF-L = neurofilament light; NOS = nitric oxide synthase; PARP = poly(ADP)ribosyl polymerase; SOD1 = copper/zinc superoxide dismutase.

REFERENCES

1. Rosen DR, Siddique T, Patterson D, et al. Mutations in Cu/Zn superoxide dismutase gene are associated with familial amyotrophic lateral sclerosis. Nature 1993;362:59–62.
2. Deng HX, Hentati A, Tainer JA, et al. Amyotrophic lateral sclerosis and structural defects in Cu, Zn superoxide dismutase. Science 1993;261:1047–1051.
3. Robberecht W, Sapp P, Viaene MK, et al. Cu/Zn superoxide dismutase activity in familial and sporadic amyotrophic lateral sclerosis. J Neurochem 1994;62:384–387.
4. Bowling AC, Barkowski EE, McKenna-Yasek D, et al. Superoxide dismutase concentration and activity in familial amyotrophic lateral sclerosis. J Neurochem 1995;64:2366–2369.
5. Puymirat J, Cossette L, Gosselin F, Bouchard JP. Red blood cell Cu/Zn superoxide dismutase activity in sporadic amyotrophic lateral sclerosis. J Neurol Sci 1994;127:121–123.
6. Tsuda T, Munthasser S, Fraser PE, et al. Analysis of the functional effects of a mutation in SOD1 associated with familial amyotrophic lateral sclerosis. Neuron 1994;13:727–736.
7. Rosen DR, Bowling AC, Patterson D, et al. A frequent ala 4 to val superoxide dismutase-1 mutation is associated with a rapidly progressive familial amyotrophic lateral sclerosis. Hum Mol Genet 1994;3:981–987.
8. Bowling AC, Schulz JB, Brown RH Jr, Beal MF. Superoxide dismutase activity, oxidative damage, and mitochondrial energy metabolism in familial and sporadic amyotrophic lateral sclerosis. J Neurochem 1993;61:2322–2325.
9. Borchelt DR, Lee MK, Slunt HS, et al. Superoxide dismutase 1 with mutations linked to familial amyotrophic lateral sclerosis possesses significant activity. Proc Natl Acad Sci USA 1993;91:8292–8296.
10. Borchelt DR, Guarnieri M, Wong PC, et al. Superoxide dismutase 1 subunits with mutations linked to familial amyotrophic lateral sclerosis do not affect wild-type subunit function. J Biol Chem 1995;270:3234–3238.
11. Reaume AG, Elliott JL, Hoffman EK, et al. Motor neurons in Cu/Zn superoxide dismutase–deficient mice develop normally but exhibit enhanced cell death after axonal injury. Nat Genet 1996;13:43–47.
12. Gurney ME, Pu H, Chiu AY, et al. Motor neuron degeneration in mice that express a human Cu, Zn superoxide dismutase mutation. Science 1994;264:1772–1775.
13. Shefner JM, Reaume AG, Flood DG, et al. Mice lacking cytosolic copper/zinc superoxide dismutase display a distinctive motor axonopathy. Neurology 1999;53:1239–1246.
14. Liu R, Althaus JS, Ellerbrock BR, et al. Enhanced oxygen radical production in a transgenic mouse model of familial amyotrophic lateral sclerosis. Ann Neurol 1998;44:763–770.
15. Beckman JS, Carson M, Smith CD, Koppenol WH. ALS, SOD and peroxynitrite. Nature 1993;364:584.
16. Estevez AG, Crow JP, Sampson JB, et al. Induction of nitric oxide–dependent apoptosis in motor neurons by zinc-deficient superoxide dismutase. Science 1999;286:2498–2500.
17. Bruijn LI, Beal MF, Becher MW, et al. Elevated free nitrotyrosine levels, but not protein-bound nitrotyrosine or hydroxyl radicals, throughout amyotrophic lateral sclerosis (ALS)–like disease implicate tyrosine nitration as an aberrant in vivo property of one familial ALS-linked superoxide dismutase 1 mutant. Proc Natl Acad Sci USA 1997;94:7606–7611.
18. Ferrante RJ, Browne SE, Shinobu LA, et al. Evidence of increased oxidative damage in both sporadic and familial amyotrophic lateral sclerosis. J Neurochem 1997;69:2064–2074.
19. Beal MF, Ferrante RJ, Browne SE, et al. Increased 3-nitrotyrosine in both sporadic and familial amyotrophic lateral sclerosis. Ann Neurol 1997;42:644–654.
20. Andrus PK, Fleck TJ, Gurney ME, Hall ED. Protein oxidative damage in a transgenic mouse model of familial amyotrophic lateral sclerosis. J Neurochem 1998;71:2041–2048.
21. Bruijn LI, Houseweart MK, Kato S, et al. Aggregation and motor neuron toxicity of an ALS-linked SOD1 mutant independent from wild-type SOD1. Science 1998;281:1851–1854.
22. Jaarsma D, Haasdijk ED, Grashorn JA, et al. Human Cu/Zn superoxide dismutase (SOD1) overexpression in mice causes mitochondrial vacuolization, axonal degeneration, and premature motoneuron death and accelerates motoneuron disease in mice expressing a familial amyotrophic lateral sclerosis mutant SOD1. Neurobiol Dis 2000;7:623–643.
23. Ghadge GD, Lee JP, Bindokas VP, et al. Mutant superoxide dismutase-1-linked familial amyotrophic lateral sclerosis: molecular mechanisms of neuronal death and protection. J Neurosci 1997;17:8756–8766.
24. Lee M, Hyun D, Jenner P, Halliwell B. Effect of overexpression of wild-type and mutant Cu/Zn-superoxide dismutases on oxidative damage and antioxidant defenses: relevance to Down's syndrome and familial amyotrophic lateral sclerosis. J Neurochem 2001;76:957–965.

25. Cookson MR, Menzies FM, Manning P, et al. Cu/Zn superoxide dismutase (SOD1) mutations associated with familial amyotrophic lateral sclerosis (ALS) affect cellular free radical release in the presence of oxidative stress. Amyotroph Lateral Scler Other Motor Neuron Disord 2002;3:75–85.

26. Corson LB, Strain JJ, Culotta VC, Cleveland DW. Chaperone-facilitated copper binding is a property common to several classes of familial amyotrophic lateral sclerosis–linked superoxide dismutase mutants. Proc Natl Acad Sci USA 1998;95:6361–6366.

27. Subramaniam JR, Lyons WE, Liu J, et al. Mutant SOD1 causes motor neuron disease independent of copper chaperone–mediated copper loading. Nat Neurosci 2002;5:301–307.

28. Wang J, Xu G, Gonzales V, et al. Fibrillar inclusions and motor neuron degeneration in transgenic mice expressing superoxide dismutase 1 with a disrupted copper-binding site. Neurobiol Dis 2002;10:128–138.

29. Parge HE, Hallewell RA, Tainer JA. Atomic structures of wild-type and thermostable mutant recombinant human Cu, Zn superoxide dismutase. Proc Natl Acad Sci USA 1992;89:6109–6113.

30. Enayat ZE, Orrell RW, Claus A, et al. Two novel mutations in the gene for copper zinc superoxide dismutase in UK families with amyotrophic lateral sclerosis. Hum Mol Genet 1995;4:1239–1240.

31. Aoki M, Abe K, Houi K, et al. Variance of age at onset in a Japanese family with amyotrophic lateral sclerosis associated with a novel Cu/Zn superoxide dismutase mutation. Ann Neurol 1995;37:676–679.

32. Azzouz M, Poindron P, Guettier S, et al. Prevention of mutant SOD1 motoneuron degeneration by copper chelators in vitro. J Neurobiol 2000;42:49–55.

33. Kato S, Sumi-Akamaru H, Fujimura H, et al. Copper chaperone for superoxide dismutase co-aggregates with superoxide dismutase 1 (SOD1) in neuronal Lewy body–like hyaline inclusions: an immunohistochemical study on familial amyotrophic lateral sclerosis with SOD1 gene mutation. Acta Neuropathol (Berl) 2001;102:233–238.

34. Shibata N, Hirano A, Kobayashi M, et al. Presence of Cu/Zn superoxide dismutase (SOD) immunoreactivity in neuronal hyaline inclusions in spinal cords from mice carrying a transgene for Gly93Ala mutant human Cu/Zn SOD. Acta Neuropathol (Berl) 1998;95:136–142.

35. Shibata N, Hirano A, Kobayashi M, et al. Intense superoxide dismutase-1 immunoreactivity in intracytoplasmic hyaline inclusions of familial amyotrophic lateral sclerosis with posterior column involvement. J Neuropathol Exp Neurol 1996;55:481–490.

36. Watanabe M, Dykes-Hoberg M, Culotta VC, et al. Histological evidence of protein aggregation in mutant SOD1 transgenic mice and in amyotrophic lateral sclerosis neural tissues. Neurobiol Dis 2001;8:933–941.

37. Wang J, Xu G, Borchelt DR. High molecular weight complexes of mutant superoxide dismutase 1: age-dependent and tissue-specific accumulation. Neurobiol Dis 2002;9:139–148.

38. Johnston JA, Dalton MJ, Gurney ME, Kopito RR. Formation of high molecular weight complexes of mutant Cu, Zn-superoxide dismutase in a mouse model for familial amyotrophic lateral sclerosis. Proc Natl Acad Sci USA 2000;97:12571–12576.

39. Koide T, Igarashi S, Kikugawa K, et al. Formation of granular cytoplasmic aggregates in COS7 cells expressing mutant Cu/Zn superoxide dismutase associated with familial amyotrophic lateral sclerosis. Neurosci Lett 1998;257:29–32.

40. Durham HD, Roy J, Dong L, Figlewicz DA. Aggregation of mutant Cu/Zn superoxide dismutase proteins in a culture model of ALS. J Neuropathol Exp Neurol 1997;56:523–530.

41. Lee JP, Gerin C, Bindokas VP, et al. No correlation between aggregates of Cu/Zn superoxide dismutase and cell death in familial amyotrophic lateral sclerosis. J Neurochem 2002;82:1229–1238.

42. Shinder GA, Lacourse MC, Minotti S, Durham HD. Mutant Cu/Zn-superoxide dismutase proteins have altered solubility and interact with heat shock/stress proteins in models of amyotrophic lateral sclerosis. J Biol Chem 2001;276:12791–12796.

43. Takeuchi H, Kobayashi Y, Yoshihara T, et al. Hsp70 and Hsp40 improve neurite outgrowth and suppress intracytoplasmic aggregate formation in cultured neuronal cells expressing mutant SOD1. Brain Res 2002;949:11–22.

44. Ince PG. Neuropathology. In RH Brown, V Meininger, M Swash (eds), Amyotrophic Lateral Sclerosis. London: Martin Dunitz Ltd, 2000;83–112.

45. Wong NK, He BP, Strong MJ. Characterization of neuronal intermediate filament protein expression in cervical spinal motor neurons in sporadic amyotrophic lateral sclerosis (ALS). J Neuropathol Exp Neurol 2000;59:972–982.

46. Bergeron C, Beric-Maskarel K, Muntasser S, et al. Neurofilament light and polyadenylated mRNA levels are decreased in amyotrophic lateral sclerosis motor neurons. J Neuropathol Exp Neurol 1994;53:221–230.

47. Menzies FM, Grierson AJ, Cookson MR, et al. Selective loss of neurofilament expression in Cu/Zn superoxide dismutase (SOD1) linked amyotrophic lateral sclerosis. J Neurochem 2002;82:1118–1128.
48. Meier J, Couillard-Despres S, Jacomy H, et al. Extra neurofilament NF-L subunits rescue motor neuron disease caused by overexpression of the human NF-H gene in mice. J Neuropathol Exp Neurol 1999;58:1099–1110.
49. Beaulieu JM, Jacomy H, Julien JP. Formation of intermediate filament protein aggregates with disparate effects in two transgenic mouse models lacking the neurofilament light subunit. J Neurosci 2000;20:5321–5328.
50. Williamson TL, Cleveland DW. Slowing of axonal transport is a very early event in the toxicity of ALS-linked SOD1 mutants to motor neurons. Nat Neurosci 1999;2:50–56.
51. Tu PH, Raju P, Robinson KA, et al. Transgenic mice carrying a human mutant superoxide dismutase transgene develop neuronal cytoskeletal pathology resembling human amyotrophic lateral sclerosis lesions. Proc Natl Acad Sci USA 1996;93:3155–3160.
52. Kong J, Xu Z. Overexpression of neurofilament subunit NF-L and NF-H extends survival of a mouse model for amyotrophic lateral sclerosis. Neurosci Lett 2000;281:72–74.
53. Couillard-Despres S, Zhu Q, Wong PC, et al. Protective effect of neurofilament heavy gene overexpression in motor neuron disease induced by mutant superoxide dismutase. Proc Natl Acad Sci USA 1998;95:9626–9630.
54. Nguyen MD, Lariviere RC, Julien JP. Deregulation of Cdk5 in a mouse model of ALS: toxicity alleviated by perikaryal neurofilament inclusions. Neuron 2001;30:135–147.
55. Julien JP, Beaulieu JM. Cytoskeletal abnormalities in amyotrophic lateral sclerosis: beneficial or detrimental effects? J Neurol Sci 2000;180:7–14.
56. Williamson TL, Bruijn LI, Zhu Q, et al. Absence of neurofilaments reduces the selective vulnerability of motor neurons and slows disease caused by a familial amyotrophic lateral sclerosis–linked superoxide dismutase 1 mutant. Proc Natl Acad Sci USA 1998;95:9631–9636.
57. Couillard-Despres S, Meier J, Julien JP. Extra axonal neurofilaments do not exacerbate disease caused by mutant Cu, Zn superoxide dismutase. Neurobiol Dis 2000;7:462–470.
58. Mourelatos Z, Adler H, Hirano A, et al. Fragmentation of the Golgi apparatus of motor neurons in amyotrophic lateral sclerosis revealed by organelle-specific antibodies. Proc Natl Acad Sci USA 1990;87:4393–4395.
59. Gonatas NK, Stieber A, Mourelatos Z, et al. Fragmentation of the Golgi apparatus of motor neurons in amyotrophic lateral sclerosis. Am J Pathol 1992;140:731–737.
60. Johnston PA, Stieber A, Gonatas NK. A hypothesis on the traffic of MG160, a medial Golgi sialoglycoprotein, from the trans-Golgi network to the Golgi cisternae. J Cell Sci 1994;107(pt 3):529–537.
61. Mourelatos Z, Gonatas NK, Stieber A, et al. The Golgi apparatus of spinal cord motor neurons in transgenic mice expressing mutant Cu, Zn superoxide dismutase becomes fragmented in early, preclinical stages of the disease. Proc Natl Acad Sci USA 1996;93:5472–5477.
62. Afifi AK, Aleu FP, Goodgold J, MacKay B. Ultrastructure of atrophic muscle in amyotrophic lateral sclerosis. Neurology 1966;16:475–481.
63. Atsumi T. The ultrastructure of intramuscular nerves in amyotrophic lateral sclerosis. Acta Neuropathol (Berl) 1981;55:193–198.
64. Hirano A, Nakano I, Kurland LT, et al. Fine structural study of neurofibrillary changes in a family with amyotrophic lateral sclerosis. J Neuropathol Exp Neurol 1984;43:471–480.
65. Nakano Y, Hirayama K, Terao K. Hepatic ultrastructural changes and liver dysfunction in amyotrophic lateral sclerosis. Arch Neurol 1987;44:103–106.
66. Okamoto K, Hirai S, Shoji M, et al. Axonal swellings in the corticospinal tracts in amyotrophic lateral sclerosis. Acta Neuropathol (Berl) 1990;80:222–226.
67. Sasaki S, Iwata M. Ultrastructural study of the synapses of central chromatolytic anterior horn cells in motor neuron disease. J Neuropathol Exp Neurol 1996;55:932–939.
68. Browne SE, Bowling AC, Baik MJ, et al. Metabolic dysfunction in familial, but not sporadic, amyotrophic lateral sclerosis. J Neurochem 1998;71:281–287.
69. Fujita K, Yamauchi M, Shibayama K, et al. Decreased cytochrome c oxidase activity but unchanged superoxide dismutase and glutathione peroxidase activities in the spinal cords of patients with amyotrophic lateral sclerosis. J Neurosci Res 1996;45:276–281.
70. Borthwick GM, Johnson MA, Ince PG, et al. Mitochondrial enzyme activity in amyotrophic lateral sclerosis: implications for the role of mitochondria in neuronal cell death. Ann Neurol 1999;46:787–790.

71. Wong PC, Pardo CA, Borchelt DR, et al. An adverse property of a familial ALS-linked SOD1 mutation causes motor neuron disease characterized by vacuolar degeneration of mitochondria. Neuron 1995;14:1105–1116.

72. Kong J, Xu Z. Massive mitochondrial degeneration in motor neurons triggers the onset of amyotrophic lateral sclerosis in mice expressing a mutant SOD1. J Neurosci 1998;18:3241–3250.

73. Menzies F, Cookson MR, Chrzanowska-Lightowlers ZMA, et al. Mitochondrial dysfunction in a cell culture model of amyotrophic lateral sclerosis. Brain 2002;125:1522–1533.

74. Okado-Matsumoto A, Fridovich I. Subcellular distribution of superoxide dismutases (SOD) in rat liver: Cu, Zn-SOD in mitochondria. J Biol Chem 2001;276:38388–38393.

75. Sturtz LA, Diekert K, Jensen LT, et al. A fraction of yeast Cu, Zn-superoxide dismutase and its metallochaperone, CCS, localize to the intermembrane space of mitochondria. A physiological role for SOD1 in guarding against mitochondrial oxidative damage. J Biol Chem 2001;276:38084–38089.

76. Jaarsma D, Rognoni F, van Duijn W, et al. CuZn superoxide dismutase (SOD1) accumulates in vacuolated mitochondria in transgenic mice expressing amyotrophic lateral sclerosis-linked SOD1 mutations. Acta Neuropathol (Berl) 2001;102:293–305.

77. Higgins CM, Jung C, Ding H, Xu Z. Mutant Cu, Zn superoxide dismutase that causes motoneuron degeneration is present in mitochondria in the CNS. J Neurosci 2002;22:1–6.

78. Okado-Matsumoto A, Fridovich I. Amyotrophic lateral sclerosis: a proposed mechanism. Proc Natl Acad Sci USA 2002;99:9010–9014.

79. Klivenyi P, Ferrante RJ, Matthews RT, et al. Neuroprotective effects of creatine in a transgenic animal model of amyotrophic lateral sclerosis. Nat Med 1999;5:347–350.

80. Li M, Ona VO, Guegan C, et al. Functional role of caspase-1 and caspase-3 in an ALS transgenic mouse model. Science 2000;288:335–339.

81. Pasinelli P, Borchelt DR, Houseweart MK, et al. Caspase-1 is activated in neural cells and tissue with amyotrophic lateral sclerosis–associated mutations in copper-zinc superoxide dismutase. Proc Natl Acad Sci USA 1998;95:15763–15768.

82. Pasinelli P, Houseweart MK, Brown RH Jr, Cleveland DW. Caspase-1 and -3 are sequentially activated in motor neuron death in Cu, Zn superoxide dismutase–mediated familial amyotrophic lateral sclerosis. Proc Natl Acad Sci USA 2000;97:13901–13906.

83. Friedlander RM, Brown RH, Gagliardini V, et al. Inhibition of ICE slows ALS in mice. Nature 1997;388:31.

84. Guegan C, Vila M, Rosoklija G, et al. Recruitment of the mitochondrial-dependent apoptotic pathway in amyotrophic lateral sclerosis. J Neurosci 2001;21:6569–6576.

85. Guegan C, Vila M, Teissman P, et al. Instrumental activation of Bid by caspase-1 in a transgenic mouse model of ALS. Mol Cell Neurosci 2002;20:553–562.

86. Vukosavic S, Stefanis L, Jackson-Lewis V, et al. Delaying caspase activation by Bcl-2: A clue to disease retardation in a transgenic mouse model of amyotrophic lateral sclerosis. J Neurosci 2000;20:9119–9125.

87. Kostic V, Jackson-Lewis V, de Bilbao F, et al. Bcl-2: prolonging life in a transgenic mouse model of familial amyotrophic lateral sclerosis. Science 1997;277:559–562.

88. Gonzalez de Aguilar JL, Gordon JW, Rene F, et al. Alteration of the Bcl-x/Bax ratio in a transgenic mouse model of amyotrophic lateral sclerosis: evidence for the implication of the p53 signaling pathway. Neurobiol Dis 2000;7:406–415.

89. Kuntz CT, Kinoshita Y, Beal MF, et al. Absence of p53: no effect in a transgenic mouse model of familial amyotrophic lateral sclerosis. Exp Neurol 2000;165:184–190.

90. Yoshihara T, Ishigaki S, Yamamoto M, et al. Differential expression of inflammation- and apoptosis-related genes in spinal cords of a mutant SOD1 transgenic mouse model of familial amyotrophic lateral sclerosis. J Neurochem 2002;80:158–167.

91. Ishigaki S, Liang Y, Yamamoto M, et al. X-Linked inhibitor of apoptosis protein is involved in mutant SOD1-mediated neuronal degeneration. J Neurochem 2002;82:576–584.

92. Hensley K, Floyd RA, Gordon B, et al. Temporal patterns of cytokine and apoptosis-related gene expression in spinal cords of the G93A-SOD1 mouse model of amyotrophic lateral sclerosis. J Neurochem 2002;82:365–374.

93. Malaspina A, Kaushik N, de Belleroche J. Differential expression of 14 genes in amyotrophic lateral sclerosis spinal cord detected using gridded cDNA arrays. J Neurochem 2001;77:132–145.

94. Olsen MK, Roberds SL, Ellerbrock BR, et al. Disease mechanisms revealed by transcription profiling in SOD1-G93A transgenic mouse spinal cord. Ann Neurol 2001;50:730–740.

95. Kirby J, Menzies FM, Cookson MR, et al. Differential gene expression in a cell culture model of SOD1-related familial motor neuron disease. Hum Mol Genet 2002;11:2061–2075.
96. Yamazaki H, Nakata T, Okada Y, Hirokawa N. KIF3A/B: a heterodimeric kinesin superfamily protein that works as a microtubule plus end-directed motor for membrane organelle transport. J Cell Biol 1995;130:1387–1399.
97. Zirngibl R, Schulze D, Mirski SE, et al. Subcellular localization analysis of the closely related Fps/Fes and Fer protein-tyrosine kinases suggests a distinct role for Fps/Fes in vesicular trafficking. Exp Cell Res 2001;266:87–94.
98. Dustin ML, Rothlein R, Bhan AK, et al. Induction by IL 1 and interferon-gamma: tissue distribution, biochemistry, and function of a natural adherence molecule (ICAM-1). J Immunol 1986;137:245–254.
99. Takayama S, Sato T, Krajewski S, et al. Cloning and functional analysis of BAG-1: a novel Bcl-2–binding protein with anti-cell death activity. Cell 1995;80:279–284.
100. Miller CC, Ackerley S, Brownlees J, et al. Axonal transport of neurofilaments in normal and disease states. Cell Mol Life Sci 2002;59:323–330.
101. Menzies FM, Ince PG, Shaw PJ. Mitochondrial involvement in amyotrophic lateral sclerosis. Neurochem Int 2002;40:543–551.
102. Ince P, Stout N, Shaw P, et al. Parvalbumin and calbindin D28k in the human motor system and in motor neuron disease. Neuropathol Appl Neurobiol 1993;19:291–299.
103. Williams TL, Day NC, Ince PG, et al. Calcium-permeable alpha-amino-3-hydroxy-5-methyl-4-isoxazole propionic acid receptors: a molecular determinant of selective vulnerability in amyotrophic lateral sclerosis. Ann Neurol 1997;42:200–207.
104. Shaw PJ, Williams TL, Slade JY, et al. Low expression of GluR2 AMPA receptor subunit protein by human motor neurons. Neuroreport 1999;10:261–265.
105. Roy J, Minotti S, Dong L, et al. Glutamate potentiates the toxicity of mutant Cu/Zn-superoxide dismutase in motor neurons by postsynaptic calcium-dependent mechanisms. J Neurosci 1998; 18:9673–9684.
106. Schiffer D, Cordera S, Cavalla P, Migheli A. Reactive astrogliosis of the spinal cord in amyotrophic lateral sclerosis. J Neurol Sci 1996;139(suppl):27–33.
107. Kawamata T, Akiyama H, Yamada T, McGeer PL. Immunologic reactions in amyotrophic lateral sclerosis brain and spinal cord tissue. Am J Pathol 1992;140:691–707.
108. Murayama S, Inoue K, Kawakami H, et al. A unique pattern of astrocytosis in the primary motor area in amyotrophic lateral sclerosis. Acta Neuropathol (Berl) 1991;82:456–461.
109. Bruijn LI, Becher MW, Lee MK, et al. ALS-linked SOD1 mutant G85R mediates damage to astrocytes and promotes rapidly progressive disease with SOD1-containing inclusions. Neuron 1997;18:327–338.
110. Howland DS, Liu J, She Y, et al. Focal loss of the glutamate transporter EAAT2 in a transgenic rat model of SOD1 mutant–mediated amyotrophic lateral sclerosis (ALS). Proc Natl Acad Sci USA 2002;99:1604–1609.
111. Pramatarova A, Laganiere J, Roussel J, et al. Neuron-specific expression of mutant superoxide dismutase 1 in transgenic mice does not lead to motor impairment. J Neurosci 2001;21:3369–3374.
112. Lino MM, Schneider C, Caroni P. Accumulation of SOD1 mutants in postnatal motoneurons does not cause motoneuron pathology or motoneuron disease. J Neurosci 2002;22:4825–4832.
113. Gong YH, Parsadanian AS, Andreeva A, et al. Restricted expression of G86R Cu/Zn superoxide dismutase in astrocytes results in astrocytosis but does not cause motoneuron degeneration. J Neurosci 2000;20:660–665.
114. Torrance CJ, Agrawal V, Vogelstein B, Kinzler KW. Use of isogenic human cancer cells for high-throughput screening and drug discovery. Nat Biotechnol 2001;19:940–945.
115. Wong PC, Cai H, Borchelt DR, Price DL. Genetically engineered mouse models of neurodegenerative diseases. Nat Neurosci 2002;5:633–639.
116. Nagano S, Ogawa Y, Yanagihara T, Sakoda S. Benefit of a combined treatment with trientine and ascorbate in familial amyotrophic lateral sclerosis model mice. Neurosci Lett 1999;265:159–162.
117. Dugan LL, Turetsky DM, Du C, et al. Carboxyfullerenes as neuroprotective agents. Proc Natl Acad Sci USA 1997;94:9434–9439.
118. Reinholz MM, Merkle CM, Poduslo JF. Therapeutic benefits of putrescine-modified catalase in a transgenic mouse model of familial amyotrophic lateral sclerosis. Exp Neurol 1999;159:204–216.
119. Andreassen OA, Dedeoglu A, Friedlich A, et al. Effects of an inhibitor of poly(ADP-ribose) polymerase, desmethylselegiline, trientine, and lipoic acid in transgenic ALS mice. Exp Neurol 2001;168:204–216.

120. Ferrante RJ, Klein AM, Dedeoglu A, Beal MF. Therapeutic efficacy of EGb761 (Gingko biloba extract) in a transgenic mouse model of amyotrophic lateral sclerosis. J Mol Neurosci 2001; 17:89–96.
121. Jiang F, DeSilva S, Turnbull J. Beneficial effect of ginseng root in SOD-1 (G93A) transgenic mice. J Neurol Sci 2000;180:52–54.
122. Cudkowicz ME, Pastusza KA, et al. Survival in transgenic ALS mice does not vary with CNS glutathione peroxidase activity. Neurology 2002;59:729–734.
123. Andreassen OA, Dedeoglu A, Klivenyi P, et al. N-acetyl-L-cysteine improves survival and preserves motor performance in an animal model of familial amyotrophic lateral sclerosis. Neuroreport 2000;11:2491–2493.
124. Facchinetti F, Sasaki M, Cutting FB, et al. Lack of involvement of neuronal nitric oxide synthase in the pathogenesis of a transgenic mouse model of familial amyotrophic lateral sclerosis. Neuroscience 1999;90:1483–1492.
125. Jung C, Rong Y, Doctrow S, et al. Synthetic superoxide dismutase/catalase mimetics reduce oxidative stress and prolong survival in a mouse amyotrophic lateral sclerosis model. Neurosci Lett 2001;304:157–160.
126. Gurney ME, Cutting FB, Zhai P, et al. Benefit of vitamin E, riluzole, and gabapentin in a transgenic model of familial amyotrophic lateral sclerosis. Ann Neurol 1996;39:147–157.
127. Liu R, Li B, Flanagan SW, et al. Increased mitochondrial antioxidative activity or decreased oxygen free radical propagation prevent mutant SOD1-mediated motor neuron cell death and increase amyotrophic lateral sclerosis–like transgenic mouse. J Neurochem 2002;80:488–500.
128. Hottinger AF, Fine EG, Gurney ME, et al. The copper chelator d-penicillamine delays onset of disease and extends survival in a transgenic mouse model of familial amyotrophic lateral sclerosis. Eur J Neurosci 1997;9:1548–1551.
129. Keep M, Elmer E, Fong KS, Csiszar K. Intrathecal cyclosporin prolongs survival of late-stage ALS mice. Brain Res 2001;894:327–331.
130. Barneoud P, Curet O. Beneficial effects of lysine acetylsalicylate, a soluble salt of aspirin, on motor performance in a transgenic model of amyotrophic lateral sclerosis. Exp Neurol 1999;155:243–251.
131. Van Den Bosch L, Tilkin P, Lemmens G, Robberecht W. Minocycline delays disease onset and mortality in a transgenic model of ALS. Neuroreport 2002;13:1067–1070.
132. Prudlo J, Koenig J, Graser J, et al. Motor neuron cell death in a mouse model of FALS is not mediated by the p53 cell survival regulator. Brain Res 2000;879:183–187.
133. Zhu S, Stavrovskaya IG, Drozda M, et al. Minocycline inhibits cytochrome c release and delays progression of amyotrophic lateral sclerosis in mice. Nature 2002;417:74–78.
134. Acsadi G, Anguelov RA, Yang H, et al. Increased survival and function of SOD1 mice after glial cell–derived neurotrophic factor gene therapy. Hum Gene Ther 2002;13:1047–1059.
135. Manabe Y, Nagano I, Gazi MS, et al. Adenovirus-mediated gene transfer of glial cell line–derived neurotrophic factor prevents motor neuron loss of transgenic model mice for amyotrophic lateral sclerosis. Apoptosis 2002;7:329–334.
136. Mohajeri MH, Figlewicz DA, Bohn MC. Intramuscular grafts of myoblasts genetically modified to secrete glial cell line–derived neurotrophic factor prevent motoneuron loss and disease progression in a mouse model of familial amyotrophic lateral sclerosis. Hum Gene Ther 1999;10: 1853–1866.
137. Wang LJ, Lu YY, Muramatsu S, et al. Neuroprotective effects of glial cell line–derived neurotrophic factor mediated by an adeno-associated virus vector in a transgenic animal model of amyotrophic lateral sclerosis. J Neurosci 2002;22:6920–6928.
138. Sun W, Funakoshi H, Nakamura T. Overexpression of HGF retards disease progression and prolongs life span in a transgenic mouse model of ALS. J Neurosci 2002;22:6537–6548.
139. Upton-Rice MN, Cudkowicz ME, Warren L, et al. Basic fibroblast growth factor does not prolong survival in a transgenic model of familial amyotrophic lateral sclerosis. Ann Neurol 1999;46:934.
140. Azari MF, Galle A, Lopes EC, et al. Leukemia inhibitory factor by systemic administration rescues spinal motor neurons in the SOD1 G93A murine model of familial amyotrophic lateral sclerosis. Brain Res 2001;922:144–147.
141. Dreibelbis JE, Brown RH Jr, Pastuszak KA, et al. Disease course unaltered by a single intracisternal injection of BMP-7 in ALS mice. Muscle Nerve 2002;25:122–123.
142. Trieu VN, Liu R, Liu XP, Uckun FM. A specific inhibitor of janus kinase-3 increases survival in a transgenic mouse model of amyotrophic lateral sclerosis. Biochem Biophys Res Commun 2000;267:22–25.
143. Trieu VN, Uckun FM. Genistein is neuroprotective in murine models of familial amyotrophic lateral sclerosis and stroke. Biochem Biophys Res Commun 1999;258:685–688.

10
Excitotoxicity and Oxidative Stress in Pathogenesis of Amyotrophic Lateral Sclerosis/Motor Neuron Disease

Philip Van Damme, Ludo Van Den Bosch, and Wim Robberecht

The role of excitotoxicity and oxidative stress in the pathogenesis of amyotrophic lateral sclerosis (ALS) has been widely studied. However, although recent data offer strong support in favor of a role for glutamate in motor neuron degeneration, the evidence for the involvement of excitotoxicity remains indirect. It is thought that the susceptibility of motor neurons to excitotoxicity may at least contribute to the selectivity of neuronal death in ALS. Similarly, although the presence of free-radical—induced damage to cellular constituents is well documented in ALS, whether oxidative stress plays a primary pathogenic role remains to be seen. Interestingly, excitotoxicity and oxidative stress are linked through various molecular and cellular mechanisms. Because both phenomena are potential targets for pharmacological interference, the understanding of the role of these mechanisms in the pathogenesis of ALS may have important therapeutic implications.

EXCITOTOXICITY

Glutamate is the main excitatory neurotransmitter in the brain, responsible for fast excitatory neurotransmission. However, excessive exposure to glutamate and other excitatory amino acids can have lethal effects on neurons. Already in 1957, it was discovered that glutamate induces neuronal degeneration in the retina.[1] Injury to neurons caused by excitatory amino acids was called *excitotoxicity* in 1978.[2] Excitotoxicity has been implicated in the pathogenesis of stroke, neurotrauma, epilepsy, and several neurodegenerative diseases.[3] Ca^{2+} entry through glutamate receptors (GluRs) appears to be the major trigger for neuronal injury by glutamate.[4] In this review, we briefly discuss the actions of glutamate on neurons and the mechanisms of excitotoxicity in general and then summarize the evidence for the role of excitotoxicity in the pathogenesis of ALS.

Glutamatergic Actions on Neurons

Glutamate Receptors

Glutamate released from presynaptic terminals acts on postsynaptic and presynaptic GluRs. GluRs are divided into inotropic GluRs, which are ligand-gated cation channels, and metabotropic GluRs, which are G-protein—coupled receptors that activate second-messenger systems. The inotropic receptors are further subdivided into three classes according to their preferred synthetic agonist:[5,6] AMPA (α-amino-3-hydroxy-5-methyl-4-isoxazole propionic acid), NMDA (N-methyl-D-aspartate), and KA (kainate) receptors. They are permeable to Na^+, K^+, and in a variable degree to Ca^{2+}. All receptor genes have been cloned. AMPA receptors are tetramers composed of four subunits (GluR1-4),[7–10] NMDA receptors are composed of NR1[11] and NR2 (NR2A-D) subunits,[12–15] and KA receptors are oligomers of the subunits GluR5-7 and KA1 and 2.[16–19] NMDA receptors are thought to mediate the late component of excitatory transmission.[20] They are highly permeable to Ca^{2+}.[21] At resting membrane potential, NMDA receptors are blocked by physiological concentrations of Mg^{2+} ions.[22,23] AMPA receptors mediate the early component of excitatory transmission. The Ca^{2+}-permeability of the AMPA receptor is largely determined by the presence of the GluR2 subunit in the receptor complex. Receptors containing GluR2 have a very low relative Ca^{2+} permeability compared with GluR2-lacking receptor channels.[24] The impermeability to Ca^{2+} of GluR2-containing AMPA receptors is due to the presence of a positively charged arginine at position 586 (Q/R site) of the GluR2 peptide instead of the genetically encoded neutral glutamine.[25,26] This arginine residue at the Q/R site is introduced by the editing of GluR2 pre–messenger RNA (mRNA),[27] which is virtually complete in most cell types. The role of KA receptors in physiological and pathological conditions is not known.

Within the family of metabotropic GluRs, eight members have been cloned (mGluR1-8).[28] On the basis of sequence homology, pharmacological profile, and second-messenger coupling, metabotropic GluRs can be divided into three groups: group I (mGluR1 and mGluR5) coupled to phospholipase C, group II (mGluR2 and mGluR3), and group III (mGluR4, mGluR6, mGluR7, and mGluR8), both negatively coupled to adenylate cyclase.

Glutamate Transport

Under normal conditions, glutamate released from presynaptic vesicles is quickly removed from the synaptic cleft by high-affinity glutamate transporters in the postsynaptic membrane of neurons and in astrocyte processes that surround the synaptic cleft. The reuptake of glutamate is Na^+-dependent. Five glutamate transporters (of which the human equivalents are called *excitatory amino acid transporters* [EAATs]) have been identified: GLAST (EAAT1),[29] GLT1 (EAAT2),[30] EAAC1 (EAAT3),[31] EAAT4,[32] and EAAT5.[33] GLT1 and GLAST appear to be restricted to astrocytes,[34,35] and EAAC1 is found in neurons.[36,37] The expression of EAAT4 and EAAT5 is limited to Purkinje cells and retinal cells, respectively.[33,38] Glutamate taken up by astrocytes is recycled in the glutamate—glutamine cycle.[39,40] Within the astrocyte, glutamine synthase converts glutamate into glutamine, which is released back into the extracellular space, taken up by nerve terminals, and reconverted into glutamate by the enzyme glutaminase.

Mechanisms of Excitotoxic Neuronal Death

Two forms of excitotoxicity have been described: primary or direct and secondary, slow or indirect excitotoxicity. In direct excitotoxicity, the extracellular glutamate concentration increases to a neurotoxic level. In secondary excitotoxicity, cell death occurs even with normal glutamate levels, due to an increased sensitivity of energetically compromised neurons to glutamate.

In the central nervous system, the extracellular glutamate concentration is kept low (approximately 0.6 micromolar[41]) in spite of a high intracellular concentration of approximately 10 millimolars[42] and frequent release of glutamate at glutamatergic synapses. Elevation of the extracellular glutamate concentration to 2 to 5 μmol/L is considered sufficient to cause degeneration of neurons through excessive stimulation of GluRs.[43,44] Acute elevations of glutamate are thought to increase neuronal damage in conditions as stroke and neurotrauma, whereas more chronic milder elevations of glutamate are believed to induce (secondary) excitotoxicity in affected neuronal populations in neurodegenerative diseases. Increased extracellular glutamate concentrations can occur when the release from presynaptic terminals is augmented or when the reuptake from the synaptic cleft is insufficient. In addition, lethal injury to neurons, astrocytes or microglia, can lead to the release of the intracellular glutamate content and result in excitotoxic death of surrounding neurons. Energy depletion can give rise to an increased release and a reduced reuptake of glutamate but renders neurons more vulnerable to excitotoxicity.[45,46]

Initially, the NMDA receptor was considered to be uniquely responsible for excitotoxicity.[47] More recently, it became apparent that the activation of AMPA receptors is at least as important.[48] The role of metabotropic GluRs in excitotoxicity needs further clarification. Stimulation of group II and III metabotropic GluRs appears to exert a neuroprotective effect in experimental models of excitotoxicity,[49,50] whereas agonists of group I can either enhance or attenuate excitotoxic neuronal death.[51]

Ca^{2+} influx through NMDA receptors, Ca^{2+}-permeable AMPA receptors, or voltage-operated Ca^{2+} channels appears to be the predominant mediator of neuronal injury.[4,52,53] However, other permeating ions such as Na^+, K^+, Zn^{2+}, and Cl^- can affect neuronal viability. Influx of Na^+ ions, which is passively followed by Cl^- influx, can induce osmotic swelling of neurons.[4] We observed that Cl^- influx during AMPA receptor stimulation enhanced AMPA receptor currents and excitotoxic cell death in cultured spinal motor neurons (unpublished observations). In addition, efflux of K^+ ions through GluRs is thought to contribute to neuronal injury[54,55] and influx of Zn^{2+} ions through Ca^{2+}-permeable AMPA receptors can also trigger neuronal death.[56–58]

How ion movements through the cell membrane and in particular Ca^{2+} entry can induce neuronal death is not yet completely understood, but several possible mechanisms have been described. Influx of Ca^{2+} ions can result in activation of several enzymes such as protein kinase C, phospholipases, lipases, endonucleases, proteases, protein phosphatases, xanthine oxidase, and nitric oxide synthase (NOS). Also, mitochondrial dysfunction due to increased Ca^{2+} uptake in mitochondria and subsequent free-radical formation may at least contribute to the mechanism of excitotoxicity.[59–61] A similar mechanism is thought to mediate the toxic influx of zinc ions.[57]

Excitotoxic neuronal cell death can occur by necrosis or apoptosis depending on the experimental model.[62] In some culture models a separate form of necrosis with DNA fragmentation has been described.[63]

Excitotoxic Motor Neuron Death

Several lines of evidence suggest that motor neurons, both in vitro and in vivo, are particularly vulnerable to excitotoxicity. Intrathecal or intraspinal administration of AMPA receptor agonists has been shown to induce motor neuron degeneration in animals,[64–69] whereas NMDA failed to damage spinal motor neurons.[67,69] A rather selective loss of motor neurons could be induced, especially when KA was used (kainate has a high affinity for KA receptors, resulting in rapidly desensitizing currents, and has a lower affinity for AMPA receptors, resulting in long-lasting currents).[66,69] Furthermore, intrathecal administration of inhibitors of glutamate uptake induces neuronal damage if co-administered with glutamate.[70]

In organotypic rat spinal cord cultures (spinal cord slices from postnatal rats that can be kept in culture for several weeks), motor neurons were also shown to be vulnerable to AMPA receptor—mediated excitotoxicity, but not to excessive NMDA receptor stimulation.[71,72] Both direct application of AMPA receptor agonists and inhibition of glutamate transport resulted in selective motor neuron loss, which could be prevented by antagonists of AMPA receptors.

Similarly, it was demonstrated by different groups that motor neurons in culture are particularly susceptible to exposure to GluR agonists, especially to AMPA receptor agonists.[52,73–78] In these models, Ca^{2+} influx through Ca^{2+}-permeable AMPA receptors has been shown to be crucial for triggering motor neuron death.[52,53,73,79,80] Again, little or no effect of agonists of NMDA receptors was seen in cultured motor neurons. The effect of different agonists of GluRs on motor neuron survival and on intracellular Ca^{2+} measurements is illustrated in Figure 10.1.

The mechanism-mediating cell death seems to be dependent on the experimental paradigm. In co-cultures of motor neurons on an astroglial feeder layer (Figure 10.2), short exposures to KA (as an agonist of AMPA receptors) result in selective motor neuron death mediated by Ca^{2+} influx through Ca^{2+}-permeable AMPA receptors: It is dependent on extracellular Ca^{2+} and can be inhibited by application of AMPA receptor blockers and of Ca^{2+}-permeable AMPA receptor antagonists.[53,80] However, exposure to glutamate induces motor

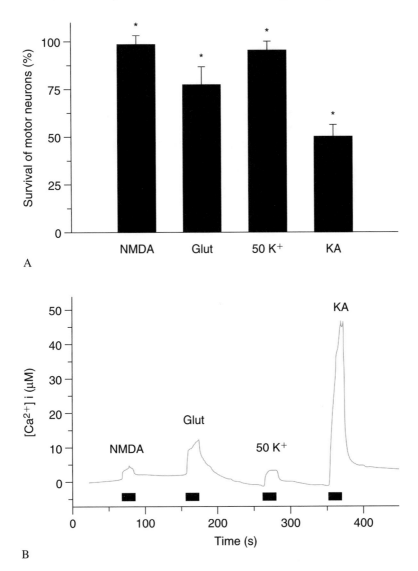

Figure 10.1 Relation between motor neuron death and changes in intracellular Ca²⁺ concentration. **(A)** Relative motor neuron survival following applications for 30 minutes of 300-micromolar N-methyl-D-aspartate, 300-micromolar glutamate, a 50-millimolar K⁺ solution (to depolarize motor neurons), and 300-micromolar kainate (KA). (For each condition, n ≥ 3; asterisk [*] denotes conditions significantly different [p < 0.05] from KA.) **(B)** Increases in intracellular Ca²⁺ concentration measured under the same conditions, using Indo-1FF as Ca²⁺ indicator.

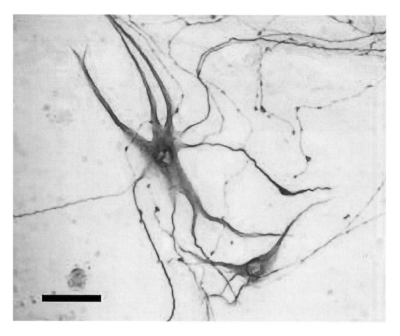

Figure 10.2   Motor neuron culture, stained with the motor neuron marker peripherin (scale bar = 40 micrometers). See color insert.

neuron degeneration that is only partially prevented by AMPA receptor antagonists and in contrast has a clear NMDA receptor—mediated component.[78]

Role of Excitotoxicity in Amyotrophic Lateral Sclerosis

Exogenous Excitotoxins Can Cause Exceptional Forms of Motor Neuron Disease

Oral intake of excitotoxins is believed to be responsible for specific forms of motor neuron disease (MND). This supports the idea that motor neurons are particularly vulnerable to excitotoxicity.

Lathyrism is a toxic upper motor neuron (UMN) disease characterized by spasticity mainly in the lower limbs caused by prolonged consumption of the chickling pea *Lathyrus sativus*.[81] The excitotoxin β-*N*-oxalyl-amino-L-alanine (BOAA), which is a potent AMPA receptor agonist[82] and abundantly present in this pea, most likely causes the motor neuron degeneration. Monkeys fed with *Lathyrus* or BOAA developed UMN signs[81,83] reminiscent of lathyrism, and intrathecal injections with BOAA were shown to induce motor neuron degeneration in the rat spinal cord.[84]

Western Pacific ALS-parkinsonism-dementia (Guam ALS) is a motor neuron syndrome originally thought to be caused by the excitotoxin β-methyl-L-alanine (BMAA) present in the seeds of false sago palm *Cycas circinalis*.[85] BMAA not only is an NMDA receptor agonist[86] but also activates AMPA receptors and metabotropic GluRs.[87] Oral administration of BMAA to monkeys resulted in a motor neuron disorder, parkinsonian features, and behavioral anomalies with predominantly degenerative changes in the motor cortex and ventral spinal cord.[88] This finding suggests that excitotoxicity is involved in the pathogenesis of the Guam complex. However, other neurotoxicological mechanisms were put forward because the concentration of BMAA in cycad flour in the Western Pacific is low and Guam disease can develop many years after the last exposure to this flour.[89] A recent study suggests that human consumption of flying foxes that also ate cycad seeds and possibly accumulated cycad toxins could be the source of BMAA intake.[90]

Abnormal Glutamate Metabolism in Amyotrophic Lateral Sclerosis

Several abnormalities in the metabolism of glutamate have been observed in patients with ALS by some groups but were disputed by others. Reductions of glutamate (and aspartate) levels have been found in brain and spinal cord tissue of patients with ALS.[91–95] Similarly, levels of *N*-acetylaspartylglutamate (NAAG), an acidic dipeptide that can be converted to glutamate, and *N*-acetylaspartate (NAA) by *N*-acetylated-α–linked amino dipeptidase (NAAL-ADase), and NAA were found to be reduced, whereas NAALDase was elevated in brain and spinal cord tissue of patients with ALS.[93,94] A proton magnetic resonance spectroscopy (^{1}H-MRS) study found evidence of reduced levels of NAA and NAAG and elevated levels of glutamate in the medulla of patients with ALS.[96] In the SOD1^{G93A} mouse model, elevated levels of extracellular glutamate have been found using microdialysis.[97] Elevated levels of glutamate (and NAAG, NAA, and aspartate) in the cerebrospinal fluid (CSF) of patients with ALS have been detected in some,[93,98] but not in all, studies.[99] Elevated plasma levels of glutamate during fasting and after oral glutamate loading were reported in one study[100] but could not be confirmed by others.[98,99] A similar controversy exists about the glutamate dehydrogenase (GDH) activities in ALS. GDH, a key enzyme in the glutamate metabolism, reversibly converts 2-oxoglutarate into glutamate. GDH activities in leukocytes from patients with ALS were found to be decreased in one study,[101] but normal in another.[100] GDH activities measured in the lumbar spinal cord from patients with ALS were increased in several spinal cord areas but were normal in the ventral horns.[95]

These findings remain difficult to interpret and their significance remains to be demonstrated. Undoubtedly, part of the contradictory results for glutamate can be explained by the technical difficulty encountered when measuring glutamate levels in different specimens.[102] In any case, these reports have greatly stimulated research into defects in glutamate transport in ALS.

Loss of Excitatory Amino Acid Transporter Type 2 in Amyotrophic Lateral Sclerosis

In 1992, diminished glutamate transport in synaptosomes from affected brain areas and spinal cord of sporadic ALS patients was reported by Rothstein et al[103] In addition, the number of [^{3}H]d-aspartate—binding sites, a measure for the density of glutamate transporters, was shown to be reduced in the spinal cords from sporadic ALS patients.[104] This reduction in glutamate transport was found to be due to a selective loss of the astroglial glutamate transporter EAAT2 protein in the motor cortex and spinal cord.[105] This loss of EAAT2 was observed not only in sporadic ALS patients[105–107] but also in familial cases.[105]

Both in vitro and in vivo experiments demonstrated that loss of EAAT2 function may give rise to selective motor neuron degeneration. Treatment of organotypic spinal cord cultures with antisense oligonucleotides to EAAT2 and EAAT1, resulting in diminished transporter protein expression, was shown to induce progressive motor neuron loss, which could be antagonized by an AMPA receptor antagonist.[108] Chronic intraventricular administration of these antisense oligonucleotides in rats resulted in a rise of extracellular glutamate levels and a progressive motor syndrome.[108] A loss of EAAT2 immunoreactivity has also been described in the ventral horn of transgenic SOD1^{G93A} and SOD1^{G37R} mice[109,110] and more recently in transgenic SOD1^{G93A} rats.[111] However, this finding could not be reproduced by others[112,113] who found no change in EAAT2 expression or only a retarded mobility on gels. The strong expression of EAAT2 in glial cells surrounding motor neuron populations that are preferentially affected in ALS and the lower expression of EAAT2 around more resistant motor neurons such as those in the oculomotor nucleus[114] suggest that disease-affected motor neurons have a higher glutamatergic input and are thus more vulnerable to elevated glutamate levels.

The mechanism explaining the loss of EAAT2 protein has been the subject of intense research, at the DNA, the mRNA, and the protein level. Mutations in the EAAT2 gene have been looked for, but no clear disease-associated mutations were found. Interestingly, in one sporadic ALS patient, a point mutation in exon 5 of EAAT2 was detected.[115] This N206S mutation resulted in deficient glycosylation of the protein, which affected transport of EAAT2 to the cell membrane. It thus gave rise to a loss of glutamate transport capacity resulting from decreased availability of the transporter in the plasma membrane. In addition, it exerted a dominant negative effect on wild type EAAT2.[116] In two patients with familial ALS not linked to SOD1, a mutation in intron 7 and a silent G-to-A transition in exon 5 were found.[115] No such mutations were detected by others,[117,118] so their significance awaits clarification.

At the mRNA level, no explanation for the loss of EAAT2 was identified either. No reductions in EAAT2 mRNA levels were found.[119] Aberrant transcripts of EAAT2 in disease-affected areas were reported in sporadic ALS patients[120] but were later found to be nonspecific.[118,121,122] Oxidative damage to the EAAT2 protein resulting in decreased glutamate transport has been implicated in both sporadic and familial ALS and is discussed later.

Whether the loss of EAAT2 represents a primary mechanism remains uncertain, but recent data provide strong evidence for the pathogenic role of EAAT2 in ALS. Mice overexpressing EAAT2 have been generated and crossbred with SOD1^{G93A} mice. Overexpression of EAAT2 would be expected to compensate for the loss of EAAT2 and slow down disease progression if this loss is pathogenetically relevant. Preliminary results suggest that the disease progression in these double transgenic animals is delayed.[123]

Excitotoxicity and SOD1 Mutations

The closest link between SOD1 mutations and excitotoxicity comes from the finding that EAAT2 can be oxidatively damaged in the presence of mutated SOD1;[124] this is discussed later. The inter-relation between the toxicity of mutant SOD1 and excitotoxicity was also studied in an in vitro model of intranuclear injections of mutant SOD1 in cultured motor neurons.[125] These injections induce progressive motor neuron death, which is dependent on extracellular glutamate and is inhibited by joro spider toxin (an antagonist of Ca^{2+}-permeable AMPA receptors) and coexpression of calbindin, but not affected by application of free-radical scavengers. This suggests that the toxicity of mutant SOD1 is induced or at least aggravated by glutamatergic stimulation.

In a different in vitro model, motor neurons in mixed spinal cord cultures from SOD1[G93A] mice were shown to be more sensitive to glutamate, which resulted in a higher free-radical production.[126] This suggests that SOD1 mutations would render motor neurons more vulnerable to excitotoxicity, which could explain why only motor neurons degenerate in mutant SOD1—induced ALS, in spite of the mutated protein being expressed ubiquitously in the organism. Despite many attempts, we have never been able to find such enhanced sensitivity in the motor neuron/glial cell co-culture system that we described.

Immune-Related Excitotoxic Motor Neuron Death

Excitotoxicity also appears to contribute to the toxicity of immunoglobulin G (IgG) present in the CSF of patients with ALS. In 1992, a high proportion of sporadic ALS patients were found to have IgG antibodies against L-type Ca^{2+} channels in the CSF.[127] CSF or purified IgG from CSF of patients with ALS were shown to be toxic to motor neuron cultures and to a hybridoma cell line.[128,129] The toxicity of these immunoglobulins might be due to their stimulatory effect on N/P-type voltage-gated Ca^{2+} channels,[129] but Ca^{2+} influx through GluRs might also be involved because this toxicity can be diminished by application of GluR antagonists.[128,130] The antiglutamate drug riluzole also protects against this toxicity.[131]

An interesting link between immune/inflammatory mechanisms and excitotoxic motor neuron death is evolving. In ALS, as in several other neurodegenerative diseases, microglial activation is known to go together with the neural loss.[132,133] Glutamate and KA were shown to induce microglial proliferation and activation, which enhanced excitotoxic neuron death in vitro, possibly because of the release of toxic compounds like NO, interleukin-1β or glutamate itself by the activated microglia.[134,135] The antibiotic minocycline, which has been shown to inhibit microglial activation,[136] protected against excitotoxic neuron death and prolonged survival of SOD1[G93A] mice.[137,138] Furthermore, the selective motor neuron death induced by inhibition of glutamate transport in organotypic spinal cord cultures could be antagonized by the anti-inflammatory cyclooxygenase-2 (COX-2) inhibitors.[139] COX-2 inhibition also prolonged survival of SOD1[G93A] mice.[140] The actual mechanism of action of these anti-inflammatory treatments and their relation to excitotoxicity require further elucidation, and the results of clinical trials with these compounds in patients with ALS are awaited.

Enhanced Vulnerability of Motor Neurons to Excitotoxicity

Several intrinsic properties of motor neurons render these cells particularly vulnerable to excitotoxicity, a phenomenon that could at least contribute to the selective vulnerability of motor neurons in ALS.

First, the capacity of motor neurons to buffer Ca^{2+} increases in the cytoplasm is limited because of the low amount of Ca^{2+}-buffering proteins they express in their cytosol. This makes these cells susceptible to increases of the intracellular Ca^{2+} concentration. Immunocytochemical studies revealed that spinal motor neurons do not express the Ca^{2+}-binding proteins parvalbumin and calbindin D-28k,[141–143] whereas less vulnerable motor neurons such as those in the oculomotor, trochlear, abducens, and Onuf nucleus clearly express Ca^{2+}-binding proteins.[142,143] Similarly, parvalbumin mRNA expression was high in ALS-resistant motor neuron pools, whereas no measurable parvalbumin expression was found in ALS-sensitive motor neurons.[144] Electrophysiological estimation of the Ca^{2+}-buffering capacity in murine brain stem and spinal cord slices confirmed a much higher Ca^{2+}-binding ratio in oculomotor than in hypoglossal or spinal motor neurons.[145–147] Motor neurons from parvalbumin-overexpressing mice were shown to be relatively resistant to excitotoxic stimuli, because they were demonstrated to have a lower increase of intracellular Ca^{2+} and an increased survival after AMPA receptor stimulation.[148] Crossbreeding of a different strain of parvalbumin-overexpressing mice with $SOD1^{G93A}$ mice delayed disease onset by 17 percent and prolonged survival by 11 percent.[149] It should also be noted that the glutamate-dependent death of motor neurons in mixed spinal cord cultures, induced by injection of mutant SOD1, could be rescued by co-overexpression of calbindin D-28k, as mentioned earlier.[125]

Second, motor neurons have a high density of AMPA receptors[150] and appear to have a high proportion of Ca^{2+}-permeable AMPA receptors.[53,73,151] Some studies have suggested that this is due to the low expression level of GluR2 in motor neurons, giving rise to GluR2-deficient Ca^{2+}-permeable AMPA receptors,[152–156] but this could not be confirmed by others.[79,157–160] Some authors found the levels of GluR2 expression to be decreased or the editing of GluR2 mRNA to be deficient in ventral spinal cords of patients with ALS.[155,161] However, a light and electron microscopic study could not detect any difference in the expression of GluR2 between $SOD1^{G86R}$ transgenic mice and non-transgenic controls.[159]

In view of this controversy, it should be noted that small differences in GluR2 levels have a large influence on the Ca^{2+} permeability of the AMPA receptor (Figure 10.3), and that total levels of GluR2 protein or mRNA may not adequately reflect the amount of GluR2 inserted in the receptor complex in the membrane. We therefore conducted an electrophysiological study of AMPA receptor properties that are dependent on the relative abundance of GluR2 and found a clear correlation between AMPA receptor—mediated motor neuron death and GluR2-dependent properties of AMPA receptors (e.g., the relative Ca^{2+} permeability and the proportion of the current through Ca^{2+}-permeable

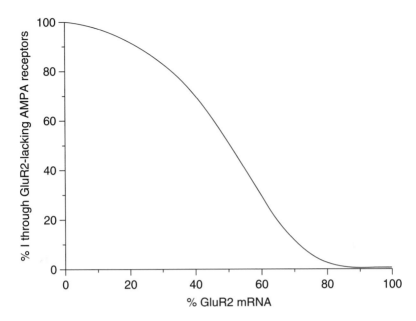

Figure 10.3 Calculation of the proportion of the current through Ca^{2+}-permeable α-amino-3-hydroxy-5-methyl-4-isoxazole propionic acid (AMPA) receptors as a function of the relative glutamate receptor subunit 2 (GluR2) messenger RNA (mRNA) content. The total current through Ca^{2+}-permeable AMPA receptors can be calculated if the following assumptions are made: The AMPA receptor is a random association of the four subunits, AMPA receptors containing a GluR2 subunit have a 15 times lower single channel conductance (<500 fS [fentosiemens] versus 7 to 8 pS [picosiemens])[253] and the regulation of GluR1-4 subunit expression occurs solely at the mRNA level. Note that most of the change of the proportion of current through Ca^{2+}-permeable AMPA receptors occurs between 40 and 60 percent GluR2 mRNA, which is close to the average GluR2 mRNA levels measured in motor neurons.[79,160]

AMPA receptors, which is the proportion of the current that can be antagonized by inhibitors of Ca^{2+}-permeable AMPA receptors),[151] suggesting that motor neurons that are vulnerable to excitotoxicity indeed express relatively more GluR2-deficient AMPA receptors than those that are less vulnerable.

In vivo evidence for the crucial role of GluR2 in motor neuron viability comes from the study of a transgenic mice that overexpress a GluR2 gene that encodes an asparagine (GluR2-N) at the Q/R site, which makes editing impossible.[162] AMPA receptor channels incorporating GluR2-N are permeable to Ca^{2+}.[26] Such mice appear to develop a motor neuron degeneration later in life.[162] However, transgenic mice that lack the GluR2 subunit, do not suffer from an MND.[163] This might be due to adaptations during development to limit excessive AMPA receptor stimulation.[164] The ultimate test for the GluR2 hypothesis in ALS would be to study the effect of GluR2 overexpression on motor neuron survival. GluR2-overexpressing mice have been generated, and the results of cross-breeding experiments with SOD1^{G93A} mice are keenly awaited.[165]

Other factors contributing to the motor neuron's vulnerability to excitotoxicity have been suggested. Motor neurons may be more sensitive to glutamate-induced NO production[76] and mitochondrial dysfunction due to increased Ca^{2+} influx in mitochondria.[60]

Role of Metabotropic Glutamate Receptors

mGluRs appear to modulate excitotoxicity in motor neurons,[166,167] but their exact role remains to be elucidated. The expression pattern of mGluRs differs between motor neuron populations that are vulnerable or resistant in ALS. Spinal and hypoglossal motor neurons mainly express mGluR1, 4, and 7, whereas motor neurons from Onuf, oculomotor, and trochlear nucleus also express mGluR5.[166,168–171] Stimulation of group I, III, and to a variable degree group II mGluRs has been shown to attenuate excitotoxic motor neuron death in vitro.[166,167] Furthermore, in spinal cords from familial and sporadic ALS patients, an upregulation of mGluRs in reactive astrocytes has been described.[170] These findings suggest a regulating role for mGluRs in motor neurons and surrounding astrocytes, but at present, the impact of these findings remains unclear.

Pharmacotherapy for Excitotoxicity in Amyotrophic Lateral Sclerosis

Riluzole, the only drug that proved effective against disease progression in patients with ALS until now,[172,173] has antiglutamate properties (among others, inhibition of glutamate release and inhibition of GluRs). This is considered indirect evidence for a pathogenic role of excitotoxicity in ALS. However, other antiglutamate treatments tested in ALS were less successful. Gabapentin, which presumably acts through inhibition of glutamate biosynthesis, prolonged survival of SOD1^{G93A} mice.[173] In spite of promising preclinical studies,[174,175] a randomized clinical trial failed to show a delay in disease progression in patients with ALS.[176] Lamotrigine, which is thought to inhibit glutamate release, had no beneficial effect on patients with ALS.[177] A clinical trial with dextromethorphan, an NMDA receptor antagonist, similarly failed.[178,179] The AMPA receptor antagonist LY300164 was tested in a small double-blind, placebo-controlled study. There was a trend toward a prolonged survival, but significance was not reached.[180] Recently, RPR 119990, a novel AMPA receptor blocker, improved motor performance and survival of SOD1^{G93A} mice, with 12.6 percent in the highest dose tested.[181] The drug has not been tested yet in patients with ALS.

OXIDATIVE STRESS

Reactive oxygen species (ROS) are highly reactive biomolecules formed during normal metabolism. The mitochondrial respiratory chain is the main source of ROS, but NOS, arachidonic acid metabolism, xanthine oxidase, monoamine oxidase, and cytochrome P-450 enzymes provide other mechanisms for endogenous ROS generation.[182] Superoxide ($O_2\cdot^-$) and hydrogen peroxide (H_2O_2) can give rise to the highly toxic hydroxyl radical ($OH\cdot$) (Fenton reaction), and $O_2\cdot^-$ and NO can generate peroxynitrite ($ONOO^-$). ROS can induce oxidative damage to proteins, lipids, and nucleic acids, resulting in cellular dysfunction and cell death. Cells are equipped with several antioxidant defenses. The enzymes superoxide dismutase (SOD), catalase, and glutathione peroxidase convert ROS into less reactive molecules, and the small molecules glutathione, vitamins C and E, and certain chemical groups of biomolecules are antioxidants. Oxidative stress arises when the generation of toxic ROS exceeds the capacity of the cellular antioxidant defenses. This can be due to an elevated production of ROS, to shortcomings in the defenses, or to a combination of both. Motor neurons are large cells with a high metabolic rate, requiring a high level of mitochondrial activity, which results in a high baseline level of ROS production. They normally contain a high level of the antioxidant enzyme SOD1.[183] Oxidative stress has been implicated in the pathogenesis of normal aging and many neurodegenerative diseases,[184] including ALS.

Oxidative Damage in Amyotrophic Lateral Sclerosis

The discovery of SOD1 mutations in some forms of familial ALS[185] fostered the belief that oxidative stress was involved in the pathogenesis of this disease, as SOD1 plays a pivotal role in free-radical metabolism. Homodimers of SOD1 convert $O_2\cdot^-$ into H_2O_2 and H_2O.[186] H_2O_2 is then further detoxified to H_2O by glutathione peroxidase or catalase. Initially, it was suggested that a decrease of enzymatic activity of mutated SOD1 could underlie the motor neuron degeneration.[187,188] It now is generally accepted that loss of dismutase activity is most likely not involved in the pathogenesis of ALS for several reasons. First, almost all mutations in SOD1 are inherited as autosomal dominant diseases. Second, SOD1 mutations cause ALS irrespective of their effect on the enzymatic activity.[189,190] Finally, transgenic mice overexpressing human familial ALS—linked mutations develop motor neuron degeneration in spite of normal endogenous SOD1 activity,[191–194] and SOD1 knockout mice retain their motor neurons.[195] This suggests that mutant SOD1 exerts its toxic actions not by a loss of dismutase activity, but through the gain of a novel cytotoxic function.

The nature of this mutation-induced function remains unknown. One of the several hypotheses put forward suggests that these mutations, which are scattered throughout the SOD1 polypeptide, all induce alterations in the enzyme's conformation so that substrates other than $O_2\cdot^-$ get access to the enzyme's active site and would give rise to an aberrant copper-dependent catalysis that converts these substrates into even more toxic-free radicals. Two substrates were particularly studied: $O_2\cdot^-$ and peroxynitrite (ONOO$^-$, the reaction product of $O_2\cdot^-$ and NO). The former may be converted into OH$^-$ radicals, the mutant SOD1 acting as a peroxidase.[196,197] The latter may react with the mutated SOD1 (having lost its zinc ion because of a mutation-induced lower affinity for zinc) to form nitronium ions, capable of damaging proteins by nitration of tyrosine residues.[198,199]

Several studies provided in vitro and in vivo evidence in favor of an aberrant enzymatic activity of mutated SOD1,[200–203] although other studies did not.[194,201] Several studies provided evidence, though circumstantial only, for the presence of oxidatively damaged nucleic acids, proteins, and lipids in patients with ALS and mutant SOD1—overexpressing mice.[204] Increased levels of markers for oxidative stress were found in the motor cortex,[205,206] spinal motor neurons,[207–211] CSF,[212–214] and serum[215] of patients with ALS. Similarly, increased levels of oxidative markers including nitrotyrosines were reported in G93A mice,[216–218] but no nitrated proteins were found.[201,219] In one study, the level of nitrated manganese—dependent SOD2 was elevated in CSF of sporadic ALS patients;[214] nitration of the tyrosine residue of this mitochondrial antioxidant enzyme is known to inactivate the enzyme.[220] 4-Hydroxynonenal (HNE), a marker of lipid peroxidation, was found to be increased in the CSF of sporadic ALS patients and was reported to induce cell death in a motor neuron hybrid cell line.[212] The primary site of generation of HNE is the plasma membrane,[221] and the major targets for HNE-induced protein damage are therefore membrane-associated proteins. Increased modification of proteins by HNE was detected in spinal motor neurons of sporadic ALS patients by immunohistochemistry and immunoblotting,[222] but not in motor neurons from familial ALS cases linked to mutations in SOD1.[210]

Although these studies demonstrate oxidative damage to be present in ALS, they do not provide evidence for its mechanism and they do not give indications about their primary or secondary pathogenic significance. In a recent study, the hypothesis of copper-mediated aberrant reactions of the mutant SOD1 was addressed directly by studying copper chaperone for SOD1 (CCS) knock-out mice.[223] CCS is required for the incorporation of copper into SOD1.[224] Ablation of the gene encoding the copper chaperone in SOD1 mutant mice led to a defect of copper incorporation in both wild type and mutant SOD1, which resulted in a dramatic decrease in SOD1 activity. Onset and progression of the MND in these mice was not significantly different than those in mutant SOD1 control mice. This suggests that at least copper-mediated aberrant enzymatic activity of mutant SOD1 is unlikely to play a role in the pathogenesis of ALS.

Oxidative Stress and Aggregates

Aggregates of mutant SOD1 are detected in motor neurons and astrocytes of mice expressing mutant SOD1 and in human ALS cases linked to SOD1[194] and formed in cultured motor neurons after microinjections of mutant but not of wild type SOD1 cDNAs.[225] The role of aggregates in the pathogenesis of ALS is discussed in Chapter 9. Recent studies on the pathogenesis of trinucleotide repeat—induced neurodegeneration suggest that oxidative stress can accompany the formation of aggregates in these conditions.[226] Conversely, oxidative stress was found to cause aggregation of SOD1 in a transgenic *Caenorhabditis elegans* model.[227] However, antioxidants did not prevent the formation of SOD1 aggregates or the motor neuron death after intranuclear injections of mutant SOD1 cDNA.[125]

Oxidative Damage and Excitotoxicity

An important target molecule of oxidative damage in SOD1-related familial ALS was suggested by Trotti et al,[124] who showed that EAAT2 is damaged by mutant SOD1—induced oxidative stress. The site of damage was shown to be located in the intracellular carboxyl-terminal and resulted in a 50 percent reduction of the glutamate uptake, possibly resulting in excitotoxic damage of motor neurons and represents a major link between oxidative stress and excitotoxicity (see later discussion).

EAAT2 was also reported to be susceptible to oxidative damage by HNE.[222] It had already been shown that the function of this transporter could be seriously compromised when damaged by HNE.[228,229] EAAT2 is equally susceptible to damage induced by other oxidants, as $ONOO^-$, H_2O_2, and $O_2^{\cdot-}$,[230,231] most likely by oxidation of cysteine sulfhydryl groups in the redox-sensing moiety of the protein.[232]

Another link between oxidative stress and excitotoxicity is of course provided by the finding that glutamate toxicity can provoke oxidative stress, as mentioned earlier. Ca^{2+} entry through GluRs resulted in a Ca^{2+} influx in mitochondria and in an increased free-radical formation in cultured motor neurons.[60,61] Furthermore, AMPA receptor—mediated excitotoxicity was attenuated by NOS inhibitors.[76] Glutamate can also bring about oxidative stress in another way, called oxidative glutamate toxicity. Increased levels of extracellular glutamate can hamper the cystine-glutamate antiporter, which results in a lower cystine uptake, intracellular glutathione depletion, and oxidative stress.[233,234] To what extent this mechanism is involved in the pathogenesis of ALS needs further clarification.

Molecular targets for oxidative stress other than EAAT2 have been suggested as well. Voltage-activated sodium channels represent another target of mutant SOD1—induced damage, resulting in a reduction of current amplitudes and a shift toward more positive potentials of the inactivation curve.[235] Similar effects on these sodium currents can be achieved by exposure to oxidants.[236,237] Oxidative damage by HNE resulted in facilitated opening of voltage-activated Ca^{2+} channels.[238] The relevance of these findings in relation to motor neuron degeneration remains unclear.

Cellular Antioxidant Defense and Antioxidant Treatment

Increased sensitivity to externally applied oxidative stress has been demonstrated in cell lines expressing mutant SOD1,[239,240] in nigral neurons from G93A mice,[241] and in fibroblasts from sporadic and SOD1-linked familial ALS patients,[242] but not in fibroblasts from patients with familial ALS not associated with SOD1 mutations.[243] Defects in the cellular responses to oxidative stress have been reported in transgenic SOD1 mice,[244] and decreased levels of the antioxidant vitamin E were found in G93A mice.[173] The cellular prion protein, which is thought to have antioxidant properties (it binds copper and has SOD activity), is downregulated in the spinal cord from early symptomatic SOD1[G86R] mice.[245]

Increasing the cellular antioxidant potential by providing it exogenously with antioxidants had beneficial effects on the disease progression in transgenic SOD1[G93A] mice. Treatment with vitamin E was shown to delay disease onset without effect on the survival.[173] Administration of the free-radical scavenger acetylcysteine improved survival in SOD1[G93A] mice with a high copy number,[246] but this was not confirmed in mice with a low copy number.[247] Treatment of male $SOD1^{G93A}$ mice with the *Ginkgo biloba* extract EGb761, which is considered to act as an NO scavenger, extended survival by approximately 10 percent.[248] Subcutaneous administration of polyamine-modified catalase, which was shown to be able to cross the blood-brain barrier, prolonged the survival by almost 12 percent.[249] Similarly, synthetic SOD/catalase mimetics were shown to increase the life span by 7 to 10 percent.[250]

Despite promising results in animal models, clinical trials of antioxidant treatments in patients with ALS have not been successful. In a randomized clinical trial of 289 patients with ALS, no beneficial effect of vitamin E was found on either motor function or survival.[251] The effect of subcutaneous administration of acetylcysteine was investigated in a randomized double-blind placebo-controlled trial.[252] The survival of patients treated with acetylcysteine was slightly prolonged, but this difference did not reach significance.

CONCLUSION

Excitotoxicity and oxidative stress are two probably interacting mechanisms of motor neuron damage that are possibly involved in the pathogenesis of ALS; the evidence for their involvement remains indirect. Because both these phenomena are targets for pharmacological interference, the understanding of their role in ALS may have important therapeutic implications.

Acknowledgments

P.V.D. is a fellow, L.V.D.B. a postdoctoral fellow, and W.R. a clinical investigator of the Fund of Scientific Research (Flanders). We are supported by the Research Council of the University of Leuven, the Fund for Scientific Research (Flanders), the American ALS Association, and the Association Belge contre les Maladies Musculaires and participate in phase V of the UIAP, Belgium (Molecular Genetics and Cell Biology).

REFERENCES

1. Lucas DR, Newhouse JP. The toxic effect of sodium L-glutamate on the inner layers of the retina. Arch Ophthalmol 1957;58:193–204.
2. Olney JW. Neurotoxicity of Excitatory Amino Acids. In EG McGeer, JW Olney, PL McGeer (eds), Kainic Acid as a Tool in Neurobiology. New York: Raven Press 1978;95–121.
3. Lipton SA, Rosenberg PA. Excitatory amino acids as a final common pathway for neurologic disorders. N Engl J Med 1994;330:613–622.
4. Choi DW. Ionic dependence of glutamate neurotoxicity. J Neurosci 1987;7:369–379.
5. Seeburg PH. The TINS/TiPS Lecture. The molecular biology of mammalian glutamate receptor channels. Trends Neurosci 1993;16:359–365.
6. Hollmann M, Heinemann S. Cloned glutamate receptors. Annu Rev Neurosci 1994;17:31–108.
7. Hollmann M, O'Shea-Greenfield A, Rogers SW, Heinemann S. Cloning by functional expression of a member of the glutamate receptor family. Nature 1989;342:643–648.

8. Keinanen K, Wisden W, Sommer B, et al. A family of AMPA-selective glutamate receptors. Science 1990;249:556–560.

9. Boulter J, Hollmann M, O'Shea-Greenfield A, et al. Molecular cloning and functional expression of glutamate receptor subunit genes. Science 1990;249:1033–1037.

10. Nakanishi N, Shneider NA, Axel R. A family of glutamate receptor genes: evidence for the formation of heteromultimeric receptors with distinct channel properties. Neuron 1990;5:569–581.

11. Moriyoshi K, Masu M, Ishii T, et al. Molecular cloning and characterization of the rat NMDA receptor. Nature 1991;354:31–37.

12. Meguro H, Mori H, Araki K, et al. Functional characterization of a heteromeric NMDA receptor channel expressed from cloned cDNAs. Nature 1992;357:70–74.

13. Monyer H, Sprengel R, Schoepfer R, et al. Heteromeric NMDA receptors: molecular and functional distinction of subtypes. Science 1992;256:1217–1221.

14. Kutsuwada T, Kashiwabuchi N, Mori H, et al. Molecular diversity of the NMDA receptor channel. Nature 1992;358:36–41.

15. Ishii T, Moriyoshi K, Sugihara H, et al. Molecular characterization of the family of the N-methyl-D-aspartate receptor subunits. J Biol Chem 1993;268:2836–2843.

16. Egebjerg J, Bettler B, Hermans-Borgmeyer I, Heinemann S. Cloning of a cDNA for a glutamate receptor subunit activated by kainate but not AMPA. Nature 1991;351:745–748.

17. Werner P, Voigt M, Keinanen K, et al. Cloning of a putative high-affinity kainate receptor expressed predominantly in hippocampal CA3 cells. Nature 1991;351:742–744.

18. Bettler B, Egebjerg J, Sharma G, et al. Cloning of a putative glutamate receptor: a low affinity kainate-binding subunit. Neuron 1992;8:257–265.

19. Herb A, Burnashev N, Werner P, et al. The KA-2 subunit of excitatory amino acid receptors shows widespread expression in brain and forms ion channels with distantly related subunits. Neuron 1992;8:775–785.

20. Collingridge GL, Lester RA. Excitatory amino acid receptors in the vertebrate central nervous system. Pharmacol Rev 1989;41:143–210.

21. Mayer ML, Westbrook GL. Permeation and block of N-methyl-D-aspartic acid receptor channels by divalent cations in mouse cultured central neurones. J Physiol 1987;394:501–527.

22. Nowak L, Bregestovski P, Ascher P, et al. Magnesium gates glutamate-activated channels in mouse central neurones. Nature 1984;307:462–465.

23. Mayer ML, Westbrook GL, Guthrie PB. Voltage-dependent block by Mg^{2+} of NMDA responses in spinal cord neurones. Nature 1984;309:261–263.

24. Hollmann M, Hartley M, Heinemann S. Ca^{2+} permeability of KA-AMPA—gated glutamate receptor channels depends on subunit composition. Science 1991;252:851–853.

25. Hume RI, Dingledine R, Heinemann SF. Identification of a site in glutamate receptor subunits that controls calcium permeability. Science 1991;253:1028–1031.

26. Burnashev N, Monyer H, Seeburg PH, Sakmann B. Divalent ion permeability of AMPA receptor channels is dominated by the edited form of a single subunit. Neuron 1992;8:189–198.

27. Sommer B, Kohler M, Sprengel R, Seeburg PH. RNA editing in brain controls a determinant of ion flow in glutamate-gated channels. Cell 1991;67:11–19.

28. Ozawa S, Kamiya H, Tsuzuki K. Glutamate receptors in the mammalian central nervous system. Prog Neurobiol 1998;54:581–618.

29. Storck T, Schulte S, Hofmann K, Stoffel W. Structure, expression, and functional analysis of a Na(+)-dependent glutamate/aspartate transporter from rat brain. Proc Natl Acad Sci USA 1992;89:10955–10959.

30. Pines G, Danbolt NC, Bjoras M, et al. Cloning and expression of a rat brain L-glutamate transporter. Nature 1992;360:464–467.

31. Kanai Y, Hediger MA. Primary structure and functional characterization of a high-affinity glutamate transporter. Nature 1992;360:467–471.

32. Fairman WA, Vandenberg RJ, Arriza JL, et al. An excitatory amino-acid transporter with properties of a ligand-gated chloride channel. Nature 1995;375:599–603.

33. Arriza JL, Eliasof S, Kavanaugh MP, Amara SG. Excitatory amino acid transporter 5, a retinal glutamate transporter coupled to a chloride conductance. Proc Natl Acad Sci USA 1997;94:4155–4160.

34. Chaudhry FA, Lehre KP, van Lookeren Campagne M, et al. Glutamate transporters in glial plasma membranes: highly differentiated localizations revealed by quantitative ultrastructural immunocytochemistry. Neuron 1995;15:711–720.

35. Lehre KP, Levy LM, Ottersen OP, et al. Differential expression of two glial glutamate transporters in the rat brain: quantitative and immunocytochemical observations. J Neurosci 1995;15: 1835–1853.
36. Torp R, Hoover F, Danbolt NC, et al. Differential distribution of the glutamate transporters GLT1 and rEAAC1 in rat cerebral cortex and thalamus: an in situ hybridization analysis. Anat Embryol (Berl) 1997;195:317–226.
37. Conti F, DeBiasi S, Minelli A, et al. EAAC1, a high-affinity glutamate transporter, is localized to astrocytes and GABAergic neurons besides pyramidal cells in the rat cerebral cortex. Cereb Cortex 1998;8:108–116.
38. Dehnes Y, Chaudhry FA, Ullensvang K, et al. The glutamate transporter EAAT4 in rat cerebellar Purkinje cells: a glutamate-gated chloride channel concentrated near the synapse in parts of the dendritic membrane facing astroglia. J Neurosci 1998;18:3606–3619.
39. Hamberger A, Jacobson I, Lindroth P, et al. Neuron-glia interactions in the biosynthesis and release of transmitter amino acids. Adv Biochem Psychopharmacol 1981;29:509–518.
40. Erecinska M, Silver IA. Metabolism and role of glutamate in mammalian brain. Prog Neurobiol 1990;35:245–296.
41. Benveniste H, Drejer J, Schousboe A, Diemer NH. Elevation of the extracellular concentrations of glutamate and aspartate in rat hippocampus during transient cerebral ischemia monitored by intracerebral microdialysis. J Neurochem 1984;43:1369–1374.
42. Kvamme E, Schousboe A, Hertz L, et al. Developmental change of endogenous glutamate and gamma-glutamyl transferase in cultured cerebral cortical interneurons and cerebellar granule cells, and in mouse cerebral cortex and cerebellum in vivo. Neurochem Res 1985;10:993–1008.
43. Meldrum B, Garthwaite J. Excitatory amino acid neurotoxicity and neurodegenerative disease. Trends Pharmacol Sci 1990;11:379–387.
44. Rosenberg PA, Amin S, Leitner M. Glutamate uptake disguises neurotoxic potency of glutamate agonists in cerebral cortex in dissociated cell culture. J Neurosci 1992;12:56–61.
45. Novelli A, Reilly JA, Lysko PG, Henneberry RC. Glutamate becomes neurotoxic via the N-methyl-D-aspartate receptor when intracellular energy levels are reduced. Brain Res 1988;451:205–212.
46. Henneberry RC, Novelli A, Cox JA, Lysko PG. Neurotoxicity at the N-methyl-D-aspartate receptor in energy-compromised neurons. An hypothesis for cell death in aging and disease. Ann N Y Acad Sci 1989;568:225–233.
47. Choi DW. Glutamate neurotoxicity and diseases of the nervous system. Neuron 1988;1:623–634.
48. Prehn JH, Lippert K, Krieglstein J. Are NMDA or AMPA/kainate receptor antagonists more efficacious in the delayed treatment of excitotoxic neuronal injury? Eur J Pharmacol 1995; 292:179–189.
49. Bruno V, Copani A, Battaglia G, et al. Protective effect of the metabotropic glutamate receptor agonist, DCG-IV, against excitotoxic neuronal death. Eur J Pharmacol 1994;256:109–112.
50. Battaglia G, Bruno V, Ngomba RT, et al. Selective activation of group-II metabotropic glutamate receptors is protective against excitotoxic neuronal death. Eur J Pharmacol 1998;356:271–274.
51. Nicoletti F, Bruno V, Catania MV, et al. Group-I metabotropic glutamate receptors: hypotheses to explain their dual role in neurotoxicity and neuroprotection. Neuropharmacology 1999;38:1477–1484.
52. Carriedo SG, Yin HZ, Weiss JH. Motor neurons are selectively vulnerable to AMPA/kainate receptor—mediated injury in vitro. J Neurosci 1996;16:4069–4079.
53. Van Den Bosch L, Vandenberghe W, Klaassen H, et al. Ca(2+)-permeable AMPA receptors and selective vulnerability of motor neurons. J Neurol Sci 2000;180:29–34.
54. Yu SP, Yeh C, Strasser U, et al. NMDA receptor—mediated K^+ efflux and neuronal apoptosis. Science 1999;284:336–339.
55. Xiao AY, Homma M, Wang XQ, et al. Role of K(+) efflux in apoptosis induced by AMPA and kainate in mouse cortical neurons. Neuroscience 2001;108:61–67.
56. Choi DW, Weiss JH, Koh JY, et al. Glutamate neurotoxicity, calcium, and zinc. Ann N Y Acad Sci 1989;568:219–224.
57. Sensi SL, Yin HZ, Carriedo SG, et al. Preferential Zn^{2+} influx through Ca^{2+}-permeable AMPA/kainate channels triggers prolonged mitochondrial superoxide production. Proc Natl Acad Sci USA 1999;96:2414–2419.
58. Yin HZ, Sensi SL, Ogoshi F, Weiss JH. Blockade of Ca^{2+}-permeable AMPA/kainate channels decreases oxygen-glucose deprivation—induced Zn^{2+} accumulation and neuronal loss in hippocampal pyramidal neurons. J Neurosci 2002;22:1273–1279.
59. Dykens JA. Isolated cerebral and cerebellar mitochondria produce free radicals when exposed to elevated Ca^{2+} and Na^+: implications for neurodegeneration. J Neurochem 1994;63:584–591.

60. Carriedo SG, Sensi SL, Yin HZ, Weiss JH. AMPA exposures induce mitochondrial Ca(2+) over-load and ROS generation in spinal motor neurons in vitro. J Neurosci 2000;20:240–250.
61. Urushitani M, Nakamizo T, Inoue R, et al. *N*-methyl-D-aspartate receptor—mediated mitochon-drial Ca(2+) overload in acute excitotoxic motor neuron death: a mechanism distinct from chronic neurotoxicity after Ca(2+) influx. J Neurosci Res 2001;63:377–387.
62. Leist M, Nicotera P. Apoptosis, excitotoxicity, and neuropathology. Exp Cell Res 1998;239:183–201.
63. Gwag BJ, Koh JY, DeMaro JA, et al. Slowly triggered excitotoxicity occurs by necrosis in corti-cal cultures. Neuroscience 1997;77:393–401.
64. Curtis DR, Malik R. A neurophysiological analysis of the effect of kainic acid on nerve fibers and terminals in the cat spinal cord. J Physiol 1985;368:99–108.
65. Pisharodi M, Nauta HJ. An animal model for neuron-specific spinal cord lesions by the microin-jection of N-methylaspartate, kainic acid, and quisqualic acid. Appl Neurophysiol 1985;48:226–233.
66. Hugon J, Vallat JM, Spencer PS, et al. Kainic acid induces early and delayed degenerative neu-ronal changes in rat spinal cord. Neurosci Lett 1989;104:258–262.
67. Urca G, Urca R. Neurotoxic effects of excitatory amino acids in the mouse spinal cord: quisqualate and kainate but not *N*-methyl-D-aspartate induce permanent neural damage. Brain Res 1990;529:7–15.
68. Nakamura R, Kamakura K, Kwak S. Late-onset selective neuronal damage in the rat spinal cord induced by continuous intrathecal administration of AMPA. Brain Res 1994;654:279–285.
69. Ikonomidou C, Qin Qin Y, Labruyere J, Olney JW. Motor neuron degeneration induced by exci-totoxin agonists has features in common with those seen in the SOD-1 transgenic mouse model of amyotrophic lateral sclerosis. J Neuropathol Exp Neurol 1996;55:211–224.
70. Hirata A, Nakamura R, Kwak S, et al. AMPA receptor—mediated slow neuronal death in the rat spinal cord induced by long-term blockade of glutamate transporters with THA. Brain Res 1997;771:37–44.
71. Rothstein JD, Jin L, Dykes-Hoberg M, Kuncl RW. Chronic inhibition of glutamate uptake pro-duces a model of slow neurotoxicity. Proc Natl Acad Sci USA 1993;90:6591–6595.
72. Saroff D, Delfs J, Kuznetsov D, Geula C. Selective vulnerability of spinal cord motor neurons to non-NMDA toxicity. Neuroreport 2000;11:1117–1121.
73. Carriedo SG, Yin HZ, Lamberta R, Weiss JH. In vitro kainate injury to large, SMI-32(+) spinal neurons is Ca^{2+} dependent. Neuroreport 1995;6:945–948.
74. Estevez AG, Stutzmann JM, Barbeito L. Protective effect of riluzole on excitatory amino acid—mediated neurotoxicity in motoneuron-enriched cultures. Eur J Pharmacol 1995;280:47–53.
75. Vandenberghe W, Van Den Bosch L, Robberecht W. Glial cells potentiate kainate-induced neu-ronal death in a motoneuron-enriched spinal coculture system. Brain Res 1998;807:1–10.
76. Urushitani M, Shimohama S, Kihara T, et al. Mechanism of selective motor neuronal death after exposure of spinal cord to glutamate: involvement of glutamate-induced nitric oxide in motor neuron toxicity and nonmotor neuron protection. Ann Neurol 1998;44:796–807.
77. Fryer HJ, Knox RJ, Strittmatter SM, Kalb RG. Excitotoxic death of a subset of embryonic rat motor neurons in vitro. J Neurochem 1999;72:500–513.
78. Van Den Bosch L, Robberecht W. Different receptors mediate motor neuron death induced by short and long exposures to excitotoxicity. Brain Res Bull 2000;53:383–388.
79. Greig A, Donevan SD, Mujtaba TJ, et al. Characterization of the AMPA-activated receptors present on motoneurons. J Neurochem 2000;74:179–191.
80. Van Den Bosch L, Van Damme P, Vleminckx V, et al. An α-mercaptoacrylic acid derivative (PD150606) inhibits selective motor neuron death via inhibition of kainate-induced Ca^{2+} influx and not via calpain inhibition. Neuropharmacology 2002;42:706–713.
81. Spencer PS, Roy DN, Ludolph A, et al. Lathyrism: evidence for role of the neuroexcitatory amino acid BOAA. Lancet 1986;2:1066–1067.
82. Bridges RJ, Stevens DR, Kahle JS, et al. Structure-function studies on *N*-oxalyl-diamino-dicar-boxylic acids and excitatory amino acid receptors: evidence that β-L-ODAP is a selective non-NMDA agonist. J Neurosci 1989;9:2073–2079.
83. Hugon J, Ludolph A, Roy DN, et al. Studies on the etiology and pathogenesis of motor neuron diseases, II: clinical and electrophysiologic features of pyramidal dysfunction in macaques fed Lathyrus sativus and IDPN. Neurology 1988;38:435–442.
84. Chase RA, Pearson S, Nunn PB, Lantos PL. Comparative toxicities of alpha- and beta-*N*-oxalyl-L-alpha, beta-diaminopropionic acids to rat spinal cord. Neurosci Lett 1985;55:89–94.

85. Spencer PS, Nunn PB, Hugon J, et al. Motor neurone disease on Guam: possible role of a food neurotoxin. Lancet 1986;1:965.
86. Ross SM, Seelig M, Spencer PS. Specific antagonism of excitotoxic action of "uncommon" amino acids assayed in organotypic mouse cortical cultures. Brain Res 1987;425:120–127.
87. Copani A, Canonico PL, Catania MV, et al. Interaction between β-*N*-methylamino-L-alanine and excitatory amino acid receptors in brain slices and neuronal cultures. Brain Res 1991;558:79–86.
88. Spencer PS, Nunn PB, Hugon J, et al. Guam amyotrophic lateral sclerosis-parkinsonism-dementia linked to a plant excitant neurotoxin. Science 1987;237:517–522.
89. Duncan MW, Steele JC, Kopin IJ, Markey SP. 2-Amino-3-(methylamino)-propanoic acid (BMAA) in cycad flour: an unlikely cause of amyotrophic lateral sclerosis and parkinsonism-dementia of Guam. Neurology 1990;40:767–772.
90. Cox PA, Sacks OW. Cycad neurotoxins, consumption of flying foxes, and ALS-PDC disease in Guam. Neurology 2002;58:956–959.
91. Perry TL, Hansen S, Jones K. Brain glutamate deficiency in amyotrophic lateral sclerosis. Neurology 1987;37:1845–1848.
92. Plaitakis A, Constantakakis E, Smith J. The neuroexcitotoxic amino acids glutamate and aspartate are altered in the spinal cord and brain in amyotrophic lateral sclerosis. Ann Neurol 1988;24:446–449.
93. Rothstein JD, Tsai G, Kuncl RW, et al. Abnormal excitatory amino acid metabolism in amyotrophic lateral sclerosis. Ann Neurol 1990;28:18–25.
94. Tsai GC, Stauch-Slusher B, Sim L, et al. Reductions in acidic amino acids and *N*-acetylaspartylglutamate in amyotrophic lateral sclerosis CNS. Brain Res 1991;556:151–156.
95. Malessa S, Leigh PN, Bertel O, et al. Amyotrophic lateral sclerosis: glutamate dehydrogenase and transmitter amino acids in the spinal cord. J Neurol Neurosurg Psychiatry 1991;54:984–988.
96. Pioro EP, Majors AW, Mitsumoto H, et al. ^{1}H-MRS evidence of neurodegeneration and excess glutamate + glutamine in ALS medulla. Neurology 1999;53:71–79.
97. Alexander GM, Deitch JS, Seeburger JL, et al. Elevated cortical extracellular fluid glutamate in transgenic mice expressing human mutant (G93A) Cu/Zn superoxide dismutase. J Neurochem 2000;74:1666–1673.
98. Shaw PJ, Forrest V, Ince PG, et al. CSF and plasma amino acid levels in motor neuron disease: elevation of CSF glutamate in a subset of patients. Neurodegeneration 1995;4:209–216.
99. Perry TL, Krieger C, Hansen S, Eisen A. Amyotrophic lateral sclerosis: amino acid levels in plasma and cerebrospinal fluid. Ann Neurol 1990;28:12–17.
100. Plaitakis A, Caroscio JT. Abnormal glutamate metabolism in amyotrophic lateral sclerosis. Ann Neurol 1987;22:575–579.
101. Hugon J, Tabaraud F, Rigaud M, et al. Glutamate dehydrogenase and aspartate aminotransferase in leukocytes of patients with motor neuron disease. Neurology 1989;39:956–958.
102. Rothstein JD, Kuncl R, Chaudhry V, et al. Excitatory amino acids in amyotrophic lateral sclerosis: an update. Ann Neurol 1991;30:224–225.
103. Rothstein JD, Martin LJ, Kuncl RW. Decreased glutamate transport by the brain and spinal cord in amyotrophic lateral sclerosis. N Engl J Med 1992;326:1464–1468.
104. Shaw PJ, Chinnery RM, Ince PG. [^{3}H]D-aspartate binding sites in the normal human spinal cord and changes in motor neuron disease: a quantitative autoradiographic study. Brain Res 1994;655:195–201.
105. Rothstein JD, Van Kammen M, Levey AI, et al. Selective loss of glial glutamate transporter GLT-1 in amyotrophic lateral sclerosis. Ann Neurol 1995;38:73–84.
106. Fray AE, Ince PG, Banner SJ, et al. The expression of the glial glutamate transporter protein EAAT2 in motor neuron disease: an immunohistochemical study. Eur J Neurosci 1998;10:2481–2489.
107. Sasaki S, Komori T, Iwata M. Excitatory amino acid transporter 1 and 2 immunoreactivity in the spinal cord in amyotrophic lateral sclerosis. Acta Neuropathol (Berl) 2000;100:138–144.
108. Rothstein JD, Dykes-Hoberg M, Pardo CA, et al. Knockout of glutamate transporters reveals a major role for astroglial transport in excitotoxicity and clearance of glutamate. Neuron 1996;16:675–686.
109. Bruijn LI, Becher MW, Lee MK, et al. ALS-linked SOD1 mutant G85R mediates damage to astrocytes and promotes rapidly progressive disease with SOD1-containing inclusions. Neuron 1997;18:327–338.
110. Bendotti C, Tortarolo M, Suchak SK, et al. Transgenic SOD1 G93A mice develop reduced GLT-1 in spinal cord without alterations in cerebrospinal fluid glutamate levels. J Neurochem 2001; 79:737–746.

111. Howland DS, Liu J, She Y, et al. Focal loss of the glutamate transporter EAAT2 in a transgenic rat model of SOD1 mutant-mediated amyotrophic lateral sclerosis (ALS). Proc Natl Acad Sci USA 2002;99:1604–1609.

112. Sasaki S, Warita H, Abe K, et al. EAAT1 and EAAT2 immunoreactivity in transgenic mice with a G93A mutant SOD1 gene. Neuroreport 2001;12:1359–1362.

113. Deitch JS, Alexander GM, Del Valle L, Heiman-Patterson TD. GLT-1 glutamate transporter levels are unchanged in mice expressing G93A human mutant SOD1. J Neurol Sci 2002;193:117–126.

114. Milton ID, Banner SJ, Ince PG, et al. Expression of the glial glutamate transporter EAAT2 in the human CNS: an immunohistochemical study. Brain Res Mol Brain Res 1997;52:17–31.

115. Aoki M, Lin CL, Rothstein JD, et al. Mutations in the glutamate transporter EAAT2 gene do not cause abnormal EAAT2 transcripts in amyotrophic lateral sclerosis. Ann Neurol 1998;43:645–653.

116. Trotti D, Aoki M, Pasinelli P, et al. Amyotrophic lateral sclerosis-linked glutamate transporter mutant has impaired glutamate clearance capacity. J Biol Chem 2001;276:576–582.

117. Meyer T, Munch C, Volkel H, et al. The EAAT2 (GLT-1) gene in motor neuron disease: absence of mutations in amyotrophic lateral sclerosis and a point mutation in patients with hereditary spastic paraplegia. J Neurol Neurosurg Psychiatry 1998;65:594–596.

118. Jackson M, Steers G, Leigh PN, Morrison KE. Polymorphisms in the glutamate transporter gene EAAT2 in European ALS patients. J Neurol 1999;246:1140–1144.

119. Bristol LA, Rothstein JD. Glutamate transporter gene expression in amyotrophic lateral sclerosis motor cortex. Ann Neurol 1996;39:676–679.

120. Lin CL, Bristol LA, Jin L, et al. Aberrant RNA processing in a neurodegenerative disease: the cause for absent EAAT2, a glutamate transporter, in amyotrophic lateral sclerosis. Neuron 1998;20:589–602.

121. Meyer T, Fromm A, Munch C, et al. The RNA of the glutamate transporter EAAT2 is variably spliced in amyotrophic lateral sclerosis and normal individuals. J Neurol Sci 1999;170:45–50.

122. Flowers JM, Powell JF, Leigh PN, et al. Intron 7 retention and exon 9 skipping EAAT2 mRNA variants are not associated with amyotrophic lateral sclerosis. Ann Neurol 2001;49:643–649.

123. Sutherland ML, Martinowich K, Rothstein JD. EAAT2 overexpression plays a neuroprotective role in the SOD1 G93A model of amyotrophic lateral sclerosis (ALS). Soc for Neurosci Abstr 2001.

124. Trotti D, Rolfs A, Danbolt NC, et al. SOD1 mutants linked to amyotrophic lateral sclerosis selectively inactivate a glial glutamate transporter. Nat Neurosci 1999;2:427–433.

125. Roy J, Minotti S, Dong L, et al. Glutamate potentiates the toxicity of mutant Cu/Zn-superoxide dismutase in motor neurons by postsynaptic calcium-dependent mechanisms. J Neurosci 1998;18:9673–9684.

126. Kruman II, Pedersen WA, Springer JE, Mattson MP. ALS-linked Cu/Zn-SOD mutation increases vulnerability of motor neurons to excitotoxicity by a mechanism involving increased oxidative stress and perturbed calcium homeostasis. Exp Neurol 1999;160:28–39.

127. Smith RG, Hamilton S, Hofmann F, et al. Serum antibodies to L-type calcium channels in patients with amyotrophic lateral sclerosis. N Engl J Med 1992;327:1721–1728.

128. Couratier P, Hugon J, Sindou P, et al. Cell culture evidence for neuronal degeneration in amyotrophic lateral sclerosis being linked to glutamate AMPA/kainate receptors. Lancet 1993; 341:265–268.

129. Smith RG, Alexianu ME, Crawford G, et al. Cytotoxicity of immunoglobulins from amyotrophic lateral sclerosis patients on a hybrid motoneuron cell line. Proc Natl Acad Sci USA 1994;91:3393–3397.

130. Tikka TM, Vartiainen NE, Goldsteins G, et al. Minocycline prevents neurotoxicity induced by cerebrospinal fluid from patients with motor neurone disease. Brain 2002;125:722–731.

131. Couratier P, Sindou P, Esclaire F, et al. Neuroprotective effects of riluzole in ALS CSF toxicity. Neuroreport 1994;5:1012–1014.

132. Kawamata T, Akiyama H, Yamada T, McGeer PL. Immunologic reactions in amyotrophic lateral sclerosis brain and spinal cord tissue. Am J Pathol 1992;140:691–707.

133. McGeer PL, Kawamata T, Walker DG, et al. Microglia in degenerative neurological disease. Glia 1993;7:84–92.

134. Tikka T, Fiebich BL, Goldsteins G, et al. Minocycline, a tetracycline derivative, is neuroprotective against excitotoxicity by inhibiting activation and proliferation of microglia. J Neurosci 2001;21:2580–2588.

135. Tikka TM, Koistinaho JE. Minocycline provides neuroprotection against N-methyl-D-aspartate neurotoxicity by inhibiting microglia. J Immunol 2001;166:7527–7533.

136. Yrjanheikki J, Keinanen R, Pellikka M, et al. Tetracyclines inhibit microglial activation and are neuroprotective in global brain ischemia. Proc Natl Acad Sci USA 1998;95:15769–15774.

137. Zhu S, Stavrovskaya IG, Drozda M, et al. Minocycline inhibits cytochrome c release and delays progression of amyotrophic lateral sclerosis in mice. Nature 2002;417:74–78.
138. Van Den Bosch L, Tilkin P, Lemmens G, Robberecht W. Minocycline delays disease onset and mortality in a transgenic model of ALS. Neuroreport 2002;13:1–4.
139. Drachman DB, Rothstein JD. Inhibition of cyclooxygenase-2 protects motor neurons in an organotypic model of amyotrophic lateral sclerosis. Ann Neurol 2000;48:792–795.
140. Frank KM, Coccia C, Drachman DB, Rothstein JD. Cox-2 inhibition prolongs survival in a transgenic mouse model for ALS (abstract). Soc Neurosci 2001.
141. Celio MR. Calbindin D-28k and parvalbumin in the rat nervous system. Neuroscience 1990;35:375–475.
142. Ince P, Stout N, Shaw P, et al. Parvalbumin and calbindin D-28k in the human motor system and in motor neuron disease. Neuropathol Appl Neurobiol 1993;19:291–299.
143. Alexianu ME, Ho BK, Mohamed AH, et al. The role of calcium-binding proteins in selective motoneuron vulnerability in amyotrophic lateral sclerosis. Ann Neurol 1994;36:846–858.
144. Elliott JL, Snider WD. Parvalbumin is a marker of ALS-resistant motor neurons. Neuroreport 1995;6:449–452.
145. Lips MB, Keller BU. Endogenous calcium buffering in motoneurons of the nucleus hypoglossus from mouse. J Physiol 1998;511:105–117.
146. Palecek J, Lips MB, Keller BU. Calcium dynamics and buffering in motoneurons of the mouse spinal cord. J Physiol 1999;520(pt 2):485–502.
147. Vanselow BK, Keller BU. Calcium dynamics and buffering in oculomotor neurones from mouse that are particularly resistant during amyotrophic lateral sclerosis (ALS)—related motoneuron disease. J Physiol 2000;525(pt 2):433–445.
148. Van Den Bosch L, Schwaller B, Vleminckx V, et al. Protective effect of parvalbumin on excitotoxic motor neuron death. Exp Neurol 2002;174:150–161.
149. Beers DR, Ho BK, Siklos L, et al. Parvalbumin overexpression alters immune-mediated increases in intracellular calcium, and delays disease onset in a transgenic model of familial amyotrophic lateral sclerosis. J Neurochem 2001;79:499–509.
150. Vandenberghe W, Ihle EC, Patneau DK, et al. AMPA receptor current density, not desensitization, predicts selective motoneuron vulnerability. J Neurosci 2000;20:7158–7166.
151. Van Damme P, Van Den Bosch L, Van Houtte E, et al. GluR2-dependent properties of AMPA receptors determine the selective vulnerability of motor neurons to excitotoxicity. J Neurophysiol 2002 88:1279–1287.
152. Williams TL, Day NC, Ince PG, et al. Calcium-permeable α-amino-3-hydroxy-5-methyl-4-isoxazole propionic acid receptors: a molecular determinant of selective vulnerability in amyotrophic lateral sclerosis. Ann Neurol 1997;42:200–207.
153. Shaw PJ, Williams TL, Slade JY, et al. Low expression of GluR2 AMPA receptor subunit protein by human motor neurons. Neuroreport 1999;10:261–265.
154. Bar-Peled O, O'Brien RJ, Morrison JH, Rothstein JD. Cultured motor neurons possess calcium-permeable AMPA/kainate receptors. Neuroreport 1999;10:855–859.
155. Takuma H, Kwak S, Yoshizawa T, Kanazawa I. Reduction of GluR2 RNA editing, a molecular change that increases calcium influx through AMPA receptors, selective in the spinal ventral gray of patients with amyotrophic lateral sclerosis. Ann Neurol 1999;46:806–815.
156. Del Cano GG, Millan LM, Gerrikagoitia I, et al. Inotropic glutamate receptor subunit distribution on hypoglossal motoneuronal pools in the rat. J Neurocytol 1999;28:455–468.
157. Tolle TR, Berthele A, Zieglgansberger W, et al. The differential expression of 16 NMDA and non—NMDA receptor subunits in the rat spinal cord and in periaqueductal gray. J Neurosci 1993;13:5009–5028.
158. Tomiyama M, Rodriguez-Puertas R, Cortes R, et al. Differential regional distribution of AMPA receptor subunit messenger RNAs in the human spinal cord as visualized by in situ hybridization. Neuroscience 1996;75:901–915.
159. Morrison BM, Janssen WG, Gordon JW, Morrison JH. Light and electron microscopic distribution of the AMPA receptor subunit, GluR2, in the spinal cord of control and G86R mutant superoxide dismutase transgenic mice. J Comp Neurol 1998;395:523–534.
160. Vandenberghe W, Robberecht W, Brorson JR. AMPA receptor calcium permeability, GluR2 expression, and selective motoneuron vulnerability. J Neurosci 2000;20:123–132.
161. Virgo L, Samarasinghe S, de Belleroche J. Analysis of AMPA receptor subunit mRNA expression in control and ALS spinal cord. Neuroreport 1996;7:2507–2511.
162. Feldmeyer D, Kask K, Brusa R, et al. Neurological dysfunctions in mice expressing different levels of the Q/R site-unedited AMPAR subunit GluR-B. Nat Neurosci 1999;2:57–64.

163. Jia Z, Agopyan N, Miu P, et al. Enhanced LTP in mice deficient in the AMPA receptor GluR2. Neuron 1996;17:945–956.
164. Harvey SC, Koster A, Yu H, et al. AMPA receptor function is altered in GLUR2-deficient mice. J Mol Neurosci 2001;17:35–43.
165. Tateno M, Tanaka M, Misawa H, et al. Generation of transgenic mice harboring GluR2 subunit of AMPA receptor driven by cholinergic neuron-specific promotor. Soc Neurosci Abstr 2001.
166. Anneser JM, Horstmann S, Weydt P, Borasio GD. Activation of metabotropic glutamate receptors delays apoptosis of chick embryonic motor neurons in vitro. Neuroreport 1998;9:2039–2043.
167. Pizzi M, Benarese M, Boroni F, et al. Neuroprotection by metabotropic glutamate receptor agonists on kainate-induced degeneration of motor neurons in spinal cord slices from adult rat. Neuropharmacology 2000;39:903–910.
168. Anneser JM, Borasio GD, Berthele A, et al. Differential expression of group I metabotropic glutamate receptors in rat spinal cord somatic and autonomic motoneurons: possible implications for the pathogenesis of amyotrophic lateral sclerosis. Neurobiol Dis 1999;6:140–147.
169. Laslo P, Lipski J, Funk GD. Differential expression of group I metabotropic glutamate receptors in motoneurons at low and high risk for degeneration in ALS. Neuroreport 2001;12:1903–1908.
170. Aronica E, Catania MV, Geurts J, et al. Immunohistochemical localization of group I and II metabotropic glutamate receptors in control and amyotrophic lateral sclerosis human spinal cord: upregulation in reactive astrocytes. Neuroscience 2001;105:509–520.
171. Tomiyama M, Kimura T, Maeda T, et al. Expression of metabotropic glutamate receptor mRNAs in the human spinal cord: implications for selective vulnerability of spinal motor neurons in amyotrophic lateral sclerosis. J Neurol Sci 2001;189:65–69.
172. Bensimon G, Lacomblez L, Meininger V. A controlled trial of riluzole in amyotrophic lateral sclerosis. ALS/Riluzole Study Group. N Engl J Med 1994;330:585–591.
173. Gurney ME, Cutting FB, Zhai P, et al. Benefit of vitamin E, riluzole, and gabapentin in a transgenic model of familial amyotrophic lateral sclerosis. Ann Neurol 1996;39:147–157.
174. Miller RG, Moore D, Young LA, et al. Placebo-controlled trial of gabapentin in patients with amyotrophic lateral sclerosis. WALS Study Group. Western Amyotrophic Lateral Sclerosis Study Group. Neurology 1996;47:1383–1388.
175. Mazzini L, Mora G, Balzarini C, et al. The natural history and the effects of gabapentin in amyotrophic lateral sclerosis. J Neurol Sci 1998;160(suppl 1):S57–S63.
176. Miller RG, Moore DH 2nd, Gelinas DF, et al. Phase III randomized trial of gabapentin in patients with amyotrophic lateral sclerosis. Neurology 2001;56:843–848.
177. Eisen A, Stewart H, Schulzer M, Cameron D. Anti-glutamate therapy in amyotrophic lateral sclerosis: a trial using lamotrigine. Can J Neurol Sci 1993;20:297–301.
178. Blin O, Azulay JP, Desnuelle C, et al. A controlled one-year trial of dextromethorphan in amyotrophic lateral sclerosis. Clin Neuropharmacol 1996;19:189–192.
179. Gredal O, Werdelin L, Bak S, et al. A clinical trial of dextromethorphan in amyotrophic lateral sclerosis. Acta Neurol Scand 1997;96:8–13.
180. Jones T. An assessment of the efficacy and safety of LY300164 in patients with ALS/MND. Abstract ALS/MND 1999.
181. Canton T, Bohme GA, Boireau A, et al. RPR 119990, a novel α-amino-3-hydroxy-5-methyl-4-isoxazole propionic acid antagonist: synthesis, pharmacological properties, and activity in an animal model of amyotrophic lateral sclerosis. J Pharmacol Exp Ther 2001;299:314–322.
182. Schulz JB, Lindenau J, Seyfried J, Dichgans J. Glutathione, oxidative stress and neurodegeneration. Eur J Biochem 2000;267:4904–4911.
183. Pardo CA, Xu Z, Borchelt DR, et al. Superoxide dismutase is an abundant component in cell bodies, dendrites, and axons of motor neurons and in a subset of other neurons. Proc Natl Acad Sci USA 1995;92:954–958.
184. Coyle JT, Puttfarcken P. Oxidative stress, glutamate, and neurodegenerative disorders. Science 1993;262:689–695.
185. Rosen DR, Siddique T, Patterson D, et al. Mutations in Cu/Zn superoxide dismutase gene are associated with familial amyotrophic lateral sclerosis. Nature 1993;362:59–62.
186. Fridovich I. Superoxide dismutases. Adv Enzymol Relat Areas Mol Biol 1986;58:61–97.
187. Deng HX, Hentati A, Tainer JA, et al. Amyotrophic lateral sclerosis and structural defects in Cu,Zn superoxide dismutase. Science 1993;261:1047–1051.
188. Robberecht W, Sapp P, Viaene MK, et al. Cu/Zn superoxide dismutase activity in familial and sporadic amyotrophic lateral sclerosis. J Neurochem 1994;62:384–387.

189. Borchelt DR, Lee MK, Slunt HS, et al. Superoxide dismutase 1 with mutations linked to familial amyotrophic lateral sclerosis possesses significant activity. Proc Natl Acad Sci USA 1994;91:8292–8296.
190. Bowling AC, Barkowski EE, McKenna-Yasek D, et al. Superoxide dismutase concentration and activity in familial amyotrophic lateral sclerosis. J Neurochem 1995;64:2366–2369.
191. Gurney ME, Pu H, Chiu AY, et al. Motor neuron degeneration in mice that express a human Cu,Zn superoxide dismutase mutation. Science 1994;264:1772–1775.
192. Ripps ME, Huntley GW, Hof PR, et al. Transgenic mice expressing an altered murine superoxide dismutase gene provide an animal model of amyotrophic lateral sclerosis. Proc Natl Acad Sci USA 1995;92:689–693.
193. Wong PC, Pardo CA, Borchelt DR, et al. An adverse property of a familial ALS-linked SOD1 mutation causes motor neuron disease characterized by vacuolar degeneration of mitochondria. Neuron 1995;14:1105–1116.
194. Bruijn LI, Houseweart MK, Kato S, et al. Aggregation and motor neuron toxicity of an ALS-linked SOD1 mutant independent from wild-type SOD1. Science 1998;281:1851–1854.
195. Reaume AG, Elliott JL, Hoffman EK, et al. Motor neurons in Cu/Zn superoxide dismutase-deficient mice develop normally but exhibit enhanced cell death after axonal injury. Nat Genet 1996;13:43–47.
196. Wiedau-Pazos M, Goto JJ, Rabizadeh S, et al. Altered reactivity of superoxide dismutase in familial amyotrophic lateral sclerosis. Science 1996;271:515–518.
197. Yim MB, Kang JH, Yim HS, et al. A gain-of-function of an amyotrophic lateral sclerosis—associated Cu,Zn-superoxide dismutase mutant: An enhancement of free radical formation due to a decrease in Km for hydrogen peroxide. Proc Natl Acad Sci USA 1996;93:5709–5714.
198. Crow JP, Sampson JB, Zhuang Y, et al. Decreased zinc affinity of amyotrophic lateral sclerosis-associated superoxide dismutase mutants leads to enhanced catalysis of tyrosine nitration by peroxynitrite. J Neurochem 1997;69:1936–1944.
199. Beckman JS, Carson M, Smith CD, Koppenol WH. ALS, SOD and peroxynitrite. Nature 1993;364:584.
200. Ghadge GD, Lee JP, Bindokas VP, et al. Mutant superoxide dismutase-1-linked familial amyotrophic lateral sclerosis: molecular mechanisms of neuronal death and protection. J Neurosci 1997;17:8756–8766.
201. Bruijn LI, Beal MF, Becher MW, et al. Elevated free nitrotyrosine levels, but not protein-bound nitrotyrosine or hydroxyl radicals, throughout amyotrophic lateral sclerosis (ALS)—like disease implicate tyrosine nitration as an aberrant in vivo property of one familial ALS-linked superoxide dismutase 1 mutant. Proc Natl Acad Sci USA 1997;94:7606–7611.
202. Bogdanov MB, Ramos LE, Xu Z, Beal MF. Elevated "hydroxyl radical" generation in vivo in an animal model of amyotrophic lateral sclerosis. J Neurochem 1998;71:1321–1324.
203. Liu R, Althaus JS, Ellerbrock BR, et al. Enhanced oxygen radical production in a transgenic mouse model of familial amyotrophic lateral sclerosis. Ann Neurol 1998;44:763–770.
204. Robberecht W. Oxidative stress in amyotrophic lateral sclerosis. J Neurol 2000;247(suppl 1):I1–I6.
205. Bowling AC, Schulz JB, Brown RH Jr, Beal MF. Superoxide dismutase activity, oxidative damage, and mitochondrial energy metabolism in familial and sporadic amyotrophic lateral sclerosis. J Neurochem 1993;61:2322–2325.
206. Ferrante RJ, Browne SE, Shinobu LA, et al. Evidence of increased oxidative damage in both sporadic and familial amyotrophic lateral sclerosis. J Neurochem 1997;69:2064–2074.
207. Abe K, Pan LH, Watanabe M, et al. Induction of nitrotyrosine-like immunoreactivity in the lower motor neuron of amyotrophic lateral sclerosis. Neurosci Lett 1995;199:152–154.
208. Shaw PJ, Ince PG, Falkous G, Mantle D. Oxidative damage to protein in sporadic motor neuron disease spinal cord. Ann Neurol 1995;38:691–695.
209. Beal MF, Ferrante RJ, Browne SE, et al. Increased 3-nitrotyrosine in both sporadic and familial amyotrophic lateral sclerosis. Ann Neurol 1997;42:644–654.
210. Shibata N, Nagai R, Miyata S, et al. Nonoxidative protein glycation is implicated in familial amyotrophic lateral sclerosis with superoxide dismutase-1 mutation. Acta Neuropathol (Berl) 2000;100:275–284.
211. Sasaki S, Shibata N, Komori T, Iwata M. iNOS and nitrotyrosine immunoreactivity in amyotrophic lateral sclerosis. Neurosci Lett 2000;291:44–48.
212. Smith RG, Henry YK, Mattson MP, Appel SH. Presence of 4-hydroxynonenal in cerebrospinal fluid of patients with sporadic amyotrophic lateral sclerosis. Ann Neurol 1998;44:696–699.
213. Tohgi H, Abe T, Yamazaki K, et al. Remarkable increase in cerebrospinal fluid 3-nitrotyrosine in patients with sporadic amyotrophic lateral sclerosis. Ann Neurol 1999;46:129–131.

214. Aoyama K, Matsubara K, Fujikawa Y, et al. Nitration of manganese superoxide dismutase in cerebrospinal fluids is a marker for peroxynitrite-mediated oxidative stress in neurodegenerative diseases. Ann Neurol 2000;47:524–527.
215. Oteiza PI, Uchitel OD, Carrasquedo F, et al. Evaluation of antioxidants, protein, and lipid oxidation products in blood from sporadic amyotrophic lateral sclerosis patients. Neurochem Res 1997;22:535–539.
216. Ferrante RJ, Shinobu LA, Schulz JB, et al. Increased 3-nitrotyrosine and oxidative damage in mice with a human copper/zinc superoxide dismutase mutation. Ann Neurol 1997;42:326–334.
217. Andrus PK, Fleck TJ, Gurney ME, Hall ED. Protein oxidative damage in a transgenic mouse model of familial amyotrophic lateral sclerosis. J Neurochem 1998;71:2041–2048.
218. Sasaki S, Warita H, Abe K, Iwata M. Inducible nitric oxide synthase (iNOS) and nitrotyrosine immunoreactivity in the spinal cords of transgenic mice with a G93A mutant SOD1 gene. J Neuropathol Exp Neurol 2001;60:839–846.
219. Williamson TL, Corson LB, Huang L, et al. Toxicity of ALS-linked SOD1 mutants. Science 2000;288:399.
220. Ischiropoulos H, Zhu L, Chen J, et al. Peroxynitrite-mediated tyrosine nitration catalyzed by superoxide dismutase. Arch Biochem Biophys 1992;298:431–437.
221. Esterbauer H, Schaur RJ, Zollner H. Chemistry and biochemistry of 4-hydroxynonenal, malonaldehyde and related aldehydes. Free Radic Biol Med 1991;11:81–128.
222. Pedersen WA, Fu W, Keller JN, et al. Protein modification by the lipid peroxidation product 4-hydroxynonenal in the spinal cords of amyotrophic lateral sclerosis patients. Ann Neurol 1998;44:819–824.
223. Subramaniam JR, Lyons WE, Liu J, et al. Mutant SOD1 causes motor neuron disease independent of copper chaperone—mediated copper loading. Nat Neurosci 2002;5:301–307.
224. Wong PC, Waggoner D, Subramaniam JR, T et al. Copper chaperone for superoxide dismutase is essential to activate mammalian Cu/Zn superoxide dismutase. Proc Natl Acad Sci USA 2000;97:2886–2891.
225. Durham HD, Roy J, Dong L, Figlewicz DA. Aggregation of mutant Cu/Zn superoxide dismutase proteins in a culture model of ALS. J Neuropathol Exp Neurol 1997;56:523–530.
226. Wyttenchach A, Sauvageot O, Carmichael J, et al. Heat shock protein 27 prevents cellular polyglutamine toxicity and suppresses the increase of reactive oxygen species caused by huntingtin. Hum Mol Genet 2002;11:1137–1151.
227. Oeda T, Shimohama S, Kitagawa N, et al. Oxidative stress causes abnormal accumulation of familial amyotrophic lateral sclerosis-related mutant SOD1 in transgenic *Caenorhabditis elegans*. Hum Mol Genet 2001;10:2013–2023.
228. Keller JN, Pang Z, Geddes JW, et al. Impairment of glucose and glutamate transport and induction of mitochondrial oxidative stress and dysfunction in synaptosomes by amyloid beta-peptide: role of the lipid peroxidation product 4-hydroxynonenal. J Neurochem 1997;69:273–284.
229. Blanc EM, Keller JN, Fernandez S, Mattson MP. 4-hydroxynonenal, a lipid peroxidation product, impairs glutamate transport in cortical astrocytes. Glia 1998;22:149–160.
230. Volterra A, Trotti D, Floridi S, Racagni G. Reactive oxygen species inhibit high-affinity glutamate uptake: molecular mechanism and neuropathological implications. Ann N Y Acad Sci 1994;738:153–162.
231. Trotti D, Danbolt NC, Volterra A. Glutamate transporters are oxidant-vulnerable: a molecular link between oxidative and excitotoxic neurodegeneration? Trends Pharmacol Sci 1998;19:328–334.
232. Trotti D, Rizzini BL, Rossi D, et al. Neuronal and glial glutamate transporters possess an SH-based redox regulatory mechanism. Eur J Neurosci 1997;9:1236–1243.
233. Murphy TH, Miyamoto M, Sastre A, et al. Glutamate toxicity in a neuronal cell line involves inhibition of cystine transport leading to oxidative stress. Neuron 1989;2:1547–1558.
234. Schubert D, Piasecki D. Oxidative glutamate toxicity can be a component of the excitotoxicity cascade. J Neurosci 2001;21:7455–7462.
235. Zona C, Ferri A, Gabbianelli R, et al. Voltage-activated sodium currents in a cell line expressing a Cu,Zn superoxide dismutase typical of familial ALS. Neuroreport 1998;9:3515–3518.
236. Rack M, Rubly N, Waschow C. Effects of some chemical reagents on sodium current inactivation in myelinated nerve fibers of the frog. Biophys J 1986;50:557–564.
237. Bhatnagar A, Srivastava SK, Szabo G. Oxidative stress alters specific membrane currents in isolated cardiac myocytes. Circ Res 1990;67:535–549.
238. Lu C, Chan SL, Fu W, Mattson MP. The lipid peroxidation product 4-hydroxynonenal facilitates opening of voltage-dependent Ca^{2+} channels in neurons by increasing protein tyrosine phosphorylation. J Biol Chem 2002;2:2.

239. Gabbianelli R, Ferri A, Rotilio G, Carri MT. Aberrant copper chemistry as a major mediator of oxidative stress in a human cellular model of amyotrophic lateral sclerosis. J Neurochem 1999;73:1175–1180.

240. Lee M, Hyun DH, Halliwell B, Jenner P. Effect of overexpression of wild-type and mutant Cu/ Zn-superoxide dismutases on oxidative stress and cell death induced by hydrogen peroxide, 4-hydroxynonenal or serum deprivation: potentiation of injury by ALS-related mutant superoxide dismutases and protection by Bcl-2. J Neurochem 2001;78:209–220.

241. Mena MA, Khan U, Togasaki DM, et al. Effects of wild-type and mutated copper/zinc superoxide dismutase on neuronal survival and l-DOPA—induced toxicity in postnatal midbrain culture. J Neurochem 1997;69:21–33.

242. Aguirre T, Van Den Bosch L, Goetschalckx K, et al. Increased sensitivity of fibroblasts from amyotrophic lateral sclerosis patients to oxidative stress. Ann Neurol 1998;43:452–457.

243. Jansen GA, Wanders RJ, Jobsis GJ, et al. Evidence against increased oxidative stress in fibroblasts from patients with non–superoxide-dismutase-1 mutant familial amyotrophic lateral sclerosis. J Neurol Sci 1996;139(suppl):91–94.

244. Dwyer BE, Lu SY, Nishimura RN. Heme oxygenase in the experimental ALS mouse. Exp Neurol 1998;150:206–212.

245. Dupuis L, Mbebi C, Gonzalez de Aguilar JL, et al. Loss of prion protein in a transgenic model of amyotrophic lateral sclerosis. Mol Cell Neurosci 2002;19:216–224.

246. Andreassen OA, Dedeoglu A, Klivenyi P, et al. *N*-acetyl-l-cysteine improves survival and preserves motor performance in an animal model of familial amyotrophic lateral sclerosis. Neuroreport 2000;11:2491–2493.

247. Jaarsma D, Guchelaar HJ, Haasdijk E, et al. The antioxidant *N*-acetylcysteine does not delay disease onset and death in a transgenic mouse model of amyotrophic lateral sclerosis. Ann Neurol 1998;44:293.

248. Ferrante RJ, Klein AM, Dedeoglu A, Beal MF. Therapeutic efficacy of EGb761 (*Ginkgo biloba* extract) in a transgenic mouse model of amyotrophic lateral sclerosis. J Mol Neurosci 2001;17: 89–96.

249. Poduslo JF, Whelan SL, Curran GL, Wengenack TM. Therapeutic benefit of polyamine-modified catalase as a scavenger of hydrogen peroxide and nitric oxide in familial amyotrophic lateral sclerosis transgenics. Ann Neurol 2000;48:943–947.

250. Jung C, Rong Y, Doctrow S, et al. Synthetic superoxide dismutase/catalase mimetics reduce oxidative stress and prolong survival in a mouse amyotrophic lateral sclerosis model. Neurosci Lett 2001;304:157–160.

251. Desnuelle C, Dib M, Garrel C, Favier A. A double-blind, placebo-controlled randomized clinical trial of alpha-tocopherol (vitamin E) in the treatment of amyotrophic lateral sclerosis. ALS riluzole-tocopherol Study Group. Amyotroph Lateral Scler Other Motor Neuron Disord 2001; 2:9–18.

252. Louwerse ES, Weverling GJ, Bossuyt PM, et al. Randomized, double-blind, controlled trial of acetylcysteine in amyotrophic lateral sclerosis. Arch Neurol 1995;52:559–564.

253. Swanson GT, Kamboj SK, Cull-Candy SG. Single-channel properties of recombinant AMPA receptors depend on RNA editing, splice variation, and subunit composition. J Neurosci 1997;17:58–69.

11

Mitochondrial Dysfunction in Amyotrophic Lateral Sclerosis

Clare Wood-Allum and Pamela J. Shaw

As the site of oxidative phosphorylation, mitochondria are responsible for generating the adenosine triphosphate (ATP) required to provide energy for the activities of the cell. In addition to this vital role, recently mitochondria have been found to play an important part in the regulation of intracellular calcium levels, and with this intracellular and intercellular signaling. Mitochondria are also now believed to be central to the commitment of the cell to apoptosis and to the normal aging process. Given these important cellular functions, it is not surprising that mitochondria are now implicated in the pathogenesis of several neurodegenerative diseases in addition to amyotrophic lateral sclerosis (ALS), including Alzheimer's disease, Friedreich's ataxia, Parkinson's disease, progressive supranuclear palsy, and Huntington's chorea.[1-4] A significant bioenergetic deficit has been demonstrated in all of these conditions, but whether this represents a primary or secondary contribution to disease pathogenesis remains to be seen.

Interest in mitochondrial dysfunction in ALS began after ultrastructural studies revealed morphological abnormalities in mitochondria from patients with the disease. The discovery that mutations in a ubiquitously expressed free-radical–scavenging enzyme called copper/zinc superoxide dismutase (SOD1) were responsible for around 20 percent of cases of familial ALS (FALS) intensified this interest, as mitochondria are the chief generator of free radicals in the cell, producing superoxide as an unavoidable byproduct of oxidative phosphorylation. Since then, considerable evidence has accumulated to show that mitochondrial morphology and function are altered in ALS. The relevance of these mitochondrial changes to the pathogenesis of the disease is the subject of current debate and an area of active research.

In this chapter, we consider normal mitochondrial structure and function, how these are altered in ALS, and what evidence there is that the resultant mitochondrial dysfunction contributes to disease pathogenesis in ALS. Investigation of the role mitochondria play in motor neuron death in ALS has taken place in a range of experimental systems. These include cell culture models, transgenic mouse models, and the study of human postmortem central nervous system

(CNS) tissue. Evidence cited here is taken from all of these experimental models of the disease and from patients with ALS. The rationale and evidence base for the use of mitochondrially acting therapeutic agents in ALS is also considered, along with promising work on the mitochondrial targeting of antioxidant agents.

NORMAL MITOCHONDRIAL FORM AND FUNCTION

Ultrastructure of Mitochondria

Mitochondria are frequently depicted as static, membrane-bound ovoids lying within the cytoplasm of the cell around the nucleus. This image is rather misleading, because mitochondrial form, location, and abundance vary markedly with cellular function and even within compartments of single cells. This structural heterogeneity is increasingly seen to be accompanied by functional heterogeneity as evidence accumulates for the fine tailoring of mitochondrial metabolic reactions to meet local demands.[5–7] Viewed with digital-video microscopy, mitochondria are seen to continuously change shape.[8] In order that mitochondria can be placed where they are most needed, they are transported around the cell in association with microtubules.[9] In the case of motor neurons, mitochondria are transported up and down motor neuron axons up to 1 meter in length. Mitochondrial numbers can be increased within a cell by the division of existing mitochondria, and mitochondria may fuse with one another to form large ramifying mitochondrial networks within the cytoplasm.[10,11]

Mitochondria are bounded by a double plasma membrane. Their most prominent ultrastructural feature is the inner of these two membranes, which is thrown into numerous folds, termed *cristae,* which act to increase inner membrane surface area. The inner mitochondrial membrane acts to split mitochondria into two compartments (Figure 11.1). The first, the intermembrane space, has a very similar chemical composition in terms of small molecules to the cellular cytoplasm. This is because the outer mitochondrial membrane is nonselectively permeable. The second compartment, termed the *matrix,* is enclosed by the far more selective inner mitochondrial membrane and is thus very different in chemical composition to the cytoplasm.[12] The proteins that make up the electron transport chain are embedded in the inner membrane, along with numerous transporter proteins and an ATP synthetase.[13] The matrix houses the mitochondrial genome, along with the enzymes that catalyze the oxidation of fatty acids and pyruvate to generate acetyl coenzyme A (acetyl CoA) to feed the citric acid cycle. It is the citric acid cycle that in turn generates reduced species such as nicotinamide adenine dinucleotide (NADH) and flavin adenine dinucleotide (FADH), which supply high-energy electrons to the electron transport chain.[14]

Oxidative Phosphorylation

Oxidative phosphorylation is an oxygen-requiring process by which high-energy electrons trapped in dietary carbohydrate or fats are converted into ATP,

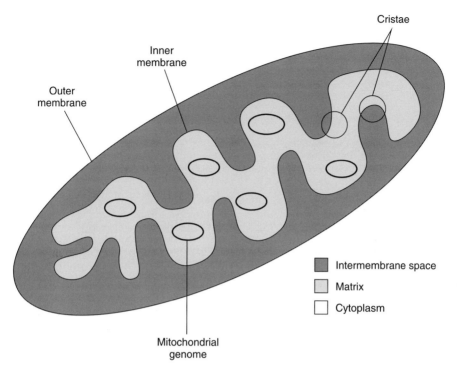

Figure 11.1   Schematic representation of normal mitochondrial ultrastructure.

the form of energy used to fuel the activities of the cell. Mitochondria use 98 percent of the oxygen taken up by the cell to generate ATP in this way.[15] In the process, they generate superoxide, an oxygen-free radical, as an unwanted but unavoidable byproduct.[16] As was discussed in Chapter 10, there is increasing evidence that oxidative damage caused by such free radicals may be important in the pathogenesis of several neurodegenerative diseases, including ALS. Figure 11.2 demonstrates how the components of oxidative phosphorylation interact and where they are sited in the mitochondrion.

Central to oxidative phosphorylation is the electron transport chain. This consists of four protein complexes, each comprising many subunits, embedded in the mitochondrial inner membrane. A schematic view of the four complexes of the mitochondrial electron transport chain is shown in Figure 11.3. Highly mobile electron carriers such as ubiquinone shuttle electrons between the complexes. Electrons at high energy are donated by NADH or FADH at specific points in the chain. Oxygen is consumed in the process. Electrons are passed protein to protein along the chain, releasing their energy as they proceed. The energy thus obtained is then used to pump protons out of the matrix and into the intermembrane space. The impermeability of the inner membrane to ions means that this generates not only a pH gradient but also an electrical potential gradient across the inner membrane of the order of 180 millivolts, inside

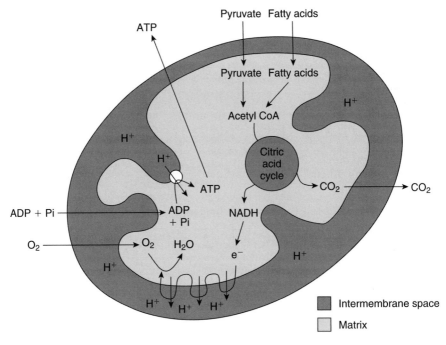

Figure 11.2 Overview of the reactions of oxidative phosphorylation. Pi = inorganic phosphate.

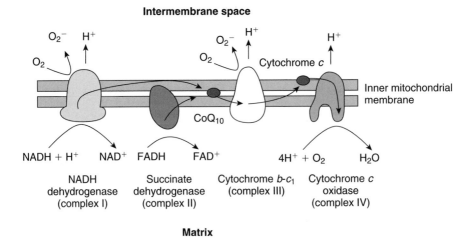

Figure 11.3 The electron transport chain. O_2^- = superoxide.

negative.[17] Mitchell[18] first postulated the existence of this so-called electro-chemical gradient in 1961. It is used to drive the synthesis of ATP from adenosine diphosphate (ADP) by a fifth protein complex also embedded in the inner mitochondrial membrane, which contains an ATP synthetase and an adenine nucleotide transporter.[13]

Oxidative phosphorylation is much more efficient than anaerobic respiration or glycolysis. For each molecule of glucose metabolized, oxidative phosphorylation can generate 36 molecules of ATP, compared with only 2 molecules generated by glycolysis.[19] Despite this efficiency, it has been estimated that 0.4 to 4.0 percent of high-energy electrons donated to the electron transport chain fail to complete the journey and instead leak out into the intermembrane space or matrix where they form the oxygen-free-radical species superoxide (O_2^-).[20–24] The chief sites where this occurs are through NADH dehydrogenase (complex I) and via ubiquinone and cytochrome *b* of complex III, as shown in Figure 11.3.[25–27] Superoxide is capable of directly inactivating important iron-sulfur–containing mitochondrial proteins[28] but also lies at the center of a cascade of reactions that may generate the even more reactive hydroxyl and peroxynitrite radicals.[26] This is discussed in more detail later in this chapter.

Mitochondrial Genome

Within the matrix of mitochondria lie multiple copies of a 16,500–base pair circular plasmid or chromosome. This mitochondrial chromosome carries the maternally inherited genetic material that makes up the mitochondrial genome. The mitochondrial genome (Figure 11.4) codes for 13 of the hundreds of subunits that make up the complexes of the electron transport chain, along with the 22 transport RNAs and 2 ribosomal RNAs that are needed to translate them.[29,30] The remaining 99 percent of mitochondrial proteins are encoded by the nuclear genome, are translated in the cytosol, and are then imported into the appropriate compartment of the mitochondrion by an elegant and complex translocation machinery.[31] Lying as it does in the mitochondrial matrix, the mitochondrial genome lies close to the electron transport chain, the chief source of free radicals in the cell. These free radicals are known to cause oxidative damage to lipids and proteins but are also damaging to DNA. Mitochondrial DNA lacks protective histones and has a high ratio of coding to noncoding sequences, making mitochondrially encoded genes more vulnerable to mutation.[32] Although the competence of DNA repair mechanisms of mitochondrial DNA (mtDNA) has recently been found to be greater than previously thought,[33] some aspects of mtDNA repair are still believed to be less sophisticated than those of the nuclear genome and mtDNA might therefore be expected to accumulate mutations over time. Increased oxidative damage to mtDNA with age has been demonstrated in human brain.[34]

Role of Mitochondria in Apoptosis

Programmed cell death or apoptosis is the means by which cell death is regulated, ensuring that excess, ectopic, or damaged cells are efficiently removed,

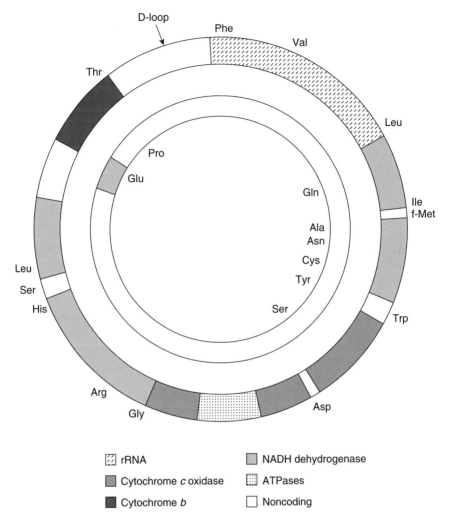

Figure 11.4   The mitochondrial genome. The outer strand is the heavy *(H)* strand. The inner strand is the light *(L)* strand. The position of tRNA genes is indicated by name.

thereby maintaining tissue homeostasis. Apoptosis is an active process that requires ATP and affects individual cells. Necrosis, an alternative way in which cells die, does not require ATP and tends to affect larger groups of cells similarly affected by a damaging event.

There is good evidence now that mitochondria are important in apoptosis. Several of the apoptosis-regulating family of Bcl-2 proteins are found anchored to the outer mitochondrial membrane. These proteins are capable of forming pores in synthetic membranes and modulate various mitochondrial events. Some are proapoptotic (Bax, Bad, Bid, Bik, Bim, and Bak), whereas others are antiapoptotic, for example, Bcl-2, Bcl_{XL}, and Bcl_{w}.[35] On receipt of a cell death stimulus, the proapoptotic protein Bax translocates to the mitochondria where it brings about the release of cytochrome *c* into the cytoplasm.[36,37] Cytochrome *c* forms part of the mammalian apoptosome comprising cytochrome *c,* apoptosis protease-activating factor-1 (Apaf-1), and procaspase-9, which serves to generate active caspase-9, an early step in the apoptotic cascade.[38] Once cytochrome *c* is released, the cell is committed irrevocably to die either by a fast apoptotic mechanism, which is Apaf-1 mediated and ATP dependent, or by a slower necrotic process secondary to the collapse of electron transport due mitochondrial cytochrome *c* depletion.[39] It is thought that mitochondria release other proapoptotic molecules as well as cytochrome *c,* including several procaspases and catabolic enzymes such as arginase.[40] Apoptosis-inducing factor (AIF) is also released and acts to activate caspases and stimulate the fragmentation of DNA.[41,42]

Mitochondrial membrane potential collapse is a feature of apoptosis triggered by some stimuli.[43] This is thought to occur because of the opening of the mitochondrial permeability transport (MPT) pore, which comprises proteins of both inner and outer mitochondrial membranes. Together they form a nonselective pore, allowing transit of all molecules smaller than 1.5 kilodaltons.[44] This results in the equilibration of hydrogen and other ions between matrix and intermembrane space, dissipating the electrochemical gradient generated by the electron transport chain. In addition, the hyperosmolarity of the matrix causes influx of water, resulting in swelling of the matrix compartment. The matrix and the inner mitochondrial membrane that contains it are together known as the *mitoplast.* The surface area of the inner membrane exceeds that of the outer membrane by some fivefold because of its cristae and therefore prevents the mitoplast from rupturing. The increase in volume of the mitoplast, however, may cause rupture of the outer membrane, allowing release of yet further caspase activators into the cytoplasm. Inhibitors of MPT opening do block apoptosis in some experimental systems.[45] Pathologically increased Ca^{2+} can cause opening of the MPT pore, as can oxidative damage to the components of the MPT.[46,47] At what stage in the apoptotic process MPT pore opening occurs is unclear, because caspases themselves can induce the MPT pore to open, resulting in a feed-forward amplification of caspase activation.[47,48]

Maintenance of Calcium Homeostasis

Increasing evidence suggests involvement of mitochondria in calcium homeostasis and cell signaling.[49,50] Calcium enters the matrix via a uniporter[51] driven by its electrochemical gradient—a combination of the electrical potential across the inner membrane generated by the electron transport chain, a locally high cytosolic $[Ca^{2+}]$ and a low matrix $[Ca^{2+}]$, which is generated by an active Na^{+}-Ca^{2+} antiporter and an Na^{+}-independent Ca^{2+} transporter, which pump calcium out of the matrix and into the intermembrane space. Interestingly, the Ca^{2+} influx modulates the rate of oxidative phosphorylation by upregulating three dehydrogenases of the citric acid cycle (pyruvate dehydrogenase, isocitrate dehydrogenase, and oxoglutarate dehydrogenase).[52,53] This increases the availability of NADH to the electron transport chain which results in the generation of more

ATP.[54] The influx also causes a transient depolarization of the inner mitochondrial membrane, which is later superseded by a hyperpolarization caused by the increased activity of the electron transport chain. Evidence exists in various neuronal cells, including at the neuromuscular junction, that mitochondria are responsible for the removal from the cytosol of calcium that has entered via voltage-gated calcium channels, thereby exerting control over the duration and kinetics of the resultant calcium signal.[55–60] A modulatory role in calcium signaling in nonexcitable cells such as astrocytes has also been shown. Inositol triphosphate (IP$_3$)–mediated release of calcium from the endoplasmic reticulum spreads in a wavelike fashion across cells and, via gap junctions, between cells. Calcium, above a threshold concentration, acts to sensitize the IP$_3$ receptor, causing yet further calcium release, serving to accelerate the propagation of the wave.[61] Mitochondria are positioned in close association with the endoplasmic reticulum and are therefore ideally placed to sense and respond to highly localized increases in calcium concentration.[62] By removing calcium released in this way, mitochondria maintain the local calcium concentration below the IP$_3$ sensitization threshold. This serves to reduce the speed at which the calcium signaling wave propagates and limits the geographical spread and duration of the signal.[63]

Threshold Effect and the Adult Onset of Amyotrophic Lateral Sclerosis

Hypotheses of ALS pathogenesis must be able to explain why disease onset is delayed into adult life, followed by inexorable disease progression. ALS is in almost all cases a disease of adult onset and this includes autosomal dominant FALS caused by mutations of SOD1, where the disease-causing genetic mutation has been present since conception. One possible explanation of this apparent "threshold effect" is the inherent decline in function of mitochondria with age. This was demonstrated some time ago by Yen et al[64] in a study of mitochondria extracted from liver biopsies from 35 people aged 31 to 76 years without liver disease. Respiratory rates and measures of the efficiency of oxidative phosphorylation all decreased linearly with increasing age. It is estimated that normal mitochondria have a life span of the order of 7 to 14 days.[65] Damaged mitochondria are degraded within lysosomes by autophagy, creating space within the cytosol for the generation of new healthy mitochondria by fission. The accumulation of damaged mitochondria in normal aged tissues, however, suggests strongly that this process is imperfect, leading to the inability of a cell to remove all ineffectively functioning mitochondria.[66] These damaged mitochondria persist, accumulating more and more damage over time, and as they do so, contribute less and less to overall mitochondrial function.

Age-related changes in mitochondrial function may then reflect the cumulative effects of oxidative damage to mitochondrial proteins and DNA. These age-related changes may be accelerated in the presence of an underlying biochemical defect such as the presence of mutations in SOD1, which may partly account for the development of an adult-onset disease phenotype.

ABNORMAL MITOCHONDRIAL MORPHOLOGY IN AMYOTROPHIC LATERAL SCLEROSIS

Evidence from Human Amyotrophic Lateral Sclerosis Tissues

As early as 1966, mitochondria of abnormal distribution, size, and shape were reported in the atrophic muscles of patients with ALS.[67] In a study of liver biopsies in 21 patients with ALS, hepatic mitochondria were also found to be morphologically abnormal and were described as having bizarre giant morphology.[68] Some of these contained paracrystalline inclusions. Siklos et al[69] studied the ultrastructure of nerve terminals of lower motor neurons and found mitochondria to be enlarged. A more recent ultrastructural study of synapses made with the cell bodies of anterior horn neurons in the lower lumbar spinal cord of patients with ALS revealed dense conglomerates of dark aggregated mitochondria with densely packed cristae in a proportion of synapses studied.[70]

Evidence from SOD1 Transgenic Mice

SOD1 transgenic mice are undoubtedly the best animal model of human ALS.[71] They are generated by the microinjection of cloned DNA of the human gene for SOD1, in either its normal or a mutant form, into the male pronucleus of the fertilized mouse egg. The human SOD1 gene then integrates into the murine genome, usually in multiple copies, and the injected egg is then implanted into a surrogate mother. This generates a single mouse carrying the human mutant SOD1 gene from which further affected mice may be bred, the trait being inherited in an autosomal dominant, mendelian fashion.

Several transgenic mouse models have been generated carrying different FALS-causing mutations of the human SOD1 gene in various copy numbers. As would be expected, mice carrying different copy numbers of the gene for mutant human SOD1 overproduce the mutant human SOD1 protein to different degrees. SOD1 transgenic mice are therefore phenotypically variable as a result of both the exact mutation of SOD1 they carry and its copy number. All, however, are born neurologically intact but go on in adulthood to develop a progressive and fatal motor dysfunction that closely mimics that seen in human ALS. Mean survival time is also dependent on which SOD1 mutation the mice carry and the number of transgene copies. It is not possible to study CNS material from patients at the presymptomatic or even early stages of ALS. A major advantage of SOD1 transgenic mice is the availability of CNS material from animals with the earliest symptoms of the disease and from presymptomatic mice identified by the polymerase chain reaction (PCR) as SOD1 transgenic mutants.

One result of this has been the identification of neuropathological correlates of early disease, the most notable of which is a prominent vacuolation within motor neurons in G93A SOD1 transgenic mice.[72] The source of these vacuoles has been the subject of several studies, and origins in endoplasmic reticulum, the Golgi apparatus, and mitochondria have all been reported. Morphological abnormalities of the Golgi apparatus are undoubtedly seen in patients with sporadic ALS (SALS) and in SOD1 transgenic mice.[73] A recent study, however, provided strong evidence that the massive vacuolation seen in G93A transgenic animals at disease onset is the result of mitochondrial degeneration. Kong and Xu[74] developed an objective assay in mice of the combined muscle strength of all four limbs and used this to follow the clinical course of wild type, normal human SOD1 transgenic mice, and G93A SOD1 transgenic mice. In parallel with this, they made a neuropathological study of the mice at defined stages of disease. By doing so, they were able to demonstrate that at the onset of muscular weakness, the vast majority of spinal motor neurons were still present and viable. This suggests strongly that the rapid decline in muscular function seen in G93A mice when compared with controls at disease onset is due not to the death of motor neurons but to their dysfunction. Loss of large motor neurons only occurred significantly at the final advanced stage of the disease when the mice were so weak that they were unable to perform the assay task. Presymptomatic G93A mice had a slight increase in the number of vacuoles identified in the ventral horns when compared with both wild type and normal SOD1 transgenic mice. At disease onset, however, ventral horn vacuolation was marked in the G93A mice compared with controls. Electron microscopy of the ventral horn from presymptomatic mice revealed dramatic morphological abnormalities of mitochondria. Mitochondria were swollen, their cristae dilated and disorganized, and there was evidence of leakage via the outer membrane or frank outer membrane breaks. Also identified were vacuoles with remnants of mitochondrial internal architecture still visible, evidence that the vacuolation seen at disease onset in G93A mice has its origin in damaged mitochondria (Figure 11.5).

Contrasting evidence from G85R SOD1 transgenic mice, however, indicates that mitochondrial vacuolation is not an invariable accompaniment of SOD1-related ALS in all lines of transgenic mice. Bruijn et al[75] carried out a neuropathological study of G85R mice and found that at no stage of disease was vacuolation a feature within the ventral horns of the spinal cord and there were no other signs of morphological abnormality of mitochondria. In these mice, early features of disease were instead Lewy body–like astrocytic inclusions strongly immunoreactive for SOD1. Vacuolation, moreover, is not a prominent feature of human FALS.[76] This, however, may be an artefactual consequence of the inevitable study of end-stage disease in humans (postmortem studies). Interestingly, the vacuolation observed in G93A mice is a transient effect, and by the time animals have reached advanced stages of their disease, vacuolization is not a prominent feature in residual spinal motor neurons. One further point worth making is that patients with autosomal dominant FALS carry only one copy of the mutant gene, whereas both transgenic mouse models cited here carry multiple copies. It is possible that differences in mitochondrial morphology between these two mouse strains is at least partially a function of differences of mutant gene copy number.

Evidence from Cell Culture Models of Amyotrophic Lateral Sclerosis

Several cellular models of SOD1-related FALS have been generated to facilitate investigation of the mechanisms by which SOD1 exerts its toxic gain of function. These models are generally based on immortalized murine or human

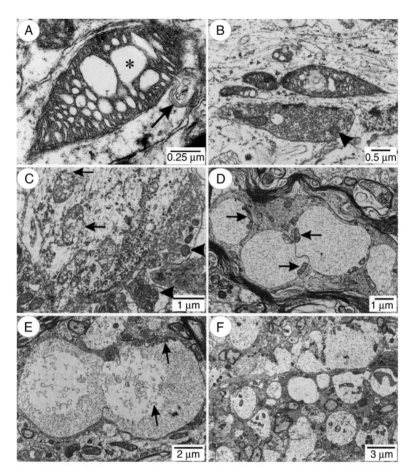

Figure 11.5 Damaged mitochondria within anterior horn cells from G93A SOD1 transgenic mice at the premuscle weakness stage viewed by transmission electron microscopy. (**A**) A swollen dendritic mitochondrion with dilated cristae *(asterisk)* and leaking outer membrane *(arrow)*. (**B**) Swollen dendritic mitochondria with dilated and disorganized cristae. A synaptic terminal on the dendrite contains normal mitochondria *(arrowhead)*. (**C**) A proximal dendrite containing mitochondria with broken outer membranes *(arrows)*. Adjacent synaptic terminals contain normal mitochondria *(arrowheads)*. (**D**) Early vacuoles in a proximal axon *(arrows* point to mitochondrial remnants). (**E**) Early vacuoles in a dendrite *(arrows* point to mitochondrial remnants). (**F**) Massive dendritic vacuolation in a motor neuron of a newly symptomatic transgenic G93A SOD1 mouse. (Reprinted with permission from Kong J, Xu Z. Massive mitochondrial degeneration in motor neurons triggers the onset of amyotrophic lateral sclerosis in mice expressing a mutant SOD1. J Neurosci 1998;18:3241–3250. Copyright 1998 by the Society of Neuroscience.)

motor neuron–like cells into which the mutated gene for human SOD1 is transfected. One such model is the neuroblastoma–spinal cord 34 (NSC34) cell line.[77] These cells were generated by the fusion of murine neuroblastoma cells and embryonic spinal motor neurons. The resultant cells are monoclonal and immortal, allowing them to be readily cultured, but they retain some key characteristics of their parental motor neurons; for example, the ability to propagate action potentials; extend neurites; and synthesize, store, and release acetylcholine. These cells have been stably transfected with the human gene for SOD1. Several NSC34 cell lines have been established including control cells expressing the transfection vector only, cells expressing normal human SOD1, and cells expressing human SOD1 carrying the G93A or the G37R mutation known to cause SOD1-related FALS in humans. Transmission electron microscopy of NSC34 cells expressing human G93A mutant SOD1 showed their mitochondria to be swollen and vacuolated (Figure 11.6).[78] Their outer membranes remained intact in most cases, but only remnants of cristae could be seen. These abnormalities were not evident in the mitochondria of NSC34 cells expressing transfection vector only or those expressing normal human SOD1.

In conclusion, mitochondrial morphological abnormalities have been demonstrated in several neural and non-neural tissues from patients with ALS and in both mouse and cell culture models of the disease. This morphological evidence of mitochondrial involvement in ALS prompted a search for functional abnormalities of mitochondria. These studies are reviewed in the following section.

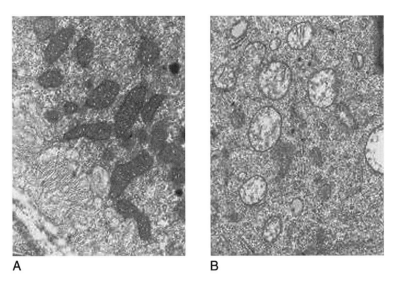

A   B

Figure 11.6 Transmission electron microscopy of mitochondria from neuroblastoma-spinal cord 34 (NSC34) cells transfected with (**A**) vector only and (**B**) human G93A SOD1. Mitochondria from cells expressing mutant SOD1 show marked morphological abnormalities not seen in control cells. (Published with the permission of Dr. FM Menzies.)

ABNORMAL MITOCHONDRIAL BIOCHEMISTRY IN AMYOTROPHIC LATERAL SCLEROSIS

Mitochondrial Antioxidant Defense System

As discussed earlier, mitochondria consume about 98 percent of the oxygen obtained by the cell to generate ATP via oxidative phosphorylation. As electrons are passed from a high-energy to a low-energy state between the complexes of the electron transport chain there is electron leakage at two main points, resulting in the generation of superoxide. The superoxide ($O_2^{\bullet-}$) thus generated may react directly with mitochondrial proteins containing iron-sulfur (Fe-S) centers such as the NADH dehydrogenase of complex I, aconitase, and succinate dehydrogenase to cause both enzymatic inactivation and the release of ferrous iron (Fe^{2+}).[26] Ferrous iron in turn may then react with hydrogen peroxide to produce the even more highly reactive hydroxyl radical in a process known as the Fenton reaction:

$$H_2O_2 + Fe^{2+} = OH^{--} + OH^{\bullet} + Fe^{3+}$$

Superoxide may also react with NO to form another damaging free radical, peroxynitrite ($ONOO^-$). The oxidative damage these and other free radicals cause to protein, lipid, and DNA when present in excess is termed *oxidative stress.*

The considerable evidence for the presence of oxidative stress in ALS has been presented in Chapter 10. In light of this and increasing evidence of oxidative stress in other neurodegenerative disorders, it is not surprising that there has been an interest in the role of mitochondrially located antioxidant systems. Manganese-containing superoxide dismutase (SOD2) is the chief antioxidant enzyme present in mitochondria. It is present at high concentrations in the mitochondrial matrix and catalyzes the same dismutation reaction as SOD1, converting superoxide to hydrogen peroxide:

$$2O_2^{\bullet} + 2H^+ = 2H_2O_2 + O_2$$

Homozygous SOD2 knockout mice, in which the expression of SOD2 is completely eliminated, die as neonates, developing a dilated cardiomyopathy, lactic acidosis, and basal ganglia degeneration. Detailed examination of mitochondrial function in these mice revealed deficits of function of complex I, complex III, and aconitase, in keeping with oxidative damage to enzymes containing Fe-S centers. Increased markers of oxidative damage to DNA were also demonstrated.[79] In a study by Melov et al,[80] homozygous SOD2 knockout mice were treated with synthetic SOD-catalase mimetics. This extended their life span by threefold, rescued the spongiform encephalopathy developed by untreated mice, and attenuated the mitochondrial defects. Heterozygous SOD2 knockout mice produce only 50 percent of the usual amount of SOD2. These mice are phenotypically normal but show an increase in biochemical indices of oxidative stress in the liver.[81] Andreasson et al[82] generated a strain of dual transgenic mice by crossing heterozygous SOD2 knockouts with G93A SOD1 transgenic mice. Half of the resultant offspring carried the mutant human SOD1 gene in multiple copies and had a 50-percent reduction in SOD2 production. These dual transgenic mice were then compared with normal G93A mice, which express a normal amount of SOD2. The dual transgenics had reduced motor skills and survived for a significantly shorter time than the G93A mice. When their spinal cords were examined neuropathologically, the dual transgenics were noted to have reduced numbers of large motor neurons than the G93A mice and those large motor neurons that were present showed more microvesiculation. It seems that an additional deficit in SOD2 made G93A transgenic mice more vulnerable to the effects of the mutated human SOD1, implying that at least some of the effects of the SOD1 mutation are mediated by an increase in oxidative stress.

Hydrogen peroxide is a source of highly reactive free hydroxyl radicals generated via the Fenton reaction. Catalase, an enzyme usually important in the removal of hydrogen peroxide from the cytosol, is not thought to be present in the mitochondria of most tissues. The glutathione peroxidases, however, also act to convert hydrogen peroxide to water and are present in mitochondria. Glutathione peroxidase itself seems to be present only in the mitochondrial matrix. There is a lipid hydroperoxide glutathione peroxidase inserted into the inner mitochondrial membrane,[83] but overall there appears to be less glutathione peroxidase activity in the intermembrane space than there is in the matrix. An additional mitochondrial peroxide-destroying system has recently been discovered. This comprises peroxiredoxin III, a protein that acts to reduce hydrogen peroxide using a reduced form of nicotinamide adenine dinucleotide phosphate (NADPH) as the source of electrons, together with a mitochondrial thioredoxin and a mitochondrial thioredoxin reductase, which serve to regenerate peroxiredoxin III. Both peroxiredoxin III and the mitochondrial thioredoxin have been shown to be induced in conditions of oxidative stress.[84]

SOD1 as a Mitochondrial Antioxidant

It had been thought that superoxide generated by the electron transport chain was released from the inner side of the inner membrane into the mitochondrial matrix where it would be dealt with by SOD2. More recent work, however, indicates that superoxide is also generated at the outer face of the inner membrane from where it can be released into the intermembrane space.[85] SOD1 was thought to be an exclusively cytoplasmic enzyme until more recently, convincing evidence from yeast[86] and rat liver[87] was presented to suggest that 1 to 5 percent of this protein is present in the intermembrane space of mitochondria. This clearly makes it well placed to deal with superoxide generated in the intermembrane space. Moreover, work on transgenic SOD1 mice has confirmed that normal human SOD1 is present in the intermembrane space of mitochondria from mice transfected with the gene for normal human SOD1, but more interestingly, mutant human SOD1 accumulates in the intermembrane space of mitochondria from G93A mice.[88] At disease onset, G93A mice were shown to have defective functioning of the electron transfer chain and ATP synthesis, along with evidence of oxidative damage to mitochondrial proteins (increased brain and spinal cord protein carbonylation) and lipids (increased brain lipid hydroperoxides). These deficiencies were not evident in presymptomatic G93A mice or in mice expressing normal human SOD1.[89] These experiments provide some support for the hypothesis that mutant SOD1 exercises at least part of its toxic gain of function by allowing the generation of excess reactive oxygen species in the mitochondrion that damage the machinery of oxidative phosphorylation, resulting in an energy deficit that subsequently compromises the survival of the cell.

Changes in Activity of the Electron Transport Chain Complexes

Several studies have provided evidence that the activities of the electron transport chain complexes are altered in ALS. Reductions in the efficiency with which the electron transport chain operates will affect the adequacy of the mitochondrial membrane potential it supports, the supply of ATP it is able to generate, and the production of damaging free-radical species. Motor neurons are large, electrically active cells and might be expected to be particularly vulnerable to energy deficits produced by dysfunctional mitochondria. Indeed, the in vitro chronic inhibition of complexes II and IV of mixed spinal cord cultures has been shown to cause a selective vulnerability to cell death of motor neurons compared with other neuronal cells, for example, interneurons, present in the culture.[90]

Evidence from Human Amyotrophic Lateral Sclerosis Studies

Several studies have investigated the activities of electron transport chain complexes obtained from muscle biopsy and postmortem CNS material from patients with ALS. Complex IV activity was found to be reduced in the postmortem spinal cord of patients with ALS, most markedly in the ventral horn where lower motor neurons are found.[91] Using an immunohistochemical technique to measure enzyme activity within individual motor neurons from postmortem patients with ALS, Borthwick et al[92] also demonstrated a decrease in complex IV activity. In a study of skeletal muscle from patients with SALS, Vielhaber et al[93] compared muscle biopsies from 17 patients with SALS with carefully defined disease to those of 21 controls. Of the 17 patients with SALS 11 showed heterogeneous defects in respiratory chain function tested in individual muscle fibers, and this was shown to be secondary to reduced activities of NADH:Q oxidoreductase (complex I) and cytochrome *c* oxidase (complex IV) in SALS muscle. Yet further studies on other brain regions (e.g., motor cortex, parietal cortex, frontal cortex, and cerebellum) have shown increases in the activities of complexes I and II/III. Interpretation of these differing results is difficult, especially given the wide range of experimental substrates used to obtain them. It does, nevertheless, seem that in ALS the activities of respiratory chain enzymes are altered and the balance of evidence favors a decrease in at least complex IV activity in ALS motor neurons.

Evidence from SOD1 Transgenic Mice

Decreases in the activity of the electron transport chain have also been reported by Browne et al[94] in G93A transgenic mice. These findings were recently confirmed by Mattiazi et al,[89] who used spectrophotometric methods to assay the activities of complexes of the respiratory transport chain from G93A transgenic mouse spinal cord. Statistically significant reductions were seen in complexes I + III, II + III, and IV from 17-week-old mice when compared with those measured in non-transgenic controls. Histochemical staining for cytochrome *c* oxidase of lumbar spinal cord from 17-week-old G93A transgenic and non-transgenic control animals also showed that G93A motor neurons were less intensely stained than the majority of non-transgenic motor neurons.

Jung et al used spectrophotometry, in situ histochemical enzyme assay, and blue native page electrophoresis to assess the activities of complexes of the electron transport chain in G93A SOD1 transgenic mice. Assays were done at five different time points from presymptomatic to late-stage disease. The activities of three electron transport chain complexes were found to be reduced, particularly in the ventral horn, early in the disease course and this decrease persisted thereafter. This decrease was not seen in wild-type mice or in mice expressing normal human SOD1.[95]

Evidence from Cell Culture Models

Spectrophotometric measurement of the activities of electron transport chain complexes in the NSC34 cell culture model of SOD1-related FALS, previously described, showed reductions in the activities of complexes II and IV in cells expressing human G93A or G37R SOD1 when compared with control cells expressing empty transfection vector or normal human SOD1.[78] These reductions in activity were not due simply to a reduction in the levels of the complexes present but may have been due to post-translational modifications resulting in impaired activity. There was also evidence of an accompanying bioenergetic defect; cells expressing mutant SOD1 were more susceptible to cell death in the presence of pharmacological inhibitors of glycolysis. Interestingly, similar decreases in the activities of complexes II and IV were seen in control cells exposed to oxidative stress by serum withdrawal.

ABNORMALITIES OF CALCIUM HANDLING

A relative lack of calcium-binding proteins has previously been invoked in an attempt to explain the specificity of cell death in ALS. Spinal motor neurons and those of the hypoglossal nucleus do not express the calcium-buffering protein calbindin D-28k or parvalbumin. Oculomotor neurons and those motor neurons within Onuf's nucleus, which are relatively spared in ALS, do express these calcium-binding proteins.[96,97] Curti et al[98] studied peripheral lymphocytes from patients with SALS and found that basal cytoplasmic calcium concentrations were elevated over controls. To demonstrate the biochemical consequences of abnormalities of ALS mtDNA, Swerdlow et al[99] created cybrid cell lines in which platelets from ALS and control patients, which contain mtDNA but no nuclear DNA, were fused with a neuroblastoma cell line lacking mitochondria. The cybrid cells from SALS cases reiterated changes observed previously in other models of ALS. A proportion of the mitochondria were morphologically abnormal; there was a statistically significant reduction in complex I activity; levels of free-radical–scavenging enzymes were raised (SOD2, SOD1, catalase, glutathione reductase, glutathione peroxidase) and mitochondria derived from ALS patient platelets showed a reduced capacity to sequester calcium. Given the role of calcium as an inducer of the citric acid cycle dehydrogenases, and thereby the electron transport chain, this deficiency of calcium uptake into the matrix may compromise the ability of the cell to generate ATP. Anything else that acts to reduce the mitochondrial membrane potential by a direct effect on the activity of the electron transport chain (e.g., oxidative damage to its components) will have its effects potentiated by the reduction of calcium sequestration. The excitotoxic hypothesis of the pathogenesis of ALS discussed in detail elsewhere in this book suggests that overstimulation of α-amino-3-hydroxy-5-methyl-4-isoxazole propionic acid (AMPA) receptors could result in an abnormally large influx of calcium into the cytoplasm, resulting in the triggering of a cascade of potentially harmful intracellular events including the opening of the MPT and commitment of the cell to apoptosis. If a compromised ability to sequester calcium in the matrix were proven to be a feature of motor neurons in vivo, this would serve to exacerbate the harmful effects of excitotoxicity.

GENETIC ABNORMALITIES

Of the approximately 10 percent of all ALS cases that are inherited, only 20 percent are due to mutations in the SOD1 gene. A handful of autosomal recessive, juvenile-onset ALS and primary lateral sclerosis cases have recently been attributed to mutations to a gene on chromosome 2, which codes a novel protein named *alsin*.[100,101] The genes responsible for the remaining 80 percent of FALS cases, however, remain unknown, although linkage has been established to other sites. Prompted by the evidence previously presented implicating mitochondria in the pathogenesis of ALS, mutations to mtDNA and to nuclear DNA, which codes the remaining 99 percent of mitochondrial proteins, have been sought in patients with FALS.

Search for Causative Mutations

Given the incontrovertible evidence for the involvement of oxidative stress in ALS, the gene for SOD2, the major mitochondrial free-radical–scavenging enzyme, was a logical place to look for ALS-causing mutations. Tomkins et al[102] searched the entirety of the coding regions of the SOD2 gene for mutations in 70 patients with ALS using single-stranded conformational polymorphism (SSCP) analysis and heteroduplex analysis. No mutations were found and no polymorphisms were found that could be shown to be associated with the disease. In a search for mutations in genes coding antioxidant enzymes other than SOD1 in non–SOD1-related FALS, Parboosingh et al[103] also used SSCP to examine three of the five predicted exons of the gene for SOD2 (66% of the gene) in a group of 73 unrelated patients with FALS who are known not to have mutations in SOD1. No mutations were identified. Tomblyn et al[104] sequenced the whole SOD2 gene in 20 patients with SALS and 10 control patients. Homozygosity for a structural dimorphism A9V in the mitochondrial targeting sequence of the SOD2 gene was found to be overrepresented among the patients with SALS, although the study group was not in Hardy-Weinberg equilibrium, limiting the significance of this finding. Homozygosity for the A9 allele, in contrast, was found to be an independent risk factor for SALS in a study of 72 patients and 136 controls from Sweden.[105]

Comi et al[106] reported an interesting case of a patient with an early onset, predominantly upper motor neuron ALS-like syndrome found to have a heteroplasmic, out-of-frame 5–base pair truncating deletion to the 5′ end of the mtDNA-encoded subunit I of cytochrome *c* oxidase (COX). This patient presented at age 29 years with a spastic paraparesis, which progressed over a year to involve his upper limbs. By age 33 years, he had a spastic tetraparesis and had developed mild dysarthria and dysphagia. At this time, sparse fasciculations were evident in all limbs. He died at age 35 years from pneumonia complicating his worsening dysphagia. Muscle biopsies performed at ages 32 and 33 revealed pronounced cytochrome *c* oxidase deficiency, along with some ragged red fibers, indicating severe mitochondrial impairment. The mutated mtDNA made up 47 and 68.7 percent of total mtDNA from the two muscle biopsies. A close correlation was demonstrated between COX deficiency, COX-I expression, and the percentage of mtDNA carrying the mutation. His mother and three sisters were all healthy over 5 years of follow-up and had normal mtDNA and muscle biopsy results.

Role of Secondary Damage to Mitochondrial DNA

Other workers have investigated the role secondary damage to mtDNA might play in the development of ALS. Because a proportion of subunits of the electron transport chain are coded by mtDNA, excessive mtDNA mutation rates might be expected to reduce the efficiency of oxidative phosphorylation. As discussed earlier, the mitochondrial genome is particularly vulnerable to mutation. This vulnerability appears to be further exaggerated in ALS. When levels of the "common deletion," a 4977–base pair deletion of mtDNA, were measured in motor and temporal cortices of patients with SALS and controls, levels of the common deletion were found to be higher in the motor cortex in both groups. More importantly, the relative difference between the levels of the deletion in the motor and the temporal cortex was more than 11-fold higher in the brains of patients with ALS than in the brains of control patients.[107]

In a study discussed earlier, Vielhaber et al[93] found reductions in the activities of complexes I and IV in skeletal muscle biopsies from patients with SALS when compared with controls. One patient with SALS was found to have multiple deletions of mtDNA, and levels of total mtDNA measured using Southern blotting were found to be reduced in the SALS biopsies when compared with controls. They additionally found that levels of citrate synthase, a non–electron transport chain mitochondrial matrix enzyme used as a mitochondrial marker, were not significantly different than those of controls, implying that the deficits observed in complex I and IV activities and the reduction in total mtDNA they observed must have been secondary to specific mitochondrial damage rather than to the loss of mitochondria in SALS muscle. An assay of membrane-bound SOD2, moreover, showed a reduction in patients with SALS compared with controls. The authors therefore postulated that oxidative damage to mtDNA was responsible for the heterogeneous deficits in electron transport chain complex activities observed.

Wiedeman et al[108] further tested the hypothesis that oxidative damage to mtDNA could result in randomly distributed point mutations throughout the mitochondrial genome, which might in turn result in reduction to electron transport chain complex activities using eight SALS and four FALS postmortem spinal cords. They found a statistically significant, though modest, increase in point mutations to the two areas of the mitochondrial genome screened, but unlike the previous study, they were unable to correlate this with the decrease in respiratory enzyme function also observed. Although the overall level of mtDNA was reduced in ALS cases compared with controls, this was accompanied by reductions in the activity of citrate synthase. They therefore suggested that the recorded reductions in electron transport chain function may have been secondary to a generalized loss of mitochondria in the anterior spinal cord, rather than to direct effects on the expression of components of the respiratory chain brought about by mutation to mtDNA.

It remains unclear therefore whether oxidative damage to mtDNA, which has been demonstrated by several groups, can be said to be the main cause of the decreases in electron transport chain complex activities also shown by several groups. Even assuming this were the case, the exact role played by the resultant energy deficit in motor neuron dysfunction and death will need to be further investigated before oxidative damage to mtDNA can be claimed as a primary event in the pathogenesis of ALS.

MITOCHONDRIA, APOPTOSIS, AND AMYOTROPHIC LATERAL SCLEROSIS

Several lines of evidence exist for cell death via apoptosis in ALS,[109] and as has already been discussed, mitochondria are now believed to be important in the commitment of the cell to apoptosis. Firstly, alterations in compartmental levels of the Bcl-2 family of proteins, which serve as apoptotic modulators, have been noted in transgenic mice and in patients with ALS, which would be expected to favor apoptosis.[110–112] Overexpression of the antiapoptotic protein Bcl-2 in transgenic mouse models of SOD1-related FALS, moreover, delays disease progression but has no effect on overall disease duration.[113] Changes in other markers of apoptosis have been found in ALS. In a study of the expression of the carbohydrate Le^Y antigen, believed to correlate with the occurrence of apoptosis, positive expression was observed in motor neurons from high cervical cord sections of patients with ALS but not from those of controls.[114] Expression of the Par-4 protein, a further marker of apoptosis was found to be increased in the lumbar spinal cords of patients with ALS when compared with expression in the lumbar cords of control patients without neurological disease.[115] There is increased activity of the proapoptotic caspases 1 and 3 in spinal cord of both transgenic mice and patients with ALS.[116,117] Finally, in postmortem spinal cord from patients with ALS, dying motor neurons can be seen displaying the characteristic morphological features of apoptosis, namely membrane blebbing, cytoplasmic condensation, compaction of organelles, chromatin condensation, and nuclear fragmentation in the absence of an inflammatory response.[118] The role of apoptosis in ALS is considered in further detail in Chapter 14.

THERAPEUTIC APPROACHES TO MITOCHONDRIAL DYSFUNCTION IN AMYOTROPHIC LATERAL SCLEROSIS

The only drug currently licensed for use as a disease-modifying agent in ALS is riluzole, an antiglutamate drug that modestly lengthens survival by approximately 3 to 4 months. Patients with ALS typically die 3 to 5 years after diagnosis and are significantly functionally impaired well before this. The need for further, more effective disease-slowing agents is therefore pressing. On the basis of evidence of mitochondrial dysfunction in the pathogenesis of ALS, it has been suggested that agents interacting with the bioenergetic status of the cell might prove to be neuroprotective and so serve to slow progression of the disease. Several potential candidates exist including nicotinamide, a substrate for complex I of the electron transport chain; riboflavin, a precursor of coenzymes of complexes I and II; carnitine, which facilitates entry of long-chain fatty acids into mitochondria and the exit of short- and medium-chain fatty acids; Ginkgo biloba extract; coenzyme Q_{10}; and creatine.[119]

Ginkgo biloba extract is a mixture of compounds obtained from the plant of the same name, which seems to act to reduce mitochondrial damage by reactive oxygen species. Ferrante and Beal[120] reported a small but statistically significant prolongation of life in SOD1 transgenic mice whose diet was supplemented by ginkgo extract. This substance has not yet been evaluated in patients with ALS.

Coenzyme Q_{10}

Coenzyme Q_{10} (CoQ_{10}), the electron transport chain electron carrier, signaling molecule and antioxidant (Figure 11.7), has also been suggested as potential therapy in mitochondrial disease and neurodegenerative diseases such as ALS, Parkinson's disease, Huntington's chorea, and Friedreich's ataxia in which mitochondrial dysfunction is believed to play a part.[121,122]

The very rare instances of primary CoQ_{10} deficiency, which is inherited in an autosomal recessive fashion, demonstrate the importance of adequate CoQ_{10} to normal neurological functioning. There are three main phenotypes in this disorder: a myopathic form including myopathy, myoglobinuria, epilepsy, and ataxia; an infantile form consisting of severe encephalopathy and renal disease; and an ataxic variant featuring ataxia, seizures, and cerebellar atrophy. CoQ_{10} supplementation has been used to some effect in certain of these individuals.[123] Benefit has also been reported in single case studies of patients with mitochon-

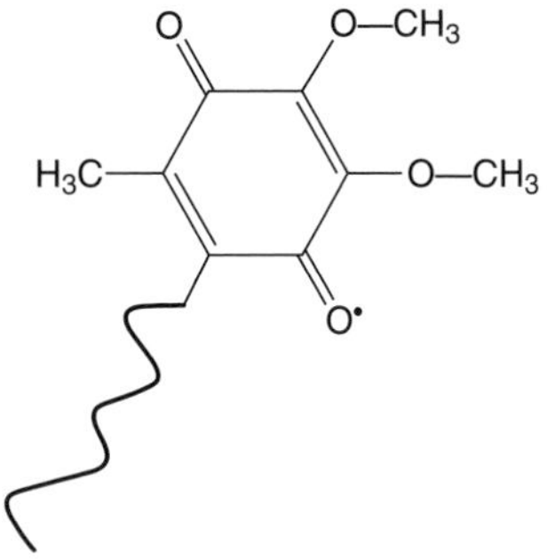

Figure 11.7 Coenzyme Q_{10} comprises a redox-active quinoid moiety to which is attached a long hydrophobic isoprenoid tail that anchors the molecule in the hydrophobic core of the inner mitochondrial membrane.

drial disease treated with CoQ_{10}.[124] In response to positive findings in animal models of Huntington's disease, The Huntington Study Group performed a randomized placebo-controlled trial of CoQ_{10}, remacemide (an NMDA receptor antagonist), and CoQ_{10} + remacemide in early Huntington's disease. There was no significant effect of any of the interventions on the primary endpoint of decline of total functional capacity, but those patients receiving CoQ_{10} did show a trend toward a slowing of decline (nonsignificant) and a trend toward slowing of the decline in an independence score (also nonsignificant) assessed after 30 months of treatment.[125]

Oral CoQ_{10} supplementation from 50 days of age at a dose of 200 milligrams per day has been carried out in a small group of G93A transgenic mice. Supplementation produced a modest but statistically significant increase in survival, from a mean of 135 days for unsupplemented mice to a mean of 141 days for mice receiving CoQ_{10}.[126] A study of CoQ_{10} levels in serum from patients with ALS showed no significant differences from levels in controls.[127] No study on the effect of CoQ_{10} in patients with ALS has yet been reported.

Creatine

The normal daily requirement of creatine is about 2 grams, of which half is generated endogenously by the liver, pancreas, and kidneys. The remainder is largely obtained by the ingestion of meat. Rare patients exist with inborn errors of the biosynthetic reactions needed to generate creatine. These patients suffer developmental delay, extrapyramidal symptoms, hypotonia, and seizures, demonstrating the importance of creatine to normal neurological function.

Creatine and phosphocreatine coexist within the cell. Phosphocreatine acts as a temporal buffer of ATP supply, allowing the rephosphorylation of ADP to ATP at times of high energy demand in a reaction catalyzed by creatine kinase. It also acts as a spatial energy buffer between mitochondria and cytosol. Mitochondrial creatine kinase exists in an octameric form and a dimeric form. The octamer is a component of complex V, the ATP synthetase. It is positioned within the intermembrane space at points of contact between the inner and outer membranes. Creatine stabilizes the octameric variety, which acts to inhibit the opening of the MPT pore.

Exogenous creatine comes in the form of creatine monohydrate, which has been shown to be both well tolerated and safe when taken as a dietary supplement. There is evidence that oral creatine crosses the blood-brain barrier and accumulates in the CNS.[128] Creatine is used extensively by "body builders" in whom it acts to increase lean muscle bulk. Trials of creatine have been carried out both in healthy volunteers and in patients with various other neuromuscular disorders,[129,130] and trials are ongoing in patients with ALS on the basis of modestly encouraging trials of creatine supplementation in SOD1 transgenic mice and the wobbler mouse model of ALS.

Klivenyi et al[131] administered a dietary supplement of 1 or 2 percent creatine monohydrate orally to G93A SOD1 transgenic mice. A statistically significant dose-dependent improvement of motor performance and improved survival resulted, along with a reduction of the loss of motor neurons at 120 days, when comparison was made with G93A SOD1 transgenic mice fed unsupplemented diets. Mean survival of unsupplemented mice was 143.7 ± 2.3 days compared with 157.2 ± 2.8 days for mice who were supplemented with 1 percent of creatine monohydrate and 169.3 ± 4.7 days for mice supplemented with 2 percent, representing an extension of survival of 13 days and 26 days, respectively. Riluzole extended survival in this model by 13 days. Counting of ventral horn neurons showed, as expected, that large motor neurons were the most profoundly affected, with a 95-percent loss in G93A SOD1 transgenic mice when compared with non-transgenic litter-mate controls. In G93A SOD1 transgenic mice fed a diet supplemented by 1 percent of creatine monohydrate, this loss of large ventral horn motor neurons did not seem to occur and cell counts were not significantly different than those of control mice. The increase in levels of 3-nitrotyrosine—a marker of oxidative damage—usually seen in the spinal cords of G93A SOD1 transgenic mice was not seen in G93A SOD1 transgenic mice whose diet was supplemented with 1 percent of creatine monohydrate; levels of 3-nitrotyrosine in spinal cord were not significantly different than those of control mice at age 120 days.

Wobbler mice are a naturally occurring model of motor neuron degeneration. The condition is inherited in an autosomal recessive fashion, with affected animals developing progressive forelimb weakness at 3 to 4 weeks of age. Animals die at approximately 12 months of age. Neuropathology, however, has shown the condition to primarily involve the cervical spinal cord, with less involvement of the lumbar cord or cortical motor neurons. This makes the wobbler mouse a poorer model of human ALS than the SOD1 transgenic mouse. A study reported by Ikeda, Iwasaki, and Kinoshita[132] demonstrated slowing of progression of disease in wobbler mice whose diet was supplemented from diagnosis aged 3 to 4 weeks for 4 weeks with 5 or 50 grams of creatine monohydrate, when compared with similar mice whose diet was not supplemented. Those wobbler mice fed the higher dose of creatine had greater grip strength, less forelimb contracture, and heavier biceps muscles than control mice. Neuropathological evaluation showed that mice fed the higher dose of creatine also showed reduced loss of spinal motor neurons and less atrophy of muscle compared with controls. No comment was made on whether survival was prolonged.

Creatine supplementation has also been shown to affect levels of metabolites in the motor cortex in ALS. Vielhaber et al[133] performed in vivo proton magnetic resonance spectroscopy on 15 patients with clinically definite SALS shown to have respiratory chain enzyme deficiencies in their skeletal muscle and 15 healthy control subjects before and after a month's creatine monohydrate supplementation. They found that the baseline *N*-acetylaspartate-to-creatine ratio (NAA/Cr) was lower in the patients with ALS than in controls. After a month's supplementation with high-dose creatine monohydrate (5 grams three times a day), the control group showed a decrease in the NAA/Cr ratio, interpreted as an increase in brain creatine level with unchanged NAA level. The NAA/Cr ratio of the patients with ALS, however, remained the same after supplementation. Because NAA is synthesized in an energy-dependent fashion within mitochondria, the authors postulated that the creatine had ameliorated a deficit of respiratory chain enzyme activity in the motor cortex of the patients with ALS, thereby allowing increased generation of NAA.

Preliminary results of a small study of creatine supplementation in 28 patients with ALS have now been published.[134] Patients were classified as having clinically probable or definite ALS. Supplementation was high dose (20 grams per day) for a week and lower dose (3 grams per day) for 3 and 6 months. Dynamometric measurements of the maximal voluntary isometric muscular contraction (MVIC) in ten muscle groups were made and a high-intensity intermittent effort protocol was used to assess fatigue. The MVIC was increased significantly in knee extensors (70% of patients) and elbow flexors (53% of patients) after 7 days of high-dose supplementation. A proportion of patients also showed reduced measures of fatigue in two muscle groups. Longer term follow-up, however, showed a linear decline in the MVIC in all muscle groups. Because no untreated group was included in the study, the results do not allow assessment of whether the rate of decline was slowed by creatine supplementation. Larger studies are currently being conducted.

Although the energetic dysfunction seen in ALS might be considered a rationale for the use of the rather nonspecific bioenergetic modifiers discussed here in patients with ALS, the preliminary findings of the one small trial of creatine in patients with ALS are not encouraging. Results of larger scale trials in patients are yet to be reported. Even the studies in transgenic animals suggest that only small improvements to longevity and modest slowing of disease progression occur when bioenergetic modifiers are used therapeutically. Given this, it seems unreasonable to recommend the use of any of the agents discussed as disease-modifying agents in ALS. Many of these substances are, however, readily available as nutraceuticals sold by health-food outlets, gymnasia, and over the Internet. Tarnopolsky and Beal[119] point out that sold in this way, as dietary supplements, these substances are much less tightly regulated than pharmaceuticals whose manufacture, purity, dosage, claims for efficacy, interactions, and adverse effects are all closely monitored. Despite this potential risk, in practice there seems to be little evidence that creatine and CoQ_{10} are harmful when taken as dietary supplements by healthy people or patients with various neuromuscular disorders. Patients with ALS who independently choose to supplement their diets in this way are therefore unlikely to significantly benefit but are also unlikely to suffer significant harm.

FUTURE DIRECTIONS

Whether the damage to mitochondria seen in patients and in models of the disease is a primary or secondary event in the pathogenesis of ALS, mitochondrially targeted protective agents designed to ameliorate oxidative damage are possible candidates for new disease-modifying agents. The bioenergetic modifiers tested in models of the disease thus far and discussed in the section "Therapeutic Approaches to Mitochondrial Dysfunction in Amyotrophic Lateral Sclerosis" have been tried on the basis that each should theoretically interact positively with the machinery of oxidative phosphorylation to improve the bioenergetics of the motor neuron. Although an energy deficit has been clearly demonstrated in ALS, no deficit in either creatine or CoQ_{10} has been conclusively demonstrated. These agents are not therefore acting in an ALS-specific fashion. Delineation in much more detail of the changes to mitochondria in ALS may reveal targets for more specific mitochondrial protective agents. The technology to target such therapeutic agents, including antioxidants, to the mitochondria is already in development.[135,136]

REFERENCES

1. Schapira AHV. Mitochondrial involvement in Parkinson's disease, Huntington's disease, hereditary spastic paraplegia and Friedreich's ataxia. Biochim Biophys Acta 1999;1410:159–170.
2. Lodi R, Taylor DJ, Schapira AH. Mitochondrial dysfunction in Friedreich's ataxia. Biol Signals Recept 2001;10:263–270.
3. Albers DS, Beal MF. Mitochondrial dysfunction in progressive supranuclear palsy. Neurochem Int 2002;40:559–564.
4. Bonilla E, Tanji K, Hirano M, et al. Mitochondrial involvement in Alzheimer's disease. Biochim Biophys Acta 1999;1410:171–182.
5. Sonnewald U, Leif H, Shousboe A. Mitochondrial heterogeneity in the brain at the cellular level. J Cereb Blood Flow Metab 1998;18:231–237.
6. Vijayasarathy C, Biunno I, Lenka N, et al. Variations in the subunit content and catalytic activity of the cytochrome *c* oxidase complex from different tissues and different cardiac compartments. Biochim Biophys Acta 1998;1371:71–82.
7. Eaton S, Barlett K. Tissue specific differences in intramitochondrial control of beta-oxidation. Adv Exp Med Biol 1999;466:161–168.
8. Margineantu D, Capaldi RA, Marcus AH. Dynamics of the mitochondrial reticulum in live cells using Fourier imaging correlation spectroscopy and digital video microscopy. Biophys J 2000;79: 1833–1849.
9. Ligon LA, Steward O. Role of microtubules and actin filaments in the movement of mitochondria in the axons and dendrites of cultured hippocampal neurons. J Compar Neurol 2000;427: 351–361.
10. Egner A, Jakobs S, Hell SW. Fast 100-nm resolution three-dimensional microscope reveals structural plasticity of mitochondria in live yeast. Proc Natl Acad Sci USA 2002;99:3370–3375.
11. De Giorgi F, Lartigue L, Ichas F. Electrical coupling and plasticity of the mitochondrial network. Cell Calcium 2000;28:365–370.
12. Bernardi P. Mitochondrial transport of cations: channels, exchangers and permeability transition. Physiol Rev 1999;79:1127–1155.
13. Saraste M. Oxidative phosphorylation at the fin de siècle. Science 1999:283;1488–1493.
14. Krebs HA, Johnson WA. The role of citric acid in intermediate metabolism in animal tissues. Enzymologia 1937;4;148–156.
15. Menzies FM, Ince PG, Shaw PJ. Mitochondrial involvement in amyotrophic lateral sclerosis. Neurochem Int 2001;1165:1–9.
16. Turrens JF. Superoxide production by the mitochondrial respiratory chain. Biosci Rep 1997;17:3–8.

17. Azzone GF, Pietrobon D, Zoratti M. Determination of the proton electrochemical gradient across biological membranes. Curr Top Bioenerg 1984;13:1–77.
18. Mitchell P. Coupling of phosphorylation to electron and hydrogen transfer by a chemi-osmotic type of mechanism. Nature 1961;191:144–148.
19. Energy Conversion: Mitochondria and Chloroplasts. In B Alberts, D Bray, J Lewis, et al (eds), Molecular Biology of the Cell. New York: Garland Publishing, 1983;483.
20. Boveris A. Determination of the production of superoxide radicals and hydrogen peroxide in mitochondria. Methods Enzymol 1984;105:429–435.
21. Chance B, Sies H, Boveris A. Hydroperoxide metabolism in mammalian organs. Physiol Rev 1979;59:527–605.
22. Turrens JF, Boveris A. Generation of superoxide anion by the NADH dehydrogenase of bovine heart mitochondria. Biochem J 1980;191:421–427.
23. Turrens JF, Alexandre A, Lehninger AL. Ubisemiquinone is the electron donor for superoxide formation by complex III of heart mitochondria. Arch Biochem Biophys 1985;237:408–414.
24. Hansford RG, Hogue BA, Mildaziene V. Dependence of H_2O_2 formation by rat heart mitochondria on substrate availability and donor age. J Bioenerg Biomembr 1997;29:89–95.
25. Zhang L, Yu L, Yu C-A. Generation of superoxide anion by succinate-cytochrome c reductase from bovine heart mitochondria. J Biol Chem 1998;273:33972–33976.
26. Beyer RE. An analysis of the role of coenzyme Q in free radical generation and as an oxidant. Biochem Cell Biol 1992;70:390–403.
27. Takashige K, Minakami S. NADH- and NADPH-dependent formation of superoxide anions by bovine heart submitochondrial particles and NADH-ubiquinone reductase preparation. Biochem J 1979;180:129–135.
28. Flint DH et al. The inactivation of Fe-S cluster containing hydrolyases by superoxide. J Biol Chem 1993;268:22369–22376.
29. Taanman J-W. The mitochondrial genome: structure, transcription, translation and replication. Biochim Biophys Acta 1999;1410:103–123.
30. Anderson S, Bankier AT, Barrell BG, et al. Sequence and organization of the human mitochondrial genome. Nature 1981;290:457–465.
31. Pfanner N, Geissler A. Versatility of the mitochondrial protein import machinery. Nat Rev 2001;2: 339–349.
32. Richter C, Park JW, Ames BN. Normal oxidative damage to mitochondrial and nuclear DNA is extensive. Proc Nat Acad Sci USA 1988;85:6465–6467.
33. Bohr VA, Anson RM. Mitochondrial DNA repair pathways. J Bioenerg. Biomembr 1999;31:391–398.
34. Mecocci P, MacGarvey U, Kaufman AE, et al. Oxidative damage to mitochondrial DNA shows marked age-dependent increases in human brain. Ann Neurol 1993;34:609–616.
35. Strasser A, O'Connor L, Dixit VM. Apoptosis signaling. Ann Rev Biochem 2000;69:217–245.
36. Jurgensmeier JM, Xie Z, Deveraux Q, et al. Bax directly induces release of cytochrome c from isolated mitochondria. Proc Natl Acad Sci USA 1998;95:4997–5002.
37. Shimizu S, Narita M, Tsujimoto Y. Bcl-2 family proteins regulate the release of apoptogenic cytochrome c by the mitochondrial channel VDAC. Nature 1999;399:483–487.
38. Li P, Nijhawan D, Budihardjo I, et al. Cytochrome c and dATP-dependent formation of Apaf-1/caspase-9 complex initiates an apoptotic protease cascade. Cell 1997;91:479–489.
39. Green DR, Reed JC. Mitochondria and apoptosis. Science 1998;28:1309–1312.
40. Susin SA, Lorenzo HK, Zamzami N, et al. Mitochondrial release of caspase-2 and -9 during the apoptotic process. J Exp Med 1999;189:381–394.
41. Susin SA, Lorenzo HK, Zamzami N, et al. Molecular characterization of mitochondrial apoptosis-inducing factor. Nature 1999;397:441–446.
42. Lorenzo HK. Apoptosis-inducing factor (AIF): a phylogenetically old, caspase independent activator of cell death. Cell Death Differ 1999;6:516–524.
43. Petit PX, Susin SA, Zamzami N, et al. Mitochondria and programmed cell death: back to the future. FEBS Lett 1996;396:7–13.
44. Bernardi P, Broekemeier KM, Pfeiffer DR. Recent progress on regulation of the mitochondrial permeability transition pore; a cyclosporin-sensitive pore in the inner mitochondrial membrane. J Bioenerg Biomembr 1994;26:509–517.
45. Zamzami N, Marchetti P, Castedo M, et al. Inhibitors of permeability transition interfere with the disruption of the mitochondrial transmembrane potential during apoptosis. FEBS Lett 1996;384:53–57.
46. Susin SA, Zamzami N, Castedo M, et al. Bcl-2 inhibits the mitochondrial release of an apoptogenic protease. J Exp Med 1996:184:1331–1341.

47. Susin SA, Zamzami N, Castedo M, et al. The central executioner of apoptosis: multiple connections between protease activation and mitochondria in Fas/APO-1/CD95- and ceramide-induced apoptosis. J Exp Med 1997;186:25–37.
48. Marzo I, Brenner C, Zamzami N, et al. The permeability transition pore complex: a target for apoptosis regulation by caspases and bcl-2–related proteins. J Exp Med 1998;187:1261–1271.
49. Duchen MR. Mitochondria and calcium: from cell signaling to cell death. J Physiol 2000; 529.1:57–68.
50. Rizzuto R, Bernardi P, Pozzan. Mitochondria as all-round players of the calcium game. J Physiol 2000;529.1:37–47.
51. McCormack JG, Halestrap AP, Denton RM. Role of calcium ions in regulation of mammalian intramitochondrial metabolism. Phys Rev 1990;70:391–425.
52. Maechler P, Wollheim CB. Mitochondrial signals in glucose-stimulated insulin secretion in the beta cell. J Physiol 2000;529:49–56.
53. Bragadin M, Pozzan T, Azzone GF. Kinetics of Ca^{2+} carrier in rat liver mitochondria. Biochemistry 1979;18:5972–5978.
54. Jouaville LS, Pinton P, Bastianutto C, et al. Regulation of mitochondrial ATP synthesis by calcium: evidence for a long-term metabolic priming. Proc Natl Acad Sci USA 1999;96:13807–13812.
55. Friel DD, Tsien RW. An FCCP-sensitive Ca^{2+} store in bullfrog sympathetic neurons and its participation in stimulus-evoked changes in $[Ca^{2+}]_i$. J Neurosci 1994;14:4007–4024.
56. Werth JL, Thayer SA. Mitochondria buffer physiological calcium loads in cultured rat dorsal root ganglion neurons. J Neurosci 1994;14:348–356.
57. Wang GJ, Thayer SA. Sequestration of glutamate-induced Ca^{2+} loads by mitochondria in cultured rat hippocampal neurons. J Neurophys 1996;76:1611–1621.
58. Wang Z, Haydon PG, Yeung ES. Direct observation of calcium-independent intercellular ATP signaling in astrocytes. Anal Chem 2000;72:2001–2007.
59. David G, Barrett JN, Barrett EF. Evidence that mitochondria buffer physiological Ca^{2+} loads in lizard motor nerve terminals. J Phys 1998;509:59–65.
60. Babcock DF, Herrington J, Goodwin PC, et al. Mitochondrial participation in the intracellular Ca^{2+} network. J Cell Biol 1997;136:833–844.
61. Peuchen S, Clark JB, Duchen MR. Mechanisms of intracellular calcium regulation in adult astrocytes. Neuroscience 1996;71:871–883.
62. Rizzuto R, Pinton P, Carrington W, et al. Close contacts with the endoplasmic reticulum as determinants of mitochondrial Ca^{2+} responses. Science 1988;280:1763–1766.
63. Boitier E, Rea R, Duchen MR. Mitochondria exert a negative feedback on the propagation of intracellular Ca^{2+} waves in rat cortical astrocytes. J Cell Biol 1999;145:795–808.
64. Yen T-C, Chen Y-S, King K-L, et al. Liver mitochondrial respiratory functions decline with age. Biochem Biophys Res Comm 1989;165:994–1003.
65. Sadun AA. Mitochondrial optic neuropathies. J Neurol Neurosurg Psychiatry 2002;72:424–426.
66. Brunk UT, Terman A. The mitochondrial-lysosomal axis theory of aging. Accumulation of damaged mitochondria as a result of imperfect autophagocytosis. Eur J Biochem 2002;269:1996–2002.
67. Affifi AK, Aleu FP, Goodgold J, MacKay B. Ultrastructure of atrophic muscle in amyotrophic lateral sclerosis. Neurology 1966;16:475–481.
68. Nakano Y, Hirayama K, Terao K. Hepatic ultrastructural changes and liver dysfunction in amyotrophic lateral sclerosis. Arch Neurol 1987;44:103–106.
69. Siklos L, Engelhardt J, Harati Y, et al. Ultrastructural evidence for altered calcium in motor nerve terminals in amyotrophic lateral sclerosis. Ann Neurol 1996;39:203–216.
70. Sasaki S, Iwata M. Ultrastructural study of synapses in the anterior horn neurons of patients with amyotrophic lateral sclerosis. Neurosci Lett 1996;204:53–56.
71. Doble A, Kennel P. Animal models of amyotrophic lateral sclerosis. Amyotroph Lateral Scler Other Motor Neuron Disord 2000;1:301–312.
72. Dal Canto MC, Gurney ME. Development of central nervous system pathology in a murine transgenic model of human amyotrophic lateral sclerosis. Am J Pathol 1994;145:1271–1279.
73. Mourelatos Z, Gonatas NK, Stieber A, et al. The Golgi apparatus of spinal cord motor neurons in transgenic mice expressing mutant Cu,Zn superoxide dismutase becomes fragmented in early, preclinical stages of the disease. Proc Natl Acad Sci USA 1996;93:5472–5477.
74. Kong J, Xu Z. Massive mitochondrial degeneration in motor neurons triggers the onset of amyotrophic lateral sclerosis in mice expressing a mutant SOD1. J Neurosci 1998;18:3241–3250.
75. Bruijn LI, Becher MW, Lee MK, et al. ALS-linked SOD1 mutant G85R mediates damage to astrocytes and promotes rapidly progressive disease with SOD1-containing inclusions. Neuron 1997;18: 327–338.

76. Ince PG. Neuropathology. In RH Brown, V Meininger, M Swash (eds), Amyotrophic Lateral Sclerosis. London: Martin Dunitz, 2000;106–107.
77. Cashman NR, Durham HD, Blusztajn JK, et al. Neuroblastoma × spinal cord (NSC) hybrid cell lines resemble developing motor neurons. Dev Dyn 1992;194:209–221.
78. Menzies FM, Cookson MR, Taylor RW, et al. Mitochondrial dysfunction in a cell culture model of familial amyotrophic lateral sclerosis. Brain 2002;125:1522–1533.
79. Melov S, Coskun P, Patel M, et al. Mitochondrial disease in superoxide dismutase 2 mutant mice. Proc Natl Acad Sci USA 1999;96:846–851.
80. Melov S, Doctrow SR, Schneider JA, et al. Lifespan extension and rescue of spongiform encephalopathy in superoxide dismutase 2 nullizygous mice treated with superoxide dismutase-catalase mimetics. J Neurosci 2001;21:8348–8353.
81. Williams MD, Van Remmen H, Conrad CC, et al. Increased oxidative damage is correlated to altered mitochondrial function in heterozygous knockout mice. J Biol Chem 1998;273:28510–28515.
82. Andreasson OA, Ferrante RJ, Klivenyi P, et al. Partial deficiency of manganese superoxide dismutase exacerbates a transgenic mouse model of amyotrophic lateral sclerosis. Ann Neurol 2000;47:447–455.
83. Arai M, Imai H, Koumura T, et al. Mitochondrial phospholipid hydroperoxide glutathione peroxidase plays a major role in preventing oxidative injury to cells. J Biol Chem 1999;274:4924–4933.
84. Rabilloud T, Heller M, Rigobello M-P, et al. The mitochondrial antioxidant defense system and its response to oxidative stress. Proteomics 2001;1:1105–1110.
85. Han D, Williams E, Cadenas E. Mitochondrial respiratory chain-dependent generation of superoxide anion and its release into the intermembrane space. J Biochem 2001;353:411–416.
86. Sturtz L, Diekert K, Jensen LT, et al. A fraction of yeast Cu,Zn-superoxide dismutase and its metallochaperone, CCS, localize to the intermembrane space of mitochondria. J Biol Chem 2001;276:38084–38089.
87. Okado-Matsumoto A, Fridovich I. Subcellular distribution of superoxide dismutases (SOD) in rat liver. J Biol Chem 2001;276:38388–38393.
88. Jaarsma D, Haasdijk ED, Grashorn JAC, et al. Human Cu/Zn superoxide dismutase (SOD1) overexpression in mice causes mitochondrial vacuolization, axonal degeneration and premature motoneuron death and accelerates motoneuron disease in mice expressing a familial amyotrophic lateral sclerosis mutant SOD1. Neurobiol Dis 2000;7:623–643.
89. Mattiazi M, D'Aurelio M, Gajewski GD, et al. Mutated human SOD1 causes dysfunction of oxidative phosphorylation in mitochondria of transgenic mice. J Biol Chem 2002;277:29626–29633.
90. Kaal E, Vlug A, Versleijen M, et al. Chronic mitochondrial inhibition induces selective motor neuron death in vitro: a new model for amyotrophic lateral sclerosis. J Neurochem 2000;74:1158–1165.
91. Fujita K, Yamauchi M, Shibayama K, et al. Decreased cytochrome c oxidase activity but unchanged superoxide dismutase and glutathione peroxidase activities in the spinal cords of patients with amyotrophic lateral sclerosis. J Neurosci Res 1996;45:276–281.
92. Borthwick GM, Johnson MA, Ince PG, et al. Mitochondrial enzyme activity in motor neuron disease: implications for the role of mitochondria in neuronal cell death. Ann Neurol 1999;46:787–791.
93. Vielhaber S, Kunz D, Winkler K, et al. Mitochondrial DNA abnormalities in skeletal muscle of patients with sporadic amyotrophic lateral sclerosis. Brain 2000;123:1339–1348.
94. Browne SE, Bowling AC, Baik MJ, et al. Metabolic dysfunction in familial, but not sporadic, amyotrophic lateral sclerosis. J Neurochem 1998;71:281–287.
95. Jung C, Higgins CJ, Xu Z. Mitochondrial electron transport chain complex dysfunction in a transgenic mouse model for amyotrophic lateral sclerosis. J Neurochem 2002;83:535–545.
96. Alexianu ME, Ho BK, Mohamed AH, et al. The role of calcium-binding proteins in selective motor neuron vulnerability in amyotrophic lateral sclerosis. Ann Neurol 1994;36:846–858.
97. Ince PG, Stout N, Shaw PJ. Parvalbumin and calbindin D-28k in the human motor system and in motor neurone disease. Neuropathol Appl Neurobiol 1993;19:291–299.
98. Curti D, Malaspina A, Facchetti G, et al. Amyotrophic lateral sclerosis: oxidative energy metabolism and calcium homeostasis in peripheral blood lymphocytes. Neurology 1996;47:1060–1064.
99. Swerdlow RH, Parks JK, Cassarino DS, et al. Mitochondria in sporadic amyotrophic lateral sclerosis. Exp Neurol 1998;153:135–142.
100. Yang Y, Hentati A, Deng H-X, et al. The gene encoding alsin, a protein with three guanine-nucleotide exchange factor domains, is mutated in a form of recessive amyotrophic lateral sclerosis. Nat Genet 2001;29:160–165.

101. Hadano S, Hand C, Osuga H, et al. A gene encoding a putative GTPase regulator is mutated in familial amyotrophic lateral sclerosis 2. Nat Genet 2001;29:166–173.
102. Tomkins J, Banner SJ, McDermott CJ, Shaw PJ. Mutation screening of manganese superoxide dismutase in amyotrophic lateral sclerosis. Neuroreport 2001;12:2319–2322.
103. Parboosingh JS, Rouleau GA, Meininger V, et al. Absence of mutations in the Mn superoxide dismutase or catalase genes in familial amyotrophic lateral sclerosis. Neuromusc Disord 1995;5:7–10.
104. Tomblyn M, Kasarkis EJ, Xu Y, St. Clair DK. Distribution of MnSOD polymorphisms in sporadic ALS patients. J Mol Neurosci 1998;10:65–66.
105. Van Landeghem GF, Tabatabaie P, Beckman G, et al. Manganese-containing superoxide dismutase signal sequence polymorphism associated with sporadic motor neuron disease. Eur J Neurol 1999;6:639–644.
106. Comi GP, Bordoni A, Salani S, et al. Cytochrome oxidase subunit I microdeletion in a patient with motor neuron disease. Ann Neurol 1998;43:110–116.
107. Dhaliwal GK, Grewal RP. Mitochondrial DNA deletion mutation levels are elevated in ALS brains. Neuroreport 2002;11:2507–2509.
108. Wiedeman FR, Manfredi G, Mawrin C, et al. Mitochondrial DNA and respiratory chain function in spinal cords of ALS patients. J Neurochem 2002;80:616–625.
109. Sathasivam S, Ince PG, Shaw PJ. Apoptosis in amyotrophic lateral sclerosis: a review of the evidence. Neuropathol Appl Neurobiol 2001;27:257–274.
110. Vukosavic S, Dubois-Dauphin M, Romero N, Przedborski S. Bax and Bcl-2 interaction in a transgenic mouse model of familial amyotrophic lateral sclerosis. J Neurochem 1999;73:2460–2468.
111. De Aguilar J-LG, Gordon JW, Rene F. Alteration of the Bcl_x/Bax ratio in a transgenic mouse model of amyotrophic lateral sclerosis: evidence for the implication of the p53 signaling pathway. Neurobiol Dis 2000;7:406–415.
112. Mu X, He J, Anderson DW, et al. Altered expression of bcl-2 and bax mRNA in amyotrophic lateral sclerosis spinal cord motor neurons. Ann Neurol 1996;40:379–386.
113. Kostic V, Jackson-Lewis V, de Bilbao F, et al. Bcl-2: prolonging life in a transgenic mouse model of familial amyotrophic lateral sclerosis. Science 1997;277:559–562.
114. Yoshiyama Y, Yamada T, Asanuma K, Asahi T. Apoptosis related antigen. Le^Y and nick-end labelling are positive in spinal motor neurons in amyotrophic lateral sclerosis. Acta Neuropathol 1994;88:207–211.
115. Pedersen WA, Luo H, Kruman I, et al. The prostate apoptosis response-4 protein participates in motor neuron degeneration in amyotrophic lateral sclerosis. FASEB J 2000;14:913–924.
116. Pasinelli P, Borchelt DR, Houseweart MK, et al. Caspase-1 is activated in neural cells and tissue with amyotrophic lateral sclerosis–associated mutations in copper-zinc superoxide dismutase. Proc Natl Acad Sci USA 1998;95:15763–15768.
117. Li M, Ona VO, Guegan C, et al. Functional role of caspase-1 and caspase-3 in an ALS transgenic mouse model. Science 2000;288:335–339.
118. P Martin LJ. Neuronal death in amyotrophic lateral sclerosis is apoptosis: possible contribution of a programmed cell death mechanism. J Neuropathol Exp Neurol 1999;58:459–471.
119. Tarnopolsky MA, Beal MF. Potential for creatine and other therapies targeting cellular energy dysfunction in neurological disorders. Ann Neurol 2001;49:561–574.
120. Ferrante RJ, Beal MF. Neuroprotective Effects of Ginkgo Biloba Extract in ALS Transgenic Mice. In Y Christen (ed), Effects of Ginkgo Biloba Extract on the Central Nervous System. Paris: Elsevier (in press).
121. Strong MJ, Patee GL. Creatine and coenzyme Q_{10} in the treatment of ALS. Amyotroph Lateral Scler Other Motor Neuron Disord 2000;1(suppl 4):17–20.
122. Shults CW, Schapira AHV. A cue to queue for CoQ? Neurology 2001;57:375–376.
123. Di Giovanni S, Mirabella M, Spinazzola A, et al. Coenzyme Q_{10} reverses pathological phenotype and reduces apoptosis in familial CoQ_{10} deficiency. Neurology 2001;57:515–518.
124. Cortelli P, Montagna P, Pierangeli G, et al. Clinical and brain bioenergetics improvement with idebenone in a patient with Leber's hereditary optic neuropathy: a clinical and ^{31}P-MRS study. J Neurol Sci 1997;148:25–31.
125. The Huntington Study Group. A randomized, placebo-controlled trial of coenzyme Q_{10} and remacemide in Huntington's disease. Neurology 2001;57:397–404.
126. Matthews RT, Yang L, Browne S, et al. Coenzyme Q_{10} administration increases brain mitochondrial concentrations and exerts neuroprotective effects. Proc Natl Acad Sci USA 1998;95:8892–8897.
127. Molina JA, de Bustos F, Jimenez-Jimenez FJ, et al. Serum levels of coenzyme Q_{10} in patients with amyotrophic lateral sclerosis. J Neural Transm 2000;107:1021–1026.

128. Dechent P, Pouwels P, Wilken B, et al. Increase of total creatine in human brain after oral supplementation of creatine-monohydrate. Am J Physiol 1999;277:R698–R704.
129. Tarnapolsky M, Martin J. Creatine monohydrate increases strength in patients with neuromuscular disease. Neurology 1999;52:854–857.
130. Walter MC, Lochmuller H, Reilich P, et al. Creatine monohydrate in muscular dystrophies: a double-blind, placebo-controlled clinical study. Neurology 2000;54:1848–1850.
131. Klivenyi P, Ferrante RJ, Matthews RT, et al. Neuroprotective effects of creatine in a transgenic animal model of amyotrophic lateral sclerosis. Nat Med 1999;5:347–350.
132. Ikeda K, Iwasaki Y, Kinoshita M. Oral administration of creatine monohydrate retards progression of motor neuron disease in the wobbler mouse. Amyotroph Lateral Scler Other Motor Neuron Disord 2000;1:207–212.
133. Vielhaber S, Kaufmann J, Kanowski M, et al. Effect of creatine supplementation on metabolite levels in ALS motor cortices. Exp Neurol 2001;172:377–382.
134. Mazzini L, Balzarini C, Colombo R, et al. Effects of creatine supplementation on exercise performance and muscular strength in amyotrophic lateral sclerosis: preliminary results. J Neurol Sci 2001;191:139–144.
135. Coulter C, Kelso GF, Lin T-K, et al. Mitochondrially targeted antioxidants and thiol reagents. Free Radic Biol Med 2000;28:1547–1554.
136. Kelso GF, Porteous CM, Coulter CV, et al. Selective targeting of a redox-active ubiquinone to mitochondria within cells. J Biol Chem 2001;276:4588–4596.

12

Cytoskeletal Abnormalities in Amyotrophic Lateral Sclerosis/Motor Neuron Disease

Janice Robertson and Jean-Pierre Julien

Amyotrophic lateral sclerosis (ALS) is an adult-onset and heterogeneous neurological disorder that affects primarily large motor neurons in the brain and spinal cord. The degeneration of motor neurons leads to denervation, atrophy of skeletal muscles, and ultimately to paralysis and death. Current evidence suggests that multiple genetic and environmental factors may be implicated in ALS pathogenesis.[1] Approximately 90 percent of patients with ALS are diagnosed as having sporadic ALS (SALS) and little is known about the genetic defects that cause or predispose to ALS (Table 12.1). Mutations in the gene coding for the copper/zinc superoxide dismutase (SOD1) are responsible for about 20 percent of familial cases, but for the vast majority of ALS cases, the etiology remains unknown.[2,3] A common pathological finding in ALS is the presence of abnormal accumulations of 10-nanometer filaments in the perikaryon and axon of motor neurons.[4-6] A central question to understanding disease pathogenesis in ALS is whether these filamentous accumulations are actively involved in the neurodegenerative mechanism, innocent bystanders occurring as a response to neuronal injury or indeed, a mechanism of neuroprotection acting by sequestering toxic molecules from their intended target(s). This chapter focuses on the role of neurofilaments (NFs) and other cytoskeletal proteins in motor neuron disease (MND) with particular emphasis on recent transgenic mouse studies.

NEURONAL CYTOSKELETON

Within the cytoplasm of all eukaryotic cells, there is a complex network of filaments known as the *cytoskeleton*. In addition to providing the cell with a structural framework, the cytoskeleton participates in many dynamic cellular

315

Table 12.1 Genetic causes of amyotrophic lateral sclerosis

Adult
  SOD1 on chromosome 21 (20% FALS)
  NF-H on chromosome 22
  Chromosome 9q21–q35 with frontotemporal dementia
  Chromosome 17q21 with frontotemporal dementia and parkinsonism
  Excitatory amino acid transporter type 2 RNA processing errors
  Cytochrome *c* oxidase: mitochondrial DNA microdeletion in one case
Juvenile
  ALS2 (alsin) chromosome 2q33–q35 autosomal recessive
  Chromosome 15q15–q24 autosomal recessive
  Chromosome 9q34 autosomal dominant

DNA = deoxyribonucleic acid; FALS = familial amyotrophic lateral sclerosis; NF-H = high molecular weight neurofilament subunit protein; RNA = ribonucleic acid; SOD1 = superoxide dismutase.

functions such as cell movement, changes in cell shape, and intracellular trafficking of organelles and other proteins. Most neuronal proteins are synthesized in the perikaryon and are delivered to their targets by a process known as *axonal transport*. Axonal transport is critically dependent on the functioning of the cytoskeleton. This is particularly crucial to motor axons, which can be up to 1 meter in length.

The neuronal cytoskeleton is made up of three filament types that can be distinguished on the basis of their diameter: microtubules, actin filaments, and intermediate filaments (IFs). These filaments are linked through numerous associated proteins and adaptor molecules to form an integrated network that can respond in a concerted manner to intracellular and extracellular cues.

Microtubules

Microtubules are 24-nanometers in diameter and are formed by the reversible polymerization of α-subunits and β-subunits of tubulin. The tubulins are encoded by a multigene family, with at least six isoforms of α-tubulin and β-tubulin, each encoded by a separate gene. Microtubules are polar structures, with a rapidly growing plus end and a slower growing minus end. In axons, microtubules are oriented with their plus ends oriented way from the cell body, whereas in dendrites, microtubules are oriented in both directions. These distinct orientations may be regulated in part by microtubule-associated proteins (MAPs). A number of MAPs co-purify with microtubules through repeated cycles of assembly and disassembly in vitro. The two most predominant MAPs in neurons are MAP2 and tau, with MAP2 being expressed in dendrites and tau expressed in axons.[7–9] One of the major functions of MAP2 and tau is to promote microtubule stability.[10] The binding of MAP2 or tau to microtubules is regulated by phosphorylation, a post-translational modification key to regulating a multitude of signaling pathways necessary for neuronal function.[11–13]

The axonal transport of organelles, trophic factors, and of neuronal proteins synthesized in the perikaryon is dependent on microtubules. Transport along microtubules is bidirectional, with anterograde transport directed toward nerve terminals (the plus end of microtubules) and retrograde transport directed toward the perikaryon (the minus end of microtubules). Axonal transport is driven by two major families of motor proteins: kinesin, which is responsible for anterograde transport, and dynein, which is responsible for retrograde transport.[14–16] Anterograde transport is classically divided into three components that depend on the rate of transport: fast component, slow component a (SCa), and slow component b (SCb).[17] Most organelles and membrane-bound vesicles are transported in the fast component, microtubules and NFs in SCa, and microfilaments and other cytoplasmic proteins in SCb. These different rates of transport appear to be determined by the amount of time the cargo remains associated with the motor; the longer the time the faster the apparent transport rate.[16,18,19]

Microfilaments

Microfilaments or actin filaments are 5 to 9 nm in diameter and are formed by the reversible polymerization of actin monomers. Like microtubules, microfilaments are polar structures, having a plus and a minus end. A number of associated proteins are involved in promoting actin polymerization or depolymerization, such as profilin and cofilin, and this dynamic rearrangement of the actin cytoskeleton is responsible for neuronal properties such as axonal growth and dendritic elaboration.[20] The response of the actin cytoskeleton to extracellular signals is mediated by the Rho family of small guanosine triphosphatases (GTPases), the most characterized of which are Rho, Rac, and Cdc42.[21]

Intermediate Filaments

IFs are 10 nanometers in diameter and are so called because they are intermediate in size between microtubules and actin filaments. IFs are in fact a large family of proteins that exhibit tissue-specific expression, with, for example, keratin filaments expressed in epithelial cells, desmin filaments expressed in muscle cells, and NFs expressed in neuronal cells.[22,23] The IF protein family is classified into six types based on sequence homology and intron-exon organization within their respective genes. However, this number is growing as new family members are identified.

All IF proteins share the same tripartite structure of an α-helical rod domain flanked by non–α-helical N-terminal "head" and C-terminal "tail" domains. The rod domains of IF proteins are highly conserved, both in sequence and length, having approximately 310 amino acid residues (~352 for the nuclear lamins). IF protein diversity is derived from the variability of the N-terminal head and C-terminal tail domains. These domains are where most post-translational modifications occur and are responsible for the interactions of IF proteins with other neuronal components. IFs are assembled by the formation of dimers in which the central rod domains of two IF proteins are wound around each other to form coiled coils. The dimers then associate in a staggered, antiparallel arrangement to form tetramers, which form the building blocks of IFs, associating laterally and longitudinally to form the final filament.[22,23] In contrast to microtubules and microfilaments, IFs have no polarity.

Three major IF types are expressed in adult neurons: NFs, α-internexin, and peripherin. NFs are the most abundant neuronal IF proteins, being expressed in most neurons of the central nervous system (CNS) and the peripheral nervous system (PNS).[24,25] They include three protein subunits: NF of low molecular weight (NF-L) of 68 to 70kd, NF of medium molecular weight (NF-M) of 150 to 160kd, and NF of high molecular weight (NF-H) of 200 to 210kd, commonly known as the NF triplet. α-Internexin, a 66-kilodalton protein, is expressed mainly in the CNS.[26,27] Peripherin, a 58-kilodalton protein, is expressed mostly in the PNS and in some neuronal populations of the CNS.[28–30] Compared with NFs, much less is known of the specific functions and properties of α-internexin and peripherin.

Neurofilaments

NF proteins, together with α-internexin, belong to type IV of the IF gene superfamily.[24] NFs are obligate heteropolymers, with filament assembly contingent on the presence of NF-L, together with NF-M, and/or NF-H.[31,32] Under defined conditions, NFs can be formed from purified NF subunits, demonstrating that other proteins are not required for filament assembly. Although NFs composed only of NF-L and NF-M or NF-L and NF-H have been demonstrated in fibroblasts transfected with the respective complementary DNAs (cDNAs),[31,32] it is considered that filaments composed of all three NF subunits represent the most abundant form in vivo (Figure 12.1).

There is much sequence homology in the overlapping regions of the NF triplet, particularly in the α-helical rod domain, which is highly conserved among all IF proteins. The major variability between the NF triplet proteins is found in the length and sequence of the C-terminal tail domain, which for NF-H comprises as much as two thirds of its total size. Ultrastructurally, the C-terminal domains of NF-H and NF-M project laterally from the filament core, forming cross-bridges between neighboring NFs and microtubules.[33,34] The C-terminal domains of NF-M and NF-H have numerous phosphorylation sites, predominantly serine-proline residues, sites for proline-directed kinases. NF-L in contrast is minimally phosphorylated, with consensus sites for protein kinase A and protein kinase C located in the N-terminal head domain. Phosphorylation at these sites of NF-L is thought to regulate filament assembly. Numerous candidate kinases have been shown to directly phosphorylate NFs in vitro. These include cyclin-dependent kinase-5 (Cdk5),[35,36] glycogen synthase kinase-3 (GSK-3),[37,38] casein kinase I and II (CKI and II),[39–41] and members of the mitogen-activated protein kinase family, ERK-1,2[42] and stress-activated protein kinases (SAPKs), or c-Jun kinase.[43–45] The function of NF phosphorylation is unknown but is believed to regulate numerous NF interactions, particularly of the C-terminal tail domain. Moreover, numerous studies have linked the NF axonal transport rate to the degree of NF phosphorylation. The more phosphorylated NFs being associated with the slowest, or stationary phase, and those that are less phosphorylated having a higher mobility. It is likely that these

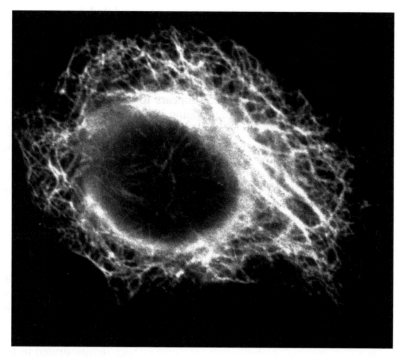

Figure 12.1 The neurofilament network in SW13 cells that have been co-transfected with expression plasmids encoding neurofilament of low and high molecular weight (NF-L, NF-H). Transfected cells are labeled by indirect immunofluorescence with antibody to NF-L.

differences in transport rates are determined by the amount of time NFs are associated with the transport motor.[19]

Peripherin

Peripherin belongs to type III of the IF gene superfamily. Peripherin is so called because of its predominant expression in the PNS, although it is also expressed at low levels in defined neuronal populations of the CNS, including spinal motor neurons. Peripherin is encoded by a single gene located within the q12–q13 region of human chromosome 12.[46–49] There are three potential AUG start codons within the pre-messenger RNA (mRNA) transcript, with translation preferentially occurring from the second of these.[50] Peripherin is unique compared with the other neuronal IF proteins in that three alternative splice variants have been detected in mouse neuroblastoma cells.[51,52] These variants have molecular weights of 56, 58, and 61 kd. The 58-kilodalton isoform corresponds to the species most readily recognized on SDS-polyacrylamide gels of extracts from peripheral nerve. The 56-kilodalton isoform is shorter due to a cryptic acceptor site in exon 9 of the peripherin gene transcript, leading to a frameshift and the replacement of the C-terminal 21 amino acids of the 58-kilodalton protein with a unique 8 amino acid sequence. The 61-kilodalton isoform contains a 96-base pair insertion within the α-helical rod domain, corresponding to the use of intron four of the peripherin gene as an exon.[51,52] The human equivalent of these mouse peripherin isoforms has not yet been detected.

The phosphorylation of tyrosine represents another unique property of peripherin compared to NFs, which are phosphorylated only on serine or threonine residues, or α-internexin, which appears to be nonphosphorylated.[53–55] The function of this tyrosine phosphorylation is unknown.

As mentioned, peripherin expression is found predominantly in neurons of the PNS. However, after neuronal injury, peripherin expression is increased in neurons of the CNS and in neurons of the PNS. This has been demonstrated in spinal motor neurons and large dorsal root ganglion (DRG) neurons after sciatic nerve crush,[56,57] in cortical neurons after stab injury, and in hippocampal neurons after transient focal ischemia.[58] The functional significance of this increased peripherin expression is unknown and has been associated with both neuronal regeneration and neurotoxicity. Interestingly, peripherin expression can be induced by proinflammatory cytokines such as interleukin-6 (IL-6) and leukemia inhibitory factor acting through the JAK-STAT pathway of transcription.[59–61] The significance of these observations will be relevant to our discussion on cytoskeletal pathology in ALS involving peripherin.

Peripherin is capable of self-assembly and co-assembly with the NF subunits.[62,63] There is some evidence that peripherin can interact with neurofilaments in vivo, including observations by immune electron microscopy in PC12 cells and rat peripheral nerve[64] and biochemical studies of DRG neuronal extracts.[65] However, whether filaments formed from both NF subunits and peripherin exist in humans is not known.

CYTOSKELETAL CHANGES IN HUMAN AMYOTROPHIC LATERAL SCLEROSIS

Abnormal Intermediate Filament Accumulations

A pathological hallmark of both SALS and familial ALS (FALS) is the presence of abnormal NF accumulations in the perikaryon and axon of motor neurons.[5,6] Peripherin is another type of IF protein detected with NF proteins in most axonal inclusion bodies, called spheroids, in motor neurons of patients with ALS (Figure 12.2).[66,67] Many factors can potentially lead to the accumulation of IF proteins including deregulation of IF protein synthesis, defective axonal transport, abnormal phosphorylation and proteolysis, and other protein modifications. There is evidence of deregulated expression of NF genes in ALS. In situ hybridization studies revealed considerable reduction in levels of NF-L mRNA in degenerating spinal motor neurons of patients with ALS.[68,69] Moreover, the decrease in mRNA levels is selective for NF-L because no significant changes were detected in NF-M and NF-H mRNA levels of patients with ALS.[69] It seems paradoxical that the reduction of NF-L mRNA levels (~87%) is even more pronounced in neurons with NF accumulations. However, because of its requirement for proper NF assembly and transport, a deficiency in NF-L can

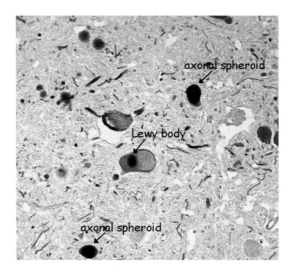

Figure 12.2   Labeling of amyotrophic lateral sclerosis lumbar spinal cord section with antibody-recognizing peripherin (×40). In addition to the generalized increase in peripherin immunoreactivity in perikarya and neuritic processes of spinal motor neurons, peripherin is associated with both axonal spheroids and Lewy body–like inclusions.

provoke the sequestration of NF-M and NF-H proteins in the cell bodies of motor neurons, as revealed from the analysis of NF-L knockout mice.[70] In addition, disorganized filaments and intracellular transport defects could result from post-translational protein modifications. Indeed a major indicator of degenerating motor neurons in ALS is the abnormal localization of phosphorylated NF epitopes in motor neuron perikaryon. Of particular interest are the recent findings that excitotoxicity can induce hyperphosphorylation of the KSP C-terminal tail domain of NF-H, which correlates with a slowing of NF transport.[71] The phosphorylation of NFs induced by increased glutamate may occur via members of the MAP kinase (MAPK) family, including ERK-1,2 and SAPKs. Other post-translational protein modifications may also be involved in disorganization of NFs. Advanced glycation products and nitration of tyrosine residues are detected in NF inclusions of ALS.[72,73] However, the extent of nitration in the NF-L protein from the spinal cord of patients with SALS does not differ from that of age-matched controls.[74]

Neurofilament Gene Mutations

Codon deletions or insertion in the KSP repeat motif of NF-H gene has been identified in a small number of patients with SALS (~1%),[75–77] whereas no such NF-H mutants have been detected in more than 1000 control DNA samples. So far, the search for mutations in all coding regions of the three NF genes has failed to reveal additional mutations linked to ALS cases.[78,79] Nonetheless, mutations in the rod domain of the NF-L and NF-M genes have recently been

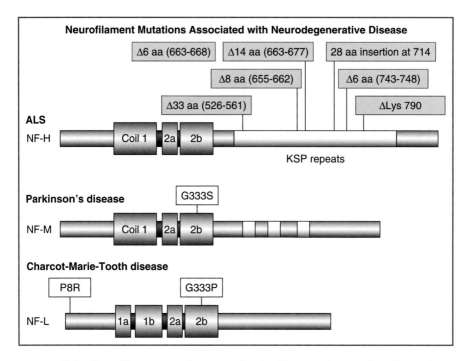

Figure 12.3 Neurofilament mutations associated with neurodegenerative disease. The mutations in neurofilament (NF) of high molecular weight are either insertions or deletions within the KSP phosphorylation domain.[75–77] These mutations are associated mainly with sporadic amyotrophic lateral sclerosis (ALS) cases (10/1047), with only one case reported so far for familial ALS (1/295). For Parkinson's disease and Charcot-Marie-Tooth disease, the mutations to NFs of medium and low molecular weight (Q333P) are located within coil 2B of the α-helical rod domain, a "hot spot" for mutations in other intermediate filament—related diseases.[80–82]

reported in cases of Charcot-Marie-Tooth disease type 2 and Parkinson's disease, respectively (Figure 12.3).[80,81] Even though the combined results support the view that NF abnormalities can induce pathogenesis, it is clear that mutations in NF genes as primary causes of disease can account for only a small proportion of cases in these neurodegenerative diseases.

TRANSGENIC MICE WITH INTERMEDIATE FILAMENT ABNORMALITIES

Neurofilament Knockout Mice

Remarkably, knockout mice for any of the type IV IF genes, that is, the three NF genes and α-internexin gene, did not develop overt phenotypes and gross developmental defects.[70,83–88] In addition, double-knockout mice deficient for both α-internexin and NF-L also exhibited no overt phenotypes.[88] The analysis of these knockout mice provided useful information on NF protein functions. The targeted disruption of the NF-L gene in mice confirmed the importance of NF-L in IF assembly. Mice lacking NF-L had a scarcity of IF structures and exhibited a severe axonal hypotrophy.[70] In the absence of NF-L, the NF-M and NF-H subunits were unable to assemble into IFs and they accumulate as protein aggregates in some neurons such as spinal motor neurons. Whereas the NF-L subunit is an absolute requirement for NF assembly, the NF-H subunit is dispensable for the formation of NF structures and for the radial growth of motor axons during development.[83,86,87] NF-M turned out to be more important than NF-H for NF assembly and transport into axons. The absence of NF-M in mice caused important decreases in NF-L levels and in NF content, resulting in axonal atrophy.[85,89] In addition, the absence of both NF-M and NF-H subunits resulted in the sequestering of unassembled NF-L proteins in neuronal perikarya and in a reduction of axonal caliber similar to the NF-L null mice.[85] The combined results suggest a requirement of heterodimerization of NF-L to NF-M or to NF-H subunits to achieve efficient assembly and translocation of NF proteins into the axonal compartment.

Although the type IV IFs are not required for nervous system development, deficiencies in NF proteins are not completely innocuous. The reduction in caliber of myelinated axons lacking NFs is accompanied by up to 50-percent reduction in conduction velocity,[90] a feature very detrimental for large animal species. Significant loss of motor axons has also been detected in the NF-L null mice[70] and in double NF-M/NF-H knockout mice.[85] Regeneration studies showed delayed maturation of regenerating myelinated axons in NF-L$^{-/-}$ mice,[70] whereas in either NF-M or NF-H null mice, the velocity of transport of slow components in the axon was increased and alterations occurred in the neuronal cytoskeleton such as a higher abundance of microtubules.[83,85] A striking feature of the NF-L knockout mice is the accumulation of NF-M and NF-H proteins in the perikaryon of motor neurons even though the absence of NF-L provoked about a 90-percent reduction of NF-H and NF-M protein levels in nervous system tissue. This emphasizes the importance of subunit stoichiometry for correct NF assembly, stability, and transport.

Neurofilament Overexpressers

The overexpression in mice of any of the three wild-type NF subunits alone can induce the formation of NF accumulations in neuronal cell bodies.[91–93] Such perikaryal accumulations of NFs are relatively well tolerated by motor neurons. For example, high-level expression of human NF-H proteins caused large perikaryal NF accumulations, resulting in atrophy of motor axons and altered axonal conductances but without motor neuron death even in 2-year-old mice.[94,95] Overexpression of NF-L in NF-H transgenic mice reduced the perikaryal swellings and rescued the motor neuron dysfunction, illustrating again the importance of subunit stoichiometry for proper NF assembly and transport.[96]

The proof that NF abnormalities can induce neuronal death in vivo came from transgenic mouse studies in which an assembly-disrupting NF-L mutant having a leucine-to-proline substitution near the end of the conserved rod domain was expressed.[97] Expression of this NF-L mutant at only 50 percent of the endogenous NF-L level led to a massive death of motor neurons within 4 weeks of birth. Although no such NF-L mutations have been reported in human ALS, similar mutations in keratins cause severe forms of skin diseases. However, the mechanism of toxicity of mutant NF-L is not fully understood. Increasing the levels of Bcl-2 did not protect the large motor neurons from the toxicity of mutant NF-L.[98] A plausible mechanism is that axonal NF accumulations can somehow interfere with axonal transport, leading to degeneration of the neuron. This is the so-called "strangulation of axonal transport hypothesis."[99,100]

Peripherin Overexpressers

As shown in the Figure 12.2, peripherin immunoreactivity is associated with the major cytoskeletal abnormalities found in ALS, that is, axonal spheroids, increased immunoreactivity in perikarya and neuritic processes, and less frequent Lewy bodies. These pathological changes are most often associated with NF abnormalities and consequently much research has focused on the potential contribution of NFs to motor neuron degeneration, with peripherin being largely overlooked. However, unlike other types of neuronal IF proteins, the sustained overexpression of wild type peripherin in mice caused the selective death of motor neurons during aging.[101] Moreover, it induced formation of perikaryal and axonal IF inclusions resembling spheroids found in human ALS. Death of neurons is exacerbated by the absence of NF-L, as shown by cross-breeding with NF-L knockout mice. This is reminiscent of the findings in ALS, described earlier, in which there is a reduction of NF-L mRNA levels in affected motor neurons.[68,69]

Even though the toxicity of peripherin overexpression may be related in part to the axonal localization of IF aggregates, other mechanisms likely contribute to pathogenesis. The detrimental effects of peripherin overexpression on motor neuron viability has also been demonstrated in vitro using cultured motor neurons intranuclearly microinjected with expression of plasmid containing peripherin (Figure 12.4).[102] Peripherin toxicity in cultured motor neurons is attenuated by coexpression of NF-L, providing additional evidence that stoichiometric ratios of peripherin and NF proteins are important to neuronal survival. An important correlate in both peripherin transgenic mice and motor neurons overexpressing peripherin in culture is that of peripherin aggregation and cell death. As described already, peripherin aggregation in the form of spheroids and Lewy bodies is a feature of motor neuron degeneration in ALS. Whether peripherin aggregation in motor neurons of the models we have described is a prerequisite to cell death is unclear.

Interestingly, peripherin aggregates are also present in DRG neurons of peripherin transgenic mice, but no loss of this cell type is detected in vivo (Figure 12.5).[102] Studies in vitro, however, have shown that DRG neurons from peripherin transgenic embryos die when grown in a proinflammatory CNS culture environment rich in activated microglia (Figure 12.6). Death of DRG neurons containing peripherin aggregates was mediated by tumor necrosis factor (TNF), a major proinflammatory cytokine released by activated microglia.[102] This experiment suggests that peripherin aggregates might predispose neurons to the detrimental effects of a proinflammatory environment. In ALS, proinflammatory markers, such as activated microglia, are associated with degenerating motor neurons.[1] Because microglia are specific to the CNS, this may in part account for the neuronal selectivity in ALS. Another consideration, mentioned earlier, is that proinflammatory cytokines can induce peripherin

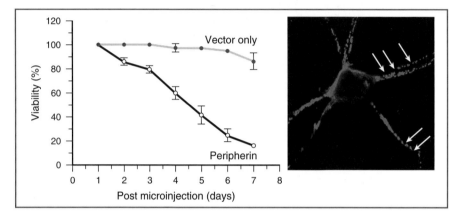

Figure 12.4 Intranuclear microinjection of mammalian expression plasmid-encoding peripherin induces death of motor neurons in culture. The viability of motor neurons expressing peripherin was compared to those microinjected with carrier plasmid alone (pRcCMV; control). The inset shows immunolabeling of a motor neuron microinjected with peripherin expression plasmid. The arrows indicate peripherin aggregates in neuronal processes.

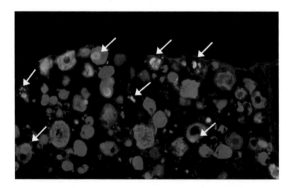

Figure 12.5 Peripherin aggregates are present in dorsal root ganglion (DRG) neurons of peripherin transgenic mice. Cryostat section from L4-L5 DRG of a peripherin transgenic mouse double labeled by indirect immunofluorescence with antibodies to peripherin and neurofilaments. Labeling reveals both large DRG neurons (expressing only neurofilaments; green); small DRG neurons (expressing only peripherin;); and mid-sized DRG neurons (expressing both neurofilaments and peripherin; yellow). Aggregates are indicated by arrows.

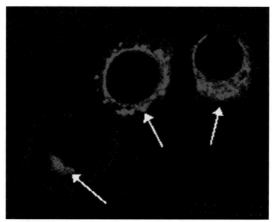

Peripherin

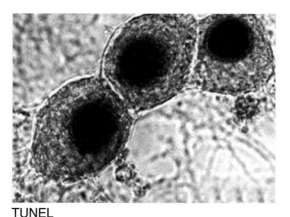

TUNEL

Figure 12.6 In dissociated spinal cord cultures, dorsal root ganglion neurons cultured from peripherin transgenic mice die when exposed to a proinflammatory extracellular environment. The double labeling using peripherin antibody (red) and TUNEL shows the presence of peripherin aggregates *(arrows)* in apoptotic cells.

expression.[60,61] Therefore cytokines released by activated microglia may not only induce death of neurons containing peripherin aggregates but also actively participate in forming aggregates by further stimulating increased expression of peripherin (Figure 12.7). A noteworthy feature of this disease model is that no gene mutation is required for neurodegeneration.

Another unique characteristic of peripherin compared with NFs is the existence, at least in the mouse, of several alternatively spliced variants of peripherin.[51,52] Abnormalities in alternative splicing is proving to be an important mechanism underlying several neurodegenerative diseases, in particular tauopathies such as frontotemporal dementia with parkinsonism linked to

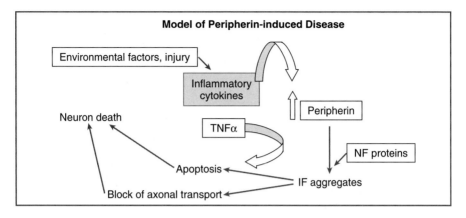

Figure 12.7   Model of peripherin-induced disease.

chromosome 17 (FTDP-17).[103] Of particular interest are our findings that differential expression of these variants occurs in a transgenic mouse model of ALS and that the Per61 species is distinctly assembly incompetent and neurotoxic when expressed in cultured primary neurons (our unpublished observation). Future studies are needed to determine whether splice variants of peripherin also exist in humans.

OTHER TRANSGENIC MOUSE MODELS

Mice Expressing Mutant SOD1

Missense mutations in the SOD1 gene account for about 20 percent of FALS cases[3] for review.[99,100] So far, more than 100 mutations have been discovered spanning all exons of the SOD1 gene, but unraveling the toxicity of SOD1 mutants has been particularly challenging. Some studies have focused on aberrant copper-mediated catalysis as a potential source of toxicity.[104,105] One hypothesis was that misfolding of SOD1 induced by mutations would allow the access of abnormal substrates such as peroxynitrite to the catalytic site, leading to the nitration of tyrosine residues.[106] Another proposal suggested that SOD1 mutants have enhanced ability to use hydrogen peroxide as substrate to generate toxic hydroxyl radicals that can damage cellular targets including DNA, protein, and lipid membranes.[107] However, neither the peroxynitrite nor the peroxidase activity hypothesis was supported by transgenic mouse studies. First, the elimination of endogenous SOD1 or addition of wild type SOD1 did not affect disease progression in SOD1^{G85R} mice.[108] Second, the gene knockout for the copper chaperone for SOD1 (CCS) that delivers copper to the SOD1 catalytic site did not affect disease progression in ALS mice.[104]

Currently, the most prevailing hypothesis is that the toxicity of SOD1 mutants is related to the propensity of misfolded protein mutants to form aggregates.[108,109] Yet, the toxicity of these protein aggregates is still poorly understood. Detrimental effects could result from the co-sequestering of essential cellular components and from overwhelming the capacity of the protein-folding chaperones and/or of ubiquitin proteasome pathway to degrade important cellular regulatory factors. Somehow, the noxious property of mutant SOD1 also affects the transport machinery. Thus transgenic mice expressing mutant SOD1 exhibit reduced rates of slow axonal transport.[110,111] Such transport defects may explain the presence of abnormal IF accumulations in human ALS cases with SOD1 mutations[6] and in transgenic mice expressing SOD1 mutants.[95,112,113]

Mating experiments to generate mice expressing mutant SOD1 in a context of NF-L deficiency provide compelling evidence that the presence of axonal NFs is not a prerequisite for pathogenesis. Yet, the absence of NF-L led to about a 15-percent extension of life span in mice expressing either $SOD1^{G85R}$ or $SOD1^{G37R}$.[114,115] Even more surprising, the overexpression of human NF-H or to a lesser extent mouse NF-H proteins, which raises perikaryal NF content and lowers axonal levels, extended the life span of mutant SOD1 mice by 65 percent and 15 percent, respectively.[116,117] From these experiments, we can see that it remains unclear whether the slowing down of disease in ALS mice is due to a reduction of NF burden in motor axons or an accumulation of NF proteins in the cell bodies of motor neurons. To further address this issue, $SOD1^{G37R}$ mice were generated in a context of one disrupted allele for each NF gene, thereby reducing the NF content and caliber of motor axons without altering the normal subunit stoichiometry and morphological distribution of NFs.[115] Motor axons with reduced calibers remained equally vulnerable to degeneration and a 40-percent decrease in the content of intact NFs did not extend the life span of $SOD1^{G37R}$ mice. This experiment suggests that the burden of intact NFs in the axon is not a key factor contributing to the selective vulnerability of motor neurons in ALS caused by mutant SOD1, and that the slowing down of disease, for instance, by NF-H overexpression, is likely the result of protective effects of perikaryal IF accumulations.

By what mechanism do perikaryal NF accumulations confer protection? We have proposed, based on the finding of deregulation of Cdk5 activity in $SOD1^{G37R}$ mice, that perikaryal NF accumulations may act as a phosphorylation sink for Cdk5 activity, thereby reducing the detrimental hyperphosphorylation of tau and other neuronal substrates.[118] The abnormal subcellular localization of Cdk5 has been observed in several neurodegenerative diseases including ALS,[119] Alzheimer's disease,[120,121] Parkinson's disease,[122] as well as in canine MND.[123] In addition, recent studies suggest that a deregulation of Cdk5 activity may directly contribute to pathogenesis of Alzheimer's disease.[124] In 1999, Patrick et al[124] reported the accumulation of p25, a truncated form of p35, in the brains of patients with Alzheimer's disease. Unlike p35, p25 is not targeted to the plasma membrane sequestering Cdk5 away from normal compartments of p35/Cdk5 and it deregulates its activity. Expression of the p25/Cdk5 complex in cultured cortical neurons induced cytoskeletal abnormalities and apoptosis.[124,125] Moreover, the overexpression of p25 in the CNS of transgenic mice caused hyperphosphorylation of tau and NFs, cytoskeletal disruption, and behavioral deficits.[126]

Another potential beneficial effect of perikaryal NF accumulations may be through the trapping of noxious components. For example, our transgenic studies revealed a rescue of peripherin-mediated degeneration of motor neurons by NF-H overexpression (J.M. Beaulieu and J.P. Julien, unpublished observation). Our analysis suggests that the protective effect of extra NF-H proteins is related to the sequestration of peripherin into the perikaryon of motor neurons, thereby abolishing the development of axonal IF inclusions that might block transport.

Tau Transgenics

As mentioned earlier, tau is an MAP that is most known for its ability to stabilize microtubules. Tau comprises six isoforms of 55 to 62 kd that are derived from a single gene via alternative splicing of the primary gene transcript. All six isoforms are expressed in normal adult human brain. Two other higher molecular weight forms of tau also exist and these are expressed mainly in the PNS. In the carboxyl half of tau, there is a highly conserved region that contains three or four consecutive repeats of 31 or 32 amino acids. This region, also present in MAP2, is involved in the binding of tau to microtubules, with the four-repeat form binding more strongly than the three-repeat form. Both the three-repeat and the four-repeat form may contain an additional 29 or 58 amino acid insert toward the N-terminus, which results in six alternatively spliced variants of tau. The expression of these tau isoforms is developmentally regulated, with the three-repeat isoform lacking N-terminal inserts being the only form of tau expressed in fetal cells.

Abnormalities of tau in human disease are collectively known as *tauopathies,* the major of which are Alzheimer's disease, FTDP-17, progressive supranuclear palsy (PSP), and ALS/parkinsonism-dementia complex.[103] The neuropathological hallmarks of tauopathies are aggregates of paired helical filaments or straight filaments found in widespread regions of the CNS. Paired helical filaments (PHFs) and straight filaments are composed of abnormally phosphorylated tau protein and is collectively known as *PHF-tau.* PHF-tau can be detected immunocytochemically using phosphorylation-dependent antibodies. The perikaryal labeling of neurons with phospho-tau antibodies is an early marker of diseased neurons.

A potential involvement of tau in ALS pathogenesis is supported by two studies. First, as described earlier, abnormal hyperphosphorylation of tau due to Cdk5 deregulation has been detected in motor neurons of SOD1^{G37R} transgenic mice and a decrease of tau hyperphosphorylation by NF-H overexpression correlated with a slowing down of disease.[118] Second, in transgenic mice overexpressing the shortest tau isoform (three-repeat isoform lacking N-terminal inserts), the earliest abnormality occurs in spinal neurons, resulting in axonal degeneration and motor weakness.[127,128] These tau transgenic mice are characterized at an early age by insoluble filamentous aggregates of hyperphosphorylated tau in spinal neurons that occur mostly as axonal spheroids. NFs are also associated with these aggregates, demonstrating that abnormalities in tau protein can directly affect NFs. Interestingly, tau-mediated disease can be attenuated in the absence of NFs as revealed by breeding experiments involving tau transgenic mice and NF-L knockout mice.[129] This has led to the proposal that NFs act as chaperones in the development of tau spheroids, supporting a role for NFs in the pathogenesis of some forms of tauopathies.

Interestingly, tau inhibits transport along microtubules in the plus-end direction so that transport by dynein-like motors, toward the cell body, becomes dominant.[130] In transfection experiments of cultured neuroblastoma cells and cortical neurons, it has been shown that the overexpression of tau induces the accumulation of NFs and of organelles such as mitochondria and peroxisomes in cell bodies by inhibiting their association with the axonal transport motor.[131] Consequently, this could explain the NF accumulations observed in motor neurons of transgenic mice overexpressing tau. As mentioned earlier, tau binding to microtubules is mediated by phosphorylation, with increased phosphorylation promoting dissociation of tau from microtubules. In cross-breeding studies of tau transgenic mice with mice overexpressing glycogen synthase kinase-3b, there is a rescue of tau-mediated NF accumulation and of the associated motor axonopathy.[132,133] This rescue is related to the increased phosphorylation of tau and to the recovery of normal NF transport.

Dynamitin

Mice Overexpressing Dynamitin

Dynein is a molecular motor responsible for retrograde axonal transport of organelles along microtubules.[133] Dynein activity requires association with dynactin, a multiprotein complex that activates the motor function of dynein and participates in cargo attachment.[134,135] Inhibition of dynein-mediated processes through dissociation of dynactin can be achieved by overexpressing the dynamitin p50 subunit of dynactin.[134,136] Interestingly, transgenic mice overexpressing dynamitin develop a late-onset and progressive MND resembling ALS.[137] These mice exhibit NF accumulations that are detected in axons of affected neurons rather than in cell bodies. These results support the view that axonal transport defects may play a critical role in the pathogenesis of ALS.

Vascular Endothelial Growth Factor

Mice with a Targeted Deletion of the Hypoxia-Response Element of Vascular Endothelial Growth Factor

Vascular endothelial growth factor (VEGF) is essential to the formation of new blood vessels both during development and after neuronal damage.[138] Surprisingly, mice with a targeted deletion of the hypoxia-response element of *VEGF* develop a motor neurodegeneration with many features similar to ALS, including the accumulation of NFs in motor neurons of the brain stem and spinal cord.[139] The mechanism for this motor neuron degeneration is unclear. It is possible that VEGF may act as a survival factor for motor neurons, or alternatively, because of their size, motor neurons may be more vulnerable to diminished vascular perfusion rates, accounting for their selectivity in this model.[139] The relationship between these proposed mechanisms and the accumulation of NFs is yet to be established.

CONCLUSION

Evidence indicates that cytoskeletal abnormalities may contribute through different molecular mechanisms to the pathogenesis of MND. Experiments with transgenic mice and cultured neuronal cells suggest that certain types of neurofilamentous accumulations similar to those found in ALS can provoke neurodegeneration. However, the cascade of events underlying the formation and neurotoxicity of IF accumulations are not fully understood. Transgenic studies reveal that deleterious IF structures could result from a variety of primary causes, including NF gene mutations or overexpression of genes encoding peripherin or of proteins associated with microtubule-based transport. Severe motor neuron loss occurred frequently in transgenic mouse models exhibiting an axonal localization of IF swellings (Table 12.2). This supports the "axonal strangulation" model by which axonal IF accumulations may impede the transport machinery. Yet, other molecular mechanisms may also contribute to the detrimental effects of IF accumulations, as revealed by the apoptotic death of

Table 12.2 Mice models of motor neuron disease with neurofilament accumulations

Transgene	Properties of IF accumulations	Death of motor neurons	Defective transport	References
Mutant NF-L	Perikaryal and axonal trapped organelles	Yes, massive loss	?	97
hNF-H	Perikaryal	No, but axonal atrophy and altered conductivity	Yes	94, 140
NF-L$^{-/-}$	Perikaryal accumulation of NF-M and NF-H	Developmental loss of 20%	Yes	70
Per	Age-dependent IF aggregates in perikarya and axons	Loss at ~2 years old	?	101
Per; NF-L$^{-/-}$	Age-dependent IF aggregates in perikarya and axons	Loss at ~4 months old	?	101
hNF-H; peripherin	Large IF accumulation in perikarya	No	?	Unpublished
Mutant SOD1	IF accumulations in perikaryon and axon	Yes	Yes	101, 112, 113
hNF-H SOD1^{G37R}	Large perikaryal IF accumulations	Yes, but delayed	?	116
Tau	Perikaryal IF accumulations	Yes	Yes	127, 141, 142
Dynamitin	Axonal IF swellings	Yes	Yes	137
VEGF	IF accumulation in perikaryon and axon	Yes	Yes	139

IF = intermediate filament; NF-H = neurofilament of high molecular weight; NF-L = neurofilament of low molecular weight; NF-M = neurofilament of medium molecular weight; VEGF = vascular endothelial growth factor.

neuronal cells exhibiting peripherin aggregates when cultured in a proinflammatory CNS environment.

In certain situations, the accumulation of IF structures may be relatively innocuous, simply reflecting alterations in the axonal transport machinery or other neuronal dysfunction. For instance, the perikaryal NF accumulations were well tolerated in some mouse models and they even had beneficial effects. The perikaryal accumulation of NFs induced by NF-H overexpression attenuated the toxicity of mutant SOD1, plausibly by acting as a phosphorylation sink for deregulated Cdk5 activity.[118] The NF-H overexpression also rescued the deleterious effects of excess peripherin probably via perikaryal sequestration of IF proteins (our unpublished observation).

Defects of axonal transport arise as a common pathway in many transgenic mouse models of MND. Due to the length of their axons, motor neurons are especially vulnerable to alterations that may affect the intracellular transport machinery. Indeed, direct evidence for a key role of axonal transport in the pathogenesis of MND recently came from reports of inhibition of molecular motors in transgenic mice. The overexpression of either tau to inhibit kinesin-dependent transport or dynamitin to disrupt the dynein-dependent retrograde transport caused motor neuron degeneration. In both situations, there was formation of abnormal NF accumulations, supporting the view that the motility of NFs is in part mediated by the kinesin and dynein/dynactin motors (Figure 12.8).

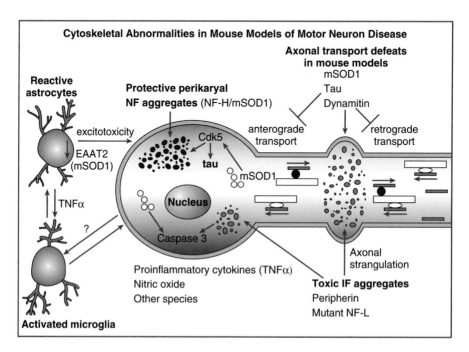

Figure 12.8 Cytoskeletal abnormalities in mouse models of motor neuron disease.

Most ALS research in the past decade has been directed toward elucidating the pathogenesis caused by SOD1 mutations. Yet, the neurodegeneration pathway triggered by mutant SOD1 is not fully understood. In light of the emerging evidence for a crucial role of axonal transport in pathogenesis, there is a need to further clarify the cytoskeletal and other molecular changes associated with the toxicity of mutant SOD1. There is also a need to identify new genes associated with ALS. A recent breakthrough was the discovery of deletion mutations in coding exons of a new gene mapping to chromosome 2q33, *ALS2,* from patients with an autosomal recessive form of juvenile ALS.[143,144] The *ALS2* gene is ubiquitously expressed and it encodes a protein having domains homologous to nucleotide exchange factors for GTPases and Db1-pleckstrin, a characteristic of Rho-type GTPases involved in various signaling cascades, membrane transport, and organization of the cytoskeleton. Hopefully, future studies with mice models of *ALS2* will provide new insights into cytoskeletal abnormalities that might cause MND.

Acknowledgments

This work was supported in part by the Canadian Institutes of Health Research (CIHR), the Neuromuscular Research Partnership (ALS Canada, MDAC and CIHR), the National Institute of Neurological Disorders and Stroke (NINDS, USA), and a grant from the Center for ALS Research at Johns Hopkins. J.-P. Julien holds a CIHR Senior Investigator Award. J.R. is funded by The Wellcome Trust, U.K., and the American ALS Association.

REFERENCES

1. Strong MJ. Progress in clinical neurosciences: the evidence for ALS as a multisystems disorder of limited phenotypic expression. Can J Neurol Sci 2001;28:283–298.
2. Cudkowicz ME, McKenna-Yasek D, Sapp PE, et al. Epidemiology of mutations in superoxide dismutase in amyotrophic lateral sclerosis. Ann Neurol 1997;41:210–221.
3. Rosen DR, Siddique T, Patterson D, et al. Mutations in Cu/Zn superoxide dismutase gene are associated with familial amyotrophic lateral sclerosis. Nature 1993;362:59–62.
4. Carpenter S. Proximal axonal enlargement in motor neuron disease. Neurology 1968;18:841–851.
5. Hirano A, Nakano I, Kurland LT, et al. Fine structural study of neurofibrillary changes in a family with amyotrophic lateral sclerosis. J Neuropathol Exp Neurol 1984;43:471–480.
6. Rouleau GA, Clark AW, Rooke K, et al. SOD1 mutation is associated with accumulation of neurofilaments in amyotrophic lateral sclerosis. Ann Neurol 1996;39:128–131.
7. Caceres A, Mautino J, Kosik KS. Suppression of MAP2 in cultured cerebellar macroneurons inhibits minor neurite formation. Neuron 1992;9:607–618.
8. Cleveland DW, Hwo SY, Kirschner MW. Purification of tau, a microtubule-associated protein that induces assembly of microtubules from purified tubulin. J Mol Biol 1977;116:207–225.
9. Goedert M, Crowther RA, Garner CC. Molecular characterization of microtubule-associated proteins tau and MAP2. Trends Neurosci 1991;14:193–199.
10. Cleveland DW, Hwo SY, Kirschner MW. Physical and chemical properties of purified tau factor and the role of tau in microtubule assembly. J Mol Biol 1977;116:227–247.
11. Bramblett GT, Goedert M, Jakes R, et al. Abnormal tau phosphorylation at Ser396 in Alzheimer's disease recapitulates development and contributes to reduced microtubule binding. Neuron 1993;10:1089–1099.

12. Goedert M, Jakes R, Crowther RA, et al. The abnormal phosphorylation of tau protein at Ser-202 in Alzheimer disease recapitulates phosphorylation during development. Proc Natl Acad Sci USA 1993;90:5066–5070.

13. Lee JH, Goedert M, Hill WD, et al. Tau proteins are abnormally expressed in olfactory epithelium of Alzheimer patients and developmentally regulated in human fetal spinal cord. Exp Neurol 1993; 121:93–105.

14. Scnapp BJ, Reese TS. Dynein is the motor for retrograde transport of organelles. Proc Natl Acad Sci USA 1989;861548–861552.

15. Martin M, Iyaduri SJ, Gassman A, et al. Cytoplasmic dynein, the dynactin complex, and kinesin are interdependent and essential for fast axonal transport. Mol Biol Cell 1999;10:3717–3728.

16. Goldstein LS. Kinesin molecular motors: transport pathways, receptors, and human disease. Proc Natl Acad Sci USA 2001;98:6999–7003.

17. Black MM, Lasek RJ. Slow components of axonal transport: two cytoskeletal networks. J Cell Biol 1980;86:616–623.

18. Shah JV, Cleveland DW. Slow axonal transport: fast motors in the slow lane. Curr Opin Cell Biol 2002;14:58–62.

19. Shea TB, Flanagan LA. Kinesin, dynein and neurofilament transport. Trends Neurosci 2001;24: 644–648.

20. Luo L. Rho GTPases in neuronal morphogenesis. Nature Reviews Neuroscience 2000;1173–1180.

21. Hall A, Nobes CD. Rho GTPases: molecular switches that control the organization and dynamics of the actin cytoskeleton. Philos Trans R Soc Lond B Biol Sci 2000;355:965–970.

22. Fuchs E, Cleveland DW. A structural scaffolding of intermediate filaments in health and disease. Science 1998;279:514–519.

23. Herrmann H, Aebi U. Intermediate filaments and their associates: multi-talented structural elements specifying cytoarchitecture and cytodynamics. Curr Opin Cell Biol 2000;12:79–90.

24. Julien JP, Mushynski WE. Neurofilaments in health and disease. Prog Nucleic Acid Res Mol Biol 1998;611–623.

25. Gotow T. Neurofilaments in health and disease. Med Electron Microsc 2000;33(4):173–199.

26. Pachter JS, Liem RK. Alpha-internexin, a 66-kD intermediate filament—binding protein from mammalian central nervous tissues. J Cell Biol 1985;101:1316–1322.

27. Chien CL, Liem RK. Characterization of the mouse gene encoding the neuronal intermediate filament protein alpha-internexin. Gene 1994;149:289–292.

28. Parysek LM, Goldman RD. Distribution of a novel 57 kDa intermediate filament (IF) protein in the nervous system. J Neurosci 1988;8:555–563.

29. Portier MM, de Nechaud B, Gros F. Peripherin, a new member of the intermediate filament protein family. Dev Neurosci 1983;6:335–344.

30. Escurat M, Djabali K, Gumpel M, et al. Differential expression of two neuronal intermediate-filament proteins, peripherin and the low-molecular-mass neurofilament protein (NF-L), during the development of the rat. J Neurosci 1990;10:764–784.

31. Lee MK, Xu Z, Wong PC, Cleveland DW. Neurofilaments are obligate heteropolymers in vivo. J Cell Biol 1993;122:1337–1350.

32. Ching GY, Liem RK. Assembly of type IV neuronal intermediate filaments in nonneuronal cells in the absence of preexisting cytoplasmic intermediate filaments. J Cell Biol 1993;122:1323–1335.

33. Gotow T, Takeda M, Tanaka T, Hashimoto PH. Macromolecular structure of reassembled neuro-filaments as revealed by the quick-freeze deep-etch mica method: difference between NF-M and NF-H subunits in their ability to form cross-bridges. Eur J Cell Biol 1992;58:331–345.

34. Hisanaga S, Hirokawa N. Structure of the peripheral domains of neurofilaments revealed by low angle rotary shadowing. J Mol Biol 1988;202:297–305.

35. Guidato S, Tsai LH, Woodgett J, Miller CC. Differential cellular phosphorylation of neurofilament heavy side-arms by glycogen synthase kinase-3 and cyclin-dependent kinase-5. J Neurochem 1996; 66:1698–1706.

36. Grant P, Sharma P, Pant HC. Cyclin-dependent protein kinase 5 (Cdk5) and the regulation of neu-rofilament metabolism. Eur J Biochem 2001;268:1534–1546.

37. Guan RJ, Khatra BS, Cohlberg JA. Phosphorylation of bovine neurofilament proteins by protein kinase FA (glycogen synthase kinase 3). J Biol Chem 1991;266:8262–8267.

38. Bajaj NP, Miller CC. Phosphorylation of neurofilament heavy-chain side-arm fragments by cyclin-dependent kinase-5 and glycogen synthase kinase-3alpha in transfected cells. J Neurochem 1997; 69:737–743.

39. Fu Z, Green CL, Bennett GS. Relationship between casein kinase I isoforms and a neurofilament-associated kinase. J Neurochem 1999;73:830–838.

40. Nakamura Y, Hashimoto R, Kashiwagi Y, et al. Casein kinase II is responsible for phosphorylation of NF-L at Ser-473. FEBS Lett 1999;455:83–86.
41. Link WT, Dosemeci A, Floyd CC, Pant HC. Bovine neurofilament-enriched preparations contain kinase activity similar to casein kinase I—neurofilament phosphorylation by casein kinase I (CKI). Neurosci Lett 1993;151:89–93.
42. Veeranna, Amin ND, Ahn NG, et al. Mitogen-activated protein kinases (Erk1,2) phosphorylate Lys-Ser-Pro (KSP) repeats in neurofilament proteins NF-H and NF-M. J Neurosci 1998;18:4008–4021.
43. Giasson BI, Mushynski WE. Study of proline-directed protein kinases involved in phosphorylation of the heavy neurofilament subunit. J Neurosci 1997;17:9466–9472.
44. Brownlees J, Yates A, Bajaj NP, et al. Phosphorylation of neurofilament heavy chain side-arms by stress activated protein kinase-1b/Jun N-terminal kinase-3. J Cell Sci 2000;113(pt 3):401–407.
45. O'Ferrall EK, Robertson J, Mushynski WE. Inhibition of aberrant and constitutive phosphorylation of the high-molecular-mass neurofilament subunit by CEP-1347(KT7515), an inhibitor of the stress-activated protein kinase signaling pathway. J Neurochem 2000;75:2358–2367.
46. Thompson MA, Ziff EB. Structure of the gene encoding peripherin, an NGF-regulated neuronal-specific type III intermediate filament protein. Neuron 1989;2:1043–1053.
47. Karpov V, Landon F, Djabali K, et al. Structure of the mouse gene encoding peripherin: a neuronal intermediate filament protein. Biol Cell 1992;76:43–48.
48. Moncla A, Landon F, Mattei MG, Portier MM. Chromosomal localization of the mouse and human peripherin genes. Genet Res 1992;59:125–129.
49. Foley J, Ley CA, Parysek LM. The structure of the human peripherin gene (PRPH) and identification of potential regulatory elements. Genomics 1994;22:456–461.
50. Ho CL, Chin SS, Carnevale K, Liem RK. Translation initiation and assembly of peripherin in cultured cells. Eur J Cell Biol 1995;68:103–112.
51. Landon F, Lemonnier M, Benarous R, et al. Multiple mRNAs encode peripherin, a neuronal intermediate filament protein. EMBO J 1989;8:1719–1726.
52. Landon F, Wolff A, de Nechaud B. Mouse peripherin isoforms. Biol Cell 2000;92:397–407.
53. Huc C, Escurat M, Djabali K, et al. Phosphorylation of peripherin, an intermediate filament protein, in mouse neuroblastoma NIE 115 cell line and in sympathetic neurons. Biochem Biophys Res Commun 1989;160:772–779.
54. Angelastro JM, Ho CL, Frappier T, et al. Peripherin is tyrosine-phosphorylated at its carboxyl-terminal tyrosine. J Neurochem 1998;70:540–549.
55. Giasson BI, Mushynski WE. Intermediate filament disassembly in cultured dorsal root ganglion neurons is associated with amino-terminal head domain phosphorylation of specific subunits. J Neurochem 1998;70:1869–1875.
56. Troy CM, Muma NA, Greene LA, et al. Regulation of peripherin and neurofilament expression in regenerating rat motor neurons. Brain Res 1990;529:232–238.
57. Wong J, Oblinger MM. Differential regulation of peripherin and neurofilament gene expression in regenerating rat DRG neurons. J Neurosci Res 1990;27:332–341.
58. Beaulieu JM, Kriz J, Julien JP. Induction of peripherin expression in subsets of brain neurons after lesion injury or cerebral ischemia. Brain Res 2002;946:153–161.
59. Djabali K, Zissopoulou A, de Hoop MJ, et al. Peripherin expression in hippocampal neurons induced by muscle soluble factor(s). J Cell Biol 1993;123:1197–1206.
60. Lecomte MJ, Basseville M, Landon F, et al. Transcriptional activation of the mouse peripherin gene by leukemia inhibitory factor: involvement of STAT proteins. J Neurochem 1998;70:971–982.
61. Sterneck E, Kaplan DR, Johnson PF. Interleukin-6 induces expression of peripherin and cooperates with Trk receptor signaling to promote neuronal differentiation in PC12 cells. J Neurochem 1996;67:1365–1374.
62. Cui C, Stambrook PJ, Parysek LM. Peripherin assembles into homopolymers in SW13 cells. J Cell Sci 1995;108(pt 10):3279–3284.
63. Beaulieu JM, Robertson J, Julien JP. Interactions between peripherin and neurofilaments in cultured cells: disruption of peripherin assembly by the NF-M and NF-H subunits. Biochem Cell Biol 1999;77:41–45.
64. Parysek LM, McReynolds MA, Goldman RD, Ley CA. Some neural intermediate filaments contain both peripherin and the neurofilament proteins. J Neurosci Res 1991;30:80–91.
65. Athlan ES, Sacher MG, Mushynski WE. Associations between intermediate filament proteins expressed in cultured dorsal root ganglion neurons. J Neurosci Res 1997;47:300–310.
66. Corbo M, Hays AP. Peripherin and neurofilament protein coexist in spinal spheroids of motor neuron disease. J Neuropathol Exp Neurol 1992;51:531–537.

67. Migheli A, Pezzulo T, Attanasio A, Schiffer D. Peripherin immunoreactive structures in amyotrophic lateral sclerosis. Lab Invest 1993;68:185–191.
68. Bergeron C, Beric-Maskarel K, Muntasser S, et al. Neurofilament light and polyadenylated mRNA levels are decreased in amyotrophic lateral sclerosis motor neurons. J Neuropathol Exp Neurol 1994;53:221–230.
69. Wong NK, He BP, Strong MJ. Characterization of neuronal intermediate filament protein expression in cervical spinal motor neurons in sporadic amyotrophic lateral sclerosis (ALS). J Neuropathol Exp Neurol 2000;59:972–982.
70. Zhu Q, Couillard-Despres S, Julien JP. Delayed maturation of regenerating myelinated axons in mice lacking neurofilaments. Exp Neurol 1997;148:299–316.
71. Ackerley S, Grierson AJ, Brownlees J, et al. Glutamate slows axonal transport of neurofilaments in transfected neurons. J Cell Biol 2000;150:165–176.
72. Chou SM, Wang HS, Taniguchi A, Bucala R. Advanced glycation endproducts in neurofilament conglomeration of motoneurons in familial and sporadic amyotrophic lateral sclerosis. Mol Med 1998;4:324–332.
73. Crow JP, Ye YZ, Strong M, et al. Superoxide dismutase catalyzes nitration of tyrosines by peroxynitrite in the rod and head domains of neurofilament-L. J Neurochem 1997;69:1945–1953.
74. Strong MJ, Sopper MM, Crow JP, et al. Nitration of the low molecular weight neurofilament is equivalent in sporadic amyotrophic lateral sclerosis and control cervical spinal cord. Biochem Biophys Res Commun 1998;248:157–164.
75. Figlewicz DA, Krizus A, Martinoli MG, et al. Variants of the heavy neurofilament subunit are associated with the development of amyotrophic lateral sclerosis. Hum Mol Genet 1994;3:1757–1761.
76. Tomkins J, Usher P, Slade JY, et al. Novel insertion in the KSP region of the neurofilament heavy gene in amyotrophic lateral sclerosis (ALS). Neuroreport 1998;9:3967–3970.
77. Al-Chalabi A, Andersen PM, Nilsson P, et al. Deletions of the heavy neurofilament subunit tail in amyotrophic lateral sclerosis. Hum Mol Genet 1999;8:157–164.
78. Rooke K, Figlewicz DA, Han FY, Rouleau GA. Analysis of the KSP repeat of the neurofilament heavy subunit in familiar amyotrophic lateral sclerosis. Neurology 1996;46:789–790.
79. Vechio JD, Bruijn LI, Xu Z, et al. Sequence variants in human neurofilament proteins: absence of linkage to familial amyotrophic lateral sclerosis. Ann Neurol 1996;40:603–610.
80. Mersiyanova IV, Perepelov AV, Polyakov AV, et al. A new variant of Charcot-Marie-Tooth disease type 2 is probably the result of a mutation in the neurofilament-light gene. Am J Hum Genet 2000; 67:37–46.
81. Lavedan C, Buchholtz S, Nussbaum RL, et al. A mutation in the human neurofilament M gene in Parkinson's disease that suggests a role for the cytoskeleton in neuronal degeneration. Neurosci Lett 2002;322:57–61.
82. De Jonghe P, Mersiyanova IV, Nelis E, et al. Further evidence that neurofilament light chain mutations can cause Charcot-Marie-Tooth disease type 2E. Ann Neurol 2001;49:245–249.
83. Zhu Q, Lindenbaum M, Levavasseur F, et al. Disruption of the NF-H gene increases axonal microtubule content and velocity of neurofilament transport: relief of axonopathy resulting from the toxin beta,beta'-iminodipropionitrile. J Cell Biol 1998;143:183–193.
84. Elder GA, Friedrich VL Jr, Margita A, Lazzarini RA. Age-related atrophy of motor axons in mice deficient in the mid-sized neurofilament subunit. J Cell Biol 1999;146:181–192.
85. Jacomy H, Zhu Q, Couillard-Despres S, et al. Disruption of type IV intermediate filament network in mice lacking the neurofilament medium and heavy subunits. J Neurochem 1999;73:972–984.
86. Rao MV, Houseweart MK, Williamson TL, et al. Neurofilament-dependent radial growth of motor axons and axonal organization of neurofilaments does not require the neurofilament heavy subunit (NF-H) or its phosphorylation. J Cell Biol 1998;143:171–181.
87. Elder GA, Friedrich VL Jr, Kang C, et al. Requirement of heavy neurofilament subunit in the development of axons with large calibers. J Cell Biol 1998;143:195–205.
88. Levavasseur F, Zhu Q, Julien JP. No requirement of alpha-internexin for nervous system development and for radial growth of axons. Brain Res Mol Brain Res 1999;69:104–112.
89. Elder GA, Friedrich VL Jr, Bosco P, et al. Absence of the mid-sized neurofilament subunit decreases axonal calibers, levels of light neurofilament (NF-L), and neurofilament content. J Cell Biol 1998; 141:727–739.
90. Kriz J, Zhu Q, Julien JP, Padjen AL. Electrophysiological properties of axons in mice lacking neurofilament subunit genes: disparity between conduction velocity and axon diameter in absence of NF-H. Brain Res 2000;885:32–44.

91. Xu Z, Cork LC, Griffin JW, Cleveland DW. Increased expression of neurofilament subunit NF-L produces morphological alterations that resemble the pathology of human motor neuron disease. Cell 1993;73:23–33.
92. Cote F, Collard JF, Houle D, Julien JP. Copy-dependent and correct developmental expression of the human neurofilament heavy gene in transgenic mice. Brain Res Mol Brain Res 1994;26:99–105.
93. Wong PC, Marszalek J, Crawford TO, et al. Increasing neurofilament subunit NF-M expression reduces axonal NF-H, inhibits radial growth, and results in neurofilamentous accumulation in motor neurons. J Cell Biol 1995;130:1413–1422.
94. Kriz J, Meier J, Julien JP, Padjen AL. Altered ionic conductances in axons of transgenic mouse expressing the human neurofilament heavy gene: a mouse model of amyotrophic lateral sclerosis. Exp Neurol 2000;163:414–421.
95. Beaulieu JM, Jacomy H, Julien JP. Formation of intermediate filament protein aggregates with disparate effects in two transgenic mouse models lacking the neurofilament light subunit. J Neurosci 2000;20:5321–5328.
96. Meier J, Couillard-Despres S, Jacomy H, et al. Extra neurofilament NF-L subunits rescue motor neuron disease caused by overexpression of the human NF-H gene in mice. J Neuropathol Exp Neurol 1999;58:1099–1110.
97. Lee MK, Marszalek JR, Cleveland DW. A mutant neurofilament subunit causes massive, selective motor neuron death: implications for the pathogenesis of human motor neuron disease. Neuron 1994;13:975–988.
98. Houseweart MK, Cleveland DW. Bcl-2 overexpression does not protect neurons from mutant neurofilament-mediated motor neuron degeneration. J Neurosci 1999;19(15):6446–6456.
99. Cleveland DW. From Charcot to SOD1: mechanisms of selective motor neuron death in ALS. Neuron 1999;24:515–520.
100. Julien JP. Amyotrophic lateral sclerosis. unfolding the toxicity of the misfolded. Cell 2001;104:581–591.
101. Beaulieu JM, Nguyen MD, Julien JP. Late onset death of motor neurons in mice overexpressing wild-type peripherin. J Cell Biol 1999;147:531–544.
102. Robertson J, Beaulieu JM, Doroudchi MM, et al. Apoptotic death of neurons exhibiting peripherin aggregates is mediated by the proinflammatory cytokine tumor necrosis factor-alpha. J Cell Biol 2001;155:217–226.
103. Lee VM, Goedert M, Trojanowski JQ. Neurodegenerative tauopathies. Annu Rev Neurosci 2001;241121–241159.
104. Subramaniam JR, Lyons WE, Liu J, et al. Mutant SOD1 causes motor neuron disease independent of copper chaperone—mediated copper loading. Nat Neurosci 2002;5:301–307.
105. Wong PC, Waggoner D, Subramaniam JR, et al. Copper chaperone for superoxide dismutase is essential to activate mammalian Cu/Zn superoxide dismutase. Proc Natl Acad Sci USA 2000;97:2886–2891.
106. Beckman JS, Crow JP. Pathological implications of nitric oxide, superoxide and peroxynitrite formation. Biochem Soc Trans 1993;21:330–334.
107. Wiedau-Pazos M, Goto JJ, Rabizadeh S, et al. Altered reactivity of superoxide dismutase in familial amyotrophic lateral sclerosis. Science 1996;271:515–518.
108. Bruijn LI, Houseweart MK, Kato S, et al. Aggregation and motor neuron toxicity of an ALS-linked SOD1 mutant independent from wild-type SOD1. Science 1998;281:1851–1854.
109. Durham HD, Roy J, Dong L, Figlewicz DA. Aggregation of mutant Cu/Zn superoxide dismutase proteins in a culture model of ALS. J Neuropathol Exp Neurol 1997;56:523–530.
110. Zhang B, Tu P, Abtahian F, et al. Neurofilaments and orthograde transport are reduced in ventral root axons of transgenic mice that express human SOD1 with a G93A mutation. J Cell Biol 1997;139:1307–1315.
111. Williamson TL, Cleveland DW. Slowing of axonal transport is a very early event in the toxicity of ALS-linked SOD1 mutants to motor neurons. Nat Neurosci 1999;2:50–56.
112. Gurney ME, Pu H, Chiu AY, et al. Motor neuron degeneration in mice that express a human Cu,Zn superoxide dismutase mutation. Science 1994;264:1772–1775.
113. Tu PH, Raju P, Robinson KA, et al. Transgenic mice carrying a human mutant superoxide dismutase transgene develop neuronal cytoskeletal pathology resembling human amyotrophic lateral sclerosis lesions. Proc Natl Acad Sci USA 1996;93:3155–3160.
114. Williamson TL, Bruijn LI, Zhu Q, et al. Absence of neurofilaments reduces the selective vulnerability of motor neurons and slows disease caused by a familial amyotrophic lateral sclerosis—linked superoxide dismutase 1 mutant. Proc Natl Acad Sci USA 1998;95:9631–9636.

115. Nguyen MD, Lariviere RC, Julien JP. Reduction of axonal caliber does not alleviate motor neuron disease caused by mutant superoxide dismutase 1. Proc Natl Acad Sci USA 2000;97: 12306–12311.

116. Couillard-Despres S, Zhu Q, Wong PC, et al. Protective effect of neurofilament heavy gene overexpression in motor neuron disease induced by mutant superoxide dismutase. Proc Natl Acad Sci USA 1998;95:9626–9630.

117. Kong J, Xu Z. Overexpression of neurofilament subunit NF-L and NF-H extends survival of a mouse model for amyotrophic lateral sclerosis. Neurosci Lett 2000;281:72–74.

118. Nguyen MD, Lariviere RC, Julien JP. Deregulation of Cdk5 in a mouse model of ALS: toxicity alleviated by perikaryal neurofilament inclusions. Neuron 2001;30:135–147.

119. Bajaj NP, Al-Sarraj ST, Anderson V, et al. Cyclin-dependent kinase-5 is associated with lipofuscin in motor neurones in amyotrophic lateral sclerosis. Neurosci Lett 1998;245:45–48.

120. Yamaguchi H, Ishiguro K, Uchida T, et al. Preferential labeling of Alzheimer neurofibrillary tangles with antisera for tau protein kinase (TPK) I/glycogen synthase kinase-3 beta and cyclin-dependent kinase 5, a component of TPK II. Acta Neuropathol (Berl) 1996;92:232–241.

121. Pei JJ, Grundke-Iqbal I, Iqbal K, et al. Accumulation of cyclin-dependent kinase 5 (cdk5) in neurons with early stages of Alzheimer's disease neurofibrillary degeneration. Brain Res 1998; 797:267–277.

122. Brion JP, Couck AM. Cortical and brainstem-type Lewy bodies are immunoreactive for the cyclin-dependent kinase 5. Am J Pathol 1995;147:1465–1476.

123. Green SL, Vulliet PR, Pinter MJ, Cork LC. Alterations in cyclin-dependent protein kinase 5 (CDK5) protein levels, activity and immunocytochemistry in canine motor neuron disease. J Neuropathol Exp Neurol 1998;57:1070–1077.

124. Patrick GN, Zukerberg L, Nikolic M, et al. Conversion of p35 to p25 deregulates Cdk5 activity and promotes neurodegeneration. Nature 1999;402:615–622.

125. Lee MS, Kwon YT, Li M, et al. Neurotoxicity induces cleavage of p35 to p25 by calpain. Nature 2000;405:360–364.

126. Ahlijanian MK, Barrezueta NX, Williams RD, et al. Hyperphosphorylated tau and neurofilament and cytoskeletal disruptions in mice overexpressing human p25, an activator of cdk5. Proc Natl Acad Sci USA 2000;97:2910–2915.

127. Ishihara T, Hong M, Zhang B, et al. Age-dependent emergence and progression of a tauopathy in transgenic mice overexpressing the shortest human tau isoform. Neuron 1999;24:751–762.

128. Ishihara T, Zhang B, Higuchi M, et al. Age-dependent induction of congophilic neurofibrillary tau inclusions in tau transgenic mice. Am J Pathol 2001;158:555–562.

129. Ishihara T, Higuchi M, Zhang B, et al. Attenuated neurodegenerative disease phenotype in tau transgenic mouse lacking neurofilaments. J Neurosci 2001;21:6026–6035.

130. Ebneth A, Godemann R, Stamer K, et al. Overexpression of tau protein inhibits kinesin-dependent trafficking of vesicles, mitochondria, and endoplasmic reticulum: implications for Alzheimer's disease. J Cell Biol 1998;143:777–794.

131. Stamer K, Vogel R, Thies E, et al. Tau blocks traffic of organelles, neurofilaments, and APP vesicles in neurons and enhances oxidative stress. J Cell Biol 2002;156:1051–1063.

132. Nuydens R, Van Den Kieboom G, Nolten C, et al. Coexpression of GSK-3beta corrects phenotypic aberrations of dorsal root ganglion cells, cultured from adult transgenic mice overexpressing human protein tau. Neurobiol Dis 2002;9:38–48.

133. Paschal BM, Vallee RB. Retrograde transport by the microtubule-associated protein MAP 1C. Nature 1987;330:181–183.

134. Echeverri CJ, Paschal BM, Vaughan KT, Vallee RB. Molecular characterization of the 50-kD subunit of dynactin reveals function for the complex in chromosome alignment and spindle organization during mitosis. J Cell Biol 1996;132:617–633.

135. King SJ, Schroer TA. Dynactin increases the processivity of the cytoplasmic dynein motor. Nat Cell Biol 2000;2:20–24.

136. Eckley DM, Gill SR, Melkonian KA, et al. Analysis of dynactin subcomplexes reveals a novel actin-related protein associated with the arp1 minifilament pointed end. J Cell Biol 1999;147: 307–320.

137. LaMonte BH, Wallace KE, Holloway BA, et al. Disruption of dynein/dynactin inhibits axonal transport in motor neurons causing late-onset progressive degeneration. Neuron 2002;34:715–727.

138. Carmeliet P. Mechanisms of angiogenesis and arteriogenesis. Nat Med 2000;6:389–395.

139. Oosthuyse B, Moons L, Storkebaum E, et al. Deletion of the hypoxia-response element in the vascular endothelial growth factor promoter causes motor neuron degeneration. Nat Genet 2001; 28:131–138.

140. Cote F, Collard JF, Julien JP. Progressive neuronopathy in transgenic mice expressing the human neurofilament heavy gene: a mouse model of amyotrophic lateral sclerosis. Cell 1993;73:35–46.

141. Spittaels K, Van den Haute C, Van Dorpe J, et al. Prominent axonopathy in the brain and spinal cord of transgenic mice overexpressing four-repeat human tau protein. Am J Pathol 1999;155: 2153–2165.

142. Probst A, Gotz J, Wiederhold KH, et al. Axonopathy and amyotrophy in mice transgenic for human four-repeat tau protein. Acta Neuropathol (Berl) 2000;99:469–481.

143. Hadano S, Hand CK, Osuga H, et al. A gene encoding a putative GTPase regulator is mutated in familial amyotrophic lateral sclerosis 2. Nat Genet 2001;29:166–173.

144. Yang Y, Hentati A, Deng HX, et al. The gene encoding alsin, a protein with three guanine-nucleotide exchange factor domains, is mutated in a form of recessive amyotrophic lateral sclerosis. Nat Genet 2001;29:160–165.

13
Role of Microglia in Amyotrophic Lateral Sclerosis

Michael J. Strong and Weiyan Wen

Although it is increasingly evident that there exists a significant interaction between motor neurons, microglia, and astrocytes in the degenerative process of amyotrophic lateral sclerosis (ALS), only recently have we begun to understand the complexity of this relationship.[1] When we are specifically considering the interactions between injured motor neurons and microglia, the assignment of a specific role to microglia becomes increasingly complex because the net effect of microglial activation may be either harmful or beneficial to the motor neuron. To compound this, there are few detailed studies of the neuroimmune response to motor neuron injury in ALS and thus conclusions regarding this relationship require some degree of extrapolation from nonhuman experimental paradigms.

Microglia are, for the most part, the central nervous system (CNS) equivalent of the macrophage. When inactive ("resting state"), microglia possess finely branched processes that extend in multiple directions. In response various pathological insults, microglia enter a "responsive state," in which multiple intracellular and surface antigens are upregulated, processes retract and hypertrophy with hyper-ramification, and the cell becomes ready to respond to a stimulus.[2,3] With further activation, microglia enter an "effector state" by becoming active secretory cells flooding the neuronal milieu with various factors—both trophic and neurotoxic. In this chapter, we review the evidence that microglia can be induced into an "effector state" in response to motor neuron injury, that this response can modulate the extent of axonal repair or regeneration, and that the process of microglial activation participates directly in the pathogenesis of neurodegeneration of ALS.

EXPERIMENTAL PARADIGMS OF MICROGLIAL ACTIVATION

Response to a Peripheral Lesion (Axotomy)

Under most circumstances, axotomized neurons do not regenerate. However, this failure to regenerate is not an absolute, but it is an age-dependent phenomenon. In the neonate, peripheral nerve injury results in extensive motor neuron losses, whereas in the adult, less extensive injury is evident. In the latter, a critical determinant of whether the neuron dies or regenerates is the proximity of the axotomy to the neuronal perikaryon, with proximal lesions giving rise to greater neuronal loss in contrast to a distal axotomy or crush injury.[4] Within 24 hours of such an injury in the adult animal, there is a prominent proliferation and migration of microglia to the perineuronal region, implying that the injured neuron possesses the inherent capacity to induce a microglial response after injury.[5,6]

Although the exact signal by which motor neurons summon this microglial response is not known, there are several candidate proteins. Granulocyte-macrophage colony-stimulating factor (GM-CSF) receptors are upregulated on microglial cells adjacent to axotomized facial motor neurons.[7] GM-CSF promotes the proliferation and differentiation of both monocytes[8] and microglia.[9] In mice lacking this factor, only a limited microglial response to peripheral nerve injury occurs.[10] Following facial axotomy, a similar loss of the early stages of microglial activation is observed in the osteopetrosis mice in which macrophage colony-stimulating factor (M-CSF) is absent.[11] In this latter model, there is a failure of microglial migration across the surface of the axotomized motor neuron (a process termed *synaptic stripping*) and a failure of microglial proliferation. Interleukin-6 (IL-6) also appears to play a role in that IL-6 knockout mice fail to demonstrate the early microglial response to motor neuron injury and show a reduced astrocytic response, in keeping with a dual role of IL-6 in both mediating motor neuron/microglial and microglial/astrocytic interactions.[12] Recently, a novel cytokine (fractalkine) has been identified as a chemoattractant in signaling the microglial response by injured motor neurons (discussed later).[13]

Having entered into an "effector state," the net result of microglial activation in the region of the injured motor neuron can vary from beneficial and promoting the survival of neurons to being overtly neurotoxic. The detrimental effect is illustrated by manipulating the microglial response to an optic nerve transection. In this, the intravitreal inoculation of a macrophage-inhibitory peptide following an optic nerve transection results in an enhanced rate of axon survival and a greater degree of axonal regeneration, whereas a macrophage-stimulating factor enhances the rate of ganglion cell degeneration.[14,15] Inhibiting microglial activation will also attenuate the extent of neuronal degeneration induced by either ischemia[16] or the excitatory neurotoxin ibotenic acid.[17]

In seeming contrast to this apparent effect of microglial activation on inhibiting the extent of neuronal degeneration, inhibiting the induction of microglial proliferation through the intraventricular administration of cytosine arabinoside (araC) did not affect the rate of target reinnervation or the loss of presynaptic terminals in the axotomized hypoglossal nucleus.[18] Moreover, the induction of an inflammatory response along a transected optic nerve resulted in an enhanced rate of neuritic growth[19] and microglial transplants will facilitate dorsal root sensory axon regeneration.[20]

Thus, although the direct axonal injury models illustrate several key aspects regarding the interactions between injured motor neurons and microglia, these experiments have also raised a number of questions. Clearly, it is not a simple phenomenon of activating microglia and then observing a single response with regards to the extent of cell death or regeneration. One potential mechanism by which such varying results can be explained relates to whether the neuronal perikarya or the axonal process is directly involved in the glial response or whether it is the degenerating tracts that are the primary target. In addition, the perineuronal microglial response to a peripheral axotomy appears to be enhanced in motor neurons harboring a preexisting pathology. For instance, in response to a facial nerve axotomy, copper/zinc superoxide dismutase (SOD1) G93A (SOD1^{G93A}) transgenic mice exhibit a considerably more robust microglial proliferative response than observed in control mice, suggesting a potential for "priming" this response.[21] As will become apparent, this is a concern in ALS in which microglial responses to both tract degeneration and direct neuronal injury are present.

RESPONSE OF MOTOR NEURONS TO CENTRAL INJURY (UPPER MOTOR NEURON LESION)

In ALS, there is not only a direct insult to the lower motor neuron through the primary degenerative process but an indirect insult mediated through the degeneration of the descending supraspinal tracts (upper motor neurons [UMNs]), including the corticospinal tracts. In the latter, trans-synaptic degeneration may also induce a neuronal injury and thus might be expected to induce a microglial response. This latter process has been well illustrated in a number of experimental paradigms, including the observation of a microglial proliferative response within the lumbosacral ventral horn in response to a contralateral middle cerebral artery occlusion.[22–24] In this paradigm, a moderate increase in the number of activated microglia in the contralateral lumbar ventral horn is observed within 48 hours. By 5 days later, microglial activation is prominent, motor neurons appear to be degenerating, and many motor neurons are engulfed by reactive microglia. By day 7, an astrocytic response begins to replace the microglial response. The entire process can be inhibited using an inhibitor of microglial phosphodiesterase activity (1-[5′-oxohexyl]-3-methyl-7-propylxanthine; propentofylline).[22]

The microglial response within the ventral horn of the lumbosacral cord caudal to an experimental spinal cord injury has also been characterized, although the extent of this response remains controversial. In the immediate region of the lesion, resting microglia are rapidly transformed into macrophage-like cells.[25] Ultimately, astrocytic proliferation results in the formation of a fibrotic cap. For several weeks following the lesioning, microglial proliferation in the caudal spinal cord continues. Within 3 days of a mid-thoracic hemisection of rat spinal cord, lumbar motor neuron synaptophysin immunostaining (a marker of synaptic terminals) is significantly reduced.[26] Concomitant with this, microglial phagocytosis of degenerating axon terminals is evident. However, from 42 to 90 days, few motor neurons degenerate and most of those that remain possess intact synaptophysin immunostaining patterns. Although Eidelberg et al[27] in 1989 described significant motor neuron loss at the L4-5 level within 24 hours of a complete thoracic cord transection, there are no other reports of such a dramatic early loss. This may reflect the variability among differing strains of rats or the method used in measuring the number of motor neurons lost. Similarly, although Koshinaga and Whittemore[28] in 1995 observed that the duration of microglial proliferation in the corticospinal tracts caudal to a mid-thoracic ischemic lesion was limited to within 12 days following the injury, they did not comment on the ventral horn pathology.

These morphological changes are associated with the induction of a neurochemical response. Concomitant with the induction of the lumbar microglia activation following a posterior spinal cord (T9) transection, a defined pattern of cytokine release is evident.[29] By 1 hour, tumor necrosis factor-α (TNF-α) messenger RNA (mRNA) levels are increased at the injury epicenter. Peak levels are evident by 6 hours, with little remaining by 24 hours. A "wave" of increased TNF-α mRNA expression spreads caudal to the epicenter of the lesion. IL-1β mRNA elevation follows a similar time course to that of TNF-α, although there is no clear evidence of caudal spread. IL-1α mRNA levels follow a similar topographical distribution, with peak mRNA levels evident by 12 hours at a time that coincides with the onset of monocyte migration. Little IL-1α and IL-1β mRNA elevation is still evident at 48 hours, with none at 72 hours. IL-6 mRNA levels are low or absent at the site of the lesion, with no detectable rostral caudal gradient.

Thus the act of acutely interrupting the UMN pathways appears to result in a response of the lumbar spinal motor neurons, presumably mediated through the trans-synaptic degeneration of the spinal motor neuron, which in turn recruits a perineuronal microglial response. Although the spinal cord transection model is perhaps a dramatic means in comparison to a chronic neurodegenerative state such as that which occurs in ALS, the principal that the perineuronal microglia response in ALS is mediated by both direct injury to the motor neuron and an indirect injury through trans-synaptic degeneration seems reasonable.

RESPONSE TO AN INTRINSIC DISTURBANCE OF MOTOR NEURON FUNCTION

The issue of whether the chronic degeneration of motor neurons is accompanied by a microglial response has been addressed through a number of transgenic models. The motor neuron dysfunction first observed by week 3 in the wobbler mouse *(wr/wr)* is preceded by significant perineuronal microglial activation with ensheathment of otherwise healthy appearing motor neurons by microglia.[30] Both brain and spinal cord demonstrate elevated TNF-α levels coincident with the onset of motor neuron dysfunction in the motor neuron disease (*mnd*) mouse in which the intraneuronal accumulation of a lipofuscin-like material results in a late-onset MND.[31] The development of motor neuron dysfunction in the SOD1[G93A] transgenic model of familial ALS (FALS) is preceded by an early alteration in the expression and upregulation of proinflammatory factors in the presymptomatic phase, with a prominent and sustained microglial response throughout the active phase of the disease progression.[32–35] Both transforming growth factor β1 (TGF-β1) and M-CSF expression are upregulated in presymptomatic mice, with TNF-α expression being increased by month 4, well in advance of the appearance of motor deficits.[33] By month 6, a significant increase in microglia numbers is observed. This process is associated with an increased level of cyclooxygenase-2 (COX-2) mRNA and protein, and an increase in prostaglandin E_2 (PGE_2) content only within the regions associated with motor neuron pathology, further confirming a role for microglial activation.[36] The latter observation is consistent with prior in vitro findings that the motor neuron death induced by chronic glutamate excitotoxicity in organotypic spinal cord cultures can be inhibited by COX-2 inhibition.[37]

Support for the role of microglia in motor neuron degeneration is also gained from the observation that the administration of minocycline, a tetracycline derivative, prolongs the symptom-free interval before the onset of motor dysfunction in the SOD1[G93A] transgenic mice.[38,39] The site of action of microglia appears to be both at the level of the microglia in which the upregulation of inducible nitric oxide synthase (iNOS) is inhibited and at the target cell where the release of mitochondrial cytochrome *c* (and thus the initiation of a proapoptotic pathway) is inhibited.[40–42]

Microglia have also been suggested to be the primary determinants of neuronal recovery following the experimental induction of chronic motor neuron degeneration. In this model, the monthly administration of aluminum chloride to young adult New Zealand white rabbits will induce a chronic motor neuron degeneration that is reversible upon cessation of the aluminum inoculum.[43,44] This reversibility/recovery appeared to relate to the absence of a microglial proliferative response based on morphological criteria.[45] In vitro, both organic and inorganic aluminum compounds inhibit microglial activation in the absence of microglial death and inhibit microglial-mediated motor neuron death.[46] This suggests that the inhibition of microglial activation by aluminum chloride in vivo allows for a neuronal milieu permissive to motor neuron recovery by inhibiting microglial activation. To confirm this, we used an immortalized murine motor neuron hybridoma (neuroblastoma-spinal cord 34 [NSC34])[47] to demonstrate that activated microglial cells can kill motor neurons by a mechanism that is dependent on the microglial release of factor(s) that act synergistically with TNF-α.[48] This process can be fully inhibited by inhibiting microglial activation. Using the same cell line, Pedersen, Cashman, and Mattson[49] observed that NSC34 cell death could be triggered by oxidative injury mediated through 4-hydroxynonenal (HNE) formation and the triggering of apoptosis, suggesting that another potential pathway of microglial-mediated motor neuron injury could be through the release of reactive oxygen species.

MECHANISMS OF MICROGLIA–NEURON INTERACTIONS

As alluded to in the previous discussion, the net effect of microglial activation can be either neuroprotective or neurotoxic. In part, this response is dependent on the nature of the signal triggering the microglial response. There are thus two pathways of interest in understanding the nature of the microglial response in ALS: first, that which relates to the nature of the signaling from motor neurons to microglia, and second, that which relates to the subsequent effect of microglia on motor neuron function.

Nature of the Neuronal Signal to Microglia

The exact nature of the signaling between motor neurons and microglia is not yet fully understood. However, a recently described cytokine (fractalkine) may function in this role. This chemokine can exist in either a soluble or a membrane-bound form and is expressed predominantly by neurons, although both microglial and astrocytic expression has been shown.[13,50,51] The receptor for fractalkine, CX3CR1, is expressed on both microglia and neurons.[52] It appears that the interaction between fractalkine and its receptor serves a neuroprotective function in that, through activation of the phosphatidylinositol-3 kinase/protein kinase B pathway, fractalkine will inhibit Fas ligand–induced microglial apoptosis through downregulation of the proapoptotic function of Bad and upregulation of the antiapoptotic activity of Bcl_{XL}.[51] A similar effect of fractalkine upon hippocampal neurons exposed to the human immunodeficiency virus (HIV) envelope protein glycoprotein 120 (gp120) has been observed and attributed to activation of the protein kinase Akt and the nuclear translocation of KF-κB.[52,53] Thus, the expression of fractalkine may represent a mechanism by which neurons inhibit the activation of microglia.

Nature of the Microglia Activation on Neuronal Viability

A number of proinflammatory cytokines (e.g., IL-1, IL-6, and TNF-α) are produced by activated microglia and have been found to be elevated following either spinal cord injury or direct brain injury.[54–56] Both IL-1 and TNF-α have similar biological properties in that at higher concentrations both are cytotoxic. IL-1 mediates a general inflammatory response that recruits the further secretion of proinflammatory cytokines (e.g., IL-6, IL-8, colony stimulating factors [CSFs], interferon-α/β [IFN-α/β]) and can also have a trophic effect. The use of a recombinant IL-1 receptor antagonist (r-Hu-met IL-1RA) significantly reduces the volume of damage following brain injury.[57] When IL-1RA–expressing cells are implanted into the wound of spinal cord–injured rats, a significant suppression of the extent of both microglial proliferation and nerve growth factor upregulation is observed.[58] When IL-1 is added to mixed astrocytic/neuronal cultures, a fivefold to sevenfold increase in astrocytes is observed.[16]

Ascribing a crisp role to TNF-α is less clear, because depending on the TNF receptor being activated, the effect of TNF can vary significantly from neurotoxic to neuroprotective.[59] When signaling through the TNFR1, TNFR1 recruits a TNF receptor–associated death domain that then interacts with the Fas-associated death domain to activate caspase-8, leading to downstream activation of effector caspases (Figure 13.1). However, the interaction of TNF-α or TNF-β with TNFR2 leads to the activation of nuclear factor-κB (NF-κB) and the transcription of a number of possible protective cytokines or neurotrophic factors. Of particular interest, knockout mice lacking TNFR2 show a failure to limit the immune response in experimental autoimmune encephalitis and the use of p74 TNF receptor (TNFR2) antisense oligonucleotides increases the extent of a hypoxic injury.[60,61] Following an ischemic injury, the severity and extent of brain injury is increased in transgenic mice lacking the TGF-α receptor.[62] Microglia can also inhibit nitric oxide (NO)–donor (SNP)–induced neuronal apoptosis in vitro through a TNF-α–dependent mechanism, whereas IL-3, IL-6, basic fibroblast growth factor (bFGF), and M-CSF are ineffective in the same experimental paradigm.[63] Hence, the role of TNF-α as a mediator of microglia–motor neuron interactions is complex and not a simple effect of inducing cell death.

Microglia also secrete a number of potent neurotrophic factors, including plasminogen, TGF-β, bFGF, NFG, and neurotrophin-3 (NT-3).[64] The potential role of such secretion was clearly demonstrated by Rabchevsky and Streit[65] in the use of Gelfoam bridges across injured spinal cord in an attempt to induce neuronal growth across the lesion. When microglia were initially grown within the Gelfoam bridges, a prominent neuritic outgrowth was observed. When astrocyte/microglia co-cultures were used, the results were less striking. When astrocytes alone were used, little neuritic growth was observed. Similarly, the addition of either TGF-β or microglia to the site of a spinal cord injury promotes axonal outgrowth from reimplanted dorsal roots.[20] The application of activated macrophages into the site of spinal cord transection in a rat results in an increased rate of axonal growth across the transection site.[66]

EVIDENCE FOR MICROGLIA ACTIVATION IN AMYOTROPHIC LATERAL SCLEROSIS

The proliferation and activation of microglia is a prominent histological feature of sALS[67–72] and the western Pacific variant of ALS[73] (Figure 13.2). Within the spinal cord, this microglial response can be imaged using [³H]PK11195 (isotopic labeling of activated microglial cells).[74] The receptor of M-CSF (CSF-1R) is constitutively expressed in human brain but appears to be expressed to a greater degree in ALS precentral gyrus, suggesting that this increase in microglial cells may relate in part to the presence of neuronal injury.[75]

There are few neurochemical studies of either the peripheral or the central immune system in ALS. Those that exist provide a somewhat confusing picture. Given the preceding discussions regarding the complexity of the microglial response, this might not be unexpected. In addition, there needs to be a differentiation between studies that have undertaken an analysis using serum or cerebrospinal fluid, and those that have used in vivo verses in vitro biological assays as the reporting systems for microglial activation. Immunoglobulin G

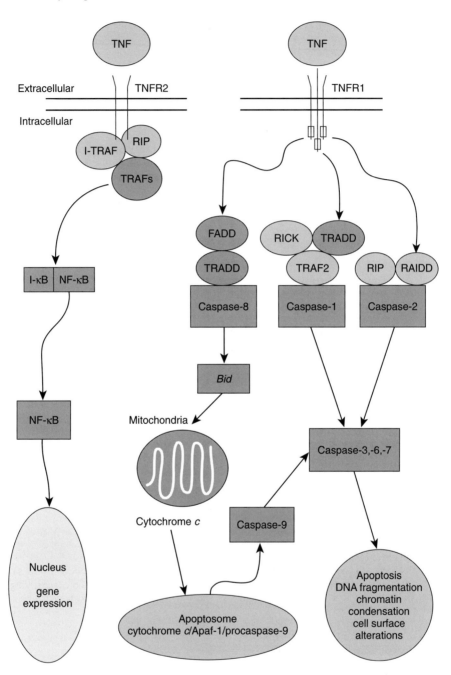

Figure 13.1   The roles of tumor necrosis factor-α (TNF-α) in both the induction of cell death and the induction of cell survival. Microglial originating TNF-α can participate in the induction of cell death by binding to TNF receptor 1 (TNFR1; also known as CD120α) to activate TNFR1-associated death domain (TRADD) protein to interact with Fas-associated death domain (FADD). This complex interacts with and activates procaspase-8, leading to the induction of apoptosis through a mitochondria-dependent pathway. Binding to TNFR1 can also lead to activation of either caspase-1 or caspase-2, leading to apoptosis through mitochondrial-independent pathways. If however TNF interacts with TNF receptor 2 (TNFR2; also known as CD120β), then the interaction of TNFR2 with TNF receptor–associated factor 2 (TRAF2) and receptor-interacting protein (RIP) leads to the phosphorylation of nuclear factor-κB (NF-κB) inhibitory protein (IκB), which is then ubiquitinated and proteolyzed, leading to free NF-κB. NF-κB is then free to translocate to the nucleus where it induces altered gene expression, some portion of which plays a role in cell survival and an antiapoptotic role.

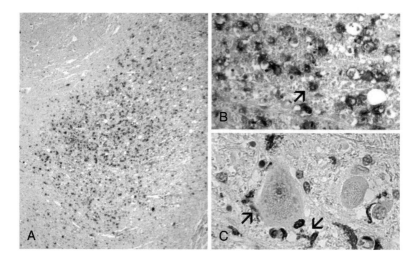

Figure 13.2   Microglial activation in the lumbosacral spinal cord of a patient with sporadic amyotrophic lateral sclerosis. Within regions of degenerating corticospinal tracts **(A)**, microglia proliferation is prominent and can be seen to largely replace the tract (×4, before reproduction). At higher magnification **(B)**, these microglia are seen to have become phagocytotic and are largely responsible for clearing the myelin debris of the degenerating tract (×20, before reproduction). (In both (A) and (C), microglial immunostained with a mouse monoclonal antibody to HLA-DR3 and localized with alkaline phosphatase, giving rise to the red coloration.) In contrast, in the perineuronal milieu **(C)**, activated microglia are seen to cluster around the motor neurons, and to extend processes to the neuronal perikaryon (×40, before reproduction; microglia immunostained with RCA and localized with 3,4-DAB giving rise to the brown coloration). Noteworthy is that normal appearance of the motor neuron, showing no evidence of degeneration at a time when microglial activation, is apparent. See color insert.

(IgG) from the sera of patients with ALS, when injected intraperitoneally into 6-week-old Balb/c mice, induced a significant ventral horn microglial response with activated microglia surrounding motor neurons, whereas no effect was observed from other neurological disease controls.[76] Both TNF-α and the soluble extracellular domains of its receptors TNF-RI and TNF-RII are increased in ALS serum, suggesting that the TNF pathway is activated in ALS, although there is no evidence of an increased cytotoxicity of ALS serum and the observed changes do not correlate with disease state (disease severity, duration, or extent of weight loss).[77] Whether serum levels of TNF-α are reflective of the cerebrospinal fluid levels is not known. Relevant to the prior discussion of the use of minocycline in transgenic murine models of ALS, an increased expression of proinflammatory cytokines, COX-2,[36,78,79] and microglia-mediated protein oxidative pathology[80] is observed in ALS.

Regardless of the evidence suggesting a role for the neuroimmune system in ALS, to date pharmacological trials using immunomodulating medications have been largely ineffective. These have included cyclophosphamide alone or in combination with either intravenous immunoglobulin or prednisone, plasmapheresis with/without azathioprine, total lymph node irradiation, cyclosporine, or intrathecal IFN-α.[81–90] A recent trial of recombinant IFN-β1a failed to demonstrate efficacy in ALS.[91]

CONCLUSION

The function of microglial activation in response to neuronal injury is complex and as it relates to ALS is only now beginning to be addressed. In spite of this, it is clear that the degeneration of motor neurons, whether induced by trauma, experimental neurotoxins, or in transgenic mice models, is accompanied by profound changes in the neuronal milieu. This change in milieu is modulated, to a significant extent, by microglia. Direct microglial/motor neuron contact does not seem to be required for this, although it is noteworthy that contact between microglia and neurons has been proposed to result in a shift in microglial function from neurotoxicity to neuroprotection.[92] Whether such a process occurs in ALS is uncertain, although it would be reasonable to expect that a spectrum of microglial interactions will be present at any given time. It is also likely that the effect of microglial activation upon motor neuron viability will be at multiple levels, and moreover that not all effects of microglial activation will be detrimental (Figure 13.3). Those that are, however, are likely critical and include a prominent upregulation of iNOS activity with the generation of NO,[93–96] increased generation of reactive oxygen species and glutamate,[97] and the release of IL-1 resulting in astrocytic activation. In the latter, IL-1 participates as wide range of factors that upregulate the expression of COX-2 and the subsequent production of proinflammatory cytokines and PGE_2.[2]

Experiments suggesting that the passive transfer of motor neuron injury is possible via microglia are of importance in bringing forward a potential mechanism of disease propagation in ALS. Further studies of this process are desperately needed given the failure of the overwhelming majority of therapies to have an impact on this devastating illness.

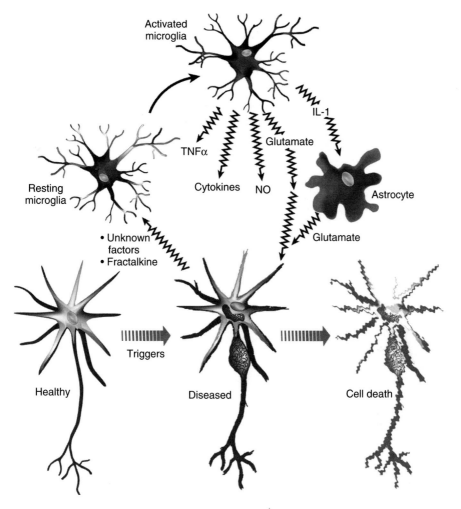

Figure 13.3 A theoretical framework for the interactions between microglia, motor neurons, and astrocytes. In this concept, the etiology of the initial motor neuron injury is a distinct process from that propagating the disease. In the former, such diverse factors as the environment, genetics, aging, and hormonal status may all contribute to reaching a threshold of motor neuron injury beyond which the biological process of amyotrophic lateral sclerosis is triggered. Once initiated, motor neuron injury signals, through unknown mechanisms, the activation of resting microglia into ramified (activated) microglia capable of mediating further neuronal injury through the release of a number of soluble factors, including tumor necrosis factor-α, proinflammatory cytokines, nitric oxide, and glutamate. The latter, which is excitotoxic at higher concentrations, fails to be taken up by astrocytes deficient in excitatory amino acid transporter type 2 transporters, resulting in the exposure of the motor neuron to chronic glutamate toxicity. The subsequent dysregulation of intracellular calcium metabolism, the inability of the motor neuron to buffer excess free calcium, the disruption of cytoskeletal metabolism, and the generation of reactive oxygen species all conspire to lead to a fulminant motor neuron death. (Reprinted with permission from Strong MJ. The basic aspects of therapeutics in amyotrophic lateral sclerosis. Pharmacol Ther 2003;5542:1–36.)

Acknowledgments

M.J.S. is supported by research grants from the ALS Society of Canada (CIHR/NRP), ALSA, and the Scottish Rite Heritage fund.

REFERENCES

1. Strong MJ. The evidence for ALS as a multisystems disorder of limited phenotypic expression. Can J Neurol Sci 2001;28:283–298.
2. Levi G, Minghetti L, Aloisi F. Regulation of prostanoid synthesis in microglial cells and effects of prostacyclin E_2 on microglial functions. Biochimie 1998;80:899–904.
3. Streit WJ, Walter SA, Pennell NA. Reactive microgliosis. Prog Neurobiol 1999;57:563–581.
4. Gu Y, Spasic Z, Wu W. The effects of remaining axons on motoneuron survival and NOS expression following axotomy in the adult rat. Dev Neurosci 1997;19:255–259.
5. Barron KD, Marciano FF, Amundson R, Mankes R. Perineuronal glial response after axotomy of central and peripheral axons. A comparison. Brain Res 1990;523:219–229.
6. Streit WJ. Microglial-neuronal interactions. J Chem Neuroanat 1993;6:261–266.
7. Raivich G, Gehrmann J, Kreutzberg GW. Increase in macrophage colony-stimulating factor and granulocyte-macrophage colony-stimulating factor receptors in the regenerating rat facial nucleus. J Neurosci Res 1991;30:682–686.
8. Lee SC, Liu W, Roth P, et al. Macrophage colony-stimulating factor in human fetal astrocytes and microglia. J Immunol 1993;150:594–604.
9. Fischer HG, Nitzgen B, Germann T, et al. Differentiation driven by granulocyte-macrophage colony-stimulating factor endows microglia with interferon-gamma–independent antigen presentation function. J Neuroimmunol 1993;42:87–96.
10. Raivich G, Moreno-Flores MT, Möller JC, Kreutzberg GW. Inhibition of posttraumatic microglial proliferation in a genetic model of macrophage colony-stimulating factor deficiency in the mouse. Eur J Neurosci 1994;6:1615–1618.
11. Kalla R, Liu Z, Xu S, et al. Microglia and the early phase of immune surveillance in the axotomized facial motor nucleus: impaired microglial activation and lymphocyte recruitment but no effect on neuronal survival or axonal regeneration in macrophage-colony stimulating factor–deficient mice. J Comp Neurol 2001;436:182–201.
12. Galiano M, Liu ZQ, Kalla R, et al. Interleukin-6 (IL6) and cellular response to facial nerve injury: effects on lymphocyte recruitment, early microglial activation and axonal outgrowth in IL6-deficient mice. Eur J Neurosci 2001;14:327–341.
13. Harrison JK, Jiang Y, Chen S, et al. Role for neuronally derived fractalkine in mediating interactions between neurons and CX3CR1-expressing microglia. Proc Natl Acad Sci USA 1998;95:10896–10901.
14. Thanos S, Mey J, Wild M. Treatment of the adult retina with microglia-suppressing factors retards axotomy-induced neuronal degradation and enhances axonal regeneration in vivo and in vitro. J Neurosci 1993;13:455–466.
15. Thanos S. The relationship of microglial cells to dying neurons during natural neuronal cell death and axotomy-induced degeneration of the rat retina. Eur J Neurosci 1991;3:1189–1207.
16. Giulian D, Roberston C. Inhibition of mononuclear phagocytes reduces ischemic injury in the spinal cord. Ann Neurol 1990;27:33–42.
17. Coffey PJ, Perry VH, Rawlins JNP. An investigation into the early stages of the inflammatory response following ibotenic acid–induced neuronal degeneration. Neuroscience 1990;35:121–132.
18. Svensson M, Aldskogius H. Infusion of cytosine-arabinoside into the cerebrospinal fluid of the rat brain inhibits the microglial cell proliferation after hypoglossal nerve injury. Glia 1993;7:286–298.
19. David S, Bouchard C, Tsatas O, Giftochristos N. Macrophages can modify the nonpermissive nature of the adult mammalian central nervous system. Neuron 1990;5:463–469.
20. Prewitt CMF, Niesman IR, Kane CJM, Houlé JD. Activated macrophage/microglial cells can promote the regeneration of sensory axons into the injured spinal cord. Exp Neurol 1997;148:433–443.
21. Mariotti R, Bentivoglio M. Activation and response to axotomy of microglia in the facial motor nuclei of G93A superoxide dismutase transgenic mice. Neurosci Lett 2000;285:87–90.

22. Wu Y-P, McRae A, Rudolphi K, Ling E-A. Propentofylline attenuates microglial reaction in the rat spinal cord induced by middle cerebral artery occlusion. Neurosci Lett 1999;260:17–20.
23. Wu Y-P, Ling E-A. Transsynaptic changes of neurons and associated microglial reaction in the spinal cord of rats following middle cerebral artery occlusion. Neurosci Lett 1998;256:41–44.
24. Wu Y-P, Ling E-A. Induction of microglial and astrocytic response in the adult rat lumbar spinal cord following middle cerebral artery occlusion. Exp Brain Res 1998;118:235–242.
25. Watanabe T, Yamamoto T, Yoshinori A, et al. Differential activation of microglia after experimental spinal cord injury. J Neurotrauma 1999;16:255–265.
26. Nacimiento W, Sappok T, Brook GA, et al. Structural changes of anterior horn neurons and their synaptic input caudal to a low thoracic spinal cord hemisection in the adult rat: a light and electron microscopic study. Acta Neuropathol 1995;90:552–564.
27. Eidelberg E, Nguyen LH, Polich R, Walden JG. Transsynaptic degeneration of motoneurons caudal to spinal cord lesions. Brain Res Bull 1989;22:39–45.
28. Koshinaga M, Whittemore SR. The temporal and spatial activation of microglia in fiber tracts undergoing anterograde and retrograde degeneration following spinal cord lesion. J Neurotrauma 1995;12:209–222.
29. Bartholdi D, Schwab ME. Expression of pro-inflammatory cytokine and chemokine mRNA upon experimental spinal cord injury in mouse: an in situ hybridization study. Eur J Neurosci 1997;9:1422–1438.
30. Boillée S, Viala L, Peschanski M, Dreyfus PA. Differential microglial response to progressive neurodegeneration in the murine mutant Wobbler. Glia 2001;33:277–287.
31. Ghezzi P, Bernardini R, Giuffrida R, et al. Tumor necrosis factor is increased in the spinal cord of an animal model of motor neuron degeneration. Eur Cytokine Network 1998;9:139–144.
32. Hall ED, Oostveen JA, Gurney ME. Relationship of microglial and astrocytic activation to disease onset and progression in a transgenic model of familial ALS. Glia 1998;23:249–256.
33. Elliott JL. Cytokine upregulation in a murine model of familial amyotrophic lateral sclerosis. Mol Brain Res 2001;95:172–178.
34. Alexianu ME, Kozovska M, Appel SH. Immune reactivity in a mouse model of familial ALS correlates with disease progression. Neurology 2001;57:1282–1289.
35. Yoshihara H, Ishigaki S, Yamamoto M, et al. Differential expression of inflammation- and apoptosis-related genes in spinal cords of a mutant SOD1 transgenic mouse model of familial amyotrophic lateral sclerosis. J Neurochem 2002;80:158–167.
36. Almer G, Guégan C, Teismann P, et al. Increased expression of the pro-inflammatory enzyme cyclooxygenase-2 in amyotrophic lateral sclerosis. Ann Neurol 2001;49:176–185.
37. Drachman DB, Rothstein JD. Inhibition of cyclooxygenase-2 protects motor neurons in an organotypic model of amyotrophic lateral sclerosis. Ann Neurol 2000;48:792–795.
38. Kriz J, Nguyen MD, Julien J-P. Minocycline slows disease progression in a mouse model of amyotrophic lateral sclerosis. Neurobiol Dis 2002;10:268–278.
39. Zhu S, Stavrovskaya IG, Drozda M, et al. Minocycline inhibits cytochrome *c* release and delays progression of amyotrophic lateral sclerosis in mice. Nature 2002;417:74–78.
40. Wu DC, Jackson-Lewis V, Vila M, et al. Blockade of microglial activation is neuroprotective in the 1-methyl-4-phenyl-1,2,3,6-tetrahydropyridine mouse model of Parkinson disease. J Neurosci 2002;22:1763–1771.
41. Yrjänheikki J, Keinänen R, Pellikka M, et al. Tetracyclines inhibit microglial activation and are neuroprotective in global brain ischemia. Proc Natl Acad Sci USA 1998;95:15769–15774.
42. Yrjänheikki J, Tikka T, Keinänen R, et al. A tetracycline derivative, minocycline, reduces inflammation and protects against focal cerebral ischemia with a wide therapeutic window. Proc Natl Acad Sci USA 1999;96:13496–13500.
43. Strong MJ, Wolff AV, Wakayama I, Garruto RM. Aluminum-induced chronic myelopathy in rabbits. Neurotoxicology 1991;12:9–22.
44. Strong MJ, Gaytan-Garcia S, Jakowec D. Reversibility of neurofilamentous inclusion formation following repeated sublethal intracisternal inoculums of AlCl₃ in New Zealand white rabbits. Acta Neuropathol 1995;90:57–67.
45. He BP, Strong MJ. A morphological analysis of the motor neuron degeneration and microglial reaction in acute and chronic in vivo aluminum chloride neurotoxicity. J Chem Neuroanat 2000;17:207–215.
46. He BP, Strong MJ. Inhibition of microglial function in vitro by aluminum. Trace Elements Med 2002;15:141–142.
47. Cashman NR, Durham H, Blusztajn JK, et al. Neuroblastoma × spinal cord (NSC) hybrid cell lines resemble developing motor neurons. Devel Dyn 1992;194:209–221.

48. He BP, Wen W, Strong MJ. Activated microglia (BV-2) facilitation of TNF-mediated motor neuron death in vitro. J Neuroimmunol 2002;128:31–38.
49. Pedersen WA, Cashman NR, Mattson MP. The lipid peroxidation product 4-hydroxynonenal impairs glutamate and glucose transport and choline acetyltransferase activity in NSC-19 motor neuron cells. Exp Neurol 1999;155:1–10.
50. Zujovic V, Benavides J, Vigé X, et al. Fractalkine modulates TNF-a secretion and neurotoxicity induced by microglial activation. Glia 2000;29:395–315.
51. Boehme SA, Lio FM, Maciejewski-Lenoir D, et al. The chemokine fractalkine inhibits Fas-mediated cell death of brain microglia. J Immunol 2000;165:397–403.
52. Meucci O, Fatatis A, Simen AA, Miller RJ. Expression of CX3CR1 chemokine receptors on neurons and their role in neuronal survival. Proc Natl Acad Sci USA 2000;97:8075–8080.
53. Meucci O, Fatatis A, Simen AA, et al. Chemokines regulate hippocampal neuronal signaling and gp120 neurotoxicity. Proc Natl Acad Sci USA 1998;95:14500–14505.
54. Woodroofe MN, Sarna GS, Wadhwa M, et al. Detection of interleukin-1 and interleukin-6 in adult rat brain, following mechanical injury, by in vivo microdialysis: evidence of a role for microglia in cytokine production. J Neuroimmunol 1991;33:227–236.
55. Knerlich F, Schilling L, Görlach C, et al. Temporal profile of expression and cellular localization of inducible nitric oxide synthase, interleukin-1β and interleukin converting enzyme after cryogenic lesion of the rat parietal cortex. Mol Brain Res 1999;68:73–87.
56. Buttini M, Sauter A, Boddeke HWGM. Induction of interleukin-1β mRNA after focal cerebral ischaemia in the rat. Mol Brain Res 1994;23:126–134.
57. Toulmond S, Rothwell NJ. Interleukin-1 receptor antagonist inhibits neuronal damage caused by fluid percussion injury in the rat. Brain Res 1995;671:261–266.
58. DeKosky ST, Styren SD, O'Malley ME, et al. Interleukin-1 receptor antagonist suppresses neurotrophin response in injured rat brain. Ann Neurol 1996;39:123–127.
59. Ghezzi P, Mennini T. Tumor necrosis factor and motoneuronal degeneration: an open problem. Neuroimmunomodulation 2001;9:178–182.
60. Shen Y, Li R, Shiosaki K. Inhibition of p75 tumor necrosis factor receptor by antisense oligonucleotides increases hypoxic injury and β-amyloid toxicity in human neuronal cell line. J Biol Chem 2002;272:3550–3553.
61. Gary DS, Bruce-Keller AJ, Kindy MS, Mattson MP. Ischemic and excitotoxic brain injury is enhanced in mice lacking the p55 tumor necrosis factor receptor. J Cereb Blood Flow Metab 1998;18:1283–1287.
62. Bruce AJ, Boling W, Kindy MS, et al. Altered neuronal and microglial responses to excitotoxic and ischemic brain injury in mice lacking TNF receptors. Nat Med 1996;2:788–794.
63. Toku K, Tanaka J, Yano H, et al. Microglial cells prevent nitric oxide–induced neuronal apoptosis in vitro. J Neurosci Res 1998;53:415–425.
64. Elkabes S, DiCicco-Bloom EM, Black IB. Brain microglia/macrophages express neurotrophins that selectively regulate microglial proliferation and function. J Neurosci 1996;16:2508–2521.
65. Rabchevsky AG, Streit WJ. Grafting of cultured microglial cells into lesioned spinal cord of adult rats enhances neurite outgrowth. J Neurosci Res 1997;47:34–48.
66. Rapalino O, Lazarov-Spiegler O, Agranov E, et al. Implantation of stimulated homologous macrophages results in partial recovery of paraplegic rats. Nat Med 1998;4:814–821.
67. Lampson LA, Kushner PD, Sobel RA. Strong expression of class II major histocompatibility complex (MHC) antigens in the absence of detectable T cell infiltration in amyotrophic lateral sclerosis (ALS) spinal cord. J Neuropathol Exp Neurol 1988;47:353.
68. Lampson LA, Kushner PD, Sobel RA. Major histocompatibility complex antigen expression in the affected tissues in amyotrophic lateral sclerosis. Ann Neurol 1990;28:365–372.
69. Troost D, van den Oord JJ, Vianney de Jong JMB. Immunohistochemical characterization of the inflammatory infiltrate in amyotrophic lateral sclerosis. Neuropathol Appl Neurobiol 1990;16:401–410.
70. Kawamata T, Akiyama H, Yamada T, McGeer PL. Immunological reactions in amyotrophic lateral sclerosis brain and spinal cord tissue. Am J Pathol 1992;140:691–707.
71. Troost D, Claessen N, van den Oord JJ, et al. Neuronophagia in the motor cortex in amyotrophic lateral sclerosis. Neuropathol Appl Neurobiol 1993;19:390–397.
72. McGeer PL, McGeer EG, Kawamata T, et al. Reactions of the immune system in chronic degenerative neurological diseases. Can J Neurol Sci 1991;18:376–379.
73. Schwab C, Steele JC, McGeer PL. Neurofibrillary tangles of Guam Parkinson-dementia are associated with reactive microglia and complement proteins. Brain Res 1998;707:196–205.

74. Sitte HH, Wanschitz J, Budka H, Berger ML. Autoradiography with [³H]PK11195 of spinal tract degeneration in amyotrophic lateral sclerosis. Acta Neuropathol 2002;101:75–78.
75. Akiyama H, Nishimura T, Kondo H, et al. Expression of the receptor for macrophage colony stimulating factor by brain microglia and its upregulation in brains of patients with Alzheimer's disease and amyotrophic lateral sclerosis. Brain Res 1994;639:171–174.
76. Obál I, Jakab JSK, Siklós L, Engelhardt JI. Recruitment of activated microglia cells in the spinal cord of mice by ALS IgG. Neuroreport 2001;12:2449–2452.
77. Poloni M, Facchetti D, Mai R, et al. Circulating levels of tumour necrosis factor-alpha and its soluble receptors are increased in the blood of patients with amyotrophic lateral sclerosis. Neurosci Lett 2000;287:211–214.
78. Krieger C, Perry TL, Ziltener HJ. Amyotrophic lateral sclerosis: interleukin-6 levels in cerebrospinal fluid. Can J Neurol Sci 1992;19:357–359.
79. Sekizawa T, Openshaw H, Ohbo K, et al. Cerebrospinal fluid interleukin 6 in amyotrophic lateral sclerosis: immunological parameter and comparison with inflammatory and non-inflammatory central nervous system diseases. J Neurol Sci 1998;154:194–199.
80. Shibata N, Nagai R, Uchida K, et al. Morphological evidence for lipid peroxidation and protein glycoxidation in spinal cords from sporadic amyotrophic lateral sclerosis patients. Brain Res 2001;917:97–104.
81. Brown RH Jr, Hauser SL, Harrington H, Weiner HL. Failure of immunosuppression with a ten- to 14-day course of high-dose intravenous cyclophosphamide to alter the progression of amyotrophic lateral sclerosis. Arch Neurol 1986;43:383–384.
82. Gourie-Devi M, Nalini A, Subbakrishna DK. Temporary amelioration of symptoms with intravenous cyclophosphamide in amyotrophic lateral sclerosis. J Neurol Sci 1997;150:167–172.
83. Tan E, Lynn J, Amato AA, et al. Immunosuppressive treatment of motor neuron syndromes. Arch Neurol 1994;51:194–200.
84. Meucci N, Nobile-Orazio E, Scarlato G. Intravenous immunoglobulin therapy in amyotrophic lateral sclerosis. J Neurol 1996;243:117–120.
85. Olarte MR, Schoenfeldt RS, McKiernan G, Rowland LP. Plasmapheresis in amyotrophic lateral sclerosis. Ann Neurol 1980;8:644–645.
86. Kelemen J, Hedlund W, Orlin JB, et al. Plasmapheresis with immunosuppression in amyotrophic lateral sclerosis. Arch Neurol 1983;40:752–753.
87. Drachman DB, Chaudhry V, Cornblath DR, et al. Trial of immunosuppression in amyotrophic lateral sclerosis using total lymphoid irradiation. Ann Neurol 1994;35:142–150.
88. Appel SH, Stewart SS, Appel V, et al. A double-blind study of the effectiveness of cyclosporine in amyotrophic lateral sclerosis. Arch Neurol 1988;45:381–386.
89. Mora JS, Munsat TL, Kao K-P, et al. Intrathecal administration of natural human interferon alpha in amyotrophic lateral sclerosis. Neurology 1986;36:1137–1140.
90. Haverkamp LJ, Smith RG, Appel SH. Trial of immunosuppression in amyotrophic lateral sclerosis using total lymph node irradiation. Ann Neurol 1994;36:253–254.
91. Beghi E, Chiò A, Inghilleri M, et al. A randomized controlled trial of recombinant interferon beta-1a in ALS. Neurology 2000;54:469–474.
92. Zietlow R, Dunnett SB, Fawcett JW. The effect of microglia on embryonic dopaminergic neuronal survival in vitro: diffusible signals from neurons and glia change microglia from neurotoxic to neuroprotective. Eur J Neurosci 1999;11:1657–1667.
93. Lockhart BP, Cressey KC, Lepagnol JM. Suppression of nitric oxide formation by tyrosine kinase inhibitors in murine N9 microglia. Br J Pharmacol 1998;123:879–889.
94. Abe K, Abe Y, Saito H. Agmatine suppresses nitric oxide production in microglia. Brain Res 2000;872:141–148.
95. Kawahara K, Gotoh T, Oyadomari S, et al. Co-induction of argininosuccinate synthetase, cationic amino acid transporter-2, and nitric oxide synthase in activated microglial cells. Mol Brain Res 2000;90:165–173.
96. Romero LI, Tatro JB, Field JA, Reichlin S. Roles of IL-1 and TNF-α in endotoxin-induced activation of nitric oxide synthase in cultured rat brain cells. Am J Physiol 1996;270:R326–R332.
97. Piani D, Frei K, Do KQ, et al. Murine brain macrophages induce NMDA receptor mediated neurotoxicity in vitro by secreting glutamate. Neurosci Lett 1991;133:159–162.
98. Strong MJ. The basic aspects of therapeutics in amyotrophic lateral sclerosis. Pharmacol Ther 2003;5542:1–36.

14

Cell Death Pathways in Amyotrophic Lateral Sclerosis

Serge Przedborski and Peter G.H. Clarke

Like other neurons, spinal cord motor neurons may die at various developmental stages and for many reasons. In most cases, the death involves sophisticated molecular processes, which are highly conserved across species. This fact has prompted many investigators to study in depth what is today called the *mode* or *mechanism* of cell death in large numbers of settings encompassing development, morphogenesis, more recently, pathological conditions. A primary impetus in studying the question of cell death in "all azimuths" with such avidity is the hope that by elucidating the key molecular factors involved in the process of death in a given disease, one may shed light on the pathogenesis of that disease and consequently devise effective neuroprotective therapies.

In this chapter, we review recent developments related to neuronal death, with particular emphasis on motor neurons, the specific cellular target of the degenerative process of amyotrophic lateral sclerosis (ALS), also called motor neuron disease (MND). In the first part of this chapter, we discuss several basic aspects related to the morphology and mechanism of neuronal death, as well as related to the fatal paralytic neurodegenerative disease that is ALS. Based on this groundwork information, in the second part of the chapter, we discuss specifically the question of neuronal death pathways in ALS through the appraisal of the rapidly growing numbers of studies using postmortem specimens or experimental models provided by cell culture systems or genetically engineered animals.

MORPHOLOGICAL TYPES OF CELL DEATH

In the nervous system, as elsewhere, different stimuli produce quite different morphological manifestations of cell death. These hallmarks are important because when considered in light of current biological understanding, they provide clues about the molecular events responsible for the cell death in a given situation. However, the diversity of cell death types is often neglected, and many authors still consider only two types, apoptosis and necrosis. The former is universally recognized to be active in the sense of being mediated by intracellular signaling pathways, and the latter is traditionally considered passive.

There is increasing evidence that this dichotomy is too narrow, especially for neurons. Even in normal development, dying neurons can adopt at least three morphological types: *apoptosis* (type 1); *autophagic cell death* (type 2); and *cytoplasmic cell death* (type 3B), with type 3A being rare and unknown in neurons.[1,2] Cytoplasmic cell death shares morphological features with necrosis, both being characterized by cytoplasmic vacuolation and relatively minor changes in the nucleus. These four types are summarized in Table 14.1. There is evidence that all four are in fact active, as is outlined in the following paragraphs.

Table 14.1   Main characteristics of the different types of neuronal death[a]

Designation	Nucleus	Cell membrane	Cytoplasm
Apoptosis	Early condensation and chromatin clumping	Early preservation and late formation of blebs containing organelles (apoptotic bodies)	Condensation, organelles preservation, loss of ribosomes from polysomes, and rough endoplasmic reticulum
Necrosis	Early swelling with scattering of chromatin along the nuclear membrane (margination); late shrinkage and diffuse condensation	Swelling of the cell followed by loss of membrane integrity	Organelle dilation and fragmentation
Autophagic death	Mild diffuse condensation; part of the nucleus may segregate or bleb	In some cases, endocytosis or blebbing	Numerous autophagic vacuoles
Cytoplasmic death	Late increased granular aspect but no margination of chromatin	Rounding of the cell	Mild organelle dilation and no loss of ribosome from rough endoplasmic reticulum

Modified from Clarke PGH. Developmental cell death: morphological diversity and multiple mechanisms. Anat Embryol 1990;181:195–213.

[a]Evidence of phagocytosis is seen in all four forms of neuronal death.

Apoptosis was initially defined in terms of its morphology—nuclear and cytoplasmic condensation, accompanied by the clumping of chromatin along the inside of the nuclear envelope but with preservation of cytoplasmic organelles until late in the death process.[3] However, current definitions are varied and even anarchical,[4] and there is a growing tendency to redefine it in terms of its signaling pathways, which have been analyzed in great detail in neuronal death, as is discussed in subsequent sections.

Autophagic cell death, characterized by the formation of numerous autophagic vacuoles (secondary lysosomes), has been reported particularly in metamorphosis but also in normal development, in disease, and in a few in vitro models.[5] Although the existence of this morphological type in neurons and other cells can scarcely be denied, little is known of its mechanistic basis, and its study is complicated by the fact that lysosomes appear to be implicated also in the triggering of standard caspase-mediated apoptosis.[6] The question arises therefore whether autophagy is causally implicated in this cell death or merely is an epiphenomenon of apoptosis. The death-mediating role of the autophagy is suggested by its very intensity, because the total volume of autophagic vacuoles can exceed that of the remaining cytosol and organelles, and even part of the nuclear DNA can be digested in these cytoplasmic vacuoles.[1] Moreover, the inhibition of autophagy with 3-methyladenine has been found to prevent autophagic cell death in several situations,[5,6] including sympathetic neurons deprived of nerve growth factor (NGF) or treated with cytosine arabinoside.[7] The distinctness of autophagic cell death with respect to apoptosis is indicated by the fact that pure cases of autophagic cell death are not prevented by classic caspase inhibitors[8] and pure cases of apoptosis are not prevented by 3-methyladenine. However, intermediate forms of cell death can occur, involving both autophagy and apoptosis, and these can be partially inhibited by both 3-methyladenine and caspase inhibitors.[6,7]

Cytoplasmic cell death is most frequently reported in immature neurons, either in normal development or following axotomy, and is characterized by dilation of the perinuclear space and organelles.[1,2] Its mechanistic basis is largely unknown, but it has recently been shown to be the main kind of cell death in axotomized retinal ganglion cells of chick embryos, and this is known to be modulated by the cellular redox state[9] and to depend on a cyclin-dependent kinase (probably Cdk5, which is not implicated in the cell cycle).[10] Cell death with a similar morphology has been reported in a non-neuronal cell line and found to depend on activation of caspase-9 by an unconventional (apoptosis protease-activating factor-1 [Apaf-1]–independent) pathway.[11]

Necrosis is generally assumed to be "passive" in the sense of not depending on intracellular signaling pathways.[12] However, there is now clear evidence that the inhibition of signaling can protect neurons against powerful excitotoxic stimuli (such as cerebral ischemia) that would normally lead to necrosis. Such protection has been provided by the inhibition or genetic deletion of poly(adenosine diphosphate-ribose) polymerase[13] and by the inhibition of c-Jun/N-terminal kinase.[14]

Our reason for emphasizing the multiplicity of cell death types is that uncritical acceptance of a rigid apoptosis/necrosis dichotomy has led to confusion and the vacuous identification as apoptosis of all cell death that was not blatantly necrotic. The word *apoptosis* should be used with caution because of inadequate definition,[4] but even on the broadest definition, its identification on the basis of in situ labeling for DNA breaks or prevention by macromolecular inhibitors can no longer be justified.[2]

Another widespread misconception relating to types of cell death is the belief that only necrosis elicits inflammation, and that apoptosis does not.[2] Although the inflammatory reaction is indeed generally stronger in regions of necrosis than of apoptosis, this may simply reflect the greater number of cells dying in necrotic regions. Moreover, those who claim that apoptosis does not elicit inflammation are referring to "exudative inflammation," whose hallmarks include the infiltration of the diseased tissue by blood-borne cells (mainly neutrophils and monocytes); they admit that apoptosis evokes a local tissue reaction. However, in the central nervous system, even to necrosis, the acute inflammatory response is largely local (by the prompt reaction of resident microglia and/or astrocytes[15]), thus resembling the phagocytic response that apoptosis is believed to evoke in peripheral tissues. The autophagic and cytoplasmic types of cell death can likewise evoke a strong microglial or astrocytic reaction.[16,17] In light of these findings, it is fair to conclude that although the intensity of the glial reaction may vary among the various forms of cell death described already, the occurrence of gliosis cannot be regarded as a hallmark of any of them. Correlatively, the glial reaction seen in affected areas of the nervous system in ALS is likely not an accurate marker of the actual type of neuronal death found in this disease.

NEURONAL DEATH IN DEVELOPMENT

ALS is not considered a neurodegenerative disease of the developing nervous system, but it is considered one of the mature nervous system. Nevertheless, the question of developmental death of motor neurons may be quite relevant to ALS, because by elucidating the exact process by which the cell death machinery regulates the fate of immature motor neurons, we may acquire a better understanding of the cascade of molecular events in the demise of adult motor neurons. The formation of the nervous system involves the proliferation of neuronal precursors within the ventricular proliferative zone, followed by the migration of postmitotic neurons to their final destinations, where they will differentiate and make synaptic connections. Cell death occurs during both phases of this process: first among the proliferating cells of the neuroepithelium and migrating neuroblasts,[18] and much later among differentiated neurons when they are forming and receiving synaptic connections.[19] We shall here discuss only the latter phase, which in most neuronal populations involves 25 to 75 percent of the initial neuronal number, although in a few populations no neurons die,[19] and in certain transient populations (such as a group of early generated "borderline cells" at the dorsolateral margin of the primate spinal cord),[20] they all die.

The roles of neuronal death appear to be multiple and may include the elimination of "wrongly" connected neurons and those with transient functions, and the adjustment of neuronal numbers.[19]

More relevant to the present context of ALS is the question of what decides between death and survival for these neurons that are in the process of making and receiving connections. The determinant signals arise mainly from the connections themselves, both afferent and efferent.

Neurotrophic factors are major carriers for the afferent and efferent signals. Historically, it was the efferent connections that were first shown to provide trophic support, through the retrograde transport of target-derived trophic factors. More recently, the afferent fibers have also been shown to exert a trophic effect[21] and to release neurotrophins.[22]

It is currently the NGF family (the *neurotrophins,* including brain-derived neurotrophic factor [BDNF], NT-3, and NT-4) whose survival role in development has been best studied.[22] The survival-promoting effects of the neurotrophins are mediated largely through binding to their high-affinity receptors, which all belong to the Trk family: TrkA binds NGF, TrkB binds BDNF or NT-4, TrkC binds NT-3. There is also a lower affinity neurotrophin receptor, which binds all of these neurotrophins, and in some cases is death mediating, notably in the early development of the retina. However, although the expression and release of neurotrophins in the neuronal death period has been well documented, as well as their survival-promoting effects when applied exogenously,[19,22] the deletion of their genes or of the corresponding *trk* family genes has caused prominent neuronal death only in the peripheral nervous system. For example, deletion of the gene for NGF or TrkA leads to the loss of an entire class of sensory neurons and all sympathetic neurons, and deletion of the gene for BDNF or TrkB leads to the loss of another class of sensory neurons, in each case during approximately the period of developmental neuronal death. But the effect of such deletions, or even a combination of them, on the survival of central neurons (including motor neurons) is slight and is manifested mainly after the period of developmental neuronal death, implying little role for these genes in normal development; however, the deletions do affect neurons in other ways such as a reduction in their size.[23,24] In contrast with this lack of effect of genetic deletion on the developmental death of central neurons, it has been shown in the visual system that increasing acutely the level of BDNF in the axonal target region reduces the developmental death, and decreasing its availability has the expected opposite effect.[25] The reason for the discrepancy between the acute experiments and the genetic deletions is unclear, but current opinion is that neurotrophins do indeed contribute to anterograde and retrograde survival signals, and that the lack of strong central effects in knockout mice may be due to the neurons' capacity to adapt their trophic needs and respond to alternative trophic molecules. Other families of neurotrophic factors may also be involved.[19]

Not all survival-modulating signals are mediated by trophic factors. Electrical activity also exerts an important influence on neuronal survival, and although this may be mediated partly by a change in the synthesis and release of trophic factors—an effect well documented in synaptic plasticity[26]—part of it occurs independently of them. In general, electrical activity in the axonal afferents promotes neuronal survival,[21] whereas electrical activity in the axonal target promotes neuronal death. The latter effect has been particularly well documented in developing motor neurons, where the pharmacological blockade of neuromuscular transmission greatly decreases naturally occurring motor neuron death.[27] In these neurons, the death-promoting effect of electrical activity appears to be due at least partly to a decrease in axonal branching, leading to reduced access to trophic factors.[27] However, experiments on the visual system suggest the existence also of a more direct effect of electrical activity independent of trophic factors, mediated by an activity-dependent retrograde death signal.[28] Because electrical activity in a neuron's afferents promotes its survival but in its axonal target promotes its death, a *global* change in electrical activity (as in anesthesia) may have little effect.

MAINTENANCE OF ADULT MOTOR NEURONS BY NEUROTROPHIC FACTORS

In view of the importance of neurotrophic factors for the survival of neurons in development, the question arises whether they are likewise important for the maintenance of adult neurons, and in particular adult motor neurons. It is well established that exogenous trophic factors can rescue axotomized adult motor neurons,[29] and attempts are being made at developing trophic factor therapies for ALS,[30] although clinical trials have so far been disappointing.[31] Moreover, most neurotrophic factors and their receptors are widely expressed in the adult nervous system, although this does not in itself prove that their adult role is to promote neuron survival (they clearly have other roles such as in synaptic plasticity). On balance, it is likely, but not absolutely proven, that adult neurons, including motor neurons, are normally dependent on a continuous supply of trophic factors, which they obtain not only from their afferents and axonal target neurons as during the period of developmental neuronal death, but also from various glia including the Schwann cells or oligodendrocytes that myelinate their axons.[19,32] The loss of neuronal dependence on targets and afferents near the end of the period of naturally occurring neuronal death may be due in large part to the incipience of these non-neuronal supplies of neurotrophic factors.

MOTOR NEURONAL DEATH IN PATHOLOGICAL SITUATIONS

Aside from their death during normal development, the selective destruction of spinal cord motor neurons also occurs abnormally in various inflammatory, genetic (e.g., SOD1 mutation), and degenerative conditions, as well as in association with metabolic defects (e.g., hexosaminidase deficiency), lymphoma, or paraproteinemia. The best known of the MNDs are acute anterior poliomyelitis, spinal muscular atrophy, and ALS, which with the prevalence of 3 to 5 of 100,000 individuals, is the most frequent paralytic disease in adults. ALS can strike anyone at any age, but generally the onset of disease is in the fourth or fifth decade of life. Common clinical features of ALS include muscle weakness, fasciculations, brisk (or depressed) reflexes, and extensor-plantar responses. Although motor deficit usually predominates in the limbs, bulbar motor neurons can be severely involved, sometimes early in the course of the disease, leading to atrophy of the tongue, dysphagia, and dysarthria. Other cranial nerves (e.g., oculomotor nerves) are usually spared. The progressive decline of muscular function results in paralysis, speech and swallowing disabilities, emotional disturbance, and ultimately, respiratory failure, causing death among the vast majority of patients with ALS within 2 to 5 years after the onset of the disease.

As in other common neurodegenerative disorders, in ALS the disease is sporadic in most patients and familial in only a few.[33] The clinical and pathological expressions of ALS are almost indistinguishable between the familial and sporadic forms, though often in the former, the age at onset is younger, the course of the disease is more rapid, and the survival after diagnosis is shorter.[33] Among the various familial forms of ALS, so far the lion's share has been given to that linked to SOD1 mutations.[34,35] To date, more than 100 point mutations in SOD1 throughout the entire gene have been identified in ALS families[36] and all but one is dominant. Most of these mutations have apparently reduced enzymatic activity,[34,37] a finding that has prompted investigators to test whether a loss of SOD1 activity can kill neurons. It was unequivocally demonstrated that reducing SOD1 activity to about 50 percent using antisense oligonucleotides kills pheochromocytoma PC-12 cells and motor neurons in spinal cord organotypic cultures.[38,39] However, mutant mice deficient in SOD1 do not develop MND[40] and the transgenic expression of different SOD1 mutants in both mice[41–43] and rats[44] causes an ALS-like syndrome in these animals regardless of whether SOD1 free-radical–scavenging catalytic activity is increased, normal, or almost absent.[41–45] These observations provide compelling evidence that the cytotoxicity of mutant SOD1 is not mediated by a loss of function, but by a gain-of-function effect.[46] Among the various proposed mechanisms, early on in the search for the nature of mutant SOD1 gained function it emerged that transfected neuronal cells expressing mutant SOD1 cDNA were dying by apoptosis.[47] Similar observations were subsequently made in transfected PC-12 cells[48] and in primary neurons grown from transgenic mice expressing mutant SOD1.[49] Collectively, these in vitro data have led many investigators to consider that mutant SOD1 may kill motor neurons by activating programmed cell death (PCD), a term that we here use in the sense of cell death mediated by specific signaling pathways. However, as we discuss later, it has been shown that inhibition of PCD in transgenic mice expressing mutant SOD1 does delay but does not permanently prevent neurodegeneration.[50,51] In our opinion, this suggests that the recruitment of PCD in this ALS model results not from a direct but from an indirect effect of the mutant protein on the PCD molecular machinery. In keeping with this view, it is, for example, well established that mutant SOD1 has the propensity to form intracellular proteinaceous aggregates whose presence in the cytosol of motor neurons may impair the microtubule-dependent axonal transport of vital nutriments or the normal turnover of intracellular proteins.[52] It may thus be possible that mutant SOD1 by stimulating, for example, a building up of protein aggregation causes major motor neuron perturbations, which in turn trigger PCD.

MORPHOLOGY OF DYING MOTOR NEURONS IN AMYOTROPHIC LATERAL SCLEROSIS

Although numerous publications report on the spinal cord neuropathology of ALS, only a handful provide fine morphological description of dying motor neurons. The classic neuropathological description of ALS specifies the characteristic loss of upper motor neurons in the cerebral cortex and of the lower motor neurons throughout the spinal cord.[53] Also indicated is the usual severe degeneration of the corticospinal tracts, which when it is present, is most evident at the level of the spinal cord. Argentophilic spheroids are often observed in the anterior horn within enlarged neuronal processes.[53] Typically, the description of residual motor neurons is limited to indicating that many are shrunken with pyknotic nuclei and others are large and pale (ghost cells).[53] Some are filled with phosphorylated neurofilament, both in their cell bodies and axons, and some contain small eosinophilic inclusions called Bunina bodies.[53] Based on morphological criteria including size, shape, and aggregates of Nissl substance, Martin[54] has arranged residual spinal cord motor neurons in ALS postmortem samples in three categories that we believe reflect different stages of degeneration. In the *chromatolysis stage,* motor neurons still resemble their normal counterparts except for the fact that the cell body appears swollen and round, the Nissl substance dispersed, and the nucleus eccentrically placed. Some chromatolytic neurons have prominent cytoplasmic hyaline body inclusions. In the *attritional stage,* the cytoplasm and the nucleus appear homogenous and condensed, and the cell body shrunken and with hazy multipolar shape. In the so-called *apoptotic stage,* the affected motor neuron is approximately one fifth of its normal diameter, the cytoplasm and nucleus are extremely condensed and the cell body adopts a fusiform or round shape devoid of any process. Notably, in none of the three stages do residual motor neurons show appreciable cytoplasmic vacuoles or nuclear condensation accompanied with round chromatin clumps. By compiling these findings, it appears that although degenerating neurons do exhibit some features reminiscent of apoptosis, none can confidently be labeled as typical apoptotic cells, whose hallmarks, as mentioned earlier, include cytoplasmic and nuclear condensation, compaction of nuclear chromatin into sharply circumscribed masses along the inside of the nuclear membrane, and structural preservation of organelles (at least until the cell is broken into membrane-bound fragments called *apoptotic bodies* that are phagocytosed).[3]

Notwithstanding the inherent limitations of ALS experimental models,[55] some have provided valuable information regarding the morphology of degenerating spinal cord motor neurons. Specifically, in the Wobbler mouse model, degenerating anterior horn motor neurons are mainly large and occupied with numerous vacuoles, whereas their nuclei appear unremarkable.[56] In equine MND,[57] some affected motor neurons are swollen and chromatolytic, whereas others are shrunken. Several careful morphological studies have also been performed in transgenic mutant SOD1 mice.[58–61] In these animals, upon reaching severe paralysis, 50 percent of anterior motor neurons still remain, among which several retain a normal appearance (Figure 14.1A), some are enlarged and hypochromatic (Figure 14.1B), resembling the chromatolytic motor neurons described in human ALS, and a few are shrunken and hyperchromatic with short or no visible processes (Figure 14.1C), resembling the atretic motor neurons also described in human ALS. In addition, most of the sick neurons have their cytoplasm occupied with vacuoles corresponding to dilated rough endoplasmic reticulum, Golgi apparatus, and mitochondria.[58] From our own ultrastructural studies in these mice (S. Przedborski, unpublished observation), we can add that many sick neurons have diffusely condensed cytoplasm and nucleus and irregular shapes. Although the actual type of this cell death remains to be determined, these dying neurons exhibit a nonapoptotic morphology with some

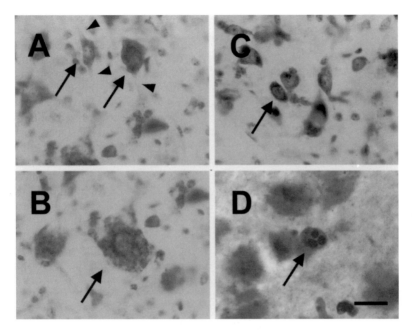

Figure 14.1 Photomicrographs illustrating the various morphological aspects of the remaining motor neurons in the anterior horn of severely paralyzed transgenic mutant SOD1 mice. (**A**) Two normal-looking motor neurons *(arrows)* with well-defined processes *(arrowheads)*. (**B**) The arrow shows a ballooned neuron that stained poorly with Nissl (i.e., hypochromatic). (**C**) Example of a condensed neuron *(arrow)*, which clearly appears shrunken and intensively stained with Nissl. (**D**) Definite apoptotic cells found in the anterior horn of an end-stage transgenic SOD1^{G93A} mouse; also visible are *(arrow)* several typical round chromatin clumps.

features reminiscent of autophagic or cytoplasmic neuronal death.[2] From our experience, definite apoptotic cells are seen but are rare in the spinal cord of affected transgenic mutant SOD1 mice (Figure 14.1D). For instance, in end-stage transgenic SOD1^{G93A} mice, which have lost about 50 percent of their anterior motor neurons, it can be estimated that about two apoptotic cells will be seen per 40-micrometer-thick section of the lumbar spinal cord. We have also observed that the vast majority of these apoptotic cells do not any longer exhibit definite morphological characteristics or express phenotypical markers allowing their identification as neurons or glia. However, some (less than 15%) of the spinal cord apoptotic cells are still immunoreactive for specific proteins such as neurofilament or glial fibrillary acid protein,[60] suggesting that both neuronal and glial cells are dying by apoptosis in the mutant SOD1 model.[61] In our opinion, the paucity of apoptotic dying motor neurons in this mouse model of ALS may stem from the difficulty in detecting them by morphological means due to the presumed low daily rate of motor neuron loss[62] and the notoriously rapid disappearance of apoptotic cells. It remains that the primary morphology of degenerating motor neurons in both human ALS and its experimental models is rather nonapoptotic.

EXPRESSION OF APOPTOTIC MARKERS IN AMYOTROPHIC LATERAL SCLEROSIS

In addition to exhibiting singular morphological features, apoptotic cells may also show various cellular alterations. Among these, the detection of internucleosomal DNA cleavage by either gel electrophoresis or in situ methods has emerged as a popular means of supporting the existence of apoptosis in all sorts of pathological situations, including ALS. However, like many of these apoptotic markers, DNA fragmentation is now well recognized as occurring in non-apoptotic cell death as well, including necrosis,[2] thus the value of DNA cleavage as a specific marker of apoptosis must be taken with caution. In addition to this caveat, the search for DNA fragmentation in ALS postmortem samples has generated conflicting results. In one study on postmortem human tissue, DNA fragmentation was detected by an in situ method in spinal cord motor neurons in ALS cases, but not at all in control cases.[63] However, in two other studies, DNA fragmentation was detected not only in motor cortex and spinal cord of patients with ALS but also, though to a lesser degree, in control cases.[64,65] In a subsequent study, internucleosomal DNA fragmentation was detected in affected (e.g., motor cortex and spinal cord) but not in spared brain regions (e.g., somatosensory cortex) of patients with ALS[54] and only in diseased motor neurons in the somatodendritic attrition and apoptotic stages, but not in the chromatolytic stage.[54] Here, the author has also documented DNA fragmentation in anterior horn gray matter of the spinal cord and motor cortex of ALS cases by gel electrophoresis,[54] a technique not frequently used in the nervous system to identify apoptosis because in many neurological situations, it is difficult to obtain samples with a sufficient high proportion of dying cells. In contrast to all these positive findings, other groups, using similar techniques and tissue samples, have failed to provide any evidence of internucleosomal cleavage of DNA in postmortem tissue from human ALS cases or from animal models of the disease.[59,65,66] Although the actual reason for these divergent results is unclear, this casts doubt about the reliability and even the specificity of such findings.

Two other apoptotic markers, the Le^Y antigen[67] and fractin,[68] were also studied in ALS and here the picture seems less ambiguous. Neither marker was detected in spinal cords of controls, but both were highly expressed in spinal cords of ALS cases[63] and transgenic SOD1^{G93A} mice, respectively.[61] Likewise, the levels of apoptosis-related protein prostate apoptosis response-4[69] were increased in spinal cord samples from both ALS patients and transgenic mutant SOD1 mice compared with their respective controls.[70] Together with the morphological data summarized earlier, these findings provide support to the view that apoptosis occurs in ALS. What all of these studies fail to do, however, is to provide definite mechanistic insights into the significance of these alterations in the pathogenesis of ALS.

ACTIVATION OF MOLECULAR CELL DEATH PATHWAYS IN AMYOTROPHIC LATERAL SCLEROSIS

Given the ambiguous results of the morphological studies, it appears that a more convincing approach to evaluating the role of apoptosis in ALS may be achieved by demonstrating whether the neurodegenerative process in transgenic mutant SOD1 mice, irrespective of the morphology of the dying cells, involves known molecular mediators of PCD and whether targeting such key factors can affect the course of the disease.

PCD is a multistep machinery (Figure 14.2) that involves a complex inter-action between survival pathways, which are activated by trophic factors, and death pathways, which are activated by various stresses. So far, the two pathways that have been most implicated in neuronal survival are the phos-phatidylinositol-3-kinase pathway, which activates Akt (also known as *protein kinase B*) to suppress the activation of proapoptotic proteins, and the extracel-lular signal-regulated kinase (ERK) mitogen-activated protein kinase pathway, which activates antiapoptotic proteins.[71]

The best-known apoptosis-mediating pathways are those involved in the activation of downstream caspases, and some authors go so far as to redefine apoptosis as caspase-mediated cell death. The caspases are a family of *cysteine-aspartate proteases* (Figure 14.2; see later for details), many of which are involved in apoptosis either at the level of upstream signaling (notably

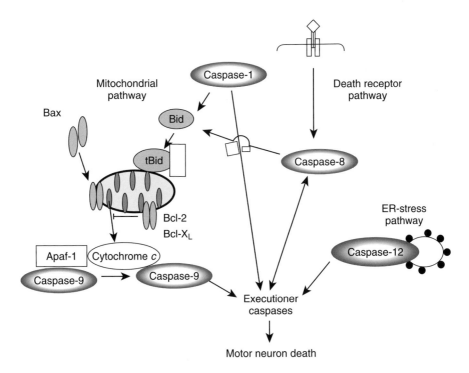

Figure 14.2 Programmed cell death molecular pathways.

caspase-8 and caspase-9) or more downstream at the effector level (notably caspase-3). Caspase-8 and caspase-9 both cleave procaspase-3 to activate it. Caspase-9 is activated by a signal derived from mitochondria under the control of the Bcl-2 family of proteins (see Figure 14.2; see below for details). Caspase-8 is activated by death receptors (members of the tumor necrosis factor [TNF] family) in the plasma membrane via the intermediary of adaptor proteins.[72] Death receptors include Fas (CD95), which seems to participate in the neurodegenerative process that affects transgenic mice expressing mutant SOD1,[73] and the low-affinity neurotrophin receptor (p75[NTR]). Other key molecules in apoptotic signaling include ceramide, mitogen-activated protein kinases (c-Jun/N-terminal kinase and p38) and the transcription factors AP-1 and nuclear factor-κB.[71,72]

In light of the presumed proapoptotic property of mutant SOD1,[47] it is tempting to suggest that the mutant protein may be a death-signaling molecule in itself, either directly by setting in motion the PCD cascade or indirectly by interacting with various intracellular targets such as trophic factors, Bcl-2 family members, or even mitochondria. The latter target is particularly appealing because mitochondria are structurally and functionally altered in transgenic mutant SOD1 mice[74,75] and play a pivotal role in PCD.[76] Also relevant to the issue of death/survival signals in the mutant SOD1 model are the Western blot and immunohistochemical demonstrations that the survival signal mediated by PI3K/AkT is weakened in spinal cords of transgenic mutant SOD1 mice even before overt neuropathological features arise.[77] Once the mutant SOD1-mediated neurodegenerative process has been initiated, several secondary alterations develop in the spinal cord of transgenic mutant SOD1 mice, including microglial cell activation[78] and T-cell infiltration,[79] both of which may release a plethora of cytokines and other pro-PCD mediators. Accordingly, although the nature of the initial death signal in transgenic mutant SOD1 mice remains elusive, in a more advanced stage of their pathology, the increased expression of several extracellular inflammation-related factors such as interleukin-1β (IL-1β), IL-6, and TNF-α[80] may amplify the death signals already reaching motor neurons in this mouse model of ALS by activating death receptors such as Fas;[73] IL-1β contents are also elevated in ALS spinal cords.[51]

PRO–CELL DEATH ALTERATIONS IN BCL-2 FAMILY MEMBERS IN AMYOTROPHIC LATERAL SCLEROSIS

Largely implicated in the regulation of PCD (see Figure 14.2), the Bcl-2 family is composed of both cell death suppressors such as Bcl-2 or Bcl-xL and promoters such as Bax, Bad, Bak, or Bcl-xS.[81] Many of these molecules are present and active within the nervous system and appear to be potent modulators of neuronal death.[82] For example, overexpression of Bcl-2 and Bcl-xL leads to increased cell survival in many neuronal systems and can protect against both experimental and genetic lesions.[83,84] Likewise, facial motor neurons in Bax null mutant mice show increased numbers at birth and resistance to death induced by neonatal axotomy.[85] Conversely, Bcl-2 knockout mice show progressive loss of a fraction of facial motor neurons and sensory neurons, and sympathetic and sensory neurons from these mice show diminished survival in culture at appropriate stages.[82] Mice deficient in Bcl-xL die at embryonic day 13 and exhibit massive death of immature postmitotic neurons throughout the brain and the spinal cord.[82]

In human ALS cases and affected transgenic SOD1[G93A] mice, *bcl2* mRNA content appears significantly decreased and that of *bax* mRNA significantly increased in the lumbar cord compared with controls.[86,87] At the protein level, spinal cord expression of the antiapoptotic proteins Bcl-2 and Bcl-xL are either unchanged[64,88] or decreased,[54,87] whereas that of the proapoptotic Bax and Bad proteins are increased[54,64,87] in both human ALS cases and symptomatic transgenic SOD1[G93A] mice. Because different SOD1 mutations do not cause the exactly same neuropathology, it is important to indicate that a very similar pattern of changes of selected pro–cell death and anti–cell death Bcl-2 family members was found in spinal cords of affected transgenic SOD1[G86R] mice compared with their wild type counterparts.[89] None of these alterations, however, is seen in young asymptomatic transgenic SOD1[G93A] mice, but they clearly become progressively more conspicuous as the neurodegenerative process progresses.[87] From a functional standpoint, it must be indicated that some key Bcl-2 family members can form homodimers (e.g., Bax/Bax) or heterodimers (e.g., Bax/Bcl-2), which alter the ability of a given Bcl-2 member to promote or inhibit cell death.[82] In keeping with this, it should be indicated that Bax in the spinal cord of both ALS patients and affected transgenic mutant SOD1 mice is not only upregulated but also expressed mainly in its deleterious homodimeric conformation.[54,87] In addition, in these animals Bax appears markedly relocated from the cytosol to the mitochondria[54,90] (Figure 14.3A), which is in many cellular settings another prerequisite to Bax activation of PCD. All of these data suggest that in ALS, during the neurodegenerative process, the finely tuned balance between cell death antagonists and agonists of the Bcl-2 family is upset toward a situation in which pro–cell death forces dominate. Consistent with this view is the demonstration that overexpression of Bcl-2, presumably by buffering some of the pro–cell death drive,[87] mitigates neurodegeneration both in in vitro and in vivo models of ALS[48,50] and prolongs survival in transgenic SOD1[G93A] mice.[50]

Other meaningful Bcl-2 family members that appear to be in play in ALS include Bid and harakiri, two potent pro-PCD peptides, which can participate in the cell death process either directly or indirectly by potentiating the effect of Bax. Bid appears highly expressed in the spinal cord of transgenic SOD1[G93A] mice and is cleaved into its most active form during the progression of the disease.[91] As for harakiri, its expression has been detected in motor neurons of ALS spinal cord specimens but not in that of controls, specifically in neurons that exhibited an abnormal morphology reminiscent of that labeled by Troost et al[88] as apoptotic.[92]

A fascinating issue concerning the deregulation of Bcl-2 family members in ALS is the elucidation of how those changes occur. As far as Bax is concerned, as in other pathological situations, it is unlikely that mutant SOD1 directly produces the observed changes in Bax. Instead, it is more likely that mutant SOD1 activates intracellular signaling pathways, which in turn cause Bax upregulation and translocation. This scenario will be in line with what we currently know about the regulation of Bax and how Bax is usually brought into action in PCD.

Relevant to the present discussion is the fact that the tumor suppressor protein p53 counts among the rare identified molecules known to regulate Bax expression.[93] In normal situations, p53 basal levels in the cell are very low, but upon activation as seen in pathological situations, there is a rapid rise in p53 mRNA and protein levels, as well as post-translational modifications that stabilize the protein.[94] Activation of the p53 pathway in ALS is evidenced by demonstrations that p53 is increased in the nuclear fraction of affected brain regions in patients with ALS[95] and by p53 immunostaining in neuron nuclei of transgenic SOD1[G86R] mice.[89] Despite the compelling evidence that p53 is activated in ALS, two independent studies have failed to provide any supportive data for an instrumental role of this transcription factor in the death of motor neurons in transgenic mutant SOD1 mice.[96]

CASPASE ACTIVATION DURING AMYOTROPHIC LATERAL SCLEROSIS NEURODEGENERATIVE PROCESS

All caspases share the ability to cleave their substrates after specific aspartic acid residues, and all are present in cells as inactive zymogens, called *procaspases*, but they differ in their primary sequences and substrate specificity.[97] An instrumental role for caspases in ALS neurodegeneration is supported by the demonstration that the irreversible broad-caspase inhibitor benzyloxycarbonyl-Val-Ala-Asp(*O*-methyl)-fluoromethylketone attenuates mutant SOD1–mediated cell death in transfected PC-12 cells[48] and in transgenic SOD1[G93A] mice.[51]

All of the identified caspases are grouped based on their function. One group includes caspase-1, -4, -5, -11, -12, and -14, which are now believed to play a role primarily in cytokine maturation. Among these, so far in ALS the lion's share has been given to caspase-1, the key enzyme responsible for the activation of IL-1β. Procaspase-1 is highly expressed in spinal cord motor neurons and its activation in spinal cord of transgenic mutant SOD1 mice coincides with the development of the glial response and with the very beginning of the loss of motor neurons in transgenic mutant SOD1 mice.[51,60,61,90,98] Despite its likely indirect role in PCD, chronic inhibition of caspase-1 by a dominant negative mutant of the enzyme has been proven effective in prolonging the life span in transgenic SOD1[G93A] mice.[99] So far, the status of the other members of the caspase-1 subfamily in ALS is unknown. Some preliminary investigations show that caspase-12, which is known to be activated following endoplasmic reticulum stress,[100] is expressed in motor neurons of non-transgenic mice and even more so in those of symptomatic transgenic SOD1[G93A] mice (C. Guégan and S. Przedborski, unpublished observation). In symptomatic transgenic SOD1[G93A] mice, most of the motor neurons immunopositive for caspase-12 appear condensed, shrunken, and vacuolized. Although more work on caspase-12 remains to be done in this model of ALS, our preliminary data argue that sick cells are the site of an endoplasmic reticulum stress whose occurrence could well contribute to the overall cascade of deleterious events that ultimately underlies the demise of spinal cord motor neurons in the mutant SOD1 model.

By contrast, caspase-2, -3, -6, -7, -8, -9, and -10 have been implicated in apoptosis per se, although their roles can be further divided into initiator and effector. Initiator caspases include procaspase-2, -8, -9, and -10, all of which have long prodomains and protein–protein interaction motifs such as the death effector domain and the caspase activation and recruitment domain that contribute to the transduction of various signals into proteolytic activity. Among these, procaspase-8 is activated after ligation of certain cell surface receptors such as the TNF receptors. Interestingly, although significant glial response and production of IL-1β occurs early in transgenic mutant SOD1 mice (see earlier), activation of caspase-8, like induction of TNF-α,[80] is only detected in spinal cords near end stage.[91] This finding suggests that in this ALS model, the TNF/caspase-8 machinery may be a late contributor to the degenerative process. Caspase-2 is another initiator of PCD whose activation also occurs in the spinal cord of affected transgenic mutant SOD1 mice (Vukosavic, Leonidas, and Przedborski, unpublished observation). Yet, ablation of caspase-2 in transgenic SOD1^{G93A} mice has been reported to have no effect on the course of the disease,[101] indicating that whatever the role of caspase-2 is in ALS, it is dispensable. A third initiator caspase is caspase-9, whose role is pivotal in the so-called mitochondrial-dependent PCD pathway.[76] Here, after a death stimulus, released mitochondrial cytochrome *c* interacts in the cytosol with Apaf-1 in the presence of dATP, which stimulates the processing of procaspase-9 into its active form, which in turn can activate the downstream executioner caspases (see later discussion). Evidence of a prominent recruitment of this mitochondrial pathway has been documented in spinal cord specimens of both patients with ALS and transgenic SOD1^{G93A} mice.[90] In this work, it is demonstrated that although cytochrome *c* is confined to the mitochondria in cells in normal control samples, it is diffusely distributed in the cytosol in several of the spared cells, especially neurons, in the pathological samples. It is also demonstrated, at least in transgenic mutant SOD1^{G93A} mice, that the mitochondrial cytochrome *c* translocation to the cytosol occurs at the same time as the cytosolic Bax translocation to the mitochondria and activation of caspase-9 and before activation of downstream caspase executioners such as caspase-3 and caspase-7 (Figure 14.3). Because caspase-9 is thought to be so critical in many cell death settings, it is predictable that the observed translocation of cytochrome *c* and activation of caspase-9 in ALS represent significant pathological events. Consistent with this view is the demonstration that preventing mitochondrial cytochrome *c* release enhances the life span of transgenic SOD1^{G93A} mice.[102] Effector caspases include procaspase-3, -6, and -7, all of which have short prodomains and lack intrinsic enzymatic activity. However, upon their cleavage, which is triggered by, for example, initiator caspases, effector caspases acquire the capacity of cleaving a large number of intracellular substrates, which probably results in the eventual death of the cell. Consistent with this scenario, it has been reported that key effector caspases such as caspase-3 and -7 (see Figure 14.3C) are indeed activated in spinal cords of transgenic mutant SOD1 mice in a time-dependent manner that parallels the time course of the neurodegenerative process[60,61]; activation of caspase-3 has also been observed in spinal cord samples from patients with ALS.[54] Yet, current data on the sequence of events in the PCD cascade indicate that once effector caspases have been activated, the cell death process, at least in certain pathological settings, has reached a point of no return. This would suggest that in these specific conditions, the death commitment point is situated upstream to these caspases, and consequently,

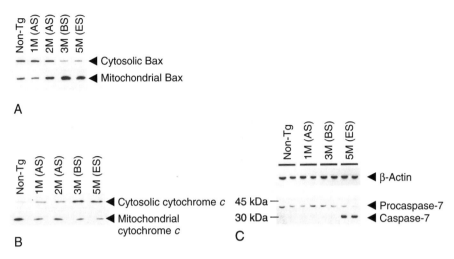

Figure 14.3 Illustrations of programmed cell death alterations in spinal cord of transgenic mutant SOD1 mice. **(A)** Western blot analysis of spinal cord extracts, demonstrating the relocation of Bax from the cytosol **(top)** to the mitochondria **(bottom)** over the course of the disease. **(B)** Coincidental changes of cytochrome *c* in the opposite direction. **(C)** Later in the disease, effector caspases such as caspase-7 are activated. 1M (AS) = 1 month asymptomatic stage; 2M (AS) = 2 months asymptomatic stage; 3M (BS) = 3 months beginning of symptoms; 5M (ES) = 5 months end stage; Non-Tg = non-transgenic litter mates. (Modified from Guégan C, Vila M, Rosoklija G, et al. Recruitment of the mitochondrial-dependent apoptotic pathway in amyotrophic lateral sclerosis. J Neurosci 2001;21:6569–6576.)

interventions aimed at inhibiting these downstream caspases may fail to provide any real neuroprotective benefit[103]; whether this applies to the demise of motor neurons in ALS remains to be determined.

CONCLUSION

We have described the evidence that numerous key molecular components of PCD are recruited in ALS. We have also shown that although precious data on PCD in ALS have been obtained thanks to the study of postmortem human samples, information regarding the temporal relationships of these changes and their significance in the pathological cascade emanates essentially from the use of transgenic mutant SOD1 mouse models. In light of the aforementioned PCD-related changes, it would appear that this active form of cell death is not the sole pathological mediator of cell demise in ALS but one key component within a coalition of deleterious factors ultimately responsible for the degenerative process. As discussed, however, the actual relationships between mutant SOD1 and the various other presumed culprits represented by protein aggregates, oxidant production, and PCD activation are still unknown and a better understanding of the pathogenic cascade in ALS will require their elucidation.

In our opinion, one of the most important take-home messages that one can extract from the body of work summarized in this chapter is that an apoptotic morphology should not be used as sole criterion of whether molecular pathways of PCD have been recruited, because this may occur in a neurodegenerative process such as that seen in ALS, even when the prevalent morphology of the dying cells is nonapoptotic.

Quite apart from the question of whether the morphology of dying neurons in ALS is apoptotic is the striking contrast found between the paucity of morphologically identified dying cells and the rather robust spinal cord molecular PCD alterations. How can this striking discrepancy be resolved? First, it is possible that the morphological expression of PCD is much more ephemeral than its molecular translation. Therefore because the degenerative process in ALS is asynchronous, small lasting differences in the expression of these markers may have a significant impact on the total number of cells that exhibit a given marker at a given time point. Second, it is also possible that because apoptotic morphological features are confined to the cell body of the dying cells and PCD molecular alterations are not, the detection of the former may be much more challenging than that of the latter. And third, it should also be considered that the molecular tools used in all of the cited studies see not only the rare truly dying cells but also the numerous sick cells, which ultimately may or may not die and thus may or may not show the typical apoptotic morphology.

Another important point that derives from the work in transgenic mutant SOD1 mice is that not only neurons but also glial cells appear to be the site of PCD cascade activation. This observation does not undermine the potential causative role of PCD in the ALS death process but raises the possibility that PCD may not kill solely neurons in this disease. Because SOD1 is expressed in all cells and not only in motor neurons, it is possible that the activation of PCD in both neurons and glia reflects the ubiquitous nature of the mutant protein expression and thus a similar situation may not be true in the forms of ALS not associated to mutant SOD1.

Clearly the overall mechanism of neurodegeneration in ALS is still incompletely known. Nevertheless, the currently available evidence indicates that PCD is in play in ALS and thus warrants further investigation of the role of the PCD cascade(s) in ALS pathogenesis and treatment. So far, the most effective therapeutic strategies in transgenic mutant SOD1 mice target distinct molecular pathways, but we predict that ultimately the best therapy for ALS will involve a pharmacological cocktail directed against multiple components of these pathways.

Acknowledgments

We wish to thank Drs. Robert E. Burke and Miquel Vila for their insightful comments on the manuscript and Ms. Pat White and Mr. Brian Jones for their help in its preparation. We wish also to acknowledge the support of the NIH/NINDS grants R29 NS37345, RO1 NS38586 and NS42269, and P50 NS38370, the U.S. Department of Defense grant (DAMD 17-99-1-9471), the Lowenstein Foundation, the Lillian Goldman Charitable Trust, the Parkinson's

Disease Foundation, the Muscular Dystrophy Association, the ALS Association, Project-ALS, and the Swiss National Science Foundation (31-61736.00).

REFERENCES

1. Clarke PGH. Developmental cell death: morphological diversity and multiple mechanisms. Anat Embryol 1990;181:195–213.
2. Clarke PGH. Apoptosis Versus Necrosis. In VE Koliatsos, RR Ratan (eds), Cell Death and Diseases of the Nervous System. New Jersey: Humana Press, 1999;3–28.
3. Kerr JFR, Wyllie AH, Currie AR. Apoptosis: a basic biological phenomenon with wide-ranging implications in tissue kinetics. Br J Cancer 1972;26:239–257.
4. Sloviter RS. Apoptosis: a guide for the perplexed. Trends Pharmacol Sci 2002;23:19–24.
5. Bursch W. The autophagosomal-lysosomal compartment in programmed cell death. Cell Death Differ 2001;8:569–581.
6. Uchiyama Y. Autophagic cell death and its execution by lysosomal cathepsins [review]. Arch Histol Cytol 2001;64:233–246.
7. Xue LZ, Fletcher GC, Tolkovsky AM. Autophagy is activated by apoptotic signaling in sympathetic neurons: an alternative mechanism of death execution. Mol Cell Neurosci 1999;14:180–198.
8. Kitanaka C, Kuchino Y. Caspase-independent programmed cell death with necrotic morphology. Cell Death Differ 1999;6:508–515.
9. Castagné V, Gautschi M, Lefèvre K, et al. Relationships between neuronal death and the cellular redox status. Focus on the developing nervous system. Prog Neurobiol 1999;59:397–423.
10. Lefèvre K, Clarke PGH, Danthe EE, Castagné V. Involvement of cyclin-dependent kinases in axotomy-induced retinal ganglion cell death. J Comp Neurol 2002;447:72–81.
11. Sperandio S, de BI, Bredesen DE. An alternative, nonapoptotic form of programmed cell death. Proc Natl Acad Sci USA 2000;97:14376–14381.
12. Wyllie AH, Kerr JF, Currie AR. Cell death: the significance of apoptosis. Int Rev Cytol 1980;68:251–306.
13. Moroni F, Meli E, Peruginelli F, et al. Poly(ADP-ribose) polymerase inhibitors attenuate necrotic but not apoptotic neuronal death in experimental models of cerebral ischemia. Cell Death Differ 2001;8:921–932.
14. Borsello T, Bonny C, Riederer BM, Clarke PGH. Cell-permeable peptides inhibit JNK action, and completely protect neurons from NMDA-induced necrotic death. Soc Neurosci Abstr 2001;27:267–215.
15. Hayward NJ, Elliott PJ, Sawyer SD, et al. Lack of evidence for neutrophil participation during infarct formation following focal cerebral ischemia in the rat. Exp Neurol 1996;139:188–202.
16. Pilar G, Landmesser L. Ultrastructural differences during embryonic cell death in normal and peripherally deprived ciliary ganglia. J Cell Biol 1976;68:339–356.
17. Cuadros MA, Martin D, Pérez-Mendoza D, et al. Response of macrophage/microglial cells to experimental neuronal degeneration in the avian isthmo-optic nucleus during development. J Comp Neurol 2000;423:659–669.
18. Blaschke AJ, Weiner JA, Chun J. Programmed cell death is a universal feature of embryonic and postnatal neuroproliferative regions throughout the central nervous system. J Comp Neurol 1998;396:39–50.
19. Burek MJ, Oppenheim RW. Cellular Interactions that Regulate Programmed Cell Death in the Developing Vertebrate Nervous System. In VE Koliatsos, RR Ratan (eds), Cell Death and Diseases of the Nervous System. New Jersey: Humana Press, 1999;145–179.
20. Knyihar E, Csillik B, Rakic P. Transient synapses in the embryonic primate spinal cord. Science 1978;202:1206–1209.
21. Catsicas M, Péquignot Y, Clarke PGH. Rapid onset of neuronal death induced by blockade of either axoplasmic transport or action potentials in afferent fibers during brain development. J Neurosci 1992;12:4642–4650.
22. von Bartheld CS. Neurotrophins in the developing and regenerating visual system. Histol Histopathol 1998;13:437–459.
23. Alcantara S, Frisen J, del Rio JA, et al. TrkB signaling is required for postnatal survival of CNS neurons and protects hippocampal and motor neurons from axotomy-induced cell death. J Neurosci 1997;17:3623–3633.

24. Woolley A, Sheard P, Dodds K, Duxson M. Alpha motoneurons are present in normal numbers but with reduced soma size in neurotrophin-3 knockout mice. Neurosci Lett 1999;272:107–110.
25. von Bartheld CS, Johnson JE. Target-derived BDNF (brain-derived neurotrophic factor) is essential for the survival of developing neurons in the isthmo-optic nucleus. J Comp Neurol 2001;433:550–564.
26. Thoenen H. Neurotrophins and activity-dependent plasticity. Prog Brain Res 2000;128:183–191.
27. Oppenheim RW, Prevette D, D'Costa A, et al. Reduction of neuromuscular activity is required for the rescue of motoneurons from naturally occurring cell death by nicotinic-blocking agents. J Neurosci 2000;20:6117–6124.
28. Primi M-P, Clarke PGH. Presynaptic initiation by action potentials of retrograde signals in developing neurons. J Neurosci 1997;17:4253–4261.
29. Li LX, Wu WT, Lin LFH, et al. Rescue of adult mouse motoneurons from injury-induced cell death by glial cell line-derived neurotrophic factor. Proc Natl Acad Sci USA 1995;92:9771–9775.
30. Eisen A, Weber M. Treatment of amyotrophic lateral sclerosis [review]. Drugs Aging 1999;14: 173–196.
31. Apfel SC. Neurotrophic factor therapy—prospects and problems. Clin Chem Lab Med 2001;39: 351–355.
32. Russell FD, Koishi K, Jiang Y, McLennan IS. Anterograde axonal transport of glial cell line–derived neurotrophic factor and its receptors in rat hypoglossal nerve. Neuroscience 2000;97:575–580.
33. Rowland LP. Hereditary and Acquired Motor Neuron Diseases. In LP Rowland (ed), Merritt's Textbook of Neurology. Philadelphia: Williams & Wilkins, 1995;742–749.
34. Deng H-X, Hentati A, Tainer JA, et al. Amyotrophic lateral sclerosis and structural defects in Cu,Zn superoxide dismutase. Science 1993;261:1047–1051.
35. Rosen DR, Siddique T, Patterson D, et al. Mutations in Cu/Zn superoxide dismutase gene are associated with familial amyotrophic lateral sclerosis. Nature 1993;362:59–62.
36. Brown RH, Jr. Amyotrophic lateral sclerosis: recent insights from genetics and transgenic mice. Cell 1995;80:687–692.
37. Przedborski S, Donaldson D, Murphy PL, et al. Blood superoxide dismutase, catalase and glutathione peroxidase activities in familial and sporadic amyotrophic lateral sclerosis. Neurodegeneration 1996;5:57–64.
38. Troy CM, Shelanski ML. Down-regulation of copper/zinc superoxide dismutase causes apoptotic death in PC12 neuronal cells. Proc Natl Acad Sci USA 1994;91:6384–6387.
39. Rothstein JD, Bristol LA, Hosler B, et al. Chronic inhibition of superoxide dismutase produces apoptotic death of spinal neurons. Proc Natl Acad Sci USA 1994;91:4155–4159.
40. Reaume AG, Elliott JL, Hoffman EK, et al. Motor neurons in Cu/Zn superoxide dismutase-deficient mice develop normally but exhibit enhanced cell death after axonal injury. Nat Genet 1996;13:43–47.
41. Gurney ME, Pu H, Chiu AY, et al. Motor neuron degeneration in mice that express a human Cu, Zn superoxide dismutase mutation. Science 1994;264:1772–1775.
42. Wong PC, Pardo CA, Borchelt DR, et al. An adverse property of a familial ALS-linked SOD1 mutation causes motor neuron disease characterized by vacuolar degeneration of mitochondria. Neuron 1995;14:1105–1116.
43. Bruijn LI, Becher MW, Lee MK, et al. ALS-linked SOD1 mutant G85R mediated damage to astrocytes and promotes rapidly progressive disease with SOD1-containing inclusions. Neuron 1997;18: 327–338.
44. Nagai M, Aoki M, Miyoshi I, et al. Rats expressing human cytosolic copper-zinc superoxide dismutase transgenes with amyotrophic lateral sclerosis: associated mutations develop motor neuron disease. J Neurosci 2001;21:9246–9254.
45. Subramaniam JR, Lyons WE, Liu J, et al. Mutant SOD1 causes motor neuron disease independent of copper chaperone-mediated copper loading. Nat Neurosci 2002;5:301–307.
46. Brown RH Jr. Superoxide dismutase in familial amyotrophic lateral sclerosis: models for gain of function. Curr Opin Neurobiol 1995;5:841–846.
47. Rabizadeh S, Gralla EB, Borchelt DR, et al. Mutations associated with amyotrophic lateral sclerosis convert superoxide dismutase from an antiapoptotic gene to a proapoptotic gene: studies in yeast and neural cells. Proc Natl Acad Sci USA 1995;92:3024–3028.
48. Ghadge GD, Lee JP, Bindokas VP, et al. Mutant superoxide dismutase-1–linked familial amyotrophic lateral sclerosis: molecular mechanisms of neuronal death and protection. J Neurosci 1997;17:8756–8766.
49. Mena MA, Khan U, Togasaki DM, et al. Effects of wild-type and mutated copper/zinc superoxide dismutase on neuronal survival and L-DOPA–induced toxicity in postnatal midbrain culture. J Neurochem 1997;69:21–33.

50. Kostic V, Jackson-Lewis V, De Bilbao F, et al. Bcl-2: Prolonging life in a transgenic mouse model of familial amyotrophic lateral sclerosis. Science 1997;277:559–562.
51. Li M, Ona VO, Guegan C, et al. Functional role of caspase-1 and caspase-3 in an ALS transgenic mouse model. Science 2000;288:335–339.
52. Cleveland DW, Rothstein JD. From Charcot to Lou Gehrig: deciphering selective motor neuron death in ALS. Nat Rev Neurosci 2001;2:806–819.
53. Hirano A. Aspects of the ultrastructure of amyotrophic lateral sclerosis. Adv Neurol 1982;36:75–88.
54. Martin LJ. Neuronal death in amyotrophic lateral sclerosis is apoptosis: possible contribution of a programmed cell death mechanism. J Neuropathol Exp Neurol 1999;58:459–471.
55. Mitsumoto H, Chad DA, Pioro EP. Amyotrophic lateral sclerosis. Philadelphia: FA Davis, 1998; 285–302.
56. Mitsumoto H, Bradley WG. Murine motor neuron disease (the Wobbler mouse): degeneration and regeneration of the lower motor neuron. Brain 1982;105(pt 4):811–834.
57. Divers TJ, Mohammed HO, Cummings JF. Equine motor neuron disease. Vet Clin North Am Equine Pract 1997;13:97–105.
58. Dal Canto MC, Gurney ME. Neuropathological changes in two lines of mice carrying a transgene for mutant human Cu,Zn SOD, and in mice overexpressing wild type human SOD: a model of familial amyotrophic lateral sclerosis (FALS). Brain Res 1995;676:25–40.
59. Migheli A, Atzori C, Piva R, et al. Lack of apoptosis in mice with ALS. Nat Med 1999;5:966–967.
60. Pasinelli P, Houseweart MK, Brown RH Jr, Cleveland DW. Caspase-1 and -3 are sequentially activated in motor neuron death in Cu,Zn superoxide dismutase–mediated familial amyotrophic lateral sclerosis. Proc Natl Acad Sci USA 2000;97:13901–13906.
61. Vukosavic S, Stefanis L, Jackson-Lewis V, et al. Delaying caspase activation by Bcl-2: a clue to disease retardation in a transgenic mouse model of amyotrophic lateral sclerosis. J Neurosci 2000; 20:9119–9125.
62. Chiu AY, Zhai P, Dal Canto MC, et al. Age-dependent penetrance of disease in a transgenic mouse model of familial amyotrophic lateral sclerosis. Mol Cell Neurosci 1995;6:349–362.
63. Yoshiyama Y, Yamada T, Asanuma K, Asahi T. Apoptosis related antigen, Le(Y) and nick-end labeling are positive in spinal motor neurons in amyotrophic lateral sclerosis. Acta Neuropathol (Berl) 1994;88:207–211.
64. Ekegren T, Grundstrom E, Lindholm D, Aquilonius SM. Upregulation of Bax protein and increased DNA degradation in ALS spinal cord motor neurons. Acta Neurol Scand 1999;100:317–321.
65. Migheli A, Cavalla P, Marino S, Schiffer D. A study of apoptosis in normal and pathologic nervous tissue after in situ end-labeling of DNA strand breaks. J Neuropathol Exp Neurol 1994;53:606–616.
66. He BP, Strong MJ. Motor neuronal death in sporadic amyotrophic lateral sclerosis (ALS) is not apoptotic. A comparative study of ALS and chronic aluminium chloride neurotoxicity in New Zealand white rabbits. Neuropathol Appl Neurobiol 2000;26:150–160.
67. Hiraishi K, Suzuki K, Hakomori S, Adachi M. Le(y) antigen expression is correlated with apoptosis (programmed cell death). Glycobiology 1993;3:381–390.
68. Suurmeijer AJ, van der Wijk J, van Veldhuisen DJ, et al. Fractin immunostaining for the detection of apoptotic cells and apoptotic bodies in formalin-fixed and paraffin-embedded tissue. Lab Invest 1999;79:619–620.
69. Rangnekar VM. Apoptosis mediated by a novel leucine zipper protein Par-4. Apoptosis 1998;3: 61–66.
70. Pedersen WA, Luo H, Kruman I, et al. The prostate apoptosis response-4 protein participates in motor neuron degeneration in amyotrophic lateral sclerosis. FASEB J 2000;14:913–924.
71. Harper SJ, LoGrasso P. Signaling for survival and death in neurones—The role of stress-activated kinases, JNK and p38. Cell Signal 2001;13:299–310.
72. Gupta S. Molecular steps of death receptor and mitochondrial pathways of apoptosis. Life Sci 2001;69:2957–2964.
73. Raoul C, Estevez A, Nishimune H, et al. Motoneuron death triggered by a specific pathway downstream of Fas. Potentiation by ALS-linked SOD1 mutations. Neuron 2002;35:1067.
74. Kong JM, Xu ZS. Massive mitochondrial degeneration in motor neurons triggers the onset of amyotrophic lateral sclerosis in mice expressing a mutant SOD1. J Neurosci 1998;18:3241–3250.
75. Browne SE, Bowling AC, Baik MJ, et al. Metabolic dysfunction in familial, but not sporadic, amyotrophic lateral sclerosis. J Neurochem 1998;71:281–287.
76. Kroemer G, Reed JC. Mitochondrial control of cell death. Nat Med 2000;6:513–519.
77. Warita H, Manabe Y, Murakami T, et al. Early decrease of survival signal-related proteins in spinal motor neurons of presymptomatic transgenic mice with a mutant SOD1 gene. Apoptosis 2001;6: 345–352.

78. Almer G, Vukosavic S, Romero N, Przedborski S. Inducible nitric oxide synthase upregulation in a transgenic mouse model of familial amyotrophic lateral sclerosis. J Neurochem 1999;72:2415–2425.

79. Alexianu ME, Kozovska M, Appel SH. Immune reactivity in a mouse model of familial ALS correlates with disease progression. Neurology 2001;57:1282–1289.

80. Nguyen MD, Julien JP, Rivest S. Induction of proinflammatory molecules in mice with amyotrophic lateral sclerosis: no requirement for proapoptotic interleukin-1beta in neurodegeneration. Ann Neurol 2001;50:630–639.

81. Chao DT, Korsmeyer SJ. Bcl-2 family: regulators of cell death. Annu Rev Immunol 1998;16: 395–419.

82. Merry DE, Korsmeyer SJ. Bcl-2 gene family in the nervous system. Annu Rev Neurosci 1997;20: 245–267.

83. Martinou J-C, Dubois-Dauphin M, Staple JK, et al. Overexpression of bcl-2 in transgenic mice protects neurons from naturally occurring cell death and experimental ischemia. Neuron 1994;13: 1017–1030.

84. Parsadanian AS, Cheng Y, Keller-Peck CR, et al. Bcl-xL is an antiapoptotic regulator for postnatal CNS neurons. J Neurosci 1998;18:1009–1019.

85. Deckwerth TL, Elliott JL, Knudson CM, et al. Bax is required for neuronal death after trophic factor deprivation and during development. Neuron 1996;17:401–411.

86. Mu X, He J, Anderson DW, et al. Altered expression of bcl-2 and bax mRNA in amyotrophic lateral sclerosis spinal cord motor neurons. Ann Neurol 1996;40:379–386.

87. Vukosavic S, Dubois-Dauphin M, Romero N, Przedborski S. Bax and Bcl-2 interaction in a transgenic mouse model of familial amyotrophic lateral sclerosis. J Neurochem 1999;73:2460–2468.

88. Troost D, Aten J, Morsink F, De Jong JMBV. Apoptosis in amyotrophic lateral sclerosis is not restricted to motor neurons. Bcl-2 expression is increased in unaffected post-central gyrus. Neuropathol Appl Neurobiol 1995;21:498–504.

89. Gonzalez de Aguilar JL, Gordon JW, Rene F, et al. Alteration of the Bcl-x/Bax ratio in a transgenic mouse model of amyotrophic lateral sclerosis: evidence for the implication of the p53 signaling pathway. Neurobiol Dis 2000;7:406–415.

90. Guégan C, Vila M, Rosoklija G, et al. Recruitment of the mitochondrial-dependent apoptotic pathway in amyotrophic lateral sclerosis. J Neurosci 2001;21:6569–6576.

91. Guégan C, Vila M, Teismann P, et al. Instrumental activation of Bid by caspase-1 in a transgenic mouse model of ALS. Mol Cell Neurosci 2002;20:553–562.

92. Shinoe T, Wanaka A, Nikaido T, et al. Upregulation of the pro-apoptotic BH3-only peptide harakiri in spinal neurons of amyotrophic lateral sclerosis patients. Neurosci Lett 2001;313:153–157.

93. Miyashita T, Krajewski S, Krajewska M, et al. Tumor suppressor p53 is a regulator of bcl-2 and bax gene expression in vitro and in vivo. Oncogene 1994;9:1799–1805.

94. Appella E, Anderson CW. Post-translational modifications and activation of p53 by genotoxic stresses. Eur J Biochem 2001;268:2764–2772.

95. Martin LJ. p53 is abnormally elevated and active in the CNS of patients with amyotrophic lateral sclerosis. Neurobiol Dis 2000;7:613–622.

96. Prudlo J, Koenig J, Graser J, et al. Motor neuron cell death in a mouse model of FALS is not mediated by the p53 cell survival regulator. Brain Res 2000;879:183–187.

97. Kaufmann SH, Hengartner MO. Programmed cell death: alive and well in the new millennium. Trends Cell Biol 2001;11:526–534.

98. Pasinelli P, Borchelt DR, Houseweart MK, et al. Caspase-1 is activated in neural cells and tissue with amyotrophic lateral sclerosis-associated mutations in copper-zinc superoxide dismutase. Proc Natl Acad Sci USA 1998;95:15763–15768.

99. Friedlander RM, Brown RH, Gagliardini V, et al. Inhibition of ICE slows ALS in mice. Nature 1997;388:31.

100. Nakagawa T, Zhu H, Morishima N, et al. Caspase-12 mediates endoplasmic-reticulum–specific apoptosis and cytotoxicity by amyloid-beta. Nature 2000;403:98–103.

101. Bergeron L, Perez GI, Macdonald G, et al. Defects in regulation of apoptosis in caspase-2–deficient mice. Genes Dev 1998;12:1304–1314.

102. Zhu S, Stavrovskaya I, Drozda M, et al. Minocycline inhibits cytochrome c release and delays progression of amyotrophic lateral sclerosis in mice. Nature 2002;417:74–78.

103. Zheng TS, Hunot S, Kuida K, et al. Deficiency in caspase-9 or caspase-3 induces compensatory caspase activation. Nat Med 2000;6:1241–1247.

15
Factors Underlying the Selective Vulnerability of Motor Neurons to Neurodegeneration

Heather D. Durham

Why are motor neurons so vulnerable to damage in amyotrophic lateral sclerosis (ALS) and other motor neuron disorders relative to other neuronal populations? Why are certain classes of motor neurons spared even late in clinical disease, that is, those in the oculomotor and abducens nucleus that control eye movements and the neurons in Onuf's nucleus controlling sphincter function? Do common physiological properties contribute to vulnerability of motor neurons in different diseases? Understanding the physiological basis of preferential vulnerability of motor neurons to damage will help in the design of therapies to assist these cells in withstanding the various stresses that precipitate motor neuron disease (MND) or contribute to the rapid progression in the later clinical stages.

All cells are continually under stress through normal metabolic activity and environmental influences. Neurons have the additional strains of neurotransmission and maintenance of extensive dendritic and axonal projections. To maintain homeostasis, cells are equipped with protective mechanisms including antioxidants, calcium-binding proteins, and calcium-sequestering organelles, stress/heat shock proteins (Hsps) to chaperone damaged proteins, and proteasomes and lysosomes to catabolize them, xenobiotic metabolizing enzymes, antiapoptotic proteins and neurotrophic factors. Different types of cells experience a particular complement of stresses, depending on their function and interaction with other cells. They also differ in the constitutive expression of cytoprotective molecules and the ability to increase expression of these proteins when under stress.

This chapter reviews the great progress researchers have made in defining the physiological profile of motor neurons that results in their reduced safety factor to survive disease-related stresses. Motor neurons are under a great deal of stress because of their size, high level of glutamatergic input, calcium-permeable receptor and ion channels, an extensive and aggregation-prone neurofilament (NF) network, and axons that extend outside the protection of

Homeostasis in motor neurons

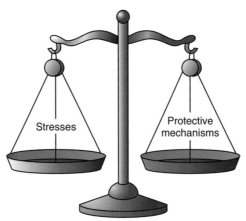

| Stresses | Protective mechanisms |

High metabolic activity
Glutamatergic input
   Quantity
   Ca^{++}-permeable receptors
Large size
   Long, large diameter processes
   Extensive dendritic tree
Neurofilaments
   Numerous and prone to aggregation
Axons extend out of CNS
Xenobiotic exposure
Mutant proteins

Calcium binding proteins* and organelles
Antioxidants
   Glutathione*
   Enzymes*
   Vitamins
Induction of stress proteins*
Catabolic pathways* (proteasomes, lysosomes)
Antiapoptotic proteins
Glial cells
   Glutamate transporters*
   Trophic factors
   Antioxidants

Figure 15.1 To maintain homeostasis, cells are equipped with protective mechanisms to counteract normal physiological stresses and added burdens imposed by expression of mutant proteins or environmental stresses. The profile of stresses and protective mechanisms varies with each cell type. Listed in this figure are (**left**) major factors contributing to vulnerability of motor neurons and (**right**) potential protective mechanisms. Asterisk (*) indicates potential deficiencies in protective mechanisms that could contribute to disease progression. (See text for details.)

the blood-brain barrier. Despite this stressful existence, motor neurons susceptible in ALS are deficient in several protective mechanisms, including cytosolic calcium-binding proteins and glutathione, and have a high threshold for inducing expression of protective molecules such as stress proteins and metallothioneins when under stress (Figure 15.1). Many of these factors also are discussed in Chapters 8 through 13 from the perspective of disease pathogenesis.

GLUTAMATERGIC INPUT

Lower motor neurons (LMNs) receive a high level of glutamatergic input from primary afferent sensory neurons, upper motor neurons (UMNs) and excitatory

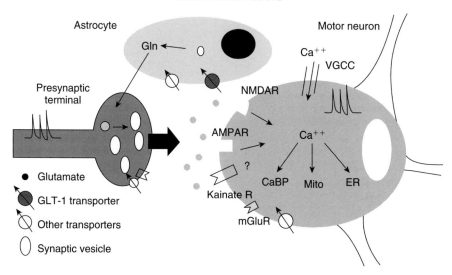

Glutamatergic neurotransmission and calcium
fluxes in motor neurons

Figure 15.2 Motor neurons are particularly vulnerable to excitotoxicity, particularly by calcium-mediated mechanisms. Excitation by the neurotransmitter, glutamate, results in Ca^{2+} entry through calcium-permeable α-amino-3-hydroxy-5-methyl-4-isoxazole propionic acid (AMPA) receptors, *N*-methyl-D-aspartate (NMDA) receptors, and voltage-gated calcium channels (VGCCs). Intracellular Ca^{2+} is sequestered by cytosolic calcium-binding protein (CaBP) and transported into mitochondria (Mito) or the endoplasmic reticulum (ER). The role of kainate receptors (kainate R) and metabotropic glutamate receptors (mGluRs) in motor neuron vulnerability is not certain. Glutamate is removed from the synaptic cleft by specific glutamate transporters on astrocytes and also neurons. In astrocytes, glutamate is converted to glutamine (Gl) and recycled to presynaptic nerve terminals. See color insert.

interneurons, which synapse onto their cell bodies and dendrites. Neurons, including motor neurons, express α-amino-3-hydroxy-5-methyl-4-isoxazole propionic acid (AMPA), kainate, *N*-methyl-D-aspartate (NMDA), and metabotropic subtypes of glutamate receptors (GluRs), with the fast current essential for neurotransmission being carried by AMPA/kainate receptors (Figure 15.2). Motor neurons are extremely vulnerable to excitotoxic cell death.[1,2] In general, the amount of Ca^{2+} influx induced by specific GluR agonists correlates with their toxicity.[3] Whereas in many types of neurons, Ca^{2+} influx through NMDA receptors is the major contributor to excitotoxic injury, AMPA/kainate receptor excitation is of paramount importance in motor neurons, particularly with long-duration low-level activation.[3–9] Even though motor neurons have a high AMPA receptor current density,[10] expression of GluRs does not by itself account for the sensitivity of motor neurons to excitotoxicity or the preferential vulnerability of motor neurons in ALS because many classes of neurons that receive glutamatergic input are more resistant to damage. However, the following evidence demonstrates that the presence of a specific subtype of AMPA receptor that is permeable to calcium ions is important.

AMPA receptors are formed by homo-oligomeric or hetero-oligomeric assembly of four receptor subunits termed *GluR1, GluR2, GluR3,* and *GluR4.*[11] When incorporated into AMPA receptors, GluR2 prevents Ca^{2+} influx during channel opening, but to do so, the subunit must undergo Q/R editing at the RNA level.[12] Although the level of expression of GluR2 in motor neurons has been somewhat controversial, immunocytochemical, electrophysiological, and pharmacological studies have demonstrated that motor neurons, both in intact spinal cord and in culture, have a significant population of AMPA receptors that lack GluR2.[3,8,9,13–25] Indeed, a specific inhibitor of Ca^{2+}-permeable AMPA receptors (the joro spider toxin) reduced both AMPA-induced death of cultured motor neurons and toxicity of mutant copper/zinc superoxide dismutase (SOD1) responsible for a familial form of ALS (FALS-1).[21] Neuroprotection in this culture model also was obtained by increasing the level of Q/R-edited, but not unedited, GluR2 in motor neurons by gene transfer.[26]

Normally, essentially all GluR2 RNA undergoes Q/R editing. In one study, reduced efficiency of Q/R editing was measured in ventral spinal cord of a subpopulation of patients with ALS, whereas editing was normal in unaffected nervous tissues.[27] Deficiencies in RNA processing in compromised cells could impair GluR2 editing, resulting in a greater percentage of AMPA receptors being calcium permeable and a further exacerbation of cytotoxicity.

The kainate receptor subunit GluR6 also undergoes Q/R editing[12] and therefore prevents Ca^{2+} influx through the receptor channel. Although GluR6 is present on embryonic motor neurons,[17,28] this subunit was not detected in adult mouse spinal cord.[28] The significance to vulnerability of motor neurons has not been established.

Other sources of intracellular Ca^{2+} include influx through voltage-gated calcium channels (VGCC) and release from intracellular stores, particularly endoplasmic reticulum. Although the VGCC blocker nifedipine was slightly protective in a culture model of FALS-1,[21] similar agents such as verapamil and nimodipine were not effective in slowing progression of sporadic ALS (SALS) in clinical trials.[29–31]

Immunoglobulin G (IgG) from serum of patients with ALS has been shown to include antibodies to L-type VGCC. In passive transfer experiments, IgG fractions increased Ca^{2+} in motor nerve terminals, suggesting another possible source of intracellular calcium in the disease state.[32,33]

As reviewed in Chapter 10, there is considerable evidence that direct excitotoxicity resulting from increased levels of GluR activation contribute to the progression of motor neuron loss in animal models of MNDs and patients with ALS. Elevated levels of excitatory amino acids have been measured in serum and cerebrospinal fluid in patients with ALS,[34–36] glutamate transport is decreased in brain and spinal cord in ALS,[37] and loss of the glial glutamate transporter (GLT-1) has been measured in human patients with SALS,[38] in transgenic mice expressing G85R mutant SOD1,[39] and in G93A mutant SOD1 transgenic rats.[40] Reuptake of glutamate from the synaptic cleft by these specific transporters is essential to control the duration of receptor stimulation following presynaptic release of the neurotransmitter. Inhibition of transporter function has been shown experimentally to induce excitotoxic death of motor neurons in culture.[41]

The aforementioned studies demonstrated the importance of excitotoxicity, at least in later stages of disease, and provided the rationale for the therapeutic use of antiglutamate drugs including riluzole in ALS. However, the clinical benefit has been disappointing.[42] This could mean that excitotoxicity is not a major contributor to motor neuron death, that other risk factors are more important, or that even physiological levels of GluR activation may be sufficient to increase the vulnerability of motor neurons to disease-related stressors. In a primary culture model of FALS, which was established by microinjection of mutant SOD1 plasmid expression vectors into nuclei of motor neurons in dissociated cultures of murine spinal cord, toxicity of mutant SOD1 was prevented by AMPA/kainate receptor antagonists.[21] These experiments demonstrated that even nonlethal levels of glutamate present in the culture were sensitizing motor neurons to the damaging effects of mutant protein. In another study, motor neurons in cultures established from mutant SOD1 mice exhibited greatly increased vulnerability to glutamate toxicity.[43] If these observations in culture are relevant in vivo, therapies that target neurotransmitter release may be of limited benefit because levels required to significantly protect motor neurons would also impair neurotransmission and motor function. If so, postsynaptic consequences of GluR activation may be more effective therapeutic targets.

CALCIUM-BINDING PROTEINS

Pools of motor neurons that are preserved in patients with ALS (e.g., oculomotor and abducens nuclei) express significant levels of one or more cytosolic calcium-binding proteins (CaBPs), whereas vulnerable populations do not.[44–48] Indeed, the calcium-buffering capacity is much larger in oculomotor compared to spinal motor neurons.[49,50] CaBPs, such as calbindin D-28k, parvalbumin, calretinin, and neurocalcin, buffer calcium ions in the cytoplasm that enter through glutamate receptors and VGCC during neurotransmission, preventing inappropriate activation of calcium-dependent proteases and signaling pathways. It appears that motoneuronal vulnerability results from the combination of the high level of Ca^{2+} influx associated with neurotransmission in motor neurons, increased GluR activation resulting from impaired glutamate transporter function, and low calcium-buffering capacity, rather than one of these factors alone.

Several studies have demonstrated the cytoprotective effect of CaBP against stresses associated with MND: Calbindin D-28k prevented toxicity of ALS IgG in a motoneuron hybrid cell line[51]; calbindin D-28k gene transfer protected cultured primary motor neurons from the toxicity of glutamate, paraquat, and mutant SOD1[21]; calbindin D-28k significantly delayed death of PC12 cells expressing V148G mutant SOD1[52]; parvalbumin overexpression delayed disease onset and slightly prolonged survival in G93A SOD1 transgenic mice[53]; and motor neurons from parvalbumin transgenic mice were more resistant to kainate-induced excitotoxicity than were neurons from non-transgenic litter mates.[54] A potential therapeutic strategy in MND would be to upregulate CaBP by gene therapy or pharmacological agents, but these treatments could have detrimental side effects. In some other neuronal types, increased levels of calbindin potentiates toxicity. For example, hippocampal neurons of calbindin

D-28k knockout mice are more susceptible to ischemia.[55] Inappropriate expression of calbindin could also affect normal physiological functions that depend on calcium transients. Low calcium-buffering capacity may be important physiologically in motor neurons to facilitate the fast recovery times of calcium transients underlying the high-frequency calcium oscillations associated with rhythmical activity in motor neurons.[50]

ANTIOXIDANTS

Most cells maintain strongly reducing conditions by the action of radical scavenging molecules such as glutathione (GSH) and associated enzymes. GSH is a tripeptide (glycine-cysteine-glutamic acid) that serves as a general, nonenzymatic, free-radical scavenger in cells, in addition to being required as a cofactor for glutathione peroxidase in the enzymatic detoxification of hydrogen peroxide generated by dismutation of superoxide. Spinal motor neurons in situ[56,57] and in culture[21] do not contain significant reserves of GSH relative to astrocytes and are particularly vulnerable to oxidative stress. In experimental models, depletion of GSH promotes oxidative stress, whereas an increasing GSH level is neuroprotective.[21,58-60] GSH may also serve as a neuromodulator. GSH-binding sites were increased in spinal cords of patients with SALS, suggesting upregulation due to decreased levels of ligand.[61] Glutathione peroxidase is at least two orders of magnitude lower in ventral spinal cord compared with erythrocytes.[62] This is not likely significant for FALS-1 because crossing mutant SOD1 transgenic mice with glutathione overexpressers failed to alter disease course.[63]

Motor neurons may be deficient in other proteins with antioxidant function. Transcripts encoding certain antioxidant proteins (metallothioneins, thioredoxin, and lysyl oxidase) were elevated in spinal cord of patients with ALS[64] and G93A SOD1 transgenic mice,[65] indicating that some cells had upregulated these proteins; however, neither the cell types responsible for these elevations, nor the ability of motor neurons to upregulate these proteins, has been established. Preliminary studies from our laboratory indicate that cultured motor neurons do not significantly upregulate metallothionein I, II, or III in response to oxidative stress or altered metal homeostasis (Taylor and Durham, unpublished observations).

Neuronal cells have increased exposure to pro-oxidants because of high metabolic activity associated with neurotransmission and higher availability of certain substrates such as unsaturated lipid in neuronal membranes. Glutamate excitotoxicity is mediated by generation of reactive oxygen species (ROS) and through increased Ca^{2+} levels.[66,67] Not only is the restoration of the resting membrane potential and ionic distribution by Na^+/K^+-ATPase metabolically demanding, but an increased intracellular Ca^{2+} level can lead to increased ROS production by perturbing function of mitochondria (a major storage sink for Ca^{2+} loads in cells) and activating calcium-dependent enzymes including neuronal nitric oxide synthase (nNOS), which catalyzes production of nitric oxide.

The evidence for mitochondrial involvement in ALS has been reviewed recently by Menzies, Ince, and Shaw.[68] Structural changes and functional impairment include paracrystallin inclusions, abnormal shapes, increased activity complex I of the electron transport chain, decreased complex IV activity, and increased mitochondrial DNA mutations. In transgenic mice expressing human SOD1 with disease-associated mutations, mitochondrial swelling is evident during the symptomatic phase.[69] Although SOD1 is primarily considered a cytosolic enzyme, recent studies establishing its presence in the inter-mitochondrial membrane space indicate a normal function in detoxifying superoxide generated in mitochondria.[70,71] Thus, regardless of the actual toxic gain of function to SOD1 conferred by disease-causing mutations, compromise of mitochondrial function and resulting oxidative stress may promote cellular damage and contribute significantly to motor neuron loss.

There is evidence that oxidative stress contributes to motor neuron loss in both FALS and SALS, at least as a secondary mechanism, if not the primary cause, which is reviewed in more detail in Chapter 10. Unmanaged, ROS can damage proteins, nucleic acids, and lipids. Pathways that protect these macromolecules from damage or promote their turnover once damaged are extremely important. Certainly cells with strong antioxidant capacity would be more resistant to oxidative stress, but motor neurons may not be in that category. Certain antioxidants (carboxyfullerenes[72] vitamin E and selenium,[73] creatine,[74] putrescine-modified catalase,[75] and SOD2[76]) have produced small protective effects in mutant SOD1 transgenic mice, although others have not.[77] Nevertheless, there is sufficient evidence of the involvement of oxidative stress, at least in the progression of the disease, to support evaluation of antioxidants as combination therapies along with other types of drugs in patients with ALS.

METABOLISM

Motor neurons are large cells with extensive dendritic and axonal processes. They are susceptible to oxidative stress and require energy to support the high metabolic activity associated with neurotransmission. Oxidative metabolism must be supported by good blood flow and delivery of oxygen. A particular susceptibility of motor neurons to hypoxia is suggested by the observation that deletion of the hypoxia-responsive element in the vascular endothelial growth factor (VEGF) promoter causes selective degeneration of motor neurons and an ALS-like phenotype and neuropathology in mice.[78] VEGF is a critical factor in growth of blood vessels in response to metabolic demand through response to hypoxia.

Environmental exposures have been suspected of contributing to sporadic MND directly or in association with genetic predispositions. Motor neuron nerve terminals are outside the protection of the blood-brain barrier; toxins, viruses, metals, and immunoglobulins can enter by bulk or receptor-mediated endocytosis and access cell bodies by retrograde transport. The cytochrome P-450 (CYP) enzymes not only are important in the oxidative, peroxidative, and reductive metabolism of endogenous compounds, including steroids, prostaglandins, and biogenic amines, but also metabolize a wide range of xenobiotics including drugs and environmental pollutants.[79] The highest expression of these enzymes is found in liver, the major organ engaged in metabolism of foreign chemicals. However, other tissues including the nervous system may express specific CYP isoforms, although at about one-tenth the level of liver.[80] On one hand, conversion of lipophilic xenobiotics, which penetrate the blood-brain barrier, to more polar derivatives by CYP-dependent monooxygenases could be protective; it is often the metabolites that are neurotoxic. Also, ROS are byproducts of these oxidation reactions and could add to oxidative stress in cells with low levels of glutathione and other antioxidant defenses. CYP 2E1,[81] whose substrates include ethanol and other solvents with neurotoxic potential, and CYP 2B1,[82] a phenytoin-inducible enzyme, have been detected by immunolabeling in LMNs. Most studies of CYP localization in brain have been conducted in rodents by immunolabeling. One study in humans failed to detect CYP activity in cervical spinal cord by a spectrophotometric assay.[62] The role played by CYP enzymes in xenobiotic metabolism in spinal cord or on motor neuron vulnerability to chemical exposures has not been examined systematically.

STRESS RESPONSE

When cells are exposed to various stressful conditions (e.g., hyperthermia, oxidative stress, ischemia, calcium ionophore, trauma, exposure to toxic chemicals, and mutant proteins), they synthesize families of highly conserved, protective proteins called Hsps (e.g., Hsp70, Hsp40, Hsp60, Hsp90, and Hsp110; the small Hsps: heme oxygenase, ubiquitin, Hsp25/27, and αB-crystallin; and the glucose-regulated proteins: GRP75, GRP78, and GRP94).[68,72,73,83,84] The inducible Hsps and their constitutively expressed analogues, heat shock cognate proteins (Hscs), are classified as molecular chaperones: They aid in the folding and transporting of proteins, as well as in protecting cells by refolding or targeting abnormal proteins for degradation, thus preventing their interaction with inappropriate partners and precipitation into aggregates (Figure 15.3). Molecular chaperones do not work alone to rid cells of aberrant proteins, but in partnership wherein intractable proteins are shuttled to the ubiquitin-proteasomal proteolytic system for degradation (see Figure 15.3). Proteasomes are barrel-shaped, cytoplasmic structures responsible for degrading most soluble intracellular proteins and short-lived regulatory proteins, as well as damaged, incompletely translated, and mutant proteins in cells.[85,86]

Evidence suggests that a high threshold for activation of the stress response and compromise of proteasomal function could be important factors in the vulnerability of motor neurons to disease-related stresses and in disease progression. A high threshold for induction of the major stress-inducible Hsps has been documented in rabbits subjected to hyperthermia[87,88] or ischemia.[89] No expression of the major inducible Hsp, Hsp70, was detected in cultured motor neurons subjected to glutamate excitotoxicity, heat shock, oxidative stress, or expression of mutant SOD1, and inducible Hsp70 protein was not detected in spinal motor neurons of transgenic mice expressing human G93A SOD1 or in motor neurons in spinal cord from human patients with SALS or mutant SOD1–induced ALS.[90] In familial diseases resulting in expression of mutant protein, such as FALS-1 and spinobulbar muscular atrophy (SBMA), motor

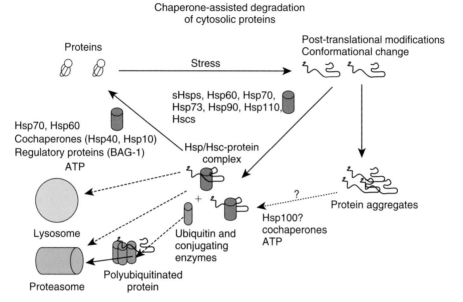

Figure 15.3 The heat shock proteins (Hsps) and heat shock cognate proteins (Hscs) function as molecular chaperones to bind to proteins with altered conformation (through transcriptional errors, genetic mutations or post-translational modifications) to prevent them from forming aggregates in the cell. Under some circumstances, the normal conformation of proteins can be restored in an adenosine triphosphate (ATP)–dependent process involving the cooperative action of chaperones and regulatory proteins. Otherwise, the proteins are targeted to proteasomes, usually following polyubiquitination, but in some cases in a ubiquitin-independent fashion. Lysosomes are the other major organelle for proteolysis in cells. One pathway to lysosomal degradation is chaperone-dependent microautophagy by which Hsp73 delivers proteins to lysosomes. See color insert.

neurons are particularly vulnerable to depletion of Hsps because of the requirement for chaperoning to proteasomes for degradation.[91–93]

Examination of postmortem tissues has revealed microscopic cytoplasmic inclusions in FALS and SALS and in the trinucleotide repeat disease, SBMA (Kennedy's disease).[94,95] Aggregation of abnormal proteins commonly occurs in stressed cells,[96,97] eventually resulting in the formation of larger inclusions called aggresomes.[98] Hsps are protective in cell culture models of FALS-1,[99] but Hsp70 alone is not protective in animal models. Crossing three different lines of mutant SOD1 transgenic mice with Hsp70 overexpressers failed to alter disease progression.[100] However, protection in animal models may require upregulation of multiple Hsps and proteasomes. Whereas Hsps can interact with abnormal proteins to prevent them from inflicting damage, long-term protection would depend on either regenerating a normally folded protein (requires ATP and co-chaperones) or degrading them. That abrogation of proteasomal function upregulates both Hsps and proteasomes indicates their co-regulation and complementary function.[101,102] Therefore cells that have a high threshold for inducing chaperones may also end up with insufficient proteasomes to keep up with the demand under stressed conditions. Proteasome inhibitors induce apoptosis, and neurons are particularly sensitive.[103–105]

Abrogation of proteasomal function may be a general property of mutant proteins associated with neurodegenerative diseases. Proteins with expanded polyglutamine repeats, including the androgen receptor protein in SBMA, are degraded by the proteasome and impair proteasomal function in proportion to repeat length.[93] Many mutant SOD1 proteins have decreased half-lives relative to wild type SOD1[106]; however, mutant proteins accumulate and form inclusions when proteasomal activity is compromised by treatment with chemical inhibitors.[91,107] Degradation of reporter peptides is inhibited in cell lines stably expressing mutant SOD1 protein (Kabashi, Agar, and Durham, unpublished observations). Aside from any other toxicity of mutant SOD1 and downstream effects, cellular function might be disrupted by accumulation of other proteins including transcription factors, cell cycle proteins, DNA repair enzymes, kinases, and proteases that are controlled by proteasomal degradation.

Cells expressing mutant SOD1 are more sensitive to oxidative stress and this manifests at the level of the proteasome. Proteins modified as a result of high levels of oxidative stress (*vide supra*) require Hsps as chaperones to deliver them to proteasomes for catabolism and to sequester them until they can be processed. This requirement is illustrated by a study in SH-SY5Y neural cells. Cells stably expressing the human HDJ-1 Hsp were more resistant to oxidative injury. These transfectants experienced similar degrees of ROS formation as non-transfected cells but had greater preservation of both proteasomal activity and mitochondrial function following exposure to oxidative stressors.[108] Competition for chaperones and proteasomes by oxidatively modified proteins and disease-associated mutant protein could significantly impair catabolism of both, as well as normal regulatory proteins whose levels are controlled by proteasomal degradation. This possibility is supported by a study in which *Caenorhabditis elegans* transgenic for mutant SOD1 proteins were subjected to oxidative stress by treatment with paraquat. Proteasomal activity was reduced relative to nonstressed cells, and mutant SOD1 accumulated and formed aggregates.[109]

UNIQUE ASPECTS OF THE CYTOSKELETON

Accumulation of NFs in perikarya and proximal axonal spheroids, hyperphosphorylation of perikaryal and dendritic NF proteins, and the presence of perikaryal inclusions immunoreactive for NF proteins are features of several MNDs including SALS and FALS,[110–112] infantile spinal muscular atrophy,[113,114] chemically induced neuropathies,[115–119] and mechanical injury.[120–122] Motor neurons have such a high content of NFs in their perikarya, dendrites, and axons that immunoreactivity with NF antibodies is used as one of the criteria for identification.[123] The high content of NFs and their particular organization in motor neurons may contribute to vulnerability of these cells.

A particular feature of both UMNs and LMNs is the presence of conspicuous bundles of NFs that course from the cell body into dendrites.[124,125] A similar pattern of dendritic NFs is observed in neurons of Clarke's column, which may be involved in ALS.[126] In contrast, the NFs in the dendrites of most other motor neurons are sparse and not arranged in bundles.[126] The high NF content in motor neuron dendrites suggested that altered transport might be responsible for the dendritic atrophy, which is a neuropathological feature of surviving motor neurons in ALS spinal cord.[127–129] The absence of NF-L dramatically reduced dendritic growth in developing, large motor neurons, demonstrating the importance of NFs for dendritic morphology in these cells.[130]

The high content of NFs in motoneuronal axons correlates with their large diameter.[131] The long large-diameter axonal projections to peripheral limb muscles and axons of UMNs projecting through the corticospinal tract to synapse on LMNs are particularly sensitive to toxicants that disrupt cytoskeletal organization or transport.[132] In mature motor neurons, NFs are composed of the NF triplet proteins (NF of light [NF-L], medium [NF-M], and high [NF-H] molecular weight). Increased NF phosphorylation of perikaryal and dendritic NFs occurs in MNDs.[133] The C-terminal extensions of NF-M and NF-H proteins contain multiple repeats of the sequence KSP arranged in particular motifs.[134] These serine residues are substrates for multiple protein kinases including those activated by stress (e.g., Jun-N-terminal kinases and cyclin-dependent kinase-5 [Cdk5]).[135–137] Hyperphosphorylation of NFs was proposed to affect their transport.[138,139]

NFs normally run parallel to and interact with microtubules but have a tendency to self-associate when their transport is inhibited, segregating into swirling arrays.[140] NFs in motor neurons are particularly prone to this type of aggregation. Microinjection of antibodies to phosphorylated NF-H caused collapse of dendritic NF networks and proximal axonal accumulations of NFs in cultured motor neurons, but not in dorsal root ganglion neurons.[141] Accumulation of NFs in cell bodies or proximal axons occurs preferentially in motor neurons of transgenic mice overexpressing normal individual NF proteins.[142–144] Accumulation and hyperphosphorylation of NFs and selective loss of motor neurons were observed in transgenic mice overexpressing NF-L with a point mutation.[145] (For more detailed information, see Chapter 12.)

Motor neurons may be sensitive to neurofilamentous changes, but do abnormalities contribute to disease pathogenesis? Variants of the NF-H gene have been identified in a few patients with ALS, indicating that NFs can play a primary role in a small subset of cases.[146–148] In most patients with ALS, changes in the expression of cytoskeletal proteins (both identify and stoichiometry), post-translational modifications, and disruption of transport/malorientation may represent a physiological response to injury. These changes could be detrimental to motor neurons rather than protective.

It is known that stoichiometry of subunits is important for maintaining normal NF organization, because NF transport in NF-H overexpressing mice is normalized by co-expression of an NF-L transgene.[149] Changes in gene expression that could alter stoichiometry of NF subunits have been measured in ALS spinal cord, that is, decrease in messenger RNA (mRNA) encoding NF-L relative to other subunits.[150,151] The influence of NF subunit expression on MND has been tested in mutant SOD1 transgenic mouse models, but these studies have created as many questions as answers. Deletion of NF-L reduced, not enhanced, motor neuron vulnerability in G85R mutant SOD1 transgenic mice, slowing disease onset and progression, despite the fact that other NF subunits accumulated in cell bodies.[152] Also surprising was that overexpression of human NF-H, which in itself induces motor impairment, was protective when crossed into the G37R mutant SOD1 transgenic line.[153] Because NFs also contain multiple calcium-binding sites,[154] it was proposed that increased levels of NF-M/NF-H in perikarya, which occur in both the NF-L knockout and the NF-H transgenic mice, could act as a sink for Ca^{2+} to assist in maintaining calcium homeostasis.[153]

Peripherin is an intermediate filament protein expressed during development in motor neurons and re-expressed following injury. Peripherin is found associated with axonal spheroids in degenerating motor neurons of patients with ALS[155,156] and in perikaryal and axonal inclusions in transgenic mice overexpressing a mutant SOD1 linked to FALS.[157] Overexpression of peripherin in transgenic mice results in formation of peripherin-containing inclusions and selective motor neuron death.[158] In a primary cell culture model, peripherin-induced neuronal death was shown to depend on tumor necrosis factor-α (TNF-α) released by activated microglia.[159] Other studies have demonstrated that death of motor neurons, at least in mutant SOD1 transgenic mice, is a cooperative process involving the surrounding non-neuronal cells.[39,160–162] Under these circumstances, expression of peripherin could contribute to a positive feedback mechanism that ultimately destroys motor neurons.

AGING

The most obvious risk factor for ALS is aging. Motor neurons appear to develop properly and function well into adulthood, even in FALS and in SBMA where the genetic mutations causing disease are expressed throughout life. Although it has not been determined when motor neuron loss begins in adult-onset MNDs, the evolution of disease pathogenesis has been studied extensively in the transgenic mouse models. Loss of motor neurons is not gradual over the lifetime of mutant SOD1 transgenic mice; rather, it begins in adulthood before the clinically symptomatic phase, progressing rapidly in the later stages.[69]

A number of protective mechanisms become less responsive with age and likely contribute to the reduced safety factor for cells to respond to physiological and environmental stresses. The threshold for activation of the stress response increases with aging.[163] In addition, biological waste accumulates as cytoplasmic and lysosomal inclusions.[164] Decreased levels of proteasomal activity and subunit expression have been measured in aging spinal cord.[165] Other than proteasomes, the other major route for turnover of the cytoplasm is the lysosome. Macroautophagy, whereby the lysosome engulfs sections of cytoplasm including whole organelles, is particularly important for turnover of mitochondria and proteasomes.[166] Another type of autophagy that is chaperone mediated accounts for degradation of about 30 percent of cytosolic proteins.[167] Proteins containing a KFERQ sequence motif bind the 73-kilodalton Hsc73. The chaperone-substrate complex binds to lysosomal-associated membrane protein-2a (Lamp2a) receptor and a lysosomal chaperone, Ly-Hsc73, assists in transporting the substrate into the lysosome. The protein recycling machinery of lysosomes is not perfect, and undegradable byproducts accumulate as lipofuscin linearly with time, particularly in postmitotic cells such as neurons. An age-related decline in Lamp2a and chaperone-mediated autophagy has been reported.[168] In FALS-1, an increase in the levels of mutant protein occurs just before the period of motor neuron loss.[169] A decreased efficiency of protein chaperoning and protein turnover with aging also will have an impact on turnover of signaling molecules that are degraded by proteasomes or chaperone-mediated autophagy. It is interesting that Cdk5, a kinase associated with apoptosis, accumulates in degenerating motor neurons in ALS and co-localizes with lipofuscin.[170] Altered turnover of normal regulatory proteins could contribute to the progression of motor neuron disorders and should be investigated.

Increased physiological stress can occur with aging, putting further demands on proteolytic systems. Increased oxidative stress and inflammatory responses have been invoked as major contributors to aging and can result in formation of oxidatively modified macromolecules, increased intracellular calcium, and alterations in calcium signaling.[171] Inhibition of proteasomal function by oxidatively modified proteins is discussed above. Formation of lipofuscin in lysosomes also is enhanced by oxidative stress.[166] ROS-induced somatic mutations in nuclear and mitochondrial DNA accumulate with age and could further compromise cellular function and ATP production.[172]

We also need to understand more about how aging changes in glia affect motor neuron function. Astrocytes are important players in neurotransmission through, for example, reuptake of glutamate, secretion of neuromodulators and neurotrophic factors, and buffering of ions, among others.[173] The glutamate transporters and calcium-regulatory proteins are particularly sensitive to oxidative stress; thus, oxidation of these proteins could contribute to alteration in glutamate and calcium homeostasis in MNDs and in disease progression. Increased presence of GLT-1 dimers and retarded electrophoretic mobility of monomers has been reported in severely affected G93A mutant SOD1 transgenic mice, consistent with post-translational modifications to the protein.[174] Although there is some evidence for altered calcium signaling in aged astrocytes, the effect of aging, as well as glial activation, on intimate association between astrocytes and motor neurons and the feedback loops that influence each other's function need to be explored.[173]

CONCLUSION

How a cell responds to the disease-causing stresses may be as important in determining outcome as the identity of initiating factors. How a cell responds depends on the protective mechanisms at its disposal given the complement of physiological stresses with which it has to cope. Although we can expect to identify eventually all of the genes responsible for familial forms of MNDs, it may be some time before we understand the initiating factors leading to sporadic ALS. Thus therapies are likely to be based on reducing stress on neurons or propping up their defensive mechanisms. The experience with clinical trials in human patients and animal models demonstrates that multiple pathways must be targeted using a drug cocktail to achieve significant therapeutic benefit.

REFERENCES

1. Regan RF, Choi DW. Glutamate neurotoxicity in spinal cord cell culture. Neuroscience 1991;43: 585–591.
2. Stewart GR, Olney JW, Pathikonda M, et al. Excitotoxicity in the embryonic chick spinal cord. Ann Neurol 1991;30:758–766.
3. Lu YM, Yin HZ, Chiang J, et al. Ca^{2+}-permeable AMPA/kainate and NMDA channels: high rate of Ca^{2+} influx underlies potent induction of injury. J Neurosci 1996;16:5457–5465.
4. Weiss JH, Choi DW. Slow non–NMDA receptor mediated neurotoxicity and amyotrophic lateral sclerosis. Adv Neurol 1991;56:311–318.
5. Choi DW. Calcium and excitotoxic neuronal injury. Ann N Y Acad Sci 1994;747:162–171.
6. Kwak S, Nakamura R. Acute and late neurotoxicity in the rat spinal cord in vivo induced by glutamate receptor agonists. J Neurol Sci 1995;129(suppl):99–103.
7. Rothstein JD, Kuncl RW. Neuroprotective strategies in a model of chronic glutamate-mediated motor neuron toxicity. J Neurochem 1995;65:643–651.
8. Carriedo SG, Yin HZ, Weiss JH. Motor neurons are selectively vulnerable to AMPA/kainate receptor–mediated injury in vitro. J Neurosci 1996;16:4069–4079.
9. Regan RF. The vulnerability of spinal cord neurons to excitotoxic injury: comparison with cortical neurons. Neurosci Lett 1996;213:9–12.
10. Vandenberghe W, Ihle EC, Patneau DK, et al. AMPA receptor current density, not desensitization, predicts selective motoneuron vulnerability. J Neurosci 2000;20:7158–7166.
11. Hollmann M, Heinemann S. Cloned glutamate receptors. Annu Rev Neurosci 1994;17:31–108.
12. Seeburg PH. The role of RNA editing in controlling glutamate receptor channel properties. J Neurochem 1996;66:1–5.
13. Tölle TR, Berthele A, Zieglgänsberger W, et al. The differential expression of 16 NMDA and non–NMDA receptor subunits in the rat spinal cord and in periaqueductal gray. J Neurosci 1993; 13:5009–5028.
14. Jakowec MW, Fox AJ, Martin LJ, et al. Quantitative and qualitative changes in AMPA receptor expression during spinal cord development. Neuroscience 1995;67:893–907.
15. Jakowec MW, Yen L, Kalb RG. In situ hybridization analysis of AMPA receptor subunit gene expression in the developing rat spinal cord. Neuroscience 1995;67:909–920.
16. Tomiyama M, Rodriquez-Puertas R, Cortés R, et al. Differential regional distribution of AMPA receptor subunit messenger RNAs in the human spinal cord as visualized by in situ hybridization. Neuroscience 1996;75:901–915.
17. Temkin R, Lowe D, Jensen P, et al. Expression of glutamate receptor subunits in alpha-motoneurons. Mol Brain Res 1997;52:38–45.
18. Williams TL, Day NC, Ince PG, et al. Calcium-permeable α-amino-3-hydroxy-5-methyl-4-isoxazole propionic acid receptors: a molecular determinant of selective vulnerability in amyotrophic lateral sclerosis. Ann Neurol 1997;42:200–207.
19. Morrison BM, Janssen WM, Gordon JW, et al. Light and electron microscopic distribution of the AMPA receptor subunit, GluR2, in the spinal cord of control and G86R mutant superoxide dismutase transgenic mice. J Comp Neurol 1998;395:523–534.
20. Carriedo SG, Yin HZ, Sensi SL, et al. Rapid Ca^{2+} entry through Ca^{2+}-permeable AMPA/kainate channels triggers marked intracellular Ca^{2+} rises and consequent oxygen radical production. J Neurosci 1998;18:7727–7738.
21. Roy J, Minotti S, Dong L, et al. Glutamate potentiates the toxicity of mutant Cu/Zn-superoxide dismutase in motor neurons by postsynaptic calcium-dependent mechanisms. J Neurosci 1998;18: 9673–9684.
22. Bar-Peled O, O'Brien RJ, Morrison JH, et al. Cultured motor neurons possess calcium-permeable AMPA/kainate receptors. Neuroreport 1999;10:855–859.
23. Carriedo SG, Sensi SL, Yin HZ, et al. AMPA exposures induce mitochondrial Ca^{2+} overload and ROS generation in spinal motor neurons in vitro. J Neurosci 2000;20:240–250.
24. Greig A, Donevan SD, Mujtaba TJ, et al. Characterization of the AMPA-activated receptors present on motoneurons. J Neurochem 2000;74:179–191.
25. Van Damme P, Van Den BL, Van Houtte E, et al. GluR2-dependent properties of AMPA receptors determine the selective vulnerability of motor neurons to excitotoxicity. J Neurophysiol 2002;88: 1279–1287.
26. Doroudchi MM, Bianchi AA, Sowden JE, et al. Gene transfer of the GluR2 glutamate receptor subunit protects motor neurons in a model of familial ALS. Soc Neurosci Abstr 2001;29:106.11.

27. Takuma H, Kwak S, Yoshizawa T, et al. Reduction of GluR2 RNA editing, a molecular change that increases calcium influx through AMPA receptors, selective in the spinal ventral gray of patients with amyotrophic lateral sclerosis. Ann Neurol 1999;46:806–815.
28. Stegenga SL, Kalb RG. Developmental regulation of *N*-methyl-D-aspartate– and kainate-type glutamate receptor expression in the rat spinal cord. Neuroscience 2001;105:499–507.
29. Ziv I, Achiron A, Djaldetti R, et al. Can nimodipine affect progression of motor neuron disease? A double-blind pilot study. Clin Neuropharmacol 1994;17:423–428.
30. Miller RG, Shepherd R, Dao H, et al. Controlled trial of nimodipine in amyotrophic lateral sclerosis. Neuromusc Disord 1996;6:101–104.
31. Miller RG, Smith SA, Murphy JR, et al. A clinical trial of verapamil in amyotrophic lateral sclerosis. Muscle Nerve 1996;19:511–515.
32. Engelhardt JI, Siklos L, Appel SH. Altered calcium homeostasis and ultrastructure in motoneurons of mice caused by passively transferred anti-motoneuronal IgG. J Neuropathol Exp Neurol 1997; 56:21–39.
33. Mohamed HA, Mosier DR, Zou LL, et al. Immunoglobulin Fcgamma receptor promotes immunoglobulin uptake, immunoglobulin-mediated calcium increase, and neurotransmitter release in motor neurons. J Neurosci Res 2002;69:110–116.
34. Rothstein JD, Tsai G, Kuncl RW, et al. Abnormal excitatory amino acid metabolism in amyotrophic lateral sclerosis. Ann Neurol 1990;28:18–25.
35. Plaitakis A. Altered glutamatergic mechanisms and selective motor neuron degeneration in amyotrophic lateral sclerosis: possible role of glycine. Adv Neurol 1991;56:319–326.
36. Shaw PJ, Forrest V, Ince PG, et al. CSF and plasma amino acid levels in motor neuron disease: elevation of CSF glutamate in a subset of patients. Neurodegeneration 1995;4:209–216.
37. Rothstein JD, Martin LJ, Kuncl RW. Decreased glutamate transport by the brain and spinal cord in amyotrophic lateral sclerosis. N Engl J Med 1992;326:1464–1468.
38. Rothstein JD, Van Kammen M, Levey AI, et al. Selective loss of glial glutamate transporter GLT-1 in amyotrophic lateral sclerosis. Ann Neurol 1995;38:73–84.
39. Bruijn LI, Becher MW, Lee MK, et al. ALS-linked SOD1 mutant G85R mediates damage to astrocytes and promotes rapidly progressive disease with SOD1-containing inclusions. Neuron 1997; 18:327–338.
40. Howland DS, Liu J, She YJ, et al. Focal loss of the glutamate transporter EAAT2 in a transgenic rat model of SOD1 mutant–mediated amyotrophic lateral sclerosis (ALS). Proc Nat Acad Sci USA 2002;99:1604–1609.
41. Corse AM, Bilak MM, Bilak SR, et al. Preclinical testing of neuroprotective neurotrophic factors in a model of chronic motor neuron degeneration. Neurobiol Dis 1999;6:335–346.
42. Bensimon G, Lacomblez L, Meininger V, et al. A controlled trial of riluzole in amyotrophic lateral sclerosis. N Engl J Med 1994;330:585–591.
43. Kruman II, Pedersen WA, Springer JE, et al. ALS-linked Cu/Zn-SOD mutation increases vulnerability of motor neurons to excitotoxicity by a mechanism involving increased oxidative stress and perturbed calcium homeostasis. Exp Neurol 1999;160:28–39.
44. Ince P, Stout N, Shaw P, et al. Parvalbumin and calbindin D-28k in the human motor system and in motor neuron disease. Neuropathol Appl Neurobiol 1993;19:291–299.
45. Alexianu ME, Ho B-K, Mohamed AH, et al. The role of calcium-binding proteins in selective motoneuron vulnerability in amyotrophic lateral sclerosis. Ann Neurol 1994;36:846–858.
46. Elliott JL, Snider WD. Parvalbumin is a marker of ALS-resistant motor neurons. Neuroreport 1995; 6:449–452.
47. Junttila T, Koistinaho J, Reichardt L, et al. Localization of neurocalcin-like immunoreactivity in rat cranial motoneurons and spinal cord interneurons. Neurosci Lett 1995;183:100–103.
48. Reiner A, Medina L, Figueredo-Cardenas G, et al. Brainstem motoneuron pools that are selectively resistant in amyotrophic lateral sclerosis are preferentially enriched in parvalbumin: evidence from monkey brainstem for a calcium-mediated mechanism in sporadic ALS. Exp Neurol 1995;131: 239–250.
49. Palecek J, Lips MB, Keller BU. Calcium dynamics and buffering in motoneurons of the mouse spinal cord. J Physiol 1999;520(pt 2):485–502.
50. Vanselow BK, Keller BU. Calcium dynamics and buffering in oculomotor neurones from mouse that are particularly resistant during amyotrophic lateral sclerosis (ALS)–related motoneuron disease. J Physiol 2000;525(pt 2):433–445.
51. Ho BK, Alexianu ME, Colom LV, et al. Expression of calbindin-D_{28K} in motoneuron hybrid cells after retroviral infection with calbindin-D_{28K} cDNA prevents amyotrophic lateral sclerosis IgG-mediated cytotoxicity. Proc Natl Acad Sci USA 1996;93:6796–6801.

52. Ghadge GD, Lee JP, Bindokas VP, et al. Mutant superoxide dismutase-1–linked familial amyotrophic lateral sclerosis—molecular mechanisms of neuronal death and protection. J Neurosci 1997;17:8756–8766.
53. Beers DR, Ho BK, Siklos L, et al. Parvalbumin overexpression alters immune-mediated increases in intracellular calcium, and delays disease onset in a transgenic model of familial amyotrophic lateral sclerosis. J Neurochem 2001;79:499–509.
54. Van Den BL, Schwaller B, Vleminckx V, et al. Protective effect of parvalbumin on excitotoxic motor neuron death. Exp Neurol 2002;174:150–161.
55. Klapstein GJ, Vietla S, Lieberman DN, et al. Calbindin-D28k fails to protect hippocampal neurons against ischemia in spite of its cytoplasmic calcium buffering properties: evidence from calbindin-D28k knockout mice. Neuroscience 1998;85:361–373.
56. Philbert MA, Beiswanger CM, Waters DK, et al. Cellular and regional distribution of reduced glutathione in the nervous system of the rat: histochemical localization by mercury orange and o-phthalaldehyde-induced histofluorescence. Toxicol Appl Pharmacol 1991;107:215–227.
57. Beiswanger CM, Diegmann MH, Novak RF, et al. Developmental changes in the cellular distribution of glutathione and glutathione S-transferases in the murine nervous system. Neurotoxicology 1995;16:425–440.
58. Ratan RR, Murphy TH, Baraban JM. Macromolecular synthesis inhibitors prevent oxidative stress–induced apoptosis in embryonic cortical neurons by shunting cysteine from protein synthesis to glutathione. J Neurosci 1994;14:4385–4392.
59. Kruman I, Bruce-Keller AJ, Bredesen D, et al. Evidence that 4-hydroxynonenal mediates oxidative stress–induced neuronal apoptosis. J Neurosci 1997;17:5089–5100.
60. Shinpo K, Kikuchi S, Sasaki H, et al. Selective vulnerability of spinal motor neurons to reactive dicarbonyl compounds, intermediate products of glycation, in vitro: implication of inefficient glutathione system in spinal motor neurons. Brain Res 2000;861:151–159.
61. Lanius RA, Krieger C, Wagey R, et al. Increased [^{35}S]glutathione binding sites in spinal cords from patients with sporadic amyotrophic lateral sclerosis. Neurosci Lett 1993;163:89–92.
62. Fitzmaurice PS, Shaw IC, Mitchell JD. Alteration of superoxide dismutase activity in the anterior horn in motoneuron disease patients. J Neurol Sci 1995;129(suppl):96–98.
63. Cudkowicz ME, Pastusza KA, Sapp PC, et al. Survival in transgenic ALS mice does not vary with CNS glutathione peroxidase activity. Neurology 2002;59:729–734.
64. Malaspina A, Kaushik N, De Belleroche J. Differential expression of 14 genes in amyotrophic lateral sclerosis spinal cord detected using gridded cDNA arrays. J Neurochem 2001;77:132–145.
65. Olsen MK, Roberds SL, Ellerbrock BR, et al. Disease mechanisms revealed by transcription profiling in SOD1-G93A transgenic mouse spinal cord. Ann Neurol 2001;50:730–740.
66. Choi DW. Glutamate receptors and the induction of excitotoxic neuronal death. Prog Brain Res 1994;100:47–51.
67. Dugan LL, Choi DW. Excitotoxicity, free radicals, and cell membrane changes. Ann Neurol 1994;35(suppl):S17–S21.
68. Menzies FM, Ince PG, Shaw PJ. Mitochondrial involvement in amyotrophic lateral sclerosis. Neurochem Int 2002;40:543–551.
69. Kong J, Xu Z. Massive mitochondrial degeneration in motor neurons triggers the onset of amyotrophic lateral sclerosis in mice expressing a mutant SOD1. J Neurosci 1998;18:3241–3250.
70. Sturtz LA, Diekert K, Jensen LT, et al. A fraction of yeast Cu,Zn-superoxide dismutase and its metallochaperone, CCS, localize to the intermembrane space of mitochondria—a physiological role for SOD1 in guarding against mitochondrial oxidative damage. J Biol Chem 2001;276:38084–38089.
71. Okado-Matsumoto A, Fridovich I. Subcellular distribution of superoxide dismutases (SOD) in rat liver; Cu,Zn-SOD in mitochondria. J Biol Chem 2001;276:38388–38393.
72. Dugan LL, Turetsky DM, Du D, et al. Carboxyfullerenes as neuroprotective agents. Proc Natl Acad Sci USA 1997;94:9434–9438.
73. Gurney ME, Cutting FB, Zhai P, et al. Benefit of vitamin E, riluzole, and gabapentin in a transgenic model of familial amyotrophic lateral sclerosis. Ann Neurol 1996;39:147–157.
74. Klivenyi P, Ferrante RJ, Matthews RT, et al. Neuroprotective effects of creatine in a transgenic animal model of amyotrophic lateral sclerosis. Nat Med 1999;5:347–350.
75. Reinholz MM, Merkle CM, Poduslo JF. Therapeutic benefits of putrescine-modified catalase in transgenic mouse model of familial amyotrophic lateral sclerosis. Exp Neurol 1999;159:204–216.
76. Flanagan SW, Anderson RD, Ross MA, et al. Overexpression of manganese superoxide dismutase attenuates neuronal death in human cells expressing mutant (G37R) Cu/Zn-superoxide dismutase. J Neurochem 2002;81:170–177.

77. Cleveland DW, Rothstein JD. From Charcot to Lou Gehrig: deciphering selective motor neuron death in ALS [review]. Nat Rev Neurosci 2001;2:806–819.
78. Oosthuyse B, Moons L, Storkebaum E, et al. Deletion of the hypoxia-response element in the vascular endothelial growth factor promoter causes motor neuron degeneration. Nat Genet 2001;28: 131–138.
79. Silverstein FS, Nelson C. The microsomal calcium-ATPase inhibitor thapsigargin is a neurotoxin in perinatal rodent brain. Neurosci Lett 1992;145:157–160.
80. Hodgson AV, White TB, White JW, et al. Expression analysis of the mixed function oxidase system in rat brain by the polymerase chain reaction. Mol Cell Biochem 1993;120:171–179.
81. Hansson T, Tindberg N, Ingelman-Sundberg M, et al. Regional distribution of ethanol-inducible cytochrome P450 IIE1 in the rat central nervous system. Neuroscience 1990;34:451–463.
82. Volk B, Hettmannsperger U, Papp T, et al. Mapping of phenytoin-inducible cytochrome P450 immunoreactivity in the mouse central nervous system. Neuroscience 1991;42:215–235.
83. Marcuccilli CJ, Miller RJ. CNS stress response: too hot to handle? Trends Neurosci 1994;17: 135–138.
84. Morimoto RI, Kline MP, Bimston DN, et al. The heat-shock response: regulation and function of heat-shock proteins and molecular chaperones. Essays Biochem 1997;32:17–29.
85. Baumeister W, Walz J, Zuhl F, et al. The proteasome: paradigm of a self-compartmentalizing protease. Cell 1998;92:367–380.
86. Sherman MY, Goldberg AL. Cellular defenses against unfolded proteins: a cell biologist thinks about neurodegenerative diseases [review]. Neuron 2001;29:15–32.
87. Manzerra P, Brown IR. Expression of heat shock genes (hsp70) in the rabbit spinal cord: localization of constitutive and hyperthermia-inducible mRNA species. J Neurosci Res 1992;31: 606–615.
88. Manzerra P, Brown IR. The neuronal stress response: nuclear translocation of heat shock proteins as an indicator of hyperthermic stress. Exp Cell Res 1996;229:35–47.
89. Sakurai M, Aoki M, Abe K, et al. Dissociation of HSP72 and HSC73 heat shock mRNA inductions after spinal cord ischemia in rabbit. Neurosci Lett 1996;217:113–116.
90. Batulan ZB, Minotti S, Figlewicz DA, et al. High threshold for activation of the stress response in motor neurons: a source of vulnerability in ALS? Soc Neurosci Abstr 2000;26:85.15.
91. Johnston JA, Dalton MJ, Gurney ME, et al. Formation of high molecular weight complexes of mutant Cu,Zn-superoxide dismutase in a mouse model for familial amyotrophic lateral sclerosis. Proc Natl Acad Sci USA 2000;97:12571–12576.
92. Shinder GA, Lacourse MC, Minotti S, et al. Mutant Cu/Zn-superoxide dismutase proteins have altered solubility and interact with heat shock/stress proteins in models of amyotrophic lateral sclerosis. J Biol Chem 2001;276:12791–12796.
93. Bailey CK, Andriola IF, Kampinga HH, et al. Molecular chaperones enhance the degradation of expanded polyglutamine repeat androgen receptor in a cellular model of spinal and bulbar muscular atrophy. Hum Mol Genet 2002;11:515–523.
94. Goedert M, Spillantini MG, Davies SW. Filamentous nerve cell inclusions in neurodegenerative diseases. Curr Opin Neurobiol 1998;8:619–632.
95. Paulson HL, Fischbeck KH. Trinucleotide repeats in neurogenetic disorders. Annu Rev Neurosci 1998;19:79–107.
96. Kabakov AE, Gabai VL. Protein aggregation as primary and characteristic cell reaction to various stresses. Experientia 1993;49:706–713.
97. Mifflin LC, Cohen RE. Characterization of denatured protein inducers of the heat shock (stress) response in *Xenopus laevis* oocytes. J Biol Chem 1994;269:15710–15717.
98. Johnston JA, Ward CL, Kopito RR. Aggresomes: a cellular response to misfolded proteins. J Cell Biol 1998;143:1883–1898.
99. Bruening W, Roy J, Giasson B, et al. Upregulation of protein chaperones preserves viability of cells expressing toxic Cu/Zn-superoxide dismutase mutants associated with amyotrophic lateral sclerosis. J Neurochem 1999;72:693–699.
100. Ward CM, Liu J, Young DJ, et al. Increasing the protein folding chaperone HSP70 does not affect time course of SOD1-mutant–mediated amyotrophic lateral sclerosis. Soc Neurosci Abstr 2001;27: 107.12.
101. Mathew A, Mathur SK, Morimoto RI. Heat shock response and protein degradation: regulation of HSF2 by the ubiquitin-proteasome pathway. Mol Cell Biol 1998;18:5091–5098.
102. Mathew A, Mathur SK, Jolly C, et al. Stress-specific activation and repression of heat shock factors 1 and 2. Mol Cell Biol 2001;21:7163–7171.

103. Pasquini LA, Besio MM, Adamo AM, et al. Lactacystin, a specific inhibitor of the proteasome, induces apoptosis and activates caspase-3 in cultured cerebellar granule cells. J Neurosci Res 2000; 59:601–611.

104. Qiu JH, Asai A, Chi S, et al. Proteasome inhibitors induce cytochrome *c*-caspase-3–like protease-mediated apoptosis in cultured cortical neurons. J Neurosci 2000;20:259–265.

105. Suzuki Y, Nakabayashi Y, Takahashi R. Ubiquitin-protein ligase activity of X-linked inhibitor of apoptosis protein promotes proteasomal degradation of caspase-3 and enhances its anti-apoptotic effect in Fas-induced cell death. Proc Natl Acad Sci USA 2001;98:8662–8667.

106. Ratovitski T, Corson LB, Strain J, et al. Variation in the biochemical/biophysical properties of mutant superoxide dismutase 1 enzymes and the rate of disease progression in familial amyotrophic lateral sclerosis kindreds. Hum Mol Genet 1999;8:1451–1460.

107. Hoffman EK, Wilcox HM, Scott RW, et al. Proteasome inhibition enhances the stability of mouse Cu/Zn superoxide dismutase with mutations linked to familial amyotrophic lateral sclerosis. J Neurol Sci 1996;139:15–20.

108. Ding QX, Keller JN. Proteasome inhibition in oxidative stress neurotoxicity: implications for heat shock proteins. J Neurochem 2001;77:1010–1017.

109. Oeda T, Shimohama S, Kitagawa N, et al. Oxidative stress causes abnormal accumulation of familial amyotrophic lateral sclerosis–related mutant SOD1 in transgenic *Caenorhabditis elegans*. Hum Mol Genet 2001;10:2013–2023.

110. Manetto V, Sternberger NH, Perry G, et al. Phosphorylation of neurofilaments is altered in amyotrophic lateral sclerosis. J Neuropathol Exp Neurol 1988;47:642–653.

111. Murayama S, Bouldin TW, Suzuki K. Immunocytochemical and ultrastructural studies of upper motor neurons in amyotrophic lateral sclerosis. Acta Neuropathol (Berl) 1992;83:518–524.

112. Sobue G, Hashizume Y, Yasuda T, et al. Phosphorylated high molecular weight neurofilament protein in lower motor neurons in amyotrophic lateral sclerosis and other neurodegenerative diseases involving ventral horn cells. Acta Neuropathol 1990;79:402–408.

113. Kato S, Hirano A. Ubiquitin and phosphorylated neurofilament epitopes in ballooned neurons of the extraocular muscle nuclei in a case of Werdnig-Hoffmann disease. Acta Neuropathol 1990;80: 334–337.

114. Murayama S, Bouldin TW, Suzuki K. Immunocytochemical and ultrastructural studies of Werdnig-Hoffmann disease. Acta Neuropathol 1991;81:408–417.

115. Bizzi A, Gambetti P. Phosphorylation of neurofilament is altered in aluminum intoxication. Acta Neuropathol 1986;71:154–158.

116. Troncoso JC, Sternberger NH, Sternberger LA, et al. Immunocytochemical studies of neurofilament antigens in the neurofibrillary pathology induced by aluminum. Brain Res 1986;364:295–300.

117. Hugon J, Vallat JM. Abnormal distribution of phosphorylated neurofilaments in neuronal degeneration induced by kainic acid. Neurosci Lett 1990;119:45–48.

118. Watson DF, Griffin JW, Fittro KP, et al. Phosphorylation-dependent immunoreactivity of neurofilaments increases during axonal maturation and beta, beta′-iminodipropionitrile intoxication. J Neurochem 1989;53:1818–1829.

119. Watson DF, Fittro KP, Hoffman PN, et al. Phosphorylation-related immunoreactivity and the rate of transport of neurofilament in chronic 2,5-hexamidine intoxication. Brain Res 1991;539:103–109.

120. Goldstein ME, Cooper HS, Bruce J, et al. Phosphorylation of neurofilament proteins and chromatolysis following transection of rat sciatic nerve. J Neurosci 1987;7:1586–1594.

121. Mansour H, Bignami A, Labkovsky B, et al. Neurofilament phosphorylation in neuronal perikarya following axotomy: a study of rat spinal cord with central and dorsal root transection. J Comp Neurol 1989;283:481.

122. Martin JE, Mather KS, Swash M, et al. Spinal cord trauma in man—studies of phosphorylated neurofilament and ubiquitin expression. Brain 1990;113:1553–1562.

123. Carriedo SG, Yin H-Z, Lamberta R, et al. In vitro kainate injury to large, SMI-32(+) spinal neurons is Ca^{2+} dependent. Neuroreport 1995;6:945–948.

124. Wuerker R, Palay SL. Neurofilaments and microtubules in anterior horn cells of the rat. Tissue Cell 1969;1:387–402.

125. Kaiserman-Abramoff IR, Peters A. Some aspects of the morphology of Betz cells in the cerebral cortex of the cat. Brain Res 1972;43:527–546.

126. Wuerker RB, Kirkpatrick JB. Neuronal microtubules, neurofilaments, and microfilaments. Int Rev Cytol 1972;33:45–75.

127. Nakano I, Hirano A. Atrophic cell processes of large motor neurons in the anterior horn in amyotrophic lateral sclerosis: observation with silver impregnation method. J Neuropathol Exp Neurol 1987;46:40–49.

128. Carpenter S, Karpati G, Durham H. Dendritic attrition precedes motor neuron death in amyotrophic lateral sclerosis (ALS). Neurology 1988;34:252.
129. Durham HD, Karpati G, Carpenter S. The Pathogenesis and Significance of Dendritic Atrophy in Amyotrophic Lateral Sclerosis. In FC Rose, FH Norris (eds), ALS. New Advances in Toxicology and Epidemiology. London: Smith-Gordon, 1990.
130. Zhang Z, Casey DM, Julien JP, et al. Normal dendritic arborization in spinal motoneurons requires neurofilament subunit L. J Comp Neurol 2002;450:144–152.
131. Hoffman PN, Cleveland DW, Griffin JW, et al. Neurofilament gene expression: a major determinant of axonal caliber. Proc Natl Acad Sci USA 1987;84:3472–3476.
132. Spencer PS, Allen CN, Kisby GE, et al. On the etiology and pathogenesis of chemically induced neurodegenerative disorders. Neurobiol Aging 1994;15:265–267.
133. Julien JP, Mushynski WE. Neurofilaments in health and disease. Prog Nucleic Acid Res Mol Biol 1998;61:1–23.
134. Julien J-P, Mushynski WE. The distribution of phosphorylation sites among identified fragments of mammalian neurofilaments. J Biol Chem 1983;258:4019–4025.
135. Giasson BI, Mushynski WE. Aberrant stress-induced phosphorylation of perikaryal neurofilaments. J Biol Chem 1996;271:30404–30409.
136. Grant P, Sharma P, Pant HC. Cyclin-dependent protein kinase 5 (Cdk5) and the regulation of neurofilament metabolism. Eur J Biochem 2001;268:1534–1546.
137. Nguyen MD, Lariviere RC, Julien JP. Deregulation of Cdk5 in a mouse model of ALS: toxicity alleviated by perikaryal neurofilament inclusions. Neuron 2001;30:135–147.
138. Nixon RA, Sihag RK. Neurofilament phosphorylation: a new look at regulation and function. Trends Neurosci 1991;14:501–506.
139. Sanchez I, Hassinger L, Sihag RK, et al. Local control of neurofilament accumulation during radial growth of myelinating axons in vivo. Selective role of site-specific phosphorylation. J Cell Biol 2000;151:1013–1024.
140. Veronesi B, Peterson ER, Bornstein MB, et al. Ultrastructural studies of the dying-back process, VI: examination of nerve fibers undergoing giant axonal degeneration in organotypic culture. J Neuropathol Exp Neurol 1983;42:153–165.
141. Durham HD. An antibody against hyperphosphorylated neurofilament proteins collapses the neurofilament network in motor neurons but not in dorsal root ganglion cells. J Neuropathol Exp Neurol 1992;51:287–297.
142. Côté F, Collard J-F, Julien J-P. Progressive neuronopathy in transgenic mice expressing the human neurofilament heavy gene: a mouse model of amyotrophic lateral sclerosis. Cell 1993;73:35–46.
143. Xu Z, Cork LC, Griffin JW, et al. Involvement of neurofilaments in motor neuron disease. J Cell Sci 1993;106(suppl 17):101–108.
144. Wong PC, Marszalek J, Crawford TO, et al. Increasing neurofilament subunit NF-M expression reduces axonal NF-H, inhibits radial growth, and results in neurofilamentous accumulation in motor neurons. J Cell Biol 1995;130:1413–1422.
145. Lee MK, Marszalek JR, Cleveland DW. A mutant neurofilament subunit causes massive, selective motor neuron death: Implications for the pathogenesis of human motor neuron disease. Neuron 1994;13:975–988.
146. Figlewicz DA, Krizus A, Martinoli MG, et al. Variants of the heavy neurofilament subunit are associated with the development of amyotrophic lateral sclerosis. Hum Mol Genet 1994;3:1757–1761.
147. Tomkins J, Usher P, Slade JY, et al. Novel insertion in the KSP region of the neurofilament heavy gene in amyotrophic lateral sclerosis (ALS). Neuroreport 1998;9:3967–3970.
148. Al-Chalabi A, Andersen PM, Nilsson P, et al. Deletions of the heavy neurofilament subunit tail in amyotrophic lateral sclerosis. Hum Mol Genet 1999;8:157–164.
149. Meier J, Couillard-Després S, Jacomy H, et al. Extra neurofilament NF-L subunits rescue motor neuron disease caused by overexpression of the human NF-H gene in mice. J Neuropathol Exp Neurol 1999;58:1099–1110.
150. Wong NKY, He BP, Strong MJ. Characterization of neuronal intermediate filament protein expression in cervical spinal motor neurons in sporadic amyotrophic lateral sclerosis (ALS). J Neuropathol Exp Neurol 2000;59:972–982.
151. Menzies FM, Grierson AJ, Cookson MR, et al. Selective loss of neurofilament expression in Cu/Zn superoxide dismutase (SOD1) linked amyotrophic lateral sclerosis. J Neurochem 2002;82:1118–1128.
152. Williamson TL, Bruijn LI, Zhu Q, et al. Absence of neurofilaments reduces the selective vulnerability of motor neurons and slows disease caused by a familial amyotrophic lateral sclerosis-linked superoxide dismutase 1 mutant. Proc Natl Acad Sci USA 1998;95:9631–9636.

153. Couillard-Després S, Zhu Q, Wong PC, et al. Protective effect of neurofilament NF-H overexpression in motor neuron disease induced by mutant superoxide dismutase. Proc Natl Acad Sci USA 1998;95.
154. Lefebvre S, Mushynski WE. Calcium binding to untreated and dephosphorylated porcine neurofilaments. Biochem Biophys Res Commun 1987;145:1006–1011.
155. Corbo M, Hays AP. Peripherin and neurofilament protein coexist in spinal spheroids of motor neuron disease. J Neuropathol Exp Neurol 1992;51:531–537.
156. Migheli A, Pezzulo T, Attanasio A, et al. Peripherin immunoreactive structures in amyotrophic lateral sclerosis. Lab Invest 1993;68:185–191.
157. Tu PH, Raju P, Robinson KA, et al. Transgenic mice carrying a human mutant superoxide dismutase transgene develop neuronal cytoskeletal pathology resembling human amyotrophic lateral sclerosis lesions. Proc Natl Acad Sci USA 1996;93:3155–3160.
158. Beaulieu JM, Nguyen MD, Julien JP. Late onset death of motor neurons in mice overexpressing wild-type peripherin. J Cell Biol 1999;147:531–544.
159. Robertson J, Beaulieu JM, Doroudchi MM, et al. Apoptotic death of neurons exhibiting peripherin aggregates is mediated by the proinflammatory cytokine tumor necrosis factor-alpha. J Cell Biol 2001;155:217–226.
160. Pramatarova A, Laganiere J, Roussel J, et al. Neuron-specific expression of mutant superoxide dismutase 1 in transgenic mice does not lead to motor impairment. J Neurosci 2001;21:3369–3374.
161. Lino MM, Schneider C, Caroni P. Accumulation of SOD1 mutants in postnatal motoneurons does not cause motoneuron pathology or motoneuron disease. J Neurosci 2002;22:4825–4832.
162. McGeer PL, McGeer EG. Inflammatory processes in amyotrophic lateral sclerosis. Muscle Nerve 2002;26:459–470.
163. Verbeke P, Fonager J, Clark BF, et al. Heat shock response and ageing: mechanisms and applications. Cell Biol Int 2001;25:845–857.
164. Terman A. Garbage catastrophe theory of aging: imperfect removal of oxidative damage? Redox Rep 2001;6:15–26.
165. Keller JN, Huang FF, Markesbery WR. Decreased levels of proteasome activity and proteasome expression in aging spinal cord. Neuroscience 2000;98:149–156.
166. Brunk U, Terman A. Lipofuscin: mechanisms of age-related accumulation and influence on cell function. Free Radic Biol Med 2002;33:611.
167. Cuervo AM, Dice JF. Lysosomes, a meeting point of proteins, chaperones, and proteases. J Mol Med 1998;76:6–12.
168. Cuervo AM, Dice JF. Age-related decline in chaperone-mediated autophagy. J Biol Chem 2000; 275:31505–31513.
169. Andrus PK, Fleck TJ, Gurney ME, et al. Protein oxidative damage in a transgenic mouse model of familial amyotrophic lateral sclerosis. J Neurochem 1998;71:2041–2048.
170. Bajaj NP, Al Sarraj ST, Anderson V, et al. Cyclin-dependent kinase-5 is associated with lipofuscin in motor neurones in amyotrophic lateral sclerosis. Neurosci Lett 1998;245:45–48.
171. Squier TC, Bigelow DJ. Protein oxidation and age-dependent alterations in calcium homeostasis. Front Biosci 2000;5:D504–D526.
172. Wei YH, Lee HC. Oxidative stress, mitochondrial DNA mutation, and impairment of antioxidant enzymes in aging. Exp Biol Med 2002;227:671–682.
173. Cotrina ML, Nedergaard M. Astrocytes in the aging brain. J Neurosci Res 2002;67:1–10.
174. Deitch JS, Alexander GM, Del Valle L, et al. GLT-1 glutamate transporter levels are unchanged in mice expressing G93A human mutant SOD1. J Neurol Sci 2002;193:117–126.

SECTION 3

OTHER MOTOR NEURON DISORDERS

16
Spinal Muscular Atrophy

Kevin Talbot and Kay E. Davies

DEFINITION AND CLASSIFICATION OF SPINAL MUSCULAR ATROPHY

The term *spinal muscular atrophy* (SMA) was first used by 19th century neurologists to distinguish neurogenic atrophy from muscle wasting caused by a primary disorder of muscle. Subsequently there has been a degree of nosological confusion about these disorders, which is slowly being eliminated as a result of advances in molecular genetics. Although it is difficult to come up with an all-encompassing and unambiguous definition of SMA, it is usually thought of as a symmetrical, pure lower motor neuron (LMN) disorder, with sparing of sensation and absence of pyramidal tract involvement, which is slowly progressive and genetically determined. Anita Harding[1] pointed out the illogicality of the term *SMA* for a group of disorders that may involve bulbar musculature and proposed the term *hereditary motor neuronopathy* (HMN), but in practice the term *SMA* is still in widespread use. The classification scheme developed by Harding has been taken up by many. However, developments in molecular genetics will mean that this scheme will almost certainly have to be revised when the true extent of both clinical and genetic heterogeneity in these disorders is revealed. For example, new types of distal SMA have been described since Harding's classification. In addition, there remains the problem of the not infrequent adult patient with SMA in whom the condition appears to be sporadic and a genetic etiology is therefore presumed but not proven.

Although there is some logic in restricting the term to pure LMN syndromes, it is common clinical experience that families exist in which more widespread involvement is evident consistent with the notion that the molecular defect, while having a predisposition for motor neurons, may affect other classes of long neurons. In this chapter, we review the clinical forms of SMA, both recessive and dominant, using genetic linkage where it has been identified as the main basis for classification. At the risk of producing a dry catalog, we document all of the published reports of linkage because in combination with clinical descriptions, this does produce an overview of the large amount of variation in these disorders. The molecular pathogenesis of two types of recessive SMA of childhood is discussed in some detail because these diseases have revealed defects in molecular pathways, which may be of fundamental relevance to motor neurons. The possible overlap between dominant SMA and both hereditary spastic paraparesis (HSP) and hereditary motor and sensory neuropathy (HMSN) (Charcot-Marie-Tooth type 2D [CMT2D]) is also mentioned. Finally, we discuss the implications of these disorders for motor neuron biology in general.

Most cases of SMA appear to be due to mutations in a single gene segregating in a dominant, recessive, or X-linked fashion. However, as with other forms of neurodegeneration such as ataxia, there appear to be sporadic cases of SMA for which a genetic cause is less certain. This is particularly true of late-onset dominant distal SMA and the focal form of monomelic SMA referred to as Hirayama's disease, which in most cases is not associated with a family history. In addition to these syndromes in which linkage has been established, there are many families with SMA displaying different distributions that have not been linked to any genetic region. From a practical clinical point of view, it is reasonable to consider these different syndromes according to mode of inheritance, genetic linkage, and by the clinical pattern of weakness. This approach should eventually allow a comprehensive account of all of the various forms of SMA (Table 16.1).

For infantile forms of SMA, the differential diagnosis is that of the "floppy infant" and this is discussed later in this chapter. Adult-onset weakness and wasting always raises concerns about amyotrophic lateral sclerosis (ALS) and other forms of malignant motor neuron disease (MND). Some patients with

Table 16.1   Spinal muscular atrophy syndromes: genetic and clinical correlates

Disease	Genetics (OMIM number)	Clinical features
Autosomal recessive		
Proximal SMA of childhood types I through IV (synonym, Werdnig-Hoffman disease, Kugelberg-Welander syndrome)	**600354** Inactivating mutations (large scale deletions, gene conversion events, point mutations) in the SMN gene, chromosome 5q13	Onset from neonate to adult depending on type; proximal, lower limbs more than upper limbs; facial muscles and diaphragm characteristically spared; bulbar involvement mirrors severity
SMARD1	**604320** Mutations in *IGHMBP2* on chromosome 11q13; animal model *nmd* mouse	Acute presentation at birth with respiratory distress and feeding difficulty; death less than 6 months
Distal SMA	**697088** Mapped to chromosome 11q13; SMARD1 locus excluded by linkage; large consanguineous Lebanese pedigree	Variable age at onset (infancy to third decade), occasional diaphragm involvement; slowly progressive; reduced or absent reflexes, scoliosis and reduced respiratory function; no bulbar involvement

Table 16.1   (continued)

Disease	Genetics (OMIM number)	Clinical features
SMA with cerebellar hypoplasia	Not linked to 5q13	Intellectual impairment, wasting of tongue and limbs, extraocular muscle dysfunction; death in first year
SMA with arthrogryposis	**253310** LCCS linked to 9q34; some cases of 5q13 SMA have arthrogryposis	Fatal in third trimester; restricted to Finland; pathologically similar to SMN-related SMA
Jerash HMN	**605726** Cluster of Jordanian consanguineous pedigrees mapped to 9p21.1–p12	Onset in first decade (6–10 years) in distal lower limbs, pes cavus, upper limbs; pyramidal tract involvement (extensor plantars and brisk reflexes); slow progression
Autosomal dominant		
Distal SMA with upper limb predominance (distal HMN-V)	**600794** 7p15, probably allelic with CMT2D **601472**	Weakness and wasting of upper limb in adolescence, slow progression, occasional pyramidal tract involvement and mild sensory loss
SMA with vocal cord paralysis (distal HMN-VII)	**158580** 2p14	Presents in third decade in upper limb with later slow progression to lower limb; hoarse voice in all affected
Distal SMA with lower limb predominance (distal HMN-II)	**158590** 12q24	Median onset 20 years in lower limb; slowly progressive
Congenital distal SMA	**600175** 12q23–q24 in some families but genetically heterogeneous	Nonprogressive lower limb atrophy from birth; proximal and distribution and upper limbs spared
Scapuloperoneal SMA	**181405** 12q23–q24; may be allelic with congenital distal SMA	Variable onset from childhood to fifth decade, slow progression to loss of ambulation
X-linked		
SMA with arthrogryposis and congenital contractures	**301830** Xp11.3–q11.2	Neonatal hypotonia, areflexia, chest deformities, facial dysmorphic features, and congenital joint contractures
Spinobulbar muscular atrophy	**313200** Trinucleotide repeat in the androgen receptor	See Chapter 17[a]

HMN = hereditary motor neuronopathy; LCCS = lethal congenital contracture syndrome; SMA = spinal muscular atrophy; SMARD = SMA with respiratory distress; SMN = survival motor neuron.

[a]Modified from Olney RK, Aminoff MJ, So YT. Clinical and electrodiagnostic features of X-linked recessive bulbospinal neuronopathy. Neurology 1991:41;823–828.

SMA will initially have been misdiagnosed as having ALS. Some general comments about differential diagnosis are therefore relevant at this point. Adult-onset SMA is typically a very slowly progressive condition in which clinically detectable deterioration may only be evident over decades. It is generally a symmetrical process, without bulbar involvement in the majority of patients and is by definition a pure LMN syndrome (but see comments on overlap syndromes, later in this chapter). ALS is a rapidly progressive disease with a focal or asymmetrical onset, bulbar involvement, and upper motor neuron (UMN) signs. Despite these differences, the conditions are not infrequently confused by the inexperienced. Further difficulty arises when one considers rapidly progressive pure LMN diseases in which the only distinction from SMA is in the rate of progression.[2]

AUTOSOMAL RECESSIVE PROXIMAL SPINAL MUSCULAR ATROPHY

Clinical Features

A number of genetically determined syndromes of infantile onset anterior horn cells disease lead to hypotonia, respiratory distress, and often death in infancy. Of these the most common is autosomal recessive proximal SMA caused by mutations in the survival motor neuron (SMN) gene. The molecular pathogenesis of this disorder is discussed in detail. On clinical grounds, proximal recessive SMA has been divided according to motor milestones achieved[3] and this classification by severity has subsequently been shown to correlate with the molecular diathesis. Type I disease (SMA-I), previously known as Werdnig-Hoffmann disease, has onset in utero or within the first 6 months of life. This has led to speculation that it is a disorder of neuronal maturation or programmed cell death, rather than a form of neurodegenerative disease. Affected children never sit and death from respiratory failure occurs before 2 years of age in the majority, although occasional patients survive for longer periods on ventilation. Children with type II disease (SMA-II) achieve the ability to sit unaided but never stand. The ultimate prognosis depends on the degree of respiratory involvement and prolonged survival over decades is common with modern respiratory support. Type III SMA (SMA-III) generally starts in early childhood, and by definition, children achieve the ability to walk unaided. Onset in later childhood and adult life is well described, even in the fifth or sixth decade. This has led to the use of the term type IV SMA (SMA-IV) for later onset cases. All types of SMN-related SMA, regardless of age at onset and severity, share the common features of being symmetrical and proximal and of sparing the facial musculature and importantly, the diaphragm. The latter feature allows the disorder to be distinguished on clinical grounds from "SMA with respiratory distress" (SMARD), which is due to mutations in a separate gene. Intellect and other neurological functions are unaffected and neuropathology studies have not revealed significant involvement of other neurons outside of the ventral horn of the spinal cord. The cause of the deterioration in function observed in patients with SMA has long been debated. It has not been demonstrated unequivocally that patients with the milder form of SMA undergo continued and progressive motor neuron fallout. Functional decline may be due to the failure of denervated muscle to develop congruently with the growth of the axial skeleton, leading to scoliosis and contributing to subsequent respiratory insufficiency. In the milder forms, stability of motor function over many decades is common.

The prognosis of proximal recessive SMA is largely dependent on respiratory muscle weakness. With increasing use of noninvasive ventilation, survival in the more severe forms of SMA-I and SMA-II is likely to improve. In a large clinical series of 240 patients with SMA-II, the survival rate was 98.5 percent at 5 years and 68.5 percent at 25 years.[4] The authors further subdivided their patients into those with onset before the age of 3 years (SMA-IIIa) and those with onset after the age of 3 years (SMA-IIIb). The probability of being able to walk was 70.3 percent and 22 percent at 10 years and 40 years, respectively, after onset in SMA-IIIa. For SMA-IIIb, 96.7 percent were walking 10 years after onset and 58.7 percent at 40 years. Life expectancy for SMA-III is thought to be normal.

Differential Diagnosis

Several other conditions may be mistaken for SMN-related SMA. The advent of molecular testing has resolved long running uncertainty about the etiological relationship of these disorders to classic Werdnig-Hoffmann disease.[5] SMARD is dealt with in its own section, later in this chapter.

Spinal Muscular Atrophy with Pontocerebellar Hypoplasia

SMA with pontocerebellar hypoplasia is frequently confused with Werdnig-Hoffmann disease because it presents with neonatal hypotonia. However, the children are intellectually less responsive and imaging reveals poor cerebellar development. The pattern of weakness may be more generalized and involves the diaphragm.[6,7] Molecular testing has shown conclusively that this autosomal recessive disorder is not due to mutations in the SMN gene.[8–10]

Spinal Muscular Atrophy with Congenital Contractures

Few patients, mostly male, have been described in which a clinical pattern of weakness indistinguishable from Werdnig-Hoffmann disease is associated with congenital long-bone fractures.[11,12] This disorder, which may be autosomal recessive or X-linked recessive, is genetically distinct from SMN-related SMA.[13]

Spinal Muscular Atrophy and Arthrogryposis

Arthrogryposis is a nonspecific response to in utero muscle weakness of any cause and therefore occurs in a range of disorders including congenital myasthenia and typical and atypical SMA. For the purposes of linkage studies, it was proposed that arthrogryposis be used as an exclusion criterion, but it is now established that it may occur in SMN-related SMA.[13,14] Another autosomal recessive syndrome of anterior horn cell involvement with multiple congenital contractures and in utero death has mostly been reported in the Finnish population.[15] The main clinical findings include intrauterine growth retardation with marked fetal hydrops, multiple contractures, and facial abnormalities, especially micrognathia. At autopsy, pulmonary hypoplasia and muscular atrophy were present. There was a paucity of anterior horn motor neurons in the four cases studied. The syndrome has been linked to chromosome 9q34.[16] X-linked SMA/arthrogryposis is a distinct condition that has been mapped to the short arm of the X chromosome.[17] Affected individuals showed hypotonia, areflexia, chest deformities, facial dysmorphic features, and congenital joint contractures. The findings of electromyography (EMG) and muscle biopsy were consistent with loss of anterior horn cells. Most children died in infancy, although one was still alive at the age of 13 years when the linkage study was performed.

Spinal Muscular Atrophy and Congenital Heart Defects

Although complex central nervous system (CNS) degeneration and amyotrophy have been described in association with atrial septal defect (ASD) in one family, this is likely to represent a distinct genetic disorder.[18] However, there is evidence that congenital heart defects also occur in conjunction with typical SMN-related SMA.[13,19] A large number of different types of abnormality were described (ventricular septal defects, ASDs, complex structural defects), and it remains likely that this is a chance association given the high frequency of congenital heart defects in the background population (7/1000). However, the presence of a congenital heart defect should not preclude SMN testing.

Metabolic Disorders Mimicking Infantile Spinal Muscular Atrophy

A large number of metabolic disorders presenting in infancy can involve anterior horn cells and may be confused with Werdnig-Hoffman disease. There are usually clues to a metabolic disorder such as ketoacidosis. Recently a mutation in nuclear-encoded cytochrome oxidase assembly gene, SCO2, has been associated with pathological evidence of anterior horn cell loss in an infant with generalized hypotonia and cardiomyopathy who died of respiratory failure 7 weeks after birth.[20] This suggests that mitochondrial diseases can mimic SMA. Anterior horn cell involvement in hexosaminidase A deficiency is usually associated with other CNS disturbance such as ataxia, but rare cases presenting with juvenile-onset SMA have been described.[21]

Molecular Pathogenesis

Despite historical arguments about the nosological relationship between Werdnig-Hoffmann disease (SMA-I) and Kugelberg-Welander syndrome

(SMA-III), linkage analysis ultimately revealed that these disorders, differing only in age at onset and prognosis but clinically very similar, are allelic and map to chromosome 5q.[22–24] Two studies, published simultaneously in 1995 and purporting to have identified the gene for recessive proximal SMA, revealed a high level of complexity in the genomic organization of the candidate region on 5q13.[25,26] A large genomic region spanning at least 500 kilobases occurs as an inverted duplication (Figure 16.1). This duplication exists in nonhuman primates and thus occurred at least 3 million years ago, although sequence divergence since then has led to significant differences between the two copies of individual genes shown in Figure 16.1.[27] Deletions of the telomeric copies of SMN (now referred to as *SMN1*) and the neuronal apoptosis inhibitory protein (NAIP) genes were shown to be associated with 98 percent and 60 percent, respectively, of cases of SMA. However, of great significance is that intragenic mutations (i.e., missense mutations, small deletions, or insertions) causing SMA have been found only in SMN. Therefore deletion in the telomeric copy of NAIP does not seem to be a necessary or sufficient condition for the development of the disease. Its role as a modifier gene for SMA severity continues to be explored, however, because it is a caspase inhibitor and rescues motor neurons in axotomized rats.[28] Of enormous practical clinical importance is the use of SMN1 deletion testing as a robust and sensitive test for SMA and the widespread availability of prenatal diagnosis.

Subsequent to the duplication of the SMN gene, there has been sequence divergence, which allows differentiation of SMN1 from SMN2 by polymerase chain reaction (PCR). Both primary gene sequences predict identical proteins, but a translationally silent change within an exonic splice enhancer in intron 6/exon 7 of SMN2 leads to the skipping of exon 7 in 80 percent of the transcript and to a truncated protein product. The 20 percent of full-length protein

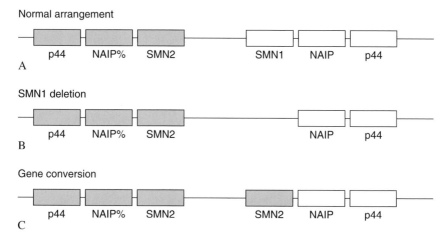

Figure 16.1 The complex genomic organization of the survival motor neuron (SMN) region of chromosomes gives rise to both gene deletions, which are severe mutations, and gene conversion events, which are mild mutations, because SMN1 is replaced with SMN2, which can provide a small amount of functional protein.

derived from SMN2 is presumed to be insufficient to rescue the SMA pheno-type when SMN1 is homozygously deleted.[29] To understand the motor neuron specificity of deletions in SMN, we must account for the fact that the approx-imately 20 percent of full-length protein derived from the SMN2 gene can provide sufficient function for all other cell types. This implies an exquisite sen-sitivity of motor neurons to lack of SMN or to a cell-specific function. The observation that motor neurons do appear to express higher levels of SMN would support either of these hypotheses.[30,31] One of the most promising exper-imental approaches to therapy for SMA comes from using synthetic exon-specific activators to block the molecular signal that induces skipping of exon 7, thereby inducing SMN2 to produce exclusively a full-length SMN trans-cript.[32] Because of the technical challenge of delivering such a therapy to the whole animal, these studies have so far been restricted to cells in culture.

The molecular basis for the variation in phenotype lies in the fact that absence of SMN1 by PCR testing can be due to complete deletion or gene conversion in which the SMN1 gene is replaced by an SMN2 copy during DNA replica-tion (see Figure 16.1B and C). This gives rise to a model in which patients with SMA are compound heterozygotes of deleted and gene-converted alleles. Carrier chromosomes can therefore consist of a single or a double copy of SMN2, and patients will have anything from one to four copies of SMN2, giving rise to a progressive increase in full-length SMN protein.[33,34] More complex pat-terns probably occur, because up to six copies of SMN2 per chromosome have been described and variations in regulatory sequences may also play a role, but the number of SMN2 copies, as measured by quantitative PCR, shows a good correlation with disease severity.[35] Therefore despite data suggesting that mutant SMN protein can exert a dominant negative effect in some cell systems,[36,37] the effect that causes SMA is likely to be due to SMN deficiency. Missense mutations occur in a minority of patients with SMA but are of inter-est because they show interesting patterns of clustering, which gives some insight into the functional domains of the protein. The SMN protein shows a remarkable degree of evolutionary conservation in specific regions at the C-terminal and N-terminal, which are identical in SMN orthologues in fission yeast and nematode and have therefore been preserved in more than a billion years of evolution. Most of the missense mutations described to date cluster in a region that has homology to RNA interacting proteins.[38]

Since the SMN gene has been identified, there has been rapid progress in identifying the complex range of proteins with which it appears to interact (Table 16.2). Most of these are known to be RNA-associated proteins and it is therefore necessary to briefly review the basic biology of messenger RNA (mRNA) processing (Figure 16.2). After transcription, pre-mRNA undergoes 5′ capping and 3′ polyadenylation, which have an effect on transcript stability and subsequent translation. Pre-mRNA is spliced in the nucleus in spliceosomes, which are aggregated protein-RNA complexes of which the principal compo-nents are U1, 2, 4/6, and 5 small nuclear ribonucleoprotein (snRNP) (uridine-rich snRNP). Heteronuclear RNPs (hnRNPs) are mRNA interacting proteins that bind to nascent transcripts and that influence interaction with spliceosomal RNPs and have a role in export of processed mRNA from the nucleus to the cytoplasm.[52] Specific mechanisms exist for the nuclear retention of unprocessed mRNA. Retroviruses have mechanisms for bypassing this to allow unspliced

Table 16.2   Survival motor neuron function

Function of SMN	Interacting proteins	Key references
Cytoplasmic assembly of snRNP	Sm core proteins; Gemin 2, 3, 4; profilin	39–45
Pre-mRNA splicing in the nucleus	U snRNPs, Sm proteins	37, 46, 47
Transcriptional regulation	RNA helicase A, RNA polymerase II, viral transcriptional activators	37, 48
Ribosomal RNA and snoRNP biogenesis	Fibrillarin, GAR1	49, 50
Motor neuron–specific RNP chaperone?	hnRNP-R, hnRNP-Q	51

hnRNP = heteronuclear RNP; mRNA = messenger ribonucleic acid; RNP = ribonucleoprotein; SMN = survival motor neuron; snoRNP = small nucleolar RNP; snRNP = small nuclear RNP; U snRNP = uridine-rich small nuclear ribonucleoprotein.

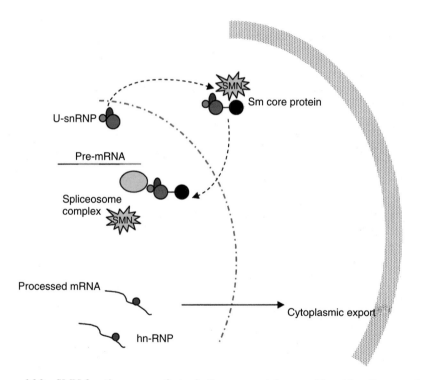

Figure 16.2   SMN functions as a cofactor in Sm core protein assembly with spliceosomal ribonucleoprotein in the cytoplasm. In addition, it appears to have critical nuclear functions in regulating splicing. See color insert.

messages to reach the cytoplasm. SMN is ubiquitously expressed and shows both punctuate nuclear and diffuse cytoplasmic staining in cells in culture, including motor neurons (Figure 16.3). SMN has been shown to cluster in intranuclear suborganelles associated with so-called "coiled bodies," first described by Cajal more than a century ago,[53] and thought to function in RNP maturation. snRNP is exported from the nucleus to be assembled in the cytoplasm into a complex that includes SMN and Sm core proteins. SMN has been found to be an important cofactor for assembly of RNP complexes before reimport into the nucleus where it participates in splicing reactions. In addition, it has some direct role in efficient splicing and in nuclear transcription. Therefore SMN appears to modulate RNP biogenesis both in the cytoplasm and in the nucleus and to directly influence splicing and transcription. The nucleolus is a subnuclear organelle containing the ribosomal RNA gene clusters and ribosome biogenesis factors. Recent studies suggest it may also have roles in RNA transport, RNA modification, and cell cycle regulation. Despite more than 150 years of research into nucleoli, many aspects of their structure and function remain uncharacterized. By analogy with nuclear RNP, nucleoli contain small nucleolar RNP (snoRNPs). Recently SMN has been identified as part of a multiprotein complex with snoRNP, further widening the number of interactions with various types of RNP (see Table 16.2).

These pathways have traditionally been considered as part of the "housekeeping" activity of cells. In contrast, there has been little progress in identifying the molecular substrate of the cellular specificity of the disease for motor neurons. Why do defects in a ubiquitous and fundamental biological pathway, involving a protein in which the key functional domains are conserved in evolution as far back as yeast, lead to such a cell-specific disease as SMA? There is a tight linkage between the severity of SMA and the amount of full-length SMN protein, either directly detected by antibody[30] or indirectly predicted from SMN2 copy number.[35] It would therefore appear that motor neurons have a "dose-dependent" requirement for SMN and that there is a threshold of protein level above which the disease is unlikely to develop. In addition, SMN might have a set of protein partners in motor neurons, which are cell specific and govern motor neuron–specific RNP metabolism. The identification of a developmentally regulated, SMN-interacting RNP, hnRNP-R, that localizes to motor axons is of particular interest in this regard.[51] Furthermore, the localization of SMN to the growth cone of developing neurons in culture provides further support that there is an important neuronal-specific function for SMN at sites distant from the nucleus.[54]

Transgenic mouse models have been difficult to engineer because of the need to replicate the multicopy nature of the human genomic organization. Mice deficient in SMN ("SMN knockout" mice) fail to implant, suggesting an obligate requirement for SMN in development.[55] Attempts to model the human disease have used several approaches. Transgenic mice with human SMN2 were crossed with heterozygous SMN-null mutant mice to create animals with varying copy numbers of SMN2[56,57] and varying degrees of motor neuron loss. An alternative approach is to use targeted inactivation of SMN in neurons, allowing normal expression in other tissues and circumventing embryonic lethality.[58] The potential value of these models can be summarized as (1) in confirming that the severity of the disease is tightly linked to SMN2 copy number,

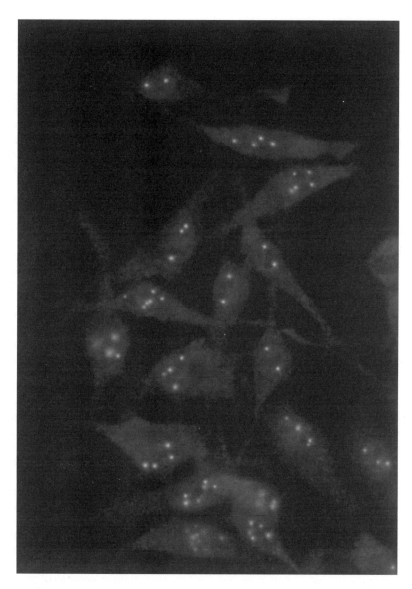

Figure 16.3 Immunostaining of HeLa cells in culture with an antibody directed against the survival motor neuron protein. There is diffuse cytoplasmic staining and punctuate nuclear staining in subnuclear organelles thought to be critical for ribonucleoprotein metabolism. See color insert. (Courtesy Dr. Kirstie Anderson, Department of Human Anatomy and Genetics, University of Oxford.)

and thus the total amount of full-length SMN protein (2) in giving insights into the early changes in gene expression and cellular morphology that occur in motor neuron death and (3) providing a biological system in which to test potential therapeutic strategies. Attempts to upregulate the expression of SMN2 in transgenic mice models using drugs is a promising approach.[59,60] However, it may be difficult to find an agent that does this without significant toxicity or in a way that is specific to the SMN gene. One of the major challenges for developing therapies in SMA is that affected individuals fall into two groups in which clinical trials may be equally difficult. Those with overwhelming motor neuron loss that probably begins in utero and leads to devastating neuromuscular paralysis evident at birth (SMA-I) probably need restorative cell therapy because rescuing the few surviving motor neurons is unlikely to have a clinically significant effect. At the other extreme is a group of patients (SMA-II and SMA-III) in which weakness and progressive disability is often so slow that it can be measured only over periods of several years. Performing clinical trials in either of these groups will be very difficult indeed.

AUTOSOMAL RECESSIVE DISTAL SPINAL MUSCULAR ATROPHY

Distal SMA is usually dominantly inherited. However, some rare recessive forms are described in the following sections.

Spinal Muscular Atrophy with Respiratory Distress due to Mutations in IGHMBP2

Less than 1% of infantile SMA is of this type, which is characterized by severe diaphragmatic weakness with exenteration of abdominal contents, leading to respiratory distress.[13] Muscle weakness is greater distally than proximally.[61] The condition is known to be genetically heterogeneous with one form (SMARD1) linked to chromosome 11p but at least one family unlinked to this locus.[62] In Harding's classification, this is referred to as *distal HMN type VI* (dHMN-VI). The clinical features resemble those of the neuromuscular degeneration *(nmd)* mouse,[63] which is due to mutation in the *IGHMBP2* gene. Intriguingly, the gene for SMARD1 has been identified as *IGHMBP2,* which is known to have RNA helicase activity, providing a further link to motor neuron degeneration and RNA metabolism. Although the exact cellular function of this gene is unknown, its helicase structure and involvement in pre-mRNA processing are in keeping with a similar function to that of SMN and provide further evidence that LMNs have a selective vulnerability to defects in RNA handling.

Distal Spinal Muscular Atrophy Linked to 11q13

Viollet et al[64] described linkage to chromosome 11q13 in a large consanguineous pedigree of Lebanese origin. Given the similarity of the distal pattern of weakness to that of SMARD, they chose to investigate linkage to the same region and demonstrated a combined logarithmic odds (LOD) score of 4.59 over a genomic region that encompasses *IGHMBP2*. However, sequencing of the gene in affected individuals revealed no mutations. The phenotype of this disorder is highly variable. In some individuals, it becomes manifest in infancy with loss of ambulation during childhood, but other individuals remain ambulant beyond the fourth decade. Distal limb weakness is combined with generalized areflexia, normal sensation, and absence of bulbar involvement. In parallel with SMARD, the more severely affected patients have shown evidence of diaphragmatic weakness and reduced vital capacity, but not the severe respiratory failure of SMARD. It remains possible that this disorder is allelic to SMARD but due to mutations in the promoter region or is due to mutations in a neighboring gene.

Jerash Hereditary Motor Neuronopathy

Jerash HMN demonstrates perfectly the problem of the overlap of SMA with disorders involving the corticospinal tract. A total of 27 individuals from 7 consanguineous families from the Jerash region of Jordan have a disorder that has been linked to chromosome 9p21.1-p12.[65] Onset is in childhood with symmetrical lower limb distal atrophy, pes cavus, and weakness of dorsiflexion. Upper limb involvement of wrist and finger flexors developed later. The disorder seems to be associated with absent ankle jerks and extensor-plantar responses in the early stages progressing to generalized hyporeflexia and loss of Babinski reflexes, although presumably the latter may just reflect severe distal weakness. What is referred to by the authors as "regression" of pyramidal tract signs does not seem to be an altogether satisfactory concept.

AUTOSOMAL DOMINANT SPINAL MUSCULAR ATROPHY

The dominantly inherited forms of SMA are rarer and clinically less well defined than the childhood recessive forms. There are significant issues about whether disorders that include involvement outside of the motor neuron should be included under the rubric of SMA. In addition, there is confusion between the term "distal SMA" and the so-called "spinal" form of CMT disease, known as CMT2D or dHMN in Harding's scheme. Whether pure motor forms of neuronopathy should be considered forms of MND or forms of neuropathy is an unresolved issue. However, there is abundant clinical and electrophysiological data in favor of the anterior horn cell being the primary site of pathology, and therefore from a biological standpoint, distal motor neuronopathies may turn out to have more in common with SMAs than with CMT neuropathies. This variation in terminology makes it difficult to compare different descriptions in the neurological literature. The classification proposed by Anita Harding in which HMN is divided into seven types seems reasonable, but it has not been universally adopted and the term *SMA* is still used in a descriptive sense. The exact incidence of dominant SMA is not known and has not been addressed since the studies by Pearn[66] in the northeast of England, where the incidence was found to be considerably lower than that of childhood recessive SMA. However, given the nosological confusion outlined earlier in this chapter, it may be more common than previously thought. None of the genes for dominant forms of SMA has yet been identified and the various types are described according to the distribution of weakness and linkage studies.

Distal Spinal Muscular Atrophy with Lower Limb Predominance (Peroneal Muscular Atrophy Like)

Distal SMA with lower limb predominance appears to be dominantly inherited in most patients, but patients with no family history are seen from time to time. This apparently sporadic form of the disease may be due to new mutations, late-onset recessive disease or a nongenetic etiology. An early study by Pearn and Hudgson[67] found a high rate of consanguinity in isolated cases of distal SMA, suggesting that recessive forms might exist. Dyck and Lambert[68] included distal neurogenic weakness with a peroneal muscular atrophy presentation in the group of "hereditary and motor and sensory neuropathies." Subsequent reports confirmed the frequent sporadic occurrence and the wide age range of presentation.[69,70] Only 10 of Harding's series of 34 cases[70] belonged to five families, the remainder being sporadic. The age at onset was mostly in the first two decades and progression was slow. Many patients had retained reflexes and occasionally they were brisk. The rationale for making the distinction between upper and lower limb predominant forms of distal SMA comes from recent linkage studies showing that these disorders, in some families at least, localize to different chromosomes. However, the situation is far from resolved and specific dominant SMA-determining genes may well turn out to be associated with considerable clinical heterogeneity.

Timmerman et al[71] described a large Belgian pedigree with onset in the second to fourth decade of lower limb distal SMA with progression to involve all muscle groups in the legs. Progression is slow and the arms were mildly affected. Subsequently this family has been linked to chromosome 12q24.[72] This is adjacent to but apparently separate from the scapuloperoneal form of SMA (SPSMA) and the congenital benign dominant SMA loci at 12q24.[73] At least one similar family has been shown to be unlinked to this locus, underlining the genetic heterogeneity of distal SMA.[74]

Distal Spinal Muscular Atrophy with Upper Limb Predominance

Early reports of distal amyotrophy affecting the hands emphasized the dominant inheritance of this disorder and the occasional appearance of affected individuals with UMN signs.[75,76] The existence of this disorder as a separate diagnostic entity from lower limb distal SMA has been justified by genetic studies that have linked this disorder to chromosome 7p in a large Bulgarian pedigree[77] and subsequently in U.S. families.[78] A further study appears to demonstrate that CMT2D and distal SMA of the upper limbs are the same disorder.[79] A recent Austrian family unlinked to 7p has provided evidence for genetic heterogeneity in this disorder.[80] This large family demonstrates onset between 10 and 34 years and a large number of individuals with pathologically brisk reflexes. The authors also demonstrated prolonged central motor conduction time in some individuals. The so-called "ALS4" locus on 9q was also excluded.

Distal Spinal Muscular Atrophy with Vocal Cord Paralysis

Young and Harper first described distal SMA with vocal cord paralysis in a four-generation British family.[81] The onset is in adolescence in the majority and upper limb involvement precedes lower limb. Wasting and weakness of distal limb muscles (especially finger extension) is accompanied by areflexia and a postural tremor. Impaired vital capacity and exertional intolerance occur. The vocal cords have reduced mobility on laryngoscopy and affected individuals have a husky voice. Despite the vocal cord involvement, this appears to be a slowly progressive and essentially benign disorder, in keeping with most other dominant forms of SMA. A genome-wide screen of this and another British family[82] has linked the disorder to chromosome 2q14[83] and suggested a common ancestral mutation. The authors have referred to this disorder as *dHMN-VII*.

The differential diagnosis of motor weakness with vocal cord paralysis in adulthood also includes forms of axonal CMT disease and distal myopathy. Few families have been described including one with sensorineural hearing loss[84] and others with sensorimotor involvement (HMSN-IIC).[85] Whether this disorder is also linked to chromosome 2q is unknown. A much more severe recessive form of axonal CMT disease with vocal cord paralysis has been described as occurring in CMT4A due to mutations in ganglioside-induced differentiation-associated protein.[86] A form of distal myopathy with vocal cord and pharyngeal involvement is linked to 5q31.[87]

Congenital Dominant Distal Spinal Muscular Atrophy

Congenital dominant distal SMA is a mild disorder that may present with congenital contractures of the lower limb or delayed motor milestones and unlike other dominant forms of SMA appears to be nonprogressive. Fleury and Hageman[88] described a Dutch family with seven affected individuals in three generations. Congenital talipes and arthrogryposis is associated with weakness of the lower limb with a distal predominance and only mild and variable involvement of the upper limb. Further pedigrees with identical clinical features have been described in the Netherlands and Canada.[89,90] Subsequently the original Dutch family has been linked to 12q23–q24.[91] This is within the same region as the localization for SPSMA. Whether these two disorders are allelic remains to be determined, but the lack of progression and distinct clinical features of this disorder justifies its inclusion as a separate disorder. Furthermore in at least one family with the clinical features of this disorder, linkage to 12q has been excluded, suggesting genetic heterogeneity.

Scapuloperoneal Spinal Muscular Atrophy

Distal muscle wasting with a scapuloperoneal distribution was first described in the 1920 and 1930s,[92,93] but these cases were heterogeneous, some being myopathic and others neurogenic in origin, with occasional sensory involvement. Several large pedigrees with EMG-verified denervation have now been described,[94–96] and this disorder has been linked, in a large New England pedigree to 12q23–q24.[97] Therefore SPSMA appears to be a distinct clinical entity. Curiously, an apparently myopathic scapuloperoneal syndrome has been linked to a neighboring region of chromosome 12.[98] Many of the families described in the literature contain individuals with both myopathic and neurogenic changes on muscle biopsy. Furthermore, this is the same region to which dominant congenital benign SMA and distal SMA with lower limb predominance have been mapped. Although the genetic and physical mapping of the region would suggest that the myopathic and neurogenic forms of scapuloperoneal syndrome are separate disorders, there is overlap between the candidate genetic loci for SPSMA and congenital dominant SMA, which may indicate that they are the same disorder.[73]

The clinical descriptions of SPSMA vary. The five-generation pedigree in a study by Kaeser[94] had onset between the ages of 30 to 50 years and inexorable progression over decades to loss of ambulation, but probably a normal life span.[94] Some of the family members appear to have had pharyngeal involvement late in the illness. The New England pedigree linked to chromosome 12 differs in having an earlier age at onset, earlier involvement of the lower limb, and in possibly showing genetic anticipation.[96] The youngest generation appears to have congenital onset with absence of individual muscles and progression to severe disability by adolescence. As with other forms of SMA, this rare syndrome of SPSMA may turn out to be a genetically heterogeneous condition.

Proximal Dominant Spinal Muscular Atrophy

Proximal symmetrical SMA occurring in adults may be due to SMN mutations if there is no history to suggest dominant inheritance.[99] Although pseudodominant inheritance has also been described,[100] clear autosomal dominant forms of adult-onset proximal SMA also exist.[101] We are currently undertaking linkage studies in one such family in which slowly progressive weakness of hip flexion is associated with marked triceps weakness and preservation of forearm flexion. Ambulation in this family is maintained until the eighth decade.

OVERLAP BETWEEN SPINAL MUSCULAR ATROPHY, HEREDITARY MOTOR AND SENSORY NEUROPATHY, AND HEREDITARY SPASTIC PARAPARESIS

The strict application of the term *SMA* to pure LMN disorders has led to a certain amount of confusion in the classification of these disorders. It is our experience that it is not rare to find that some families with dominant distal SMA have subtle (brisk reflexes) or overt (extensor-plantar responses) UMN signs. Mild to moderate reductions of vibration sense in the lower limb are also common. It is biologically plausible that there will be disorders in which the genetic defect will lead to dysfunction of long neurons and that the predilection for UMNs or LMNs will be relative. The use of the term *ALS* for slowly progressive forms of distal atrophy with variable UMN involvement masks the fact that on prognostic grounds these disorders are more akin to SMA rather than to ALS, a disease considerably more malignant in behavior. A single family from the United States in which distal amyotrophy and UMN signs occurred with onset in adolescence but in which life expectancy was normal has been linked to chromosome 9q34,[102] with the proposed diagnosis of juvenile ALS. Three families have recently been described in which the same linkage was found but the diagnostic label given was of distal SMA or the spinal form of CMT.[103] The combination of distal amyotrophy of the upper limbs and HSP has been referred to as *Silver syndrome* and linked to chromosome 11q12–q14.[104] Although this disorder appears in most patients to lead to significant disability of the type seen in HSP, it does provide further demonstration of considerable overlap between slowly progressive pyramidal tract and anterior horn cell diseases.

FOCAL FORMS OF SPINAL MUSCULAR ATROPHY

Hirayama's Disease

Monomelic amyotrophy of the upper limb has been most commonly described in the Indian subcontinent[105] and in the Japanese population, where it is variously known as Hirayama's disease[106] or the Sobue form of segmental muscular atrophy.[107] Rare patients of non-Asian origin have been reported.[108] Painless weakness and wasting of one limb generally develops over a period of months, followed by arrest or very slow progression and long-term stability.[106,107,109] Lower limb involvement is much rarer but clearly follows the same benign pattern.[108] There is a male preponderance with onset in early adult life and an absence of a positive family history. Rarely the condition can be bilateral. Magnetic resonance imaging of the cervical spine is essential to rule out compressive lesions, and if this is normal, the most important investigation is electrophysiological evaluation to rule out multifocal motor neuropathy with conduction block. The differential diagnosis includes that of a monomelic presentation of ALS, which is only formally excluded after a sufficient time has elapsed. However, in the appropriate clinical setting, the disorder is sufficiently characteristic to make it instantly recognizable. The so-called "flail-arm syndrome" or the amyotrophic brachial diplegia variant of ALS is distinguished from Hirayama's disease by bilateral symmetrical onset, greater involvement of proximal musculature, and ultimate progression to full-blown ALS, albeit with a longer than average survival.[110] The cases described by Harding, Bradbury, and Murray[111] as "chronic asymmetrical SMA" seem to be a heterogeneous group may have included some cases of Hirayama's disease, but weakness was bilateral and involved both upper and lower limbs in most patients. This study took place before conduction block neuropathies were widely recognized, and the follow-up period of only 3 years makes it difficult to be certain that some of these cases did not ultimately develop ALS.

The etiology of most cases of monomelic amyotrophy remains an enigma. Historical autopsy studies seemed to favor a primary degeneration of segmental pools of motor neurons,[112] although recent reviews have stressed the possible role of focal structural changes in the spine.[113] It has been proposed that focal venous ischaemia arises through compressive flattening of the lower cervical cord due to forward displacement of the cervical dural sac and spinal cord induced by recurrent neck flexion.[114,115] It is not clear why this should give rise to a disorder that is so frequently unilateral and is exclusively a lower motor neuronopathy, sparing the long tracts. At least one other imaging study has shown no difference between the anteroposterior cord diameter between patients and controls, supporting the notion that the etiology is a primary degeneration of motor neurons.[116]

Chronic Neurogenic Quadriceps Amyotrophy

Two reports have appeared in the literature of patients presenting with the extremely rare combination of isolated quadriceps amyotrophy associated with calf hypertrophy. One study of two patients suggested that this disorder may be inherited and associated in other family members with more widespread SMA.[117] To what extent this is an etiologically heterogeneous condition is unclear.[118]

Spinobulbar Muscular Atrophy Syndromes

A number of rare bulbar motor neuron syndromes of childhood have been described, and the clinical and genetic features suggest that these are a group of recessively inherited focal forms of SMA. Fazio-Londe syndrome was described in the last decade of the 19th century as progressive bulbar paralysis of childhood, and case reports continue to occur. The largest most recent study of five patients suggested that even within this extremely rare condition, there is genetic heterogeneity with one dominant form and possibly two recessive forms.[119] The most frequent description is of a rapidly progressive bulbar degeneration with death from respiratory tract infection.

Another rare but potentially fatal form of bulbar motor neuronopathy is Brown-Vialetto-van Laere syndrome. Progressive weakness of muscles groups associated with cranial nerves VII to XII is associated with sensorineural deafness. Most patients die of respiratory involvement, but the rapidity of progression seems to be very variable. A consanguineous Lebanese family with three affected siblings supports an autosomal recessive pattern of inheritance, although this family appears to have more widespread involvement than other cases.[120] Other families with possible dominant inheritance have been described.[121]

Hopkins Syndrome

Hopkins syndrome is an unusual condition and is mentioned here because it may be confused with other forms of monomelic amyotrophy. Most patients described have been children, although it has also been reported in adults.[122] What appears to be a focal myelitis over multiple spinal segments leads to weakness and wasting of one limb within a week of an acute severe asthmatic attack. The etiology is unknown, but most patients have been on steroids. The condition does not recover.

CONCLUSION

The SMAs represent a large number of separate single-gene disorders. The elucidation of the molecular pathogenesis will collectively tell us much about the nature of LMN development and survival. By extension, there is reason to believe that this will also shed light on the pathogenesis of ALS. The last 10 years have seen considerable progress in defining the genetic subtypes of SMA and in revealing the importance of RNA handling as a potentially important factor in determining motor neuron vulnerability. In this chapter, we have attempted to emphasize the following general points about SMA:

- The infantile recessive forms of SMA are part of a growing number of neurological disorders including fragile-X mental retardation and myotonic dystrophy, in which abnormalities of RNA handling appear to be central to the disease process. This suggests that neurons are particularly vulnerable to defects in RNA handling and this area deserves further study.
- Juvenile and adult-onset SMAs are distinguished from ALS not just by the pure LMN nature of the disease but also by the slow progression. The term *ALS* should therefore be reserved for inherited forms of MND, which behave in a similarly malignant fashion to sporadic ALS.
- There are many families in which the combination of distal amyotrophy and pyramidal tract involvement occur together. This suggests that there may be similarities in the molecular basis of disorders of long neurons such as SMA and HSP.

Acknowledgments

Dr. Talbot is funded by a Medical Research Council/GlaxoSmithKline Clinician Scientist Fellowship. We are grateful to Dr. Anderson and Dr. Michael Donaghy for comments on the manuscript.

REFERENCES

1. Harding AE. Inherited Neuronal Atrophy and Degeneration Predominantly of Lower Motor Neurones. In PJ Dyck, PK Thomas (eds), Peripheral Neuropathy. Philadelphia: WB Saunders, 1993;1051–1064.

2. Van den Berg-Vos RM, et al. Hereditary pure lower motor neuron disease with adult onset and rapid progression. J Neurol 2001;248:290–296.
3. Munsat T, Davies K. Spinal muscular atrophy. 32nd ENMC International Workshop. Naarden, The Netherlands, 10–12 March 1995. Neuromusc Disord 1996;6:125–127.
4. Zerres K, et al. A collaborative study on the natural history of childhood and juvenile onset proximal spinal muscular atrophy (type II and III SMA): 569 patients. J Neurol Sci 1997;146:67–72.
5. Zerres K, Wirth B, Rudnik-Schoneborn S. Spinal muscular atrophy—clinical and genetic correlations. Neuromusc Disord 1997;7:202–207.
6. Chou SM, et al. Infantile olivopontocerebellar atrophy with spinal muscular atrophy (infantile OPCA + SMA). Clin Neuropathol 1990;9:21–32.
7. Goutieres F, Aicardi J, Farkas E. Anterior horn cell disease associated with pontocerebellar hypoplasia in infants. J Neurol Neurosurg Psychiatry 1977;40:370–378.
8. Dubowitz V, Daniels RJ, Davies KE. Olivopontocerebellar hypoplasia with anterior horn cell involvement (SMA) does not localize to chromosome 5q. Neuromusc Disord 1995;5:25–29.
9. Rudnik-Schoneborn S, et al. Exclusion of the gene locus for spinal muscular atrophy on chromosome 5q in a family with infantile olivopontocerebellar atrophy (OPCA) and anterior horn cell degeneration. Neuromusc Disord 1995;5:19–23.
10. Muntoni F, et al. Clinical spectrum and diagnostic difficulties of infantile ponto-cerebellar hypoplasia type 1. Neuropediatrics 1999;30:243–248.
11. Kelly TE, et al. Spinal muscular atrophy variant with congenital fractures. Am J Med Genet 1999; 87:65–68.
12. Borochowitz Z, Glick B, Blazer S. Infantile spinal muscular atrophy (SMA) and multiple congenital bone fractures in sibs: a lethal new syndrome. J Med Genet 1991;28:345–348.
13. Rudnik-Schoneborn S, et al. Clinical spectrum and diagnostic criteria of infantile spinal muscular atrophy: further delineation on the basis of SMN gene deletion findings. Neuropediatrics 1996;27: 8–15.
14. Burglen L, et al. Survival motor neuron gene deletion in the arthrogryposis multiplex congenita-spinal muscular atrophy association. J Clin Invest 1996;98:1130–1132.
15. Herva R, et al. A lethal autosomal recessive syndrome of multiple congenital contractures. Am J Med Genet 1985;20:431–439.
16. Makela-Bengs P, et al. Assignment of the disease locus for lethal congenital contracture syndrome to a restricted region of chromosome 9q34, by genome scan using five affected individuals. Am J Hum Genet 1998;63:506–516.
17. Kobayashi H, et al. A gene for a severe lethal form of X-linked arthrogryposis (X-linked infantile spinal muscular atrophy) maps to human chromosome Xp11.3–q11.2. Hum Mol Genet 1995;4: 1213–1216.
18. Moller P, et al. Spinal muscular atrophy type I combined with atrial septal defect in three sibs. Clin Genet 1990;38:81–83.
19. Burglen L, et al. SMN gene deletion in variant of infantile spinal muscular atrophy. Lancet 1995;346:316–317.
20. Salviati L, et al. Cytochrome *c* oxidase deficiency due to a novel SCO2 mutation mimics Werdnig-Hoffmann disease. Arch Neurol 2002;59:862–865.
21. Rondot P, et al. Juvenile GM_2 gangliosidosis with progressive spinal muscular atrophy onset [in French]. Rev Neurol (Paris) 1997;153:120–123.
22. Brzustowicz LM, et al. Genetic mapping of chronic childhood-onset spinal muscular atrophy to chromosome 5q11.2-13.3. Nature 1990;344:540–541.
23. Gilliam TC, et al. Genetic homogeneity between acute and chronic forms of spinal muscular atrophy. Nature 1990;345:823–825.
24. Melki J, et al. Mapping of acute (type I) spinal muscular atrophy to chromosome 5q12–q14. The French Spinal Muscular Atrophy Investigators. Lancet 1990;336:271–273.
25. Lefebvre S, et al. Identification and characterization of a spinal muscular atrophy-determining gene. Cell 1995;80:155–165.
26. Roy N, et al. The gene for neuronal apoptosis inhibitory protein is partially deleted in individuals with spinal muscular atrophy. Cell 1995;80:167–178.
27. Rochette CF, Gilbert N, Simard LR. SMN gene duplication and the emergence of the SMN2 gene occurred in distinct hominids: SMN2 is unique to Homo sapiens. Hum Genet 2001;108:255–266.
28. Perrelet D, et al. IAP family proteins delay motoneuron cell death in vivo. Eur J Neurosci 2000;12:2059–2067.
29. Cartegni L, Krainer AR. Disruption of an SF2/ASF-dependent exonic splicing enhancer in SMN2 causes spinal muscular atrophy in the absence of SMN1. Nat Genet 2002;30:377–384.

30. Lefebvre S, et al. Correlation between severity and SMN protein level in spinal muscular atrophy. Nat Genet 1997;16:265–269.
31. Coovert DD, et al. The survival motor neuron protein in spinal muscular atrophy. Hum Mol Genet 1997;6:1205–1214.
32. Cartegni L, Krainer AR. Correction of disease-associated exon skipping by synthetic exon-specific activators. Nat Struct Biol 2003;10:120–125.
33. Campbell L, et al. Genomic variation and gene conversion in spinal muscular atrophy: implications for disease process and clinical phenotype. Am J Hum Genet 1997;61:40–50.
34. Lefebvre S, et al. The role of the SMN gene in proximal spinal muscular atrophy. Hum Mol Genet 1998;7:1531–1536.
35. Feldkotter M, et al. Quantitative analyses of SMN1 and SMN2 based on real-time LightCycler PCR: fast and highly reliable carrier testing and prediction of severity of spinal muscular atrophy. Am J Hum Genet 2002;70:358–368.
36. Mohaghegh P, et al. Analysis of mutations in the tudor domain of the survival motor neuron protein SMN. Eur J Hum Genet 1999;7:519–525.
37. Pellizzoni L, et al. A functional interaction between the survival motor neuron complex and RNA polymerase II. J Cell Biol 2001;152:75–85.
38. Talbot K, et al. Missense mutation clustering in the survival motor neuron gene: a role for a conserved tyrosine and glycine rich region of the protein in RNA metabolism? Hum Mol Genet 1997;6:497–500.
39. Liu Q, Dreyfuss G. A novel nuclear structure containing the survival of motor neurons protein. EMBO J 1996;15:3555–3565.
40. Fischer U, Liu Q, Dreyfuss G. The SMN-SIP1 complex has an essential role in spliceosomal snRNP biogenesis. Cell 1997;90:1023–1029.
41. Charroux B, et al. Gemin3: A novel DEAD box protein that interacts with SMN, the spinal muscular atrophy gene product, and is a component of gems. J Cell Biol 1999;147:1181–1194.
42. Charroux B, et al. Gemin4. A novel component of the SMN complex that is found in both gems and nucleoli. J Cell Biol 2000;148:1177–1186.
43. Campbell L, et al. Direct interaction of Smn with dp103, a putative RNA helicase: a role for Smn in transcription regulation? Hum Mol Genet 2000;9:1093–1100.
44. Giesemann T, et al. A role for polyproline motifs in the spinal muscular atrophy protein SMN. Profilins bind to and colocalize with smn in nuclear gems. J Biol Chem 1999;274:37908–37914.
45. Buhler D, et al. Essential role for the tudor domain of SMN in spliceosomal U snRNP assembly: implications for spinal muscular atrophy. Hum Mol Genet 1999;8:2351–2357.
46. Meister G, et al. Characterization of a nuclear 20S complex containing the survival of motor neurons (SMN) protein and a specific subset of spliceosomal Sm proteins. Hum Mol Genet 2000; 9:1977–1986.
47. Pellizzoni L, et al. A novel function for SMN, the spinal muscular atrophy disease gene product, in pre-mRNA splicing. Cell 1998;95:615–624.
48. Strasswimmer J, et al. Identification of survival motor neuron as a transcriptional activator-binding protein. Hum Mol Genet 1999;8:1219–1226.
49. Jones KW, et al. Direct interaction of the spinal muscular atrophy disease protein SMN with the small nucleolar RNA-associated protein fibrillarin. J Biol Chem 2001;16:16.
50. Pellizzoni L, et al. The survival of motor neurons (SMN) protein interacts with the snoRNP proteins fibrillarin and GAR1. Curr Biol 2001;11:1079–1088.
51. Rossoll W, et al. Specific interaction of Smn, the spinal muscular atrophy determining gene product, with hnRNP-R and gry-rbp/hnRNP-Q: a role for Smn in RNA processing in motor axons? Hum Mol Genet 2002;11:93–105.
52. Dreyfuss G, Kim VN, Kataoka N. Messenger-RNA–binding proteins and the messages they carry. Nat Rev Mol Cell Biol 2002;3:195–205.
53. Liu Q, et al. The spinal muscular atrophy disease gene product, SMN, and its associated protein SIP1 are in a complex with spliceosomal snRNP proteins. Cell 1997;90:1013–1021.
54. Fan L, Simard LR. Survival motor neuron (SMN) protein: role in neurite outgrowth and neuromuscular maturation during neuronal differentiation and development. Hum Mol Genet 2002;11: 1605–1614.
55. Schrank B, et al. Inactivation of the survival motor neuron gene, a candidate gene for human spinal muscular atrophy, leads to massive cell death in early mouse embryos. Proc Natl Acad Sci USA 1997;94:9920–9925.
56. Hsieh-Li HM, et al. A mouse model for spinal muscular atrophy. Nat Genet 2000;24:66–70.

57. Monani UR, et al. The human centromeric survival motor neuron gene (SMN2) rescues embry-onic lethality in Smn(−/−) mice and results in a mouse with spinal muscular atrophy. Hum Mol Genet 2000;9:333–339.

58. Frugier T, et al. Nuclear targeting defect of SMN lacking the C-terminus in a mouse model of spinal muscular atrophy. Hum Mol Genet 2000;9:849–858.

59. Chang JG, et al. Treatment of spinal muscular atrophy by sodium butyrate. Proc Natl Acad Sci USA 2001;98:9808–9813.

60. Andreassi C, et al. Aclarubicin treatment restores SMN levels to cells derived from type I spinal muscular atrophy patients. Hum Mol Genet 2001;10:2841–2849.

61. Bertini E, et al. Distal infantile spinal muscular atrophy associated with paralysis of the diaphragm: a variant of infantile spinal muscular atrophy. Am J Med Genet 1989;33:328–335.

62. Grohmann K, et al. Diaphragmatic spinal muscular atrophy with respiratory distress is hetero-geneous, and one form is linked to chromosome 11q13–q21. Am J Hum Genet 1999;65:1459–1462.

63. Cox GA, Mahaffey CL, Frankel WN. Identification of the mouse neuromuscular degeneration gene and mapping of a second site suppressor allele. Neuron 1998;21:1327–1337.

64. Viollet L, et al. Mapping of autosomal recessive chronic distal spinal muscular atrophy to chro-mosome 11q13. Ann Neurol 2002;51:585–592.

65. Christodoulou K, et al. A novel form of distal hereditary motor neuronopathy maps to chromo-some 9p21.1-p12. Ann Neurol 2000;48:877–884.

66. Pearn J. Autosomal dominant spinal muscular atrophy: a clinical and genetic study. J Neurol Sci 1978;38:263–275.

67. Pearn J, Hudgson P. Distal spinal muscular atrophy. A clinical and genetic study of 8 kindreds. J Neurol Sci 1979;43:183–191.

68. Dyck PJ, Lambert EH. Lower motor and primary sensory neuron diseases with peroneal muscu-lar atrophy, II: neurologic, genetic, and electrophysiologic findings in various neuronal degenera-tions. Arch Neurol 1968;18:619–625.

69. McLeod JG, Prineas JW. Distal type of chronic spinal muscular atrophy. Brain 1971;94:703–714.

70. Harding AE, Thomas PK. Hereditary distal spinal muscular atrophy. A report on 34 cases and a review of the literature. J Neurol Sci 1980;45:337–348.

71. Timmerman V, et al. Linkage analysis of distal hereditary motor neuropathy type II (distal HMN II) in a single pedigree. J Neurol Sci 1992;109:41–48.

72. Timmerman V, et al. Distal hereditary motor neuropathy type II (distal HMN type II): phenotype and molecular genetics. Ann N Y Acad Sci 1999;883:60–64.

73. Irobi J, et al. A clone contig of 12q24.3 encompassing the distal hereditary motor neuropathy type II gene. Genomics 2000;65:34–43.

74. De Angelis MV, et al. Autosomal dominant distal spinal muscular atrophy: an Italian family not linked to 12q24 and 7p14. Neuromusc Disord 2002;12:26–30.

75. Lander CM, Eadie MJ, Tyrer JH. Hereditary motor peripheral neuropathy predominantly affecting the arms. J Neurol Sci 1976;28:389–394.

76. O'Sullivan DJ, McLeod JG. Distal chronic spinal muscular atrophy involving the hands. J Neurol Neurosurg Psychiatry 1978;41:653–658.

77. Christodoulou K, et al. Mapping of a distal form of spinal muscular atrophy with upper limb pre-dominance to chromosome 7p. Hum Mol Genet 1995;4:1629–1632.

78. Ionasescu V, et al. Autosomal dominant Charcot-Marie-Tooth axonal neuropathy mapped on chro-mosome 7p (CMT2D). Hum Mol Genet 1996;5:1373–1375.

79. Sambuughin N, et al. Autosomal dominant distal spinal muscular atrophy type V (dSMA-V) and Charcot-Marie-Tooth disease type 2D (CMT2D) segregate within a single large kindred and map to a refined region on chromosome 7p15. J Neurol Sci 1998;161:23–28.

80. Auer-Grumbach M, et al. Phenotypic and genotypic heterogeneity in hereditary motor neu-ronopathy type V: a clinical, electrophysiological and genetic study. Brain 2000;123(pt 8):1612–1623.

81. Young I.D, Harper PS. Hereditary distal spinal muscular atrophy with vocal cord paralysis. J Neurol Neurosurg Psychiatry 1980;43:413–408.

82. Pridmore C, et al. Distal spinal muscular atrophy with vocal cord paralysis. J Med Genet 1992; 29:197–199.

83. McEntagart M, et al. Distal spinal muscular atrophy with vocal cord paralysis (dSMA-VII) is not linked to the MPD2 locus on chromosome 5q31. J Med Genet 2000;37:E14.

84. Boltshauser E, et al. Hereditary distal muscular atrophy with vocal cord paralysis and sensorineural hearing loss: a dominant form of spinal muscular atrophy? J Med Genet 1989;26:105–108.

85. Donaghy M, Kennett R. Varying occurrence of vocal cord paralysis in a family with autosomal dominant hereditary motor and sensory neuropathy. J Neurol 1999;246:552–555.
86. Cuesta A, et al. The gene encoding ganglioside-induced differentiation-associated protein 1 is mutated in axonal Charcot-Marie-Tooth type 4A disease. Nat Genet 2002;30:22–25.
87. Feit H, et al. Vocal cord and pharyngeal weakness with autosomal dominant distal myopathy: clinical description and gene localization to 5q31. Am J Hum Genet 1998;63:1732–1742.
88. Fleury P, Hageman G. A dominantly inherited lower motor neuron disorder presenting at birth with associated arthrogryposis. J Neurol Neurosurg Psychiatry 1985;48:1037–1048.
89. Frijns CJ, et al. Dominant congenital benign spinal muscular atrophy. Muscle Nerve 1994;17:192–197.
90. Adams C, Suchowersky O, Lowry RB. Congenital autosomal dominant distal spinal muscular atrophy. Neuromusc Disord 1998;8:405–408.
91. van der Vleuten AJ, et al. Localisation of the gene for a dominant congenital spinal muscular atrophy predominantly affecting the lower limbs to chromosome 12q23–q24. Eur J Hum Genet 1998;6:376–382.
92. Palmer H. Familial scapuloperoneal amyotrophy. Arch Neurol Psychiatry 1932;28:473–477.
93. Davidenkow S. Scapuloperoneal amyotrophy. Arch Neurol Psychiatry 1939;41:694–701.
94. Kaeser HE. Scapuloperoneal muscular atrophy. Brain 1965;88:407–418.
95. Emery ES, Fenichel GM, Eng G. A spinal muscular atrophy with scapuloperoneal distribution. Arch Neurol 1968;18:129–133.
96. DeLong R, Siddique T. A large New England kindred with autosomal dominant neurogenic scapuloperoneal amyotrophy with unique features. Arch Neurol 1992;49:905–908.
97. Isozumi K, et al. Linkage of scapuloperoneal spinal muscular atrophy to chromosome 12q24.1–q24.31. Hum Mol Genet 1996;5:1377–1382.
98. Wilhelmsen KC, et al. Chromosome 12-linked autosomal dominant scapuloperoneal muscular dystrophy. Ann Neurol 1996;39:507–520.
99. Brahe C, et al. Genetic homogeneity between childhood-onset and adult-onset autosomal recessive spinal muscular atrophy. Lancet 1995;346:741–742.
100. Talbot K, et al. Evidence for compound heterozygosity causing mild and severe forms of autosomal recessive spinal muscular atrophy. J Med Genet 1996;33:1019–1021.
101. Zellweger H, et al. Spinal muscular atrophy with autosomal dominant inheritance. Report of a new kindred. Neurology 1972;22:957–963.
102. Rabin BA, et al. Autosomal dominant juvenile amyotrophic lateral sclerosis. Brain 1999;122(pt 8):1539–1350.
103. De Jonghe P, et al. Autosomal dominant juvenile amyotrophic lateral sclerosis and distal hereditary motor neuronopathy with pyramidal tract signs: synonyms for the same disorder? Brain 2002;125(pt 6):1320–1325.
104. Patel H, et al. The Silver syndrome variant of hereditary spastic paraplegia maps to chromosome 11q12–q14, with evidence for genetic heterogeneity within this subtype. Am J Hum Genet 2001;69:209–215.
105. Gourie-Devi M, Suresh TG, Shankar SK. Monomelic amyotrophy. Arch Neurol 1984;41(4):388–394.
106. Hirayama K, et al. Juvenile muscular atrophy of unilateral upper extremity. Neurology 1963;13:373–380.
107. Sobue I, et al. Juvenile type of distal and segmental muscular atrophy of upper extremities. Ann Neurol 1978;3:429–432.
108. Uncini A, et al. Benign monomelic amyotrophy of lower limb: report of three cases. Acta Neurol Scand 1992;85:397–400.
109. Hirayama K. Non-progressive Juvenile Spinal Muscular Atrophy of the Distal Upper Limb (Hirayama's Disease). In J De Jong (ed), Handbook of Neurology. Amsterdam: Elsevier Science, 1991;107–120.
110. Hu MT, et al. Flail arm syndrome: a distinctive variant of amyotrophic lateral sclerosis. J Neurol Neurosurg Psychiatry 1998;65:950–951.
111. Harding AE, Bradbury PG, Murray NM. Chronic asymmetrical spinal muscular atrophy. J Neurol Sci 1983;59:69–83.
112. Hirayama K, et al. Focal cervical poliopathy causing juvenile muscular atrophy of distal upper extremity: a pathological study. J Neurol Neurosurg Psychiatry 1987;50:285–290.
113. Hirayama K. Juvenile muscular atrophy of distal upper extremity (Hirayama disease). Intern Med 2000;39:283–290.
114. Chen CJ, et al. Hirayama disease: MR diagnosis. AJNR Am J Neuroradiol 1998;19:365–368.

115. Hirayama K, Tokumaru Y. Cervical dural sac and spinal cord in juvenile muscular atrophy of distal upper extremity. Neurology 2000;54:1922–1926.
116. Schroder R, et al. MRI findings in Hirayama's disease: flexion-induced cervical myelopathy or intrinsic motor neuron disease? J Neurol 1999;246:1069–1074.
117. Furukawa T, Akagami N, Maruyama S. Chronic neurogenic quadriceps amyotrophy. Ann Neurol 1977;2:528–530.
118. Serratrice G, et al. Chronic neurogenic quadriceps amyotrophies. J Neurol 1985;232:150–153.
119. McShane MA, et al. Progressive bulbar paralysis of childhood. A reappraisal of Fazio-Londe disease. Brain 1992;115(pt 6):1889–1900.
120. Megarbane A, et al. Brown-Vialetto-Van Laere syndrome in a large inbred Lebanese family: confirmation of autosomal recessive inheritance? Am J Med Genet 2000;92:117–121.
121. Hawkins SA, Nevin NC, Harding AE. Pontobulbar palsy and neurosensory deafness (Brown-Vialetto-Van Laere syndrome) with possible autosomal dominant inheritance. J Med Genet 1990;27:176–179.
122. Horiuchi I, et al. Acute myelitis after asthma attacks with onset after puberty. J Neurol Neurosurg Psychiatry 2000;68:665–668.

17
Kennedy's Disease

Charlotte J. Sumner and Kenneth H. Fischbeck

In 1968, Dr. William Kennedy et al[1] described the clinical features of an X-linked inherited motor neuron disease (MND) that they called "progressive proximal spinal and bulbar muscular atrophy of late onset." In 1991, La Spada et al[2] reported the disease-causing mutation in Kennedy's disease; a trinucleotide (CAG) repeat expansion in the androgen receptor (AR) gene. Kennedy's disease thus became the first discovered member of a new class of neurological disorders, the polyglutamine diseases, which now include Huntington's disease (HD), dentatorubral-pallidoluysian atrophy, and six forms of spinocerebellar ataxia (SCA).[3]

PREVALENCE

Kennedy's disease, or spinobulbar muscular atrophy (SBMA), occurs in approximately 1 in 40,000 people. It has been documented in individuals of Caucasian and Asian descent, but not those of African or Aboriginal descent. SBMA appears to be more common in the Japanese and Finnish populations, perhaps due to a founder effect.[4,5]

CLINICAL FEATURES

SBMA is a slowly progressive, inherited neurodegenerative disorder, affecting men beginning at age 30 to 60 years.[1,6–9] Early manifestations of muscle cramps and fasciculations are followed by progressive weakness and atrophy of bulbar and limb muscles. Proximal limb muscles are generally more affected than distal muscles in a fairly symmetrical pattern (Figure 17.1). This results in progressive impairment of gait and wheelchair dependence, usually within 2 to 3 decades of disease onset. Tendon reflexes are reduced or absent, and no upper neuron features are present. Lower facial and tongue muscles are the most frequently affected bulbar muscles, causing dysarthria; however, patients may also

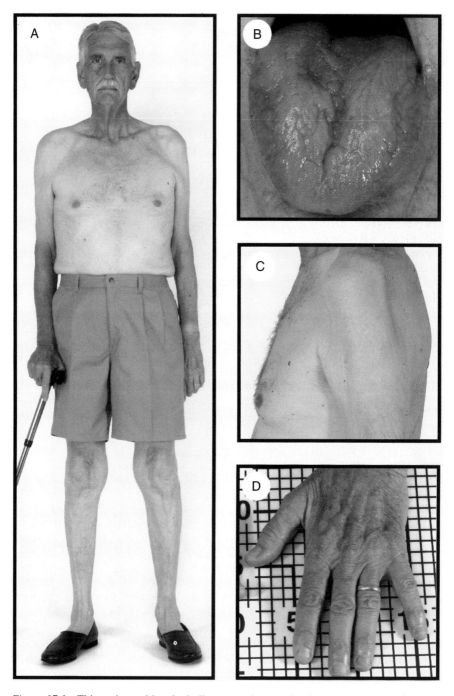

Figure 17.1 This patient with spinobulbar muscular atrophy demonstrates several typical features of the disease: **(A)** mild facial weakness, simian posture of the arms, and wasting of limb muscles; **(B)** atrophy of the tongue with a deep midline furrow; **(C)** weakness and atrophy proximally around the shoulder girdle; and **(D)** distal weakness and atrophy with loss of intrinsic hand muscle bulk, particularly in the first web space. This patient has minimal gynecomastia. See color insert.

have pharyngeal and respiratory muscle weakness, resulting in symptoms of swallowing difficulty and shortness of breath. Some patients develop severe jaw closure weakness, causing the jaw to hang open.[10] The extraocular muscles are spared. A characteristic feature of SBMA is frequent facial, particularly perioral fasciculations. In particular, patients often have "quivering" of the chin with pursing of the lips.

Patients rarely complain of sensory symptoms, and SBMA was therefore initially thought to affect motor neurons exclusively. Subsequent observations, however, revealed that mild sensory loss to vibration is frequently present in the feet, and sensory nerve conduction studies often show decreased or absent sensory nerve action potentials.[6–9,11,12] Pathology studies have confirmed dorsal root ganglion cell loss in addition to the motor neuron cell loss in the brain stem and spinal cord of patients with SBMA.[8]

Patients also show signs of mild androgen insensitivity, which may have onset in adolescence. These include gynecomastia in approximately 50 percent of patients, testicular atrophy, oligospermia, and erectile dysfunction.[13–15] Other clinical features of SBMA include postural tremor of the hands, resembling essential tremor, which may occur early or late in the course of the disease. Usually female carriers of SBMA are asymptomatic, although a minority experiences muscle cramps or tremor. Some female carriers also show mild electromyography (EMG) abnormalities.[16,17]

LABORATORY STUDIES

Serum creatine kinase levels are elevated (two to three times the normal level). Motor nerve conduction study results may be normal or show reduced-amplitude compound muscle action potentials, and sensory nerve conduction studies reveal reduced or absent sensory nerve action potentials. EMG shows widespread long-duration, large-amplitude motor units with reduced recruitment, indicating chronic denervation and partial reinnervation. Fibrillation potentials, a sign of acute denervation, are not prominent, as seen in ALS.[9,18] Some patients may have a decrement on low-frequency repetitive nerve stimulation studies.[19,20] This may be due to insecure neuromuscular transmission of collateral nerve sprouts, as has been hypothesized to occur in amyotrophic lateral sclerosis (ALS).[21] Sural nerve biopsy shows loss of large-diameter axons, and muscle biopsy usually reveals signs of chronic denervation with grouped atrophy of myofibers and fiber-type grouping. A confirmation of SBMA diagnosis can be made with genetic testing. CAG repeat number is determined by polymerase chain reaction amplification of the CAG repeat region within the AR gene (chromosomal locus Xq11-q12).[22] Early genetic testing can obviate the need for other more invasive studies.

DIFFERENTIAL DIAGNOSIS, PROGNOSIS, AND TREATMENT

Despite increased awareness of the distinguishing clinical features of SBMA, the disease may be confused with other neuromuscular disorders. Approxi-

Table 17.1   Features distinguishing spinobulbar muscular atrophy from amyotrophic lateral sclerosis

X-linked inheritance (only men affected)
Slowly progressive weakness (2 to 3 decades)
No upper motor neuron signs
Prominent perioral fasciculations
Mild sensory involvement
Signs of androgen insensitivity (gynecomastia)

mately 1 in 25 patients initially diagnosed as having ALS may have SBMA[23] (Table 17.1). Patients are also frequently misdiagnosed with myopathy or myasthenia gravis. Accurate diagnosis is important, to provide information about prognosis and genetic counseling for the patient and his or her family members and to avoid inappropriate treatment. Most patients with SBMA have a normal life span and do not die of direct consequences of their disease. Late in the course of illness, some patients are at risk of aspiration pneumonia or respiratory failure. Genetic counseling should include counseling of at-risk men in the family and daughters of affected men, who are obligate carriers and therefore have a 50-percent chance of having a son who is affected and a 50-percent chance of having a daughter who is a carrier. Treatment is principally supportive. Patients should be seen regularly for assessment of gait safety, aspiration risk, and respiratory function. Physical therapy, braces, and gait assist devices are helpful in prolonging the ability to ambulate. Unfortunately, no specific pharmacological therapy has been proven to be efficacious. Although there are anecdotal reports of improved muscle strength with testosterone therapy,[24] the results of a randomized clinical trial of testosterone were inconclusive and published in abstract form only.[25]

GENETICS

SBMA is an X-linked disease in which patients have an expansion of a trinucleotide CAG repeat (cytosine-adenine-guanine) in the AR gene from a normal length of 9 to 36 CAG repeats to a disease-associated length of 40 to 62.[2] Several studies have shown that increased repeat size correlates with earlier disease onset and increased disease severity.[26–28] Nonetheless, repeat length accounts only for a portion of the clinical variability, indicating that there are other, still unknown, factors that affect the disease course. Patients with minimally expanded repeat lengths have been reported to have unusual presentations of the disease such as very late onset,[29] isolated tremor,[30] isolated proximal limb weakness,[31] or isolated hypertrophic cardiomyopathy.[32] The length of the expanded repeat is unstable and may change when passed from one generation to the next, but unlike some trinucleotide repeat disorders such as myotonic dystrophy, anticipation (large expansion of the repeat from one generation to the next) is not a prominent feature of SBMA.

MOLECULAR PATHOPHYSIOLOGY

Androgen Receptor

The AR gene contains eight exons and spans 80 to 100 kb of DNA. The encoded protein contains approximately 900 amino acids and functions as a nuclear receptor that is a member of the steroid receptor superfamily.[33] The AR protein contains three functional domains: (1) an amino-terminal transactivation domain, which is thought to mediate transcriptional activation of target genes, (2) a centrally located DNA-binding domain, and (3) a carboxy-terminal ligand-binding domain (Figure 17.2). The polymorphic CAG repeat exists in the 5′ region of the AR gene and codes for a tract of glutamines in the amino-terminal transactivation domain of the AR protein.[34] The normal function of the polyglutamine tract is unknown, but it is not essential for transactivation of hormone-responsive genes. SBMA is due to expansion of this of polyglutamine tract.

Normally, the AR protein is produced in the cytoplasm, where it is phosphorylated and binds to heat shock proteins (Hsps). In the presence of ligand (testosterone or dihydrotestosterone), it dissociates from the Hsps and is actively transported to the nucleus, where it is free to dimerize, bind DNA at regulatory elements, and function as a transcription factor. The expanded

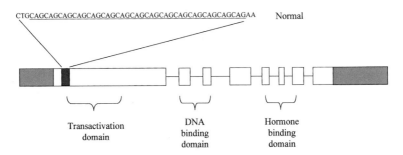

Androgen receptor gene

Figure 17.2   The functional domains of the androgen receptor gene. See color insert.

polyglutamine tract does not interfere with AR ligand binding or intracellular localization.[35] Mutant AR does result, however, in reduced target gene transactivation.[36,37] This defect may account for signs of mild androgen insensitivity in SBMA; however, loss of function of the AR does not appear to be the principal cause of motor neuron cell death.

Toxic Gain of Function

Individuals who have complete loss of function of the AR have the androgen insensitivity (testicular feminization) syndrome, a disorder that results in feminization, but no loss of motor neurons. This suggests that the primary effect of mutant AR in causing motor neuron degeneration is not loss of function, but a toxic gain of function. In other words, the structure or function of the protein is altered in such a way that it becomes deleterious to the cell. Expanded polyglutamine tracts in other genes cause degeneration of different populations of neuronal cells that result in other polyglutamine diseases, including HD and six forms of the SCAs. These disorders all exhibit autosomal dominant inheritance with a similar age at onset and rate of progression. In addition, these diseases tend to occur when the polyglutamine tract achieves a critical threshold length of approximately 40 repeats. Beyond this threshold, disease severity correlates with increasing polyglutamine length. In SBMA, women may be protected from the full expression of the disease either by X-chromosome inactivation or by having a decreased level of the AR ligand testosterone.

Experimental models provide further evidence that polyglutamine-mediated neurodegeneration results from a toxic gain of function. In the many cell culture and transgenic animal models that now exist, polyglutamine disease is recapitulated only with expression of the mutant gene, but not with knockout of expression of the gene. Mutations that cause loss of AR function result in testicular feminization syndrome in animals, as in humans, but transgenic overexpression of the AR gene with the SBMA mutation causes neurodegeneration. Initial attempts at reproducing the SBMA phenotype in transgenic mice were not successful, probably because the transgene expression levels were not high enough.[38,39] Interestingly, intergenerational instability of the expanded CAG repeat was not seen unless the mutant gene included sufficient flanking genomic DNA, indicating that the genomic context plays a role in repeat stability. Neurodegenerative phenotypes were produced with a truncated mutant AR gene under the control of neuronal promoters[40] and with a very long pure CAG repeat under control of the AR promoter.[41] Recently, a full-length AR with long repeat expansions has been expressed at high enough levels to produce a phenotype, and here the phenotype is more pronounced in males than females (G. Sobue, D. Merry, J. Morrison, and A. La Spada, personal communications). This indicates that the toxicity of the mutant AR in SBMA may be ligand dependent, that is, enhanced with the higher androgen levels that occur in males. Toxicity of mutant AR has also been demonstrated in transgenic flies (N. Bonini, personal communication) and in cell culture experiments.[42]

Inclusions and Aggregates

A common feature of the polyglutamine diseases is the presence of inclusion bodies in susceptible neurons.[43] In SBMA, AR inclusions have been identified in spinal cord motor neurons from patients[44] and in animal and cell culture models. These inclusions contain amino-terminal epitopes of the AR protein. Polyglutamine-containing fragments are more toxic than the full-length protein and may result from cleavage of mutant AR by caspases.[45] The inclusions also contain ubiquitin. *Ubiquitination* is the process by which the cell tags proteins for degradation. The presence of ubiquitinated protein inclusions suggests that there is accumulation of nondegraded protein within the cell, perhaps because of protein misfolding and aggregation. It was initially hypothesized that aggregation of mutant protein in inclusions is a central toxic event in polyglutamine-mediated neurodegeneration; however, in some models toxicity has been dissociated from the presence of inclusions.[46] Whether inclusions are toxic, protective, or simply a bystander is unresolved, but they are clearly a pathological marker of the disease.

Possible Mechanisms of Toxicity

Mutant AR and other polyglutamine-containing proteins may cause neuronal cell death through one or more mechanisms (Figure 17.3).[3] Possible targets of

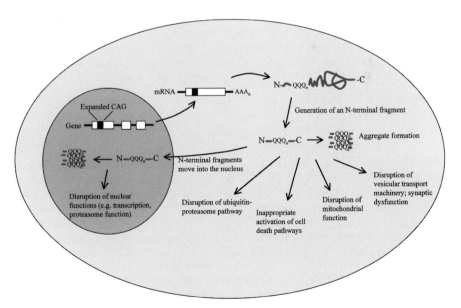

Figure 17.3 Possible mechanisms of spinobulbar muscular atrophy pathogenesis. See color insert. (Reprinted with permission from Taylor JP, Lieberman AP, Fischbeck KH. Repeat Expansion and Neurological Diseases. In AK Asbury, GM McKhann, WU McDonald, et al (eds), Diseases of the Nervous System (3rd ed). Cambridge: Cambridge University Press, 2002.)

expanded polyglutamine include the mitochondria and vesicular transport machinery.[47] Mutant polyglutamine proteins may trigger aberrant apoptosis or disrupt normal cellular function by overwhelming the ubiquitin-proteasome system (which degrades proteins) or sequestering Hsps (which stabilize and chaperone newly synthesized proteins in the cell). Other experimental evidence indicates that polyglutamine protein localization in the nucleus enhances toxicity.[48,49] One hypothesis is that mutant AR disrupts normal cellular gene transcription and RNA processing by sequestering essential transcription factors. Many transcription factors contain a polyglutamine tract that could be bound and sequestered by a mutant protein with a polyglutamine expansion. Several transcription factors have been found to co-localize with polyglutamine-containing nuclear inclusions, including CREB-binding protein (CBP) and p53.[50,51] Furthermore, altered gene transcription appears to be an early event in polyglutamine disease pathogenesis.[52,53] CBP sequestration, in particular, has been coupled with cellular toxicity.[50,54] CBP normally functions as a histone acetyltransferase. The post-translational modification of histones is an important determinant of transcriptionally active regions of chromatin; hyperacetylation of histones marks transcriptionally active regions and hypoacetylation marks transcriptionally silent regions. Sequestration of a histone acetyltransferase such as CBP might have widespread effects on gene expression that result in cellular toxicity. Restoration of the balance of histone acetylation might therefore be therapeutic. Indeed, in two different models of polyglutamine disease, histone deacetylase inhibitors have been shown to reverse the histone acetylation defect and reduce polyglutamine-induced cell death.[55,56]

CONCLUSION

Kennedy's disease is an inherited MND that is caused by a trinucleotide repeat (CAG) expansion in the AR gene. Distinct clinical features of the disease include X-linked inheritance, slow progression, limb and bulbar involvement without upper motor neuron signs, mild sensory involvement, and signs of androgen insensitivity. The mechanism of toxicity of the expanded polyglutamine stretch in the AR gene involves a toxic gain of function and is likely to be similar to that of the other known polyglutamine diseases.

REFERENCES

1. Kennedy WR, Alter M, Sung JH. Progressive proximal spinal and bulbar muscular atrophy of late onset. Neurology 1968;18:671–680.
2. La Spada AR, Wilson EM, Lubahn DB, et al. Androgen receptor gene mutations in X-linked spinal and bulbar muscular atrophy. Nature 1991;352:77–79.
3. Taylor JP, Lieberman AP, Fischbeck KH. Repeat Expansion and Neurological Diseases. In AK Asbury, GM McKhann, WU McDonald, et al (eds), Diseases of the Nervous System (3rd ed). Cambridge: Cambridge University Press, 2002.
4. Tanaka F, Doyu M, Ito Y, et al. Founder effect in spinal and bulbar muscular atrophy. Hum Mol Genet 1996;5:1253–1257.

5. Udd B, Juvonen V, Hakamies L, et al. High prevalence of Kennedy's disease in western Finland-is the syndrome underdiagnosed? Acta Neurol Scand 1998;98;128–133.

6. Harding AE, Thomas PK, Baraitser M, et al. X-linked recessive bulbospinal neuronopathy: a report of ten cases. J Neurol Neurosurg Psychiatry 1982;45:1012–1019.

7. Hausmanowa-Petrusewicz I, Borkowska J, Janczewski Z. X-linked adult form of spinal muscular atrophy. J Neurol 1983;229:175–188.

8. Sobue G, Hashizume Y, Mukai E, et al. X-linked recessive bulbospinal neuronopathy: a clinico-pathological study. Brain 1989:112;209–232.

9. Olney RK, Aminoff MJ, So YT. Clinical and electrodiagnostic features of X-linked recessive bulbospinal neuronopathy. Neurology 1991;41;823–828.

10. Suzuki T, Endo K, Igarashi S, et al. Isolated bilateral masseter atrophy in X-linked recessive bulbospinal neuronopathy. Neurology 1997;48:539–540.

11. Antonini G, Gragnani F, Romaniello A, et al. Sensory involvement in spinal-bulbar muscular atrophy (Kennedy's disease). Muscle Nerve 2000;23:252–258.

12. Polo A, Teatini F, D'Anna S, et al. Sensory involvement in X-linked spino-bulbar muscular atrophy (Kennedy's syndrome): an electrophysiological study. J Neurol 1996;243:388–392.

13. Arbizu T, Santamaria J, Gomez JM, et al. A family with adult spinal and bulbar muscular atrophy, X-linked inheritance and associated testicular failure. J Neurol Sci 1983;59:371–382.

14. Nagashima T, Seko K, Hirose K, et al. Familial bulbo-spinal muscular atrophy associated with testicular atrophy and sensory neuropathy (Kennedy-Alter-Sung syndrome). Autopsy case report of two brothers. J Neurol Sci 1988;87:141–152.

15. Warner CL, Griffin JE, Wilson JD, et al. X-linked spinomuscular atrophy: a kindred with associated abnormal androgen receptor binding. Neurology 1992;42:2181–2184.

16. Sobue G, Doyu M, Kachi T, et al. Subclinical phenotypic expressions in heterozygous females of X-linked recessive bulbospinal neuronopathy. J Neurol Sci 1993;117:74–78.

17. Mariotti C, Castellotti B, Pareyson D, et al. Phenotypic manifestations associated with CAG-repeat expansion in the androgen receptor gene in male patients and heterozygous females: a clinical and molecular study of 30 families. Neuromusc Disord 2000;10:391–397.

18. Ferrante MA, Wilbourn AJ. The characteristic electrodiagnostic features of Kennedy's disease. Muscle Nerve 1997;20:323–329.

19. Kawakami O, Takano A, Tanaka A, et al. A case of X-linked bulbar and spinal muscular atrophy with impaired neuromuscular transmission. Rinsho Shinkeigaku 1996;36:892–894.

20. Yamada M, Inaba A, Shiojiri T. X-linked spinal and bulbar muscular atrophy with myasthenic symptoms. J Neurol Sci 1997;146:183–185.

21. Bernstein LP, Antel JP. Motor neuron disease: decremental responses to repetitive nerve stimulation. Neurology 1981;31:204–207.

22. Wang Z, Thibodeau SN. A polymerase chain reaction-based test for spinal and bulbar muscular atrophy. Mayo Clin Proc 1996;71:397–398.

23. Parboosingh JS, Figlewicz DA, Krizus A, et al. Spinobulbar muscular atrophy can mimic ALS: the importance of genetic testing in male patients with atypical ALS. Neurology 1997;49:568–572.

24. Goldenberg JN, Bradley WG. Testosterone therapy and the pathogenesis of Kennedy's disease (X-linked bulbospinal muscular atrophy). J Neurol Sci 1996;135:158–161.

25. Mendell JR, Freimer M, Kissel JT. Randomized, double-blind crossover trial of androgen hormone deficiency and replacement in X-linked spinal muscular atrophy. Neurology 1996;46:A469.

26. La Spada AR, Roling DB, Harding AE, et al. Meiotic stability and genotype-phenotype correlation of the trinucleotide repeat in X-linked spinal and bulbar muscular atrophy. Nat Genet 1992;2:301–304.

27. Doyu M, Sobue G, Mukai E, et al. Severity of X-linked recessive bulbospinal neuronopathy correlates with size of the tandem CAG repeat in androgen receptor gene. Ann Neurol 1992;32:707–710.

28. Igarashi S, Tanno Y, Onodera O, et al. Strong correlation between the number of CAG repeats in androgen receptor genes and the clinical onset of features of spinal and bulbar muscular atrophy. Neurology 1992;42:2300–2302.

29. Doyu M, Sobue G, Mitsuma T, et al. Very late onset X-linked recessive bulbospinal neuronopathy: mild clinical features and a mild increase in the size of tandem CAG repeat in androgen receptor gene [letter]. J Neurol Neurosurg Psychiatry 1993;56:832–833.

30. Kaneko K, Igarashi S, Miyatake T, Tsuji S. "Essential tremor" and CAG repeats in the androgen receptor gene. Neurology 1993;43:1618–1619.

31. Igarashi S, Yonemochi Y, Tanaka K, et al. Atypical clinical presentations of X-linked spinal and bulbar atrophy in patients with mild CAG expansions in androgen receptor gene. Eur Neurol 1997:310–312.

32. Kaneko K, Igarashi S, Mayatake T, Tsuji S. Hypertrophic cardiomyopathy and increased number of CAG repeats in the androgen receptor gene. Am Heart J 1993;126:248–249.
33. Zhou ZX, Wong CI, Sar M, Wilson EM. The androgen receptor: an overview. Recent Prog Horm Res 1994;49:249–274.
34. Jenster G, van der Korput HA, van Vroonhoven C, et al. Domains of the human androgen receptor involved in steroid binding, transcriptional activation, and subcellular localization. Mol Endocrinol 1991;5:1396–1404.
35. Brooks BP, Paulson HL, Merry DE, et al. Characterization of an expanded glutamine repeat androgen receptor in a neuronal cell culture system. Neurobiol Dis 1997;4:313–323.
36. Mhatre AN, Trifio MA, Kaufman M, et al. Reduced transcriptional regulatory competence of the androgen receptor in X-linked spinal and bulbar muscular atrophy. Nat Genet 1993;5:184–187.
37. Lieberman AP, Harmison G, Strand AD, et al. Altered transcriptional regulation in cells expressing the expanded polyglutamine androgen receptor. Hum Mol Genet 2002;11:1967–1976.
38. Bingham PM, Scott MO, Wang S, et al. Stability of an expanded trinucleotide repeat in the androgen receptor gene in transgenic mice. Nat Genet 1995;9:191–196.
39. La Spada AR, Peterson KR, Meadows SA, et al. Androgen receptor YAC transgenic mice carrying CAG 45 alleles show trinucleotide repeat instability. Hum Mol Genet 1998;7:959–967.
40. Abel A, Walcott J, Woods J, et al. Expression of expanded repeat androgen receptor produces neurologic disease in transgenic mice. Hum Mol Genet 2001;10:107–116.
41. Adachi H, Kume A, Li M, et al. Transgenic mice with an expanded CAG repeat controlled by the human AR promoter show polyglutamine nuclear inclusions and neuronal dysfunction without neuronal cell death. Hum Mol Genet 2001;10:1039–1048.
42. Merry DE, Kobayashi Y, Bailey CK, et al. Cleavage, aggregation and toxicity of the expanded androgen receptor in spinal and bulbar muscular atrophy. Hum Mol Genet 1998;7:693–701.
43. Davies SW, Beardsall K, Turmaine M, et al. Are neuronal intranuclear inclusions the common neuropathology of triplet-repeat disorders with polyglutamine-repeat expansions? Lancet 1998;351:131–133.
44. Li M, Miwa S, Kobayashi Y, et al. Nuclear inclusions of the androgen receptor protein in spinal and bulbar muscular atrophy. Ann Neurol 1998;44:249–254.
45. Ellerby LM, Hackam AS, Propp SS, et al. Kennedy's disease: caspase cleavage of the androgen receptor is a crucial event in cytotoxicity. J Neurochem 1999;72:185–195.
46. Simeoni S, Mancini MA, Stenoien DL, et al. Motoneuronal cell death is not correlated with aggregate formation of androgen receptors containing elongated polyglutamine tract. Hum Mol Genet 2000;9:133–144.
47. Piccioni F, Pinton P, Simeoni S, et al. Androgen receptor with elongated polyglutamine tract forms aggregates that alter axonal trafficking and mitochondrial distribution in motor neuron processes. FASEB J 2002;16:1418–1420.
48. Klement IA, Skinner PJ, Kaytor MD, et al. Ataxin-1 nuclear localization and aggregation: role in polyglutamine-induced disease in SCA1 transgenic mice. Cell 1998;95:41–53.
49. Saudou F, Finkbeiner S, Devys D, Greenberg ME. Huntingtin acts in the nucleus to induce apoptosis but death does not correlate with the formation of intranuclear inclusions. Cell 1998;95:55–66.
50. McCampbell A, Taylor JP, Taye AA, et al. CREB-binding protein sequestration by expanded polyglutamine. Hum Mol Genet 2000;9:2197–2202.
51. Steffan JS, Kazantsev A, Spasic-Boskovic O, et al. The Huntington's disease protein interacts with p53 and CREB-binding protein and represses transcription. Proc Natl Acad Sci USA 2000;97:6763–6768.
52. Lin X, Antalffy B, Kang D, et al. Polyglutamine expansion down-regulates specific neuronal genes before pathologic changes in SCA1. Nature Neurosci 2000;3:157–163.
53. Luthi-Carter R, Strand A, Peters NL, et al. Decreased expression of striatal signaling genes in a mouse model of Huntington's disease. Hum Mol Genet 2000;9:1259–1271.
54. Nucifora FC, Sasaki M, Peters MF, et al. Interference by Huntington and atrophin-1 with CBP-mediated transcription leading to cellular toxicity. Science 2001;291:2423–2428.
55. Steffan JS, Bodai L, Pallos J, et al. Histone deacetylase inhibitors arrest polyglutamine-dependent neurodegeneration in *Drosophila*. Nature 2001;413:739–743.
56. McCampbell A, Taye AA, Whitty L, et al. Histone deacetylase inhibitors reduce polyglutamine toxicity. Proc Natl Acad Sci USA 2001;98:15179–15184.

18
Hereditary Spastic Paraparesis

Christopher J. McDermott and Pamela J. Shaw

Hereditary spastic paraparesis (HSP) is a relatively uncommon hereditary neurodegenerative disease with an incidence reported between 1 in 10,000 and 1 in 100,000. The main feature is a progressive lower limb spasticity resulting from degeneration of the corticospinal tracts within the spinal cord. The cause of the axonal degeneration in HSP is unknown. HSP is most commonly inherited in an autosomal dominant (AD) fashion. Autosomal recessive (AR) and X-linked recessive inheritance are also seen, but much less frequently. HSP may be classified with regard to phenotype, age at onset, or genetic linkage/gene mutated. The HSP phenotype may be "pure" in which the spastic paraparesis occurs in isolation or "complicated" in which the spastic paraparesis is merely one component of a much more diverse phenotype. Genetically HSP can be classified to one of 19 genetic loci, and because genes have been identified at 8 of these loci, more precise genotype-phenotype correlations are becoming possible.

PURE HEREDITARY SPASTIC PARAPARESIS

In pure HSP, progressive spastic paraparesis is the prominent feature. However, great variation in age at onset, severity, and the presence of additional features such as sensory disturbance, pes cavus, and muscle wasting is often observed. This variation was one of the earlier pointers to the genetic heterogeneity of pure HSP, and there are now ten loci identified for autosomally inherited pure HSP. Locus heterogeneity cannot alone explain the variation often seen in the same family, suggesting that further factors, genetic or environmental, are also influencing the phenotype observed in individual cases. The age at onset of pure HSP ranges from infancy to the eighth decade.[1] The severity of HSP varies between families and to a lesser extent within the same family, although life expectancy is normal. Several authors have supported the observation by Harding[1] that in early onset HSP (younger than 35 years), disease progression is slow, with most individuals remaining ambulant through most of their lives

435

and only a small proportion becoming confined to a wheelchair in elderly life. This contrasts with many cases of late-onset HSP (older than 35 years), in whom disease progression can be rapid, with many patients losing the ability to walk in their sixties and seventies.[2,3]

The most common presenting symptom is of gait disturbance noticed by the patient, a relative, or a friend. Often the patient complains of leg stiffness or balance difficulties. In children, premature wear of footwear because of toe walking is often reported. If onset is early in life, delayed motor milestones may be the first indication of a problem. The major findings on examination are to be found in the lower limbs and consist of spasticity, hyperreflexia, and extensor plantar responses, which may be accompanied by a mild pyramidal distribution of weakness. The lower limb spasticity is the prominent finding on examination, particularly in the hamstrings, quadriceps, and ankles. A characteristic feature of HSP is the marked discrepancy between the often severe spasticity and minimal muscle weakness. If the weakness is the prominent feature, the consideration of an alternative diagnosis is necessary.

Other clinical features compatible with a diagnosis of pure HSP include bladder disturbance, mild distal muscle wasting, dorsal column dysfunction, loss of ankle jerks, and mild terminal dysmetria. Cranial nerve examination and bulbar function results are normal in HSP. Other symptoms and signs that are not usually seen in pure HSP are listed in Table 18.1.[4] Pathological changes found in HSP are discussed in detail in Chapter 2.

Table 18.1   Diagnostic criteria for pure hereditary spastic paraparesis

	Clinical features
Obligatory	Family history
	Progressive gait disturbance
	Spasticity of lower limbs
	Hyperreflexia of lower limbs
	Extensor plantar responses
Common	Paresis of lower limbs
	Sphincter disturbances
	Mild dorsal column disturbance
	Pes cavus
	Hyperreflexia of upper limbs
	Mild terminal dysmetria
	Loss of ankle jerks
Uncommon	Paresis of upper limbs
	Distal amyotrophy
Diagnostic alerts	Paresis greater than spasticity
	Prominent ataxia
	Prominent amyotrophy
	Prominent upper limb involvement
	Peripheral neuropathy
	Asymmetry
	Retinal pigmentation
	Extrapyramidal signs

COMPLICATED HEREDITARY SPASTIC PARAPARESIS

In complicated HSP, the spastic paraparesis is one component of a much more varied phenotype. In contrast to pure HSP, additional features are observed co-segregating with the spastic paraparesis. The complicated phenotypes observed may be the result of mutation in a single gene, may be caused by two genes close at the same locus inherited together, or may be occurring by chance. Some of the complicated HSP phenotypes are extremely rare, being described in only single families. Interestingly at several HSP loci, heterogeneity is seen with both pure and complicated pedigrees being described. There is correlation of certain complicated phenotypes with particular HSP loci. HSP complicated with cognitive impairment is mostly associated with SPG4.[5–7] At the SPG9 locus, the HSP is complicated by a very distinct phenotype including cataracts, severe gastroesophageal reflux, and an axonal neuropathy.[8] Pigmented macular degeneration is a feature of HSP at the SPG15 locus.[9] Peripheral neuropathy has been described at several loci including SPG11 and SPG14.[10,11] The Silver variant of HSP, which is associated with marked amyotrophy and weakness of the hands, is linked to the SPG17 locus.[12] The Troyer syndrome, spastic paraparesis complicated with dysarthria, distal amyotrophy, short stature, and developmental delay, is linked to SPG20.[13]

Multiple clinical features have been described associating with spastic paraparesis in HSP pedigrees and these are summarized in Table 18.2. Several features are worthy of particular note and are discussed in the following sections.

Hereditary Spastic Paraparesis and Epilepsy

Epilepsy has increasingly been described as complicating HSP.[7,14–18] Given the high prevalence of epilepsy in the general population, a chance association must be considered. However, there are families in which the association is strong, suggesting either allelic or locus heterogeneity. Reviewing all the published pedigrees, we can find no one type of epilepsy that complicates HSP. Myoclonic jerks, simple partial, complex partial, and generalized tonic-clonic seizures have all been reported. Often different seizure types are witnessed within the same pedigree. Similarly, there is no consensus about when in the course of the HSP seizures begin. There are descriptions of seizures both predating and postdating the onset of the spastic paraparesis, again with variability being seen within the same pedigree. Recently mutations in the spastin gene (SPG4) have been associated with epilepsy and HSP.[7,18,19] In the family described by Mead et al,[18] otherwise pure HSP was complicated by epilepsy in four family members. Other family members also had spastic paraparesis alone. In this family, the seizure type varied from generalized tonic-clonic convulsions to jerks and cyanotic spells. The spastin mutation (frameshift with truncation at amino acid 437) in this family has previously been described in another HSP family with a pure HSP phenotype. Heinzlef et al[7] described a French family harboring a different spastin mutation (Q193Stop) with epilepsy and spastic paraparesis associating in certain family members. Again the seizure type varied within the family and not all who were affected by spastic paraparesis had seizures. These reports

Table 18.2 Clinical features that have been described associating with spastic paraparesis in complicated hereditary spastic paraparesis

Association	Subtypes	Comments
Amyotrophy	Peroneal muscular atrophy	Amyotrophy associated with an axonal sensory and motor neuropathy (AD)
	Silver's syndrome	Severe wasting of the small muscles of the hand with sparing of the lower limb musculature; link to SPG17 (AD)
	Troyer's syndrome	Distal wasting in the limbs with delayed development, spastic quadriparesis, pseudobulbar palsy, choreoathetosis, and short stature; linked to SPG20 (AR)
	Charlevoix–Saguenay syndrome	Similar to Troyer's syndrome with additional ataxia, described in Quebec (AR)
	Resembling juvenile FALS	Childhood onset (AR)
Cardiac defects	—	Associated with mental retardation
Cerebellar signs	—	Dysarthria with a mild upper limb ataxia
Deafness	Sensorineural	X-linked
Dementia	Subcortical or cortical pattern	Dementia can occur in isolation with HSP, when it tends to be of the subcortical type, or can be part of a much more complex phenotype (AR and AD); linked to SPG4 locus in a number of families
Endocrine dysfunction	Kallmann's syndrome	Hypogonadotrophic hypogonadism and anosmia
Epilepsy	—	Various epileptic seizure types have been described including; absence, simple/complex partial, atonic, grand mal, and myoclonic
Extrapyramidal signs	Choreoathetosis	
	Dystonia and rigidity	
	Mast syndrome	Dementia, dysarthria and athetosis in Amish people with onset in second decade (AR)
Hyperekplexia	—	Neonatal hypertonia and an exaggerated startle response (AD)
Ichthyosis	Sjögren-Larsson syndrome	Also with mental retardation and occasionally a pigmentary macular degeneration (AR)
Retinal changes	Optic atrophy	
	Retinal degeneration	Pigmentation seen in SPG15
	Kjellin's syndrome	Dysarthria, upper limb ataxia, dementia, retinal degeneration +/− amyotrophy (AR)
Sensory neuropathy	Asymptomatic	Sensory neuropathy detected only on clinical examination
	Childhood onset	With painless ulcers and deformities secondary to neuropathic bone resorption
	Adult onset	Trophic skin changes and foot ulcers
Others	SPG1	Mental retardation, aphasia, a shuffling gait and adducted thumbs; caused by mutations in L1CAM gene (X-linked)
	SPG9	Bilateral cataracts, gastroesophageal reflux and amyotrophy

AD = autosomal dominant; AR = autosomal recessive; FALS = familial amyotrophic lateral sclerosis; HSP = hereditary spastic paraparesis; L1CAM = L1 cell adhesion molecule; SPG = spastin gene.

suggest that an interaction with other genetic or environmental factors may be responsible for the manifestation of spastic paraparesis with an epilepsy phenotype in these families.

Hereditary Spastic Paraparesis and Cognitive Impairment

Dementia and cognitive impairment have been reported in complicated HSP pedigrees with additional features such as epilepsy, ataxia, parkinsonism, dysarthria, dysphagia, cardiac defects, and athetosis.[5,7,20-23] Dementia has also been described as an isolated accompaniment to spastic paraparesis in both AD and AR families.[6,24-26] In these families, the cognitive abnormalities are similar and consistent with a subcortical type of dementia, that is, impairment of attention, poor perceptual speed, poor visuomotor coordination, and forgetfulness. There is an absence of features suggesting major cortical involvement, for example, dysphasia, agnosia, and dyscalculia. A number of families with dementia complicating HSP have been linked to SPG4.[5-7] It has been suggested that affected individuals in SPG4 pedigrees with no overt cognitive problems have subclinical impairment on neuropsychometric testing, which may predate the spastic paraparesis.[27,28] Previous studies, which carefully evaluated cognitive function, demonstrated asymptomatic impairment in a number of patients with otherwise pure HSP.[29,30] It appears that as in other apparently selective motor system disorders, such as motor neuron disease (MND), there is evidence for a multisystem degenerative process, to which motor neurons are merely more susceptible.

With regard to spastic paraparesis and dementia, an alternative diagnosis to complicated HSP to consider is complicated Alzheimer's disease. There are an increasing number of families reported with spastic paraparesis and familial Alzheimer's disease. In these families, the spastic paraparesis may precede the dementia, which is modified and tends to occur later than usual for familial Alzheimer's disease, adding to the diagnostic uncertainty. In pedigrees with this complicated familial Alzheimer's phenotype, several mutations in the presenilin-1 gene have been identified.[31,32]

Hereditary Spastic Paraparesis and Amyotrophy

Distal amyotrophy is one of the most common complicating features. There is great heterogeneity, with both AD and AR inheritance being described. The mechanism of the amyotrophy is also heterogeneous, with anterior horn cell loss, axonal neuropathy, and central axonopathy contributing in different families. Several well-characterized syndromes are described in the literature.

The most common form of complicated HSP with amyotrophy is also known as peroneal muscular atrophy with pyramidal features or hereditary motor sensory neuropathy (HMSN) type V.[33-35] It tends to be transmitted as an AD trait and develops in the second decade of life or later. In addition to spastic paraparesis, affected individuals have amyotrophy associated with axonal motor and sensory neuropathy. There tends to be heterogeneity within families with regard to severity and the predominance of either neuropathy or pyramidal features. Mostacciuolo et al[35] described a large family in whom linkage to the known HSP and HMSN loci was excluded.

Silver syndrome consists of autosomal dominant HSP (AD-HSP) complicated by marked amyotrophy of the hands.[36] There is variation in age at onset (ranging from childhood to late adult) and severity. A single family has been linked to SPG17, with a further family having linkage to this locus and the other SPG loci excluded, demonstrating genetic heterogeneity even within this subtype of complicated HSP.[12]

The Troyer syndrome consists of autosomal recessive HSP (AR-HSP) complicated with amyotrophy of the hands and feet associated with pseudobulbar palsy, choreoathetosis, short stature, and mental retardation.[37,38] The original descriptions were of a childhood-onset disease in Amish people. Since originally described, further authors have attempted to broaden the Troyer phenotype, ascribing families with later onset, lack of movement disorder, atrophy or partial agenesis of the corpus callosum, and non-Amish origin to this syndrome.[39–41] The Troyer syndrome has been linked to SPG20 and the gene encodes a protein named spartin.[13] A similar syndrome with additional ataxia, Charlevoix-Saguenay disease was described in families in Quebec.[42]

A further rare phenotype of recessive HSP complicated by amyotrophy is described resembling juvenile-onset familial ALS.[38,43] In these families, childhood onset is observed with prominent wasting of the distal musculature. Neurophysiological examination shows electromyographic (EMG) denervation potentials consistent with affection of the anterior horn cells. Follow-up over 10 years revealed only slight progression.[43]

Hereditary Spastic Paraparesis and Sensory Neuropathy

HSP may be complicated by a sensory neuropathy with either childhood or adult onset. Reports describe a severe sensory neuropathy in association with HSP, with chronic painless cutaneous ulcers and neuropathic bone resorption occurring in early childhood.[44] In a less severe form, trophic skin changes and ulcers on the feet develop in adult life superimposed on a longer established spastic paraparesis.[45,46] Schady and Smith[47] reported a family with asymptomatic sensory involvement detected on clinical examination. All those within the family who underwent nerve conduction studies had decreased sensory action potentials.[47] Three patients underwent a nerve biopsy, which showed decreased numbers of large and medium-sized myelinated fibers with no evidence of demyelination, suggesting an axonal neuropathy.[47]

DIAGNOSIS

Molecular genetic testing will become increasingly relevant in the diagnosis of HSP. Although several causative genes have now been identified, for most of these, routine testing is unavailable. Therefore HSP is still often a diagnosis of exclusion. It is particularly important to exclude those diseases in which there may be a treatable cause for the spastic paraparesis, for example, vitamin B_{12}

Table 18.3 Investigation of hereditary spastic paraparesis

Investigation	Differential diagnosis
MRI	Cervical/lumbar spondylosis
	Neoplasm; primary or secondary
	Arnold Chiari malformation
MRI and CSF evaluation	Progressive multiple sclerosis
MRI and VLCFA	ALD, AMN
MRI and arylsulfatase	MLD
MRI and galactocerebroside	Krabbe leukodystrophy
MRI/birth history	Diplegic cerebral palsy
MRI/spinal angiography	Spinal cord arteriovenous malformation
EMG	Motor neuron disease
SCA genetic testing	Spinocerebellar ataxias
Vitamin B_{12}	Subacute combined degeneration of the cord
Plasma arginine, aminoaciduria	Arginase deficiency
History of *Lathyrus sativus* consumption	Neurolathyrism
Lipoprotein electrophoresis	Abetalipoproteinemia
L-dopa trial, gene analysis	Dopa responsive dystonia
Serum vitamin E level	Vitamin E deficiency
Syphilis serology	Neurosyphilis
Serum/CSF HTLV-1 antibodies	HTLV-1 infection (tropical spastic paraparesis)
HIV testing, CD4 count	AIDS

AIDS = acquired immune deficiency syndrome; ALD = adrenoleukodystrophy; AMN = adrenomyeloneuropathy; CSF = cerebrospinal fluid; EMG = electromyography; HIV = human immunodeficiency virus; HTLV-1 = human T-lymphotropic virus type 1; MLD = metachromatic leukodystrophy; MRI = magnetic resonance imaging; SCA = spinocerebellar ataxia; VLCFA = very long chain fatty acids.

deficiency, multiple sclerosis, structural spinal cord disorders, and dopa-responsive dystonia, or in which the prognosis is significantly different, for example, familial MND. Table 18.3 outlines the differential diagnosis of HSP and investigations to consider when evaluating a possible case of HSP. These investigations are useful in excluding other disorders, but they do not otherwise add to the diagnostic certainty of HSP. Central motor conduction times have been reported by several authors to show either unrecordable or delayed responses from the lower limbs, with usually normal values from the upper limbs.[48–51] Somatosensory evoked potentials have been reported to be small or absent, with the abnormality again being seen mainly in the lower limbs.[3,50,52] Nerve conduction study and EMG results are normal in most patients with pure HSP at least at the time of diagnosis.[1,3,51,53,54] Cerebrospinal fluid (CSF) analysis is usually unremarkable in HSP. However, occasional reports of abnormalities have included increased protein levels in complicated families and raised homocarnosine levels in a complicated family with spastic paraplegia, progressive mental deficiency, and retinal pigmentation.[36,55–57] Magnetic resonance imaging (MRI) may show a degree of spinal cord atrophy, but other abnormalities are not usually seen.[58] There are increasing reports, particularly in Japanese pedigrees, of mild to moderate atrophy of the corpus callosum. A number of these families have been linked to the SPG11 locus.[10] There are occasional reports of atrophy of other intracranial structures and of white matter lesions in the cerebral hemispheres.[9,49,59-61] However, marked atrophy or white matter changes on MRI require thorough exclusion of other conditions.

The most useful molecular genetic test is mutation detection in the spastin gene. Mutations in the spastin gene account for up to 40 percent of AD-HSP. The remaining 60 percent of cases are split between at least another eight AD-HSP genes. There is therefore a reasonable chance of detecting a spastin mutation in AD-HSP pedigrees. These odds are probably increased if one restricts spastin screening to pedigrees with pure HSP or HSP associated with cognitive change. Screening for mutations in the spastin gene is a costly and time-consuming affair because mutations have been identified scattered throughout the gene and therefore the whole 17 exons need to be analyzed, at least in the index cases.[19,62] However, there are significant benefits if a mutation is identified. These include being able to offer a firm diagnosis, allowing the cessation of other investigative procedures and appropriate counseling regarding prognosis and implications for the family.

A common clinical problem is that of the patient with a spastic paraparesis with apparently no family history and no cause found after extensive investigation. These patients are often labeled with "presumed HSP." In these apparently sporadic cases of spastic paraparesis, it is extremely valuable to assess the "healthy" relatives. We have on numerous occasions found subtle pyramidal signs in asymptomatic relatives, as the clincher to a diagnosis of HSP. This is perhaps not surprising given the huge intrafamilial variation reported in both age at onset and severity of the HSP phenotype. However, there are individuals given the label "presumed HSP" where no supportive clues come from examining the family members. In such cases, spastin mutations have been identified and may represent a new mutation or reduced penetrance in previous generations.[62] The percentage of sporadic spastic paraparesis caused by a spastin mutation has not been studied in detail. However, it would seem reasonable to screen those patients with a pure HSP phenotype or an HSP phenotype with additional cognitive impairment for a spastin mutation.

Mutations in the SPG3A gene, atlastin, are thought to account for approximately 15 percent of AD-HSP cases.[63] Mutation screening is worthwhile in pedigrees with a particularly young age at onset, as most reported cases have an age at onset of symptoms within the first decade.

GENETICS OF HEREDITARY SPASTIC PARAPARESIS

HSP is a disease that shows marked genetic heterogeneity. At the time of writing, 19 genetic loci have been linked to an HSP phenotype with the causative genes identified at 8 of these loci (Table 18.4). AD, AR, and X-linked inheritance are observed, with AD inheritance accounting for the majority.

Autosomal Dominant Hereditary Spastic Paraparesis

To date, ten AD-HSP loci have been identified. The genes at SPG3A, SPG4, SPG10, and SPG13 have been identified as atlastin, spastin, KIF5A, and heat shock protein 60 (Hsp60), respectively.[64-66a] The genes at the remaining loci SPG6, SPG8, SPG9, SPG12, SPG17, and SPG19 are as yet unknown.[8,12,67-71]

Table 18.4 Genetic classification of hereditary spastic paraparesis

Gene	Chromosome	Inheritance	Phenotype	Protein
SPG1	Xq28	X-linked	Complicated	L1CAM
SPG2	Xq22	X-linked	Both	PLP
SPG3	14q11.2–q24.3	AD	Pure	Atlastin
SPG4	2p21–p24	AD	Both	Spastin
SPG5	8p12–q13	AR	Pure	—
SPG6	15q11.1	AD	Pure	—
SPG7	16q24.3	AR	Both	Paraplegin
SPG8	8q24	AD	Pure	—
SPG9	10q23.3–q24.2	AD	Complicated	—
SPG10	12q13	AD	Pure	Kinesian heavy chain (KIF5A)
SPG11	15q13–q15	AR	Both	—
SPG12	19q13	AD	Pure	—
SPG13	2q24–q34	AD	Pure	Hsp60
SPG14	3q27–q28	AR	Complicated	—
SPG15	14q	AR	Complicated	—
SPG16	Xq11.2	X-linked	Pure	—
SPG17	11q12–q14	AR	Complicated	—
SPG19	9q33–q34	AD	Pure	—
SPG20	13q12.3	AR	Complicated	Spartin

AD = autosomal dominant; AR = autosomal recessive; Hsp = heat shock protein; L1CAM = L1 cell adhesion molecule; PLP = proteolipid protein.

SPG3 and Atlastin

HSP linked to SPG3 on chromosome 14q accounts for approximately 15 percent of AD-HSP.[63] HSP at this locus displays a pure phenotype.[63,72–77] The age at onset appears to be younger compared with other AD-HSP loci, with most affected individuals manifesting disease in the first decade. There are no other features to distinguish HSP at the SPG3 locus from other forms of AD-HSP. The causative gene at the SPG3 locus has been called atlastin and shares homology with several guanosine triphosphatase (GTPase) proteins.[65] The SPG3 gene consists of 14 exons, which encode a peptide of 588 amino acids, with a predicted molecular weight of 63.5 kilodaltons. All mutations detected to date are missense changes within exon 7 or exon 8. Interestingly three families share the same missense mutation in exon 7. These families were not apparently related, although haplotype studies could not rule out a distant founder effect. It may be that this area of the atlastin protein is a hot spot for mutation. Expression analysis has demonstrated atlastin to be expressed in all adult tissues examined, but it is noteworthy that the level in the brain was found to be 50 times greater than in other tissues.[65] The atlastin amino acid sequence has three conserved areas that characterize GTPase proteins; a p-loop, a DxxG motif, and an RD motif. One missense mutation, R217Q, involves the R amino acid of the conserved RD motif and is likely to alter the GTPase active site.[77] The other missense mutations identified are not predicted to effect the GTPase motifs or active site but may exert their pathogenic effect by altering secondary structure, disrupting multimerization, or disturbing protein-protein interactions.[65] Atlastin shares most homology with a particular GTPase, human guanylate binding protein-1 (GBP1).[78] Atlastin shares no homology with the other seven identified HSP genes. The homology of atlastin with GBP1 suggests that it may be a member of the dynamin family of GTPases. Dynamins are involved in a number of functions that, if disrupted, could have an adverse effect on neurons, for example, recycling of synaptic vesicles, protein trafficking, and the maintenance and distribution of mitochondria.[79–81] They have also been demonstrated to associate with cytoskeletal components including both actin and microtubules.[82]

SPG4 and Spastin

The responsible gene at the SPG4 locus, spastin, was identified in 1999, using a positional cloning strategy.[64] The gene is large, comprising 17 exons mapping to chromosome 2p21-p22, encoding a 616 amino acid protein. Spastin is ubiquitously expressed in human tissues, but in HSP, the long axons of the corticospinal tract are selectively affected. The reason for the selectivity of the neurodegenerative process is unclear.

Spastin shares homology with a large family of proteins known as the "adenosine triphosphatases (ATPases) associated with diverse cellular activities" (AAA). As the name suggests, AAA proteins are involved in a wide range of cellular processes including cell cycle regulation, gene expression, organelle biogenesis, vesicle-mediated protein transport, and as molecular chaperones co-operating in the assembly, function, and disassembly of protein complexes.[83] All the AAA proteins share a common functional domain known as the "AAA cassette," which contains highly conserved motifs including Walker A, Walker B, and the AAA minimal consensus domain. Outside the AAA cassette, there is little homology between different AAA proteins. Several subgroups of AAA proteins share closer homology. Interestingly, paraplegin, the gene responsible for SPG7, is also an AAA protein but belongs to the metalloprotease subgroup, sharing little homology with spastin outside the AAA cassette. Spastin belongs to the meiotic group, and within this group, it has particular homology with two proteins katanin and SKD1. Katanin is a microtubule severing protein, and SKD1 an endosomal morphology and trafficking protein. Katanin is involved in the dynamic regulation of the microtubule cytoskeleton throughout the cell cycle. There is evidence that spastin may also be involved in regulating the microtubule cytoskeleton.[84] When epitope-tagged wild type spastin was overexpressed in both Cos-7 and HeLa cells, it was seen to have a perinuclear/cytosolic punctate distribution. Overexpression of wild type spastin was associated with a dramatic reduction in cell tubulin content, and an increase in the amount of microtubule free ends was demonstrated. When mutant spastin was overexpressed, no decrease in cellular tubulin was seen. However, the spastin distribution changed to a filamentous pattern and co-localized with a subset of microtubules. Errico, Ballabio, and Rugarli[84] went on to demonstrate that the N-terminal domain is necessary for targeting mutant spastin to microtubules. They postulate that spastin is targeted by the N-terminus to microtubules, and once bound, it undergoes adenosine triphosphate (ATP)—dependent conformational change, which disrupts the microtubules and frees the spastin molecule. If the AAA cassette is disrupted, the conformational change does not occur and spastin remains bound to the microtubules. These data suggest that spastin, like katanin, may be acting as a microtubule severing protein.

Microtubules are dynamic polymers of α- and β-tubulin. They perform essential roles, forming the mitotic spindle in dividing cells, acting as "railways" for transport of various cellular components, organize membranous organelles, and provide architectural support in all cells. A disruption in the regulation of the microtubule transport framework in the long axons affected in HSP may underlie the pathogenesis of spastin related HSP. Recently, the gene at SPG20, to which the Troyer syndrome is linked, was identified as spartin. Interestingly spartin shares homology with the microtubule targeting N-terminal region of spastin.[13] This suggests that disruption to the microtubule cytoskeleton may be a common mechanism of axonal degeneration in HSP. Further work is needed to confirm the distribution of endogenous spastin in healthy and diseased states and to investigate the nature of the interaction of spastin with microtubules.

SPG4: Clinical Features

SPG4 is caused by mutation in the spastin gene and is the most frequent form of AD-HSP, accounting for approximately 40 percent of cases. Several authors have reported a lower frequency or have failed to identify a spastin mutation in families with tight linkage to the SPG4 locus.[28,62,85,86] This may be due to promoter or other non-coding region mutations, which are not routinely screened, and in some instances, the incomplete sensitivity of the mutation detection methodology used, for example, single-strand conformation polymorphism.

The age at onset for spastin-related HSP is highly variable, demonstrating both interfamilial and intrafamilial variation, and showing no correlation with the type or position of the mutation. The mean age at onset of symptoms ranges from 25 to 41 years old, in the published pedigrees. These mean ranges conceal the marked variation within individual families where it is not uncommon to see age at onset of symptoms ranging over 5 or more decades.

In some families, there does appear to be anticipation whereby the age at onset decreases in subsequent generations.[5,49,87,88] This is seen in other neurodegenerative diseases, such as Huntington's disease, dentatorubral-pallidoluysian atrophy, and Machado-Joseph disease. In these diseases, the younger age at onset of disease in subsequent generations correlates with the length of an abnormal trinucleotide CAG repeat expansion.[89-91] For many years before the identification of the spastin gene, there were extensive searches for evidence that SPG4 was a trinucleotide repeat disorder, to explain the apparent anticipation.[92-94] The results of these studies were never conclusive and the spastin gene does not contain an abnormally expanded CAG region. The most likely explanation for the apparent anticipation is ascertainment bias, with the disease being noticed early in the children of affected adults.

Variation is seen also in the severity of the phenotype and subsequent disability in HSP due to spastin mutations. The majority of affected people retain the ability to walk independently or with minimal support. At the extremes are asymptomatic patients with pyramidal signs in the lower limbs with a normal or only slightly abnormal gait and a few patients who are chair bound or bedridden. Indeed it is not unusual to have within the same family a severely affected individual with childhood onset and an individual in his/her seventh or eighth decade who is asymptomatic. It is estimated that up to 25 percent of HSP cases due to a spastin mutation are asymptomatic, emphasizing the importance of examining the whole family.[19] Several authors report individuals with a spastin mutation who appear to be unaffected after neurological examination.[19,28,62,86,95] One report describes a family in which there is one individual mutation carrier with childhood onset and another clinically unaffected at 78-years-old.[95] Given the huge variation in age at onset within families, it is almost impossible to decide whether these individuals represent age-dependent penetrance or perhaps true nonpenetrance.

There is evidence that disease progression and severity are worse in those with late-onset disease and that the frequency of features such as paresis, amyotrophy, dorsal column involvement, and urinary disturbance increases with disease duration.[19] These findings support the original classification of type I and II HSP made by Harding.[1] However, others have shown no correlation between severity of disease phenotype and age at onset.[96]

Gender differences may influence the timing of onset of symptoms in spastin-associated HSP.[97] In several reports, there is a tendency for asymptomatic individuals with HSP to be female.[74,87,98] This is seen in sporadic MND in which there is a male gender predominance (1.6 : 1) and onset in males occurring 5 to 10 years earlier. These differences have not been apparent in all reports, when specifically sought.[99] How gender differences produce this influence on motor neuron degeneration is unknown.

The majority of HSP cases associated with spastin mutation is of a pure phenotype.[19,62,85,95] However, there are now increasing reports of more complicated phenotypes caused by mutations in the spastin gene.[18,19,62,86]

Frank dementia has been described complicating HSP due to a spastin mutation in three families.[5-7] Webb et al[6] described a large family with 12 affected members. One patient died of a dementing illness at 62 years of age and four family members with HSP were found to have dementia of a subcortical type on neuropsychological testing. In the French family described by Heinzlef et al,[7] four out of seven affected family members had cognitive impairment, whereas one had severe dementia with cortical features such as dysphasia and visual agnosia. Three affected members also had epilepsy. In the family reported by White et al,[5] the index member with HSP died with a late-onset severe dementing illness with cortical and extrapyramidal features. Two other family members had memory impairment in old age, although detailed information on motor symptoms in these members was not available. One other family member with HSP had borderline learning difficulties with mild impairment in all aspects of memory. The pathological findings in the patient with dementia in this pedigree have been discussed earlier. There are other less detailed reports of memory problems in spastin-related HSP.[62,86]

The nature of the association of dementia with HSP in these families is unclear. It may represent co-segregation of a separate disorder such as senile dementia of the Alzheimer's disease type. If it is a direct result of the spastin mutation, there are two possible explanations as to why the cognitive changes are not seen in all affected individuals. One possibility is the expression of the dementia phenotype is influenced by other unknown genetic or environmental factors, as is postulated for the variation in age at onset of symptoms. Alternatively, cognitive impairment may be present subclinically in all spastin-related HSP but only identified when specifically sought. Supporting the latter hypothesis, McMonagle et al[28] demonstrated significantly lower Cambridge Cognitive Examination (CAMCOG) scores and increase frequency of dementia in spastin HSP compared to non spastin HSP. Their data suggest that there is evidence of cognitive impairment in all individuals with a spastin mutation when specifically sought. However, as with the rest of the phenotype, this is highly variable within and among families.

There are two families reported with HSP and epilepsy associated with spastin mutation. In the previously mentioned French family, affected family members have either spastic paraparesis alone or in addition; epilepsy, a cortical type dementia; or both.[7] The mutation in this family (Q193Stop) causes the translation of a mutant spastin protein truncated at approximately one third of the normal protein length, missing the whole AAA cassette.[19] In the second family, 4 of 24 affected with spastic paraparesis have epilepsy.[18] In this family, the mutation causes a frameshift at amino acid 427 and a premature truncation codon at 437, truncating the spastin protein within the AAA cassette. This mutation has also been described in a pure HSP pedigree with no epilepsy reported,[62] as have other truncating mutations within the same regions as both of these nonsense changes. Also, in both these families, the seizure type varies, as does the timing of the seizure onset in relation to onset of gait disturbance. These observations suggest that the epilepsy either results from a complex interaction between the effects of the spastin mutation and other as yet unknown genetic or environmental factors or is a chance phenomenon.

There are isolated reports of a variety of additional features complicating spastin-related HSP including restless legs, myoclonus, atypical seizures, dysarthria, erectile dysfunction, severe constipation, ileus, and fecal incontinence.[86,96,100] An interesting phenotype is described by Meijer et al[86] in an individual with a truncating mutation (Q434Stop) consisting of additional ataxia, footdrop, dysarthria, and nystagmus. Mead et al[18] report two siblings in a large AD spastin pedigree complicated with epilepsy (see earlier discussion) who have a combination of HSP and MS. The authors feel a chance association is unlikely and postulate that a spastin mutation may be a predisposing factor for MS. These two reports broaden the phenotype associated with a spastin mutation and suggest this gene might also be involved in other clinical entities.

SPG4: Pathogenetic Mechanism

Eighty-two mutations in the spastin gene have been published to date, 11 percent nonsense, 26 percent frameshift with consequent premature termination codon, 28 percent missense, and 35 percent splice-site mutations. The frequency of splicing mutations is higher than the 15 percent seen in other surveys of human genetic disorders.[101,102] There is no particular hot spot for mutation within the gene, with mutations throughout the length of the gene, making mutation screening a lengthy process. The majority are private mutations, with few occurring in more than one family. The majority of these mutations in some way effect the conserved AAA cassette, either by truncating the protein before or within the cassette sequence, skipping of exons within the cassette, or by causing amino acid changes within the cassette.

Given the breadth of mutations predicted to drastically alter the mutant spastin protein, haploinsufficiency has been postulated by most authors as the likely disease mechanism. Further evidence to support haploinsufficiency, rather than a dominant negative or gain of function, as a disease mechanism comes from the fact that as well as causing exon skipping, the splice-site mutations lead to the formation of unstable messenger RNA (mRNA). In these patients, the ratio of normal to mutant spastin is estimated at between 100:1[85] and 95:5.[95] Similar mutant spastin mRNA instability has been described with a missense mutation.[95] Svenson et al[103,104] describe two "leaky" or partially penetrant mutations in which both normal and mutant (deletion of exon 9 or 11) spastin is produced by the mutant alleles. Haploinsufficiency implies that a 50-percent reduction in the expression of the spastin protein causes the disease. However, the smaller reductions caused by leaky mutations or partially stable mutant transcripts suggest a much narrower interval. It seems that a critical threshold level of spastin is necessary for axonal preservation. Given the marked interfamilial and intrafamilial variation in age at onset and severity, this threshold would appear to be dynamic, interacting with as yet unknown genetic and environmental factors. A further contributing factor to the variability seen could be due to the differences in stability of the various miss spliced mRNA transcripts, which may have partial function, or the presence of "leaky" mutations described earlier.

However, the demonstration of altered microtubule regulation in cells over-expressing missense spastin mutations suggests the possibility that a dominant negative pathogenic mechanism may be involved in individuals with spastin missense mutations.[84] It is possible that more than one pathogenic mechanism may be involved, depending on the type of mutation.

In contrast to the low tolerance of nucleotide changes, several alternate mRNA transcripts have been reported in control individuals.[104] The most abundant is a transcript missing exon 4, which retains the correct reading frame. Two further, less abundant alternatively spliced mRNAs missing exon 8 or exon 15, the latter also having a subsequent frameshift, have been demonstrated. Both of these are within the conserved AAA cassette, with the exon 8 variant also missing the highly conserved Walker A motif. This would suggest a separate function for spastin not requiring the AAA cassette.

SPG4: Genotype-Phenotype Correlation

When looking at pure HSP associated with spastin mutations, several authors have found no difference in mean age at onset, severity, or a range of features such as dorsal column involvement, bladder disturbance, and upper limb involvement.[19,62,95] This is unfortunate because it means clinical features alone cannot be used to differentiate those with HSP who may be harboring a spastin mutation. Similarly no clear correlation between the type of spastin mutation and observed phenotype has been demonstrated. The interfamilial variation in age at onset for spastin-related HSP does not correlate with the type or position of the mutation within the gene. Also, the presence of complicating factors such as epilepsy or dementia does not have an obvious correlation with genotype. No difference in disease phenotype between missense and truncating mutations has been demonstrated.[19,62,95,99,105] Fonknechten et al[19] reported no difference in phenotype (e.g., age at onset or severity) between conservative and nonconservative missense changes. Indeed the presence of conservative changes, K388R L426V A556V reveals the functional importance of such residues and the low tolerance for amino acid alteration in the spastin protein.

SPG4: Polymorphisms

Very few polymorphisms have been identified in the spastin gene, with an amino acid change in almost every exon causing the HSP phenotype. This perhaps is to be expected given the highly conserved nature of much of the amino acid sequence in different species. Of the polymorphisms reported one, 1619 + 16 g→t, occurs well into intron 16 and is unlikely to have an effect on the translated protein. However, two further reported polymorphisms are more controversial. Svenson et al[104] reported a possible polymorphism G1004A, which causes no amino acid change P293P in the proband of a family with HSP; the mutation segregating with the disease in this family was in intron 9. However, a further report identified this change in a single individual with HSP and argued that the nucleotide change could possibly disrupt an exonic splicing enhancer or silencer.[86] No further family members have been analyzed in this family. Meijer et al[86] also report a possible polymorphism G1417A, which causes the missense change Arg431Glu. This change was identified in an apparently healthy spouse. It is surprising that this nonconservative change well inside the conserved AAA cassette does not cause HSP, particularly when a missense change in the same area Ser436Phe is associated with the disease phenotype.[105] Arg431Glu may represent a very rare polymorphism; however, it is possible, given the not uncommon late onset and mild HSP phenotype seen due to a spastin mutation, this spouse could still develop HSP. In their large analysis of 142 individuals, Fonknechten et al[19] found no evidence of coding region polymorphism. They report finding intronic single nucleotide polymorphisms but do not give further details.[19]

The Remaining Autosomal Dominant Hereditary Spastic Paraparesis Loci

There are eight other loci to which AD-HSP pedigrees have been linked. These remaining loci account for up to 50 percent of AD-HSP pedigrees. However, only one or two families are described linked to each of these loci. This suggests another major locus for AD-HSP is yet to be discovered. With only a few families linked to each locus, statements about a characteristic phenotype at each site must be limited. However, the phenotype at SPG6, SPG8, SPG10, SPG12, SPG13, and SPG19 is of pure HSP.[67–71,106,107] At SPG6 and SPG8, there is a suggestion that disease severity is greater with greater functional impairment reported compared with other loci. The age at onset, as with SPG3, appears younger in the families linked to SPG10 and SPG12. These observations hint at locus-specific differences in the molecular pathology of pure AD-HSP. At the SPG19 locus, the age at onset is relatively late with a benign course and a high frequency of urinary disturbance.[71]

The phenotype at both the SPG9 and the SPG17 locus is of complicated HSP. Spastic paraparesis at the SPG9 locus has been described in an Italian family in which the phenotype is complicated by bilateral cataracts, gastroesophageal reflux with vomiting, and amyotrophy.[8] A further British family has been described with cataracts, learning difficulties, and skeletal abnormalities.[108,109] In both families, anticipation of age at onset is described, suggesting that SPG9 may represent a trinucleotide repeat disorder. One family has been linked to the SPG17 locus.[12] In this family, the phenotype was of the Silver syndrome, in which HSP is complicated by amyotrophy of the small muscles of the hands.[36] A further family with a similar phenotype had linkage to this locus excluded, demonstrating genetic heterogeneity of the Silver syndrome.[12]

The gene at the SPG10 locus has been identified as KIF5A.[66a] KIF5A is expressed exclusively in neurons and forms part of the kinesin 1 motor complex, a microtubule motor responsible for anterograde travel from the neuronal cell body to the distal axon.[109a–c] The gene at the SPG13 locus has been identified as the mitochondrial chaperonin Hsp60.[66] The genes at the remaining AD-HSP loci have yet to be identified.

Autosomal Recessive Hereditary Spastic Paraparesis

AR-HSP is less common than the dominantly inherited form. AR-HSP displays similar genetic and phenotypic heterogeneity as AD-HSP. Consanguineous families have been linked to six AR-HSP loci, with both pure and complicated phenotypes described.

Pure Autosomal Recessive Hereditary Spastic Paraparesis

There are three loci for pure AR-HSP—SPG5, SPG7, and SPG11—although complicated families have also been described linking to the latter two loci.[10,110,111] There is no apparent clinical difference between pure AR-HSP and pure AD-HSP.

Complicated Autosomal Recessive Hereditary Spastic Paraparesis

Complicated AR-HSP pedigrees have been linked to five loci, SPG7, SPG11, SPG14, SPG15, and SPG20.[9–11,13,111–113] At the SPG7 locus, HSP has been associated with a variety of features: optic atrophy, cortical and cerebellar atrophy on imaging, dysphagia, slowed speech, distal amyotrophy, and sensorimotor neuropathy. Both pure and complicated HSP at the SPG7 locus have been associated with mitochondrial dysfunction (further discussion is given later in this chapter).

SPG11 is another locus at which both pure and complicated AR-HSP is linked.[10] Complicated HSP at this locus has been associated with mixed motor sensory neuropathy, cerebellar dysfunction, mental retardation, and abnormal brain imaging with MRI. The latter consisted of atrophy or agenesis of the corpus callosum in two families and periventricular white matter changes also in one of these families. In the one family linked to the SPG14 locus, the additional features co-segregating with the spastic paraparesis were a distal motor neuropathy and mild mental retardation.[11] Two families have been linked to the SPG15 locus. Pigmented macular degeneration, distal amyotrophy, mild cerebellar dysfunction, and diffuse brain atrophy on MRI scans were the complicating features described.[9]

The Troyer syndrome, which occurs in high frequency in the old-order Amish, has been linked to SPG20.[13] The Troyer syndrome is characterized by spastic paraparesis, distal atrophy, dysarthria, developmental delay, and short stature. SPG20 gene comprises nine exons spanning a distance of 43.3 kilobases on chromosome 13q12.3. SPG20 encodes a protein of 666 amino (72.7 kilodaltons) named *spartin,* which is ubiquitously expressed in adult tissues. Spartin shares homology with SNX15, VPS4, and SKD1 human proteins involved in protein trafficking, suggesting a possible similar role for spartin. Spartin also shares homology with the N-terminal region of spastin.[13] This region of spastin is thought to be responsible for targeting microtubules, suggesting that spartin may also interact with microtubules.[84]

SPG7, Paraplegin, and Mitochondrial Dysfunction in Hereditary Spastic Paraparesis

The SPG7 gene is 52 kilobases in size comprising 17 exons. The SPG7 protein, paraplegin, is a nuclear encoded mitochondrial metalloprotease. Paraplegin, like spastin (SPG4), is a member of the AAA protein family, sharing homology in the AAA cassette. However, outside of the 230 amino acid conserved AAA cassette, little homology is seen. Whereas little is known about paraplegin, other than the fact that it appears to be ubiquitously expressed, much more is known about the function of similar proteins in yeast. Afg3p and Rca1p are AAA mitochondrial metalloproteases found in yeast and each share 55 percent amino acid homology with paraplegin respectively. In yeast, Afg3p and Rca1p form a high-molecular-weight (850 kilodalton) hetero-oligomeric complex in the inner mitochondrial membrane, which is essential for mitochondrial biogenesis. They are involved in ATP synthase assembly, respiratory chain complex formation, and the degradation of incompletely synthesized mitochondrial polypeptides.[114–118] Deletion or mutation of the conserved proteolytic site of either Afg3p or Rca1p leads to dysfunction of respiratory chain activity and an impaired ability to degrade incompletely synthesized mitochondrial polypeptides. These studies show the essential role the paraplegin like genes Afg3p and Rca1p play in normal mitochondrial biogenesis in yeast. From the studies of yeast homologues, it seems likely that paraplegin functions by forming multimeric complexes that have proteolytic and chaperone-like functions in the mitochondria, essential for the normal assembly and turnover of respiratory chain complexes.

In addition to the clinical heterogeneity of SPG7 (described earlier), there is genetic heterogeneity with a different mutation described in the four families with paraplegin. All the mutations described in some way affect the conserved AAA domain, either truncating the protein or by causing an in-frame deletion. In the English pedigree described by McDermott et al,[113] the genetic story was less straightforward. The proband was a compound heterozygote with both a 9–base-pair deletion (1450–1458 del) and a missense change (1529C→T). The paraplegin missense change was inherited from a clinically normal mother. The deletion was inherited from a father who was reported to be mildly affected with spastic paraparesis. The authors argued that the father either represented a manifesting heterozygote or that the deletion he carried was behaving in a dominant-negative manner.[113] In the latter case, it may be that the deletion is affecting the ability of the translated paraplegin protein to form multimeric complexes, which in the yeast homologues appear to be necessary for normal function.

Both pure and complicated HSP at the SPG7 locus has been associated with evidence of mitochondrial dysfunction on histochemical analysis of muscle tissue.[111,113] Mutation in a further nuclear encoded mitochondrial protein, Hsp60, has recently been identified as the cause for pure AD-HSP at the SPG13 locus.[66] Whether mitochondrial dysfunction is a common feature in the pathogenesis of the HSP phenotype at the autosomal loci remains to be seen. There is evidence of further mitochondrial dysfunction in HSP. Marked respiratory chain complex I and IV deficiencies have been reported in AD-HSP and AR-HSP where both spastin and paraplegin mutations have been excluded as a cause.[119,120] However, other than at the SPG4 locus, where mitochondrial involvement has been adequately sought and not found, there has not been a thorough study in genetic subtypes of HSP. In the remaining dominant families at the SPG3, SPG6, SPG8, and SPG9 loci, only a small number of muscle biopsies have been performed (mostly only one individual for each locus) for histochemical and biochemical analysis of mitochondrial function.[8,121] The results to date suggest there is no primary role for mitochondrial dysfunction at these loci. Further studies are now required to confirm these findings and to investigate families linked to the more recently discovered dominant loci SPG10, SPG12, SPG17, SPG19, and particularly SPG13 caused by mutations in a mitochondrial chaperonin (Hsp60) gene. No studies have yet investigated mitochondrial function in the non–SPG7 AR families.

X-LINKED HEREDITARY SPASTIC PARAPARESIS

In comparison to autosomally inherited HSP, X-linked HSP is quite rare. There are three X-linked HSP loci: SPG1, SPG2, and SPG16. The genes involved at the SPG1 and SPG2 loci have been known for some time, and the molecular biology is relatively well understood and is discussed here. The gene at SPG16 is not yet known. One SPG16 family with a pure phenotype has been identified having a NOR insertion into Xq11.2.[122] Earlier, Steinmuller et al[123] reported a family in whom SPG1 and SPG2 were excluded and linkage suggested a locus within Xq11.2–q23. In this family, the phenotype was severe with additional mental retardation, upper limb involvement, visual impairment, and bladder and bowel dysfunction.[123] A further complicated pedigree has had mutation in the SPG1 gene, and SPG2 gene was excluded.[124] Whether these two additional families are both linked to SPG16, or whether there is a further X-linked locus, is yet unconfirmed.

SPG1 and L1 Cell Adhesion Molecule

SPG1 is caused by mutations in the L1 cell adhesion molecule gene (L1CAM).[125] The phenotype tends to be complicated with mental retardation and congenital musculoskeletal abnormalities, most notably the absence of extensor hallucis longus.[126] Mutations in the same gene were identified in X-linked hydrocephalus, X-linked agenesis of the corpus callosum, and the syndrome of MASA (mental retardation, aphasia, shuffling gait, and adducted thumbs). There is marked interfamilial and intrafamilial in families with L1CAM gene mutations. In a number of families, more than one of the possible L1CAM phenotypes has been observed. The diseases are now considered part of a clinical syndrome with the acronym CRASH, for corpus callosum hypoplasia, retardation, adducted thumbs, spastic paraplegia, and hydrocephalus.[127]

L1CAM is a transmembrane glycoprotein that is mainly expressed by neurons and Schwann cells.[128] It plays an essential role in the development of the nervous system, being involved neuron-neuron adhesion, axon outgrowth, and pathfinding.[129] L1CAM plays an important role in corticospinal tract formation.[130–133] In a transgenic model, loss of L1CAM disrupts the normal guidance of corticospinal axons across the midline at the level of the pyramids. The normal decussation at the pyramids is stimulated by a chemorepellent molecule secreted by the ventral spinal cord known as Sema3A.[134] L1CAM is a component of the Sema3A receptor complex, and mice deficient in L1CAM fail to respond to Sema3A in vitro.

SPG2 and Proteolipid Protein

Both pure and complicated HSP pedigrees are seen at the SPG2 locus.[135–139] Complicated HSP linked to SPG2 consists of a core phenotype of spastic paraparesis, cerebellar syndrome, and mental retardation. Interfamilial variation is seen with the core features occurring to various degrees with or without additional features such as optic atrophy. Similarly, intrafamilial variation occurs.[135,138,139]

SPG2 is caused by mutations in the proteolipid protein (PLP) gene.[140] Mutations in the PLP gene also cause Pelizaeus-Merzbacher disease (PMD). PMD is a dysmyelinating disease, the classic form having onset in infancy and death in late adolescence or young adulthood. It is characterized by nystagmus, ataxia, spasticity, abnormal movements, optic atrophy, and microcephaly. There is a more severe congenital type, which shows a rapid progression and death in infancy, as well as a transitional or intermediate form.[141] The phenotype of disease caused by mutations in the PLP gene can be considered as a continuous spectrum, with milder SPG2 at one end and the more severe PMD at the other.

PLP is the major myelin protein of the central nervous system (CNS), accounting for approximately 50 percent of total myelin protein in the adult brain. An alternatively spliced form of PLP missing 35 amino acid residues, called DM20, is also produced from the PLP gene. The function of PLP/DM20 is not confirmed. It seems likely that these proteins play a role in stabilizing the structure of CNS myelin by forming the intraperiod line. Some authors have suggested the two isoforms may have different functions. The DM20 isoform is present earlier in development and is thought to play a role in glial cell development. The PLP isoform appears later and may play a role in myelin assembly and maintenance. Mutations in the PLP gene that do not cause a reduction in the DM20 isoform are associated with the milder PMD phenotype or SPG2. Conversely mutations that affect the level of the DM20 isoform are associated with the more severe PMD phenotypes.[142] A further role for PLP/DM20 in glial-axon communication has been suggested. This followed the observation that *Plp* null mutants developed normal myelin sheaths despite lack of PLP/DM20 but subsequently went on to develop a profound axonopathy.[143–145]

CONCLUSION

With the genes identified at only 8 of the current 19 known SPG loci, there is already marked diversity in the function of genes associated with an HSP phenotype. Their functions include mitochondrial protein housekeeping, chaperoning, cytoskeleton regulation, myelin formation and maintenance, neuron outgrowth, and glial-axon communication. With the end result of mutation in any of these genes being the development of a progressive spastic paraparesis, it is tempting to speculate that these genes all feed into one common pathway essential for normal axonal function. How do mutations in these genes lead to relatively selective axonal degeneration seen at postmortem study? This is perhaps easier to explain with a protein such as PLP, which is a major myelin protein, or atlastin, which is found at high levels of expression in the CNS. However, both paraplegin and spastin are ubiquitously expressed in human tissues, and therefore differential tissue expression cannot explain the selective axonal loss seen in HSP. An explanation may come from the intrinsic properties of the neurons leading to a selective vulnerability. This pathophysiological mechanism has been suggested to explain the selective neurodegeneration seen in MND caused by mutation in the ubiquitously expressed copper/zinc superoxide dismutase (SOD1). In HSP, the longest axons of the corticospinal tract and dorsal columns undergo degeneration in their terminal portions. This degeneration proceeds proximally, but the cell body of the axon itself remains intact. These neurons have several properties that may make them selectively vulnerable. The cell bodies have to support axons of up to 1 meter. These neurons are therefore highly metabolically active and are likely therefore to be susceptible to any alteration in energy generation. Paraplegin is thought to act as a quality control for proteins within the mitochondria, removing misfolded proteins. If this function is disrupted, the mitochondria may be anticipated to become entangled with misfolded proteins, which could interfere with ATP generation. There is certainly evidence of mitochondrial dysfunction in HSP due to a paraplegin mutation and at other HSP loci. There is also increasing evidence of a role for mitochondrial dysfunction in other neurodegenerative disorders. A further vulnerability of the long axons affected in HSP is the reliance on an intact cytoskeleton and efficient transport of essential cellular components down the axon. An interruption in the transport of vital cellular components to the distal axon could be responsible for the "dying back" phenomenon observed in HSP. The identification of mutation in a kinesin motor protein (KIF5A) as the cause of AD-HSP at the SPG10 locus supports a role for impaired ascenal transport in the pathogenesis of HSP. An interruption in spastin function, which appears to involve regulating microtubules, is likely to cause disruption in the microtubule cytoskeleton, resulting in such an impairment of axonal transport. A similar disruption may occur secondary to a spartin mutation, because spartin

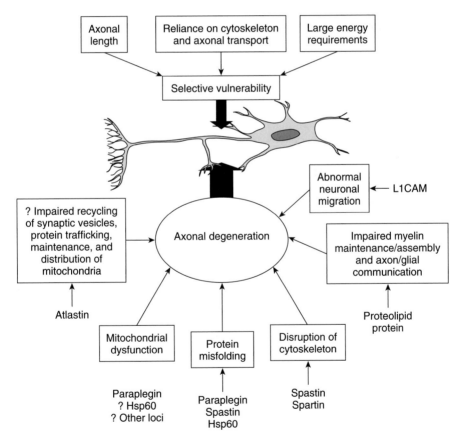

Figure 18.1 An illustration of the possible mechanisms involved in the neurodegenerative process in hereditary spastic paraparesis (HSP). Both the possible consequences of mutation in the known HSP genes and the specific properties of the neurons that may make them selectively vulnerable are illustrated.

shares homology with spastin at its N-terminal microtubule targeting region. As the proteins mutated in HSP and their functions are identified, it is likely that new opportunities to intervene in the neurodegenerative process will arise. Figure 18.1 outlines potential disease mechanisms in HSP based on current knowledge. From various genotype-phenotype studies, it is apparent that factors other than mutation in the relevant HSP gene influence the phenotype observed. Whether this influence is environmental, genetic, or both is unclear. However, there is evidence for mutation in other neuronal proteins modifying but not causing an HSP phenotype. Meyer et al[146] demonstrated that mutation in the glutamate transporter gene excitatory amino acid transporter type 2 (EAAT2) was associated with a more severe HSP phenotype. Similar modifying effects have been seen in other motor system disorders. The phenotype in MND can be influenced by mutation in the ciliary neurotrophic factor (CNTF) gene and the survival motor neuron type 2 (SMN2) gene.[147,148] Such modifiers offer potential targets for therapy.

The identification of the genes in HSP heralds a new era in terms of diagnosing the condition. In a patient with AD-HSP, the gene can now be identified in up to 40 percent of cases with spastin mutation screening. This can be increased further to 50 to 60 percent with screening of the atlastin gene. Precise diagnosis enables appropriate counseling with regard to prognosis and implications for a patient's family. However, given the huge interfamilial and intrafamilial variation in age at onset of symptoms and severity seen in SPG4, the use of prenatal screening can be less clearcut than with other inherited disorders.

Rapid progress has been made recently in our ability to accurately classify and diagnose HSP. In the coming years, there is hope that increased understanding of the neurodegenerative processes at work in HSP will lead to useful therapeutic interventions.

REFERENCES

1. Harding AE. Hereditary "pure" spastic paraplegia: a clinical and genetic study of 22 families. J Neurol Neurosurg Psychiatry 1981;44:871–883.
2. Polo JM, Calleja J, Combarros O, Berciano J. Hereditary "pure" spastic paraplegia: a study of nine families. J Neurol Neurosurg Psychiatry 1993;56:175–181.
3. Schady W, Sheard A. A quantitative study of sensory function in hereditary spastic paraplegia. Brain 1990;113:709–720.
4. McDermott CJ, White K, Bushby K, Shaw PJ. Hereditary spastic paraparesis: a review of new developments. J Neurol Neurosurg Psychiatry 2000;69:150–160.
5. White KD, Ince PG, Cookson M, et al. Clinical and pathological findings in hereditary spastic paraparesis with spastin mutation. Neurology 2000;55:89–94.
6. Webb S, Coleman D, Byrne P, et al. Autosomal dominant hereditary spastic paraparesis with cognitive loss linked to chromosome 2p. Brain 1998;121:601–609.
7. Heinzlef O, Paternotte C, Mahieux F, et al. Mapping of a complicated familial spastic paraplegia to a locus SPG4 on chromosome 2p. J Med Genet 1998;35:89–93.
8. Seri M, Cusano R, Forabosco P, et al. Genetic mapping to 10q23.3-q24.2, in a large Italian pedigree, of a new syndrome showing bilateral cataracts, gastroesophageal reflux, and spastic paraparesis with amyotrophy. Am J Hum Genet 1999;64:586–593.
9. Hughes CA, Byrne PC, Webb S, et al. SPG15, a new locus for autosomal recessive complicated HSP on chromosome 14q. Neurology 2001;56:1230–1233.
10. Murillo F, Kobayashi H, Pegoraro E, et al. Genetic localization of a new locus for recessive familial spastic paraparesis to 15q13-15. Neurology 1999;53:50–56.

11. Vazza G, Zortea M, Boaretto F, et al. A new locus for autosomal recessive spastic paraplegia associated with mental retardation and distal motor neuropathy, SPG14, maps to chromosome 3q27-q28. Am J Hum Genet 2000;67:504–509.

12. Patel H, Hart PE, Warner TT, et al. The Silver syndrome variant of hereditary spastic paraparesis maps to chromosome 11q12-q14, with evidence for genetic heterogeneity within this subtype. Am J Hum Genet 2001;69:209–215.

13. Patel H, Cross H, Proukakis C, et al. SPG20 is mutated in Troyer syndrome, an hereditary spastic paraplegia. Nat Genet 2002;31:37–38.

14. Gigli GL, Diomedi M, Bernardi G, et al. Spastic paraplegia, epilepsy and mental retardation in several members of a family: a novel genetic disorder. Am J Med Genet 1993;45:711–716.

15. Sommerfelt K, Kyllerman M, Sanner G. Hereditary spastic paraplegia with epileptic myoclonus. Acta Neurol Scand 1991;84:157–160.

16. Webb S, Flanagan N, Callaghan N, Hutchinson M. A family with spastic paraparesis and epilepsy. Epilepsia 1997;38:495–499.

17. Yih JS, Wang S-J, Su M-S, et al. Hereditary spastic paraplegia associated with epilepsy, mental retardation and hearing impairment. Paraplegia 1993;31:408–411.

18. Mead SH, Proukakis C, Wood N, et al. A large family with hereditary spastic paraparesis due to a frame shift mutation of spastin (SPG4) gene: association with multiple sclerosis in two affected siblings and epilepsy in other affected family members. J Neurol Neurosurg Psychiatry 2001;71:788–791.

19. Fonknechten N, Mavel D, Byrne P, et al. Spectrum of SPG4 mutations in autosomal dominant spastic paraplegia. Hum Mol Genet 2000;9:637–644.

20. Worster-Drought C, Greenfield JG, McMenemy W. A form of familial presenile dementia with spastic paralysis. Brain 1944;67:38–43.

21. Manson J. Hereditary spastic paraplegia with ataxia and mental defect. Br Med J 1920;2:477.

22. Sutherland JM. Familial spastic paraplegia. Its relation to mental and cardiac abnormalities. Lancet 1957;2:169–170.

23. Cross HE, McKusick VA. The Mast syndrome: a recessively inherited form of pre-senile dementia with motor disturbances. Arch Neurol 1967;16:1–13.

24. Arjundas G, Ramamurthi B, Chettur L. Familial spastic paraplegia (a review with four case reports). J Assoc Physicians India 1971;19:653–657.

25. Pridmore S, Rao G, Abusah P. Hereditary spastic paraplegia with dementia. Aust N Z J Psychiatry 1995;29:678–682.

26. Rothner AD, Yahr F, Yahr MD. Familial spastic paraparesis, optic atrophy and dementia: clinical observations of affected kindred. N Y State J Med 1976;76:756–758.

27. Byrne PC, Mc Monagle P, Webb S, et al. Age-related cognitive decline in hereditary spastic paraparesis linked to chromosome 2p. Neurology 2000;54:1510–1517.

28. McMonagle P, Byrne PC, Fitzgerald B, et al. Phenotype of AD-HSP due to mutations in the SPAST gene. Comparison with AD-HSP without mutations. Neurology 2000;55:1794–1800.

29. Reid E, Grayson C, Rubinsztein DC, et al. Subclinical cognitive impairment in autosomal dominant "pure" hereditary spastic paraplegia. J Med Genet 1999;36:797–798.

30. Tedeschi G, Allocca S, Di Costanzo A, et al. Multisystem involvement of the central nervous system in Strümpell's disease. J Neurol Sci 1991;103:55–60.

31. Crook R, Verkkoniemi A, Perez-Tur J, et al. A variant of Alzheimer's disease with spastic paraparesis and unusual plaques due to deletion of exon 9 of presenilin 1. Nat Med 1998;4:452–455.

32. Smith MJ, Kwok JBJ, McLean CA, et al. Variable phenotype of Alzheimer's disease with spastic paraparesis. Ann Neurol 2001;49:125–129.

33. Dyck PJ, Lambert EHI. Lower motor and primary sensory neuron disease with peroneal atrophy, II: neurologic, genetic, and electrophysiologic findings in various neuronal degenerations. Arch Neurol 1968;18:619–625.

34. Harding AE, Thomas PK. Peroneal muscular atrophy with pyramidal features. J Neurol Neurosurg Psychiatry 1984;47:168–172.

35. Mostacciuolo ML, Rampoldi L, Righetti E, et al. Hereditary spastic paraplegia associated with peripheral neuropathy: a distinct clinical and genetic entity. Neuromusc Disord 2000;10:497–502.

36. Silver JR. Familial spastic paraplegia with amyotrophy of the hands. J Neurol Neurosurg Psychiatry 1966;29:135–144.

37. Cross HE, McKusick VA. The Troyer syndrome. A recessive form of spastic paraplegia with distal muscle wasting. Arch Neurol 1967;16:473–485.

38. Harding AE. Hereditary spastic paraplegias. Semin Neurol 1993;13:333–336.

39. Neuhauser G, Wiffler C, Opitz JM. Familial spastic paraplegia with distal muscle wasting in the old order Amish: atypical Troyer syndrome or "new" syndrome. Clin Genet 1976;9:315–323.

40. Farag TI, El-Badramany MH, Al-Sharkawy S. Troyer syndrome: report of the first "non Amish" sibship and review. Am J Med Genet 1994;53:383–385.
41. Auer-Grumbach M, Fazekas F, Radner H, et al. Troyer syndrome: a combination of central brain abnormality and motor neuron disease? J Neurol 1999;246:556–561.
42. Bouchard JP, Barbeau A, Bouchard R, Bouchard RW. Autosomal recessive spastic ataxia of Charlevoix-Saguenay. Can J Neurol Sci 1978;5:61.
43. Bruyn RPM, Scheltens P. Autosomal recessive paraparesis with amyotrophy of the hands and feet. Acta Neurol Scand 1993;87:443–445.
44. Cavanagh NPC, Eames RA, Galvin RJ, et al. Hereditary sensory neuropathy with spastic paraplegia. Brain 1979;102:79–94.
45. Khalifeh RR, Zellweger H. Hereditary sensory neuropathy with spinal cord disease. Neurology 1963;13:406–411.
46. Koenig RH, Spiro AJ. Hereditary spastic paraparesis with sensory neuropathy. Dev Med Child Neurol 1970;12:576–581.
47. Schady W, Smith CML. Sensory neuropathy in hereditary spastic paraplegia. J Neurol Neurosurg Psychiatry 1994;57:693–698.
48. Claus D, Waddy HM, Harding AE, et al. Hereditary motor and sensory neuropathies and hereditary spastic paraplegia: a magnetic stimulation study. Ann Neurol 1990;28:43–49.
49. Nielsen JE, Krabbe K, Jennum P, et al. Autosomal dominant pure spastic paraplegia: a clinical, paraclinical and genetic study. J Neurol Neurosurg Psychiatry 1998;64:61–66.
50. Pelosi L, Lanzillo B, Perretti A, et al. Motor and somatosensory evoked potentials in hereditary spastic paraplegia. J Neurol Neurosurg Psychiatry 1991;54:1099–1102.
51. Schady W, Dick JPR, Sheard A, Crampton S. Central motor conduction studies in hereditary spastic paraplegia. J Neurol Neurosurg Psychiatry 1991;54:775–779.
52. Aalfs CM, Koelman JHTM, Posthumus Meyjes FE, Ongerboer de Visser BW. Posterior tibial and sural nerve somatosensory evoked potentials: a study in spastic paraparesis and spinal cord lesions. Electroencephalogr Clin Neurophysiol 1993;89:437–441.
53. Mcleod JG, Morgan JA, Reye C. Electrophysiological studies in familial spastic paraplegia. J Neurol Neurosurg Psychiatry 1977;40:611–615.
54. Thomas PK, Jefferys JGR, Smith IS, Loulakakis D. Spinal somatosensory evoked potentials in hereditary spastic paraplegia. J Neurol Neurosurg Psychiatry 1981;44:243–246.
55. Tyrer JH, Sutherland JM. The primary spinocerebellar atrophies and their associated defects, with a study of the foot deformity. Brain 1961;84:289–300.
56. Sjaastad O, Berstad J, Gjesdahl P, Gjessing L. Homocarsinosis. 2. A familial metabolic disorder associated with spastic paraplegia, progressive mental deficiency, and retinal pigmentation. Acta Neurol Scand 1976;53:275–290.
57. Bruyn RPM, Scheltens PH. Hereditary spastic paraparesis (Strümpell-Lorrain). In JMBV de Jong (ed), Handbook of Clinical Neurology. Amsterdam: Elsevier Science Publishers, 1991;301–317.
58. Hedera P, DiMauro S, Bonilla E, et al. Phenotypic analysis of autosomal dominant hereditary spastic paraplegia linked to chromosome 8q. Neurology 1999;53:44–50.
59. Ormerod IEC, Harding AE, Miller DH, et al. Magnetic resonance imaging in degenerative ataxic disorders. J Neurol Neurosurg Psychiatry 1994;57:51–57.
60. Kramer W. Hereditary spinal spastic paraplegia (Strümpell-Lorrain disease). Neuropathol Appl Neurobiol 1977;8:488–489.
61. Durr A, Brice A, Serdaru M, et al. The phenotype of "pure" autosomal dominant spastic paraplegia. Neurology 1994;44:1274–1277.
62. Lindsey JC, Lusher ME, McDermott CJ, et al. Mutation analysis of the spastin gene (SPG4) in patients with hereditary spastic paraparesis. J Med Genet 2000;37:759–765.
63. Rainier S, Hedera P, Alvarado D, et al. Hereditary spastic paraplegia linked to chromosome 14q11-q21: reduction of the SPG3 locus interval from 5.3 to 2.7 cM. J Med Genet 2001;38:E39.
64. Hazan J, Fonknechten N, Mavel D, et al. Spastin, a novel AAA protein, is altered in the most frequent form of autosomal dominant spastic paraplegia. Nat Genet 1999;23:296–303.
65. Zhao X, Alvarado D, Rainier S, et al. Mutations in a newly identified GTPase gene cause autosomal dominant hereditary spastic paraplegia. Nat Genet 2001;29:326–331.
66. Hansen JJ, Durr A, Cournu-Rebeix I, et al. Hereditary spastic paraplegia SPG13 is associated with a mutation in the gene encoding the mitochondrial chaperonin Hsp60. Am J Hum Genet 2002;70:1328–1332.
66a. Reid E, Kloos M, Ashley-Koch A, et al. A kinesin heavy chain (KIF5A) mutation in hereditary spastic paraparesis (SPG10). Am J Hum Genet 2002;71:1189–1194.

67. Fink JK, Wu C-TB, Jones SM, et al. Autosomal dominant familial spastic paraplegia: Tight linkage to chromosome 15q. Am J Hum Genet 1995;56:188–192.
68. Hedera P, Rainer S, Alvarado D, et al. Novel locus for autosomal dominant hereditary spastic paraplegia, on chromosome 8q. Am J Hum Genet 1999;64:563–569.
69. Reid E, Dearlove M, Rhodes M, Rubinsztein DC. A new locus for autosomal dominant "pure" hereditary spastic paraplegia mapping to chromosome 12q13, and evidence for further genetic heterogeneity. Am J Hum Genet 1999;65:757–763.
70. Reid E, Dearlove AM, Osborn O, et al. A locus for autosomal dominant "pure" hereditary spastic paraplegia maps to chromosome 19q13. Am J Hum Genet 2000;66:728–732.
71. Valente EM, Brancati F, Caputo V, et al. Novel locus for autosomal dominant pure hereditary spastic paraplegia (SPG19) maps to chromosome 9q33-q34. Ann Neurol 2002;51:681–685.
72. Hazan J, Lamy C, Melki J, et al. Autosomal dominant familial spastic paraplegia is genetically heterogeneous and one locus maps to chromosome 14q. Nat Genet 1993;5:163–167.
73. Gispert S, Santos N, Damen R, et al. Autosomal dominant familial spastic paraplegia: Reduction of the FSP1 candidate region on chromosome 14q to 7 cM and locus heterogeneity. Am J Hum Genet 1995;56:183–187.
74. Hentati A, Pericak-Vance MA, Lennon F, et al. Linkage of a locus for autosomal dominant spastic paraplegia to chromosome 2p markers. Hum Mol Genet 1994;3:1867–1871.
75. Huang S, Zhuyu, Li H, et al. Another pedigree with pure autosomal dominant spastic paraplegia (AD-FSP) from Tibet mapping to 14q11.2-q24.3. Hum Mol Genet 1997;100:620–623.
76. Lennon F, Gaskell PC, Wolpert C, et al. Linkage and heterogeneity in hereditary spastic paraparesis. Am J Hum Genet 1995;57(suppl):A217.
77. Muglia M, Magariello A, Nicoletti G, et al. Further evidence that SPG3A gene mutations cause autosomal dominant hereditary spastic paraplegia. Ann Neurol 2002;51:794–795.
78. Sever S, Muhlberg AB, Schmid SL. Impairment of dynamin's GAP domain stimulates receptor-mediated endocytosis. Nature 1999;398:481–486.
79. Nicoziani P, Vilhardt F, Llorente A, et al. Role for dynamin in late endosome dynamics and trafficking of the cation-independent mannose 6-phosphate receptor. Mol Biol Cell 2000;11:481–495.
80. Jones SM, Howell KE, Henley JR, et al. Role of dynamin in the formation of transport vesicles from the trans-Golgi network. Science 1998;279:573–577.
81. Pitts KR, Yoon Y, Krueger EW, McNiven MA. The dynamin-like protein DLP1 is essential for normal distribution and morphology of the endoplasmic reticulum and mitochondria in mammalian cells. Mol Biol Cell 1999;10:4403–4417.
82. Ochoa GC, Slepnev VI, Neff L, et al. A functional link between dynamin and the actin cytoskeleton at podosomes. J Cell Biol 2000;150:377–389.
83. Patel S, Latterich M. The AAA team: related ATPases with diverse functions. Cell Biology 1998;8:65–71.
84. Errico A, Ballabio A, Rugarli EI. Spastin, the protein mutated in autosomal dominant hereditary spastic paraplegia, is involved in microtubule dynamics. Hum Mol Genet 2002;11:153–163.
85. Burger J, Fonknechten N, Hoeltzenbein M, et al. Hereditary spastic paraplegia caused by mutations in the SPG4 gene. Eur J Hum Genet 2000;8:771–776.
86. Meijer IA, Hand CK, Cossette P, et al. Spectrum of SPG4 mutations in a large collection of North American families with hereditary spastic paraplegia. Arch Neurol 2002;59:281–286.
87. Hazan J, Fontaine B, Bruyn RPM, et al. Linkage of a new locus for autosomal dominant familial spastic paraplegia to chromosome 2p. Hum Mol Genet 1994;3:1569–1573.
88. Burger J, Metzke H, Patternote C, et al. Autosomal dominant spastic paraplegia with anticipation maps to a 4-cM interval on chromosome 2p21-p24 in a large German family. Hum Genet 1996;98:371–375.
89. Andrew SE, Goldberg YP, Kremer B, et al. The relationship between trinucleotide repeat (CAG) repeat length and clinical features of Huntington's disease. Nat Genet 1993;4:398–403.
90. Koide R, Ikeuchi T, Onodera O, et al. Unstable expansion of CAG repeat in hereditary dentatorubral-pallidoluysian atrophy (DRPLA). Nat Genet 1994;6:9–13.
91. Maciel P, Gaspar C, DeStefano AL, et al. Correlation between CAG repeat length and clinical features in Machado-Joseph Disease. Am J Hum Genet 1995;57:54–61.
92. Trottier Y, Lutz Y, Stevanin G, et al. Polyglutamine expansion as a pathological epitope in Huntington's disease and four dominant cerebellar ataxias. Nature 1995;378:403–407.
93. Nielsen JE, Koefoed P, Abell K, et al. CAG repeat expansion in autosomal dominant pure spastic paraplegia linked to chromosome 2p21-p24. Hum Mol Genet 1997;6:1811–1816.
94. Benson KF, Horwitz M, Wolff J, et al. CAG repeat expansion in autosomal dominant familial spastic paraparesis: novel expansion in subset of patients. Hum Mol Genet 1998;7:1779–1786.

95. Patrono C, Sasali C, Tessa A, et al. Missense and splice site mutations in SPG4 suggest loss-of-function in dominant spastic paraplegia. J Neurol 2002;249:200–205.
96. Namekawa M, Takiyama Y, Sakoe K, et al. A large Japanese SPG4 family with a novel insertion mutation of the SPG4 gene: a clinical and genetic study. J Neurol Sci 2001;185:63–68.
97. Morita M, Ho M, Hosler BA, et al. A novel mutation in the spastin gene in a family with spastic paraplegia. Neurosci Lett 2002;325:57–61.
98. Scott WK, Gaskell PC, Lennon F, et al. Locus heterogeneity, anticipation and reduction of the chromosome 2p minimal candidate region in autosomal dominant familial spastic paraplegia. Neurogenetics 1997;1:95–102.
99. Higgins JJ, Loveless JM, Goswami S, et al. An atypical intronic deletion widens the spectrum of mutations in hereditary spastic paraplegia. Neurology 2001;56:1482–1485.
100. Bantel A, McWilliams S, Auysh D, et al. Novel mutation of the spastin gene in familial spastic paraplegia. Clin Genet 2001;59:364–365.
101. Cooper DN, Krawczak M. Human Gene Mutation. Oxford: Bios Scientific, 1993.
102. Krawczak M, Reiss J, Cooper DN. The mutational spectrum of single base-pair substitutions in mRNA splice junctions of human genes: causes and consequences. Hum Genet 1992;90:41–54.
103. Svenson IK, Ashley-Koch AE, Pericak-Vance MA, Marchuk DA. A second leaky splice-site mutation in the spastin gene. Am J Hum Genet 2001;69:1407–1409.
104. Svenson IK, Ashley-Koch AE, Gaskell PG, et al. Identification and expression analysis of spastin gene mutations in hereditary spastic paraplegia. Am J Hum Genet 2001;68:1077–1085.
105. Hentati A, Deng H-X, Zhai H, et al. Novel mutations in spastin gene and absence of correlation with age at onset of symptoms. Neurology 2000;55:1388–1390.
106. Reid E, Dearlove AM, Whiteford ML, et al. Autosomal dominant spastic paraplegia. Refined SPG8 locus and additional genetic heterogeneity. Neurology 1999;53:1845–1849.
107. Fontaine B, Davoine C-S, Durr A, et al. A new locus for autosomal dominant pure spastic paraplegia, on chromosome 2q24-q34. Am J Hum Genet 2000;66:702–707.
108. Slavotinek AM, Pike M, Mills K, Hurst JA. Cataracts, motor system disorder, short stature, learning difficulties, and skeletal abnormalities: a new syndrome? Am J Med Genet 1996;62:42–47.
109. Nigro CL, Cusano R, Scaranari M, et al. A refined physical and transcriptional map of the SPG9 locus on 10q23.3-q24.2. Eur J Hum Genet 2000;8:777–782.
109a. Goldstein LSB. Kinesin molecular motors: transport pathways, receptors and human disease. Proc Natl Acad Sci USA 2001;98:6999–7003.
109b. Goldstein LSB, Yang Z. Micrtotubule-based transport systems in neurons: the role of kinesins and dynamins. Annu Rev Neurosci 2000;23:39–71.
109c. Xia Ch, Rahman A, Yang Z, Goldstein LS. Chromosomal localization reveals three kinesin heavy chain genes in mouse. Genomics 1998;52:209–213.
110. Hentati A, Pericak-Vance MA, Hung W-Y, et al. Linkage of "pure" autosomal recessive familial spastic paraplegia to chromosome 8 markers and evidence of genetic locus heterogeneity. Hum Mol Genet 1994;3:1263–1267.
111. Casari G, De Fusco M, Ciarmatori S, et al. Spastic paraplegia and OXPHOS impairment caused by mutations in paraplegin, a nuclear-encoded mitochondrial metalloprotease. Cell 1998;93:973–983.
112. De Michele G, De Fusco M, Cavalcanti F, et al. A new locus for autosomal recessive hereditary spastic paraplegia maps to chromosome 16q24.3. Am J Hum Genet 1998;63:135–139.
113. McDermott CJ, Dayaratne RK, Tomkins J, et al. Paraplegin gene analysis in hereditary spastic paraparesis (HSP) pedigrees in northeast England. Neurology 2001;56:467–471.
114. Tauer R, Mannhaupt G, Schnall R, et al. Yta10p, a member of a novel ATPase family in yeast, is essential for mitochondrial function. FEBS Lett 1994;353:197–200.
115. Tzagoloff A, Yue J, Jang J, Paul M-F. A new member of a family of ATPases is essential for assembly of mitochondrial respiratory chain and ATP synthetase complexes in Saccharomyces cerevisiae. Mol Cell Biol 1994;13:5418–5426.
116. Paul M-F, Tzagoloff A. Mutations in RCA1 and AFG3 inhibit F1-ATPase assembly in *Saccharomyces cerevisiae*. FEBS Lett 1995;373:66–70.
117. Langer T, Neupert W. Regulated protein degradation in mitochondria. Experimentia 1996;52:1069–1076.
118. Rep M, Grivell LA. The role of protein degradation in mitochondrial function and biogenesis. Curr Genet 1996;30:367–380.
119. Piemonte F, Casali C, Carrozzo R, et al. Respiratory chain defects in hereditary spastic paraplegias. Neuromuscul Disord 2001;11:565–569.

120. McDermott CJ, Taylor RW, Hayes C, et al. Investigation of mitochondrial function in hereditary spastic paraparesis. Neuroreport 2003;14:485–488.
121. Hedera P, DiMauro S, Bonilla E, et al. Mitochondrial analysis in autosomal dominant hereditary spastic paraplegia. Neurology 2000;55:1591–1592.
122. Tamagaki A, Shima M, Tomita R, et al. Segregation of a pure form of spastic paraplegia and NOR insertion into Xq11.2. Am J Med Genet 2000;94:5–8.
123. Steinmuller R, Lantigua-Cruz A, Garcia-Garcia R, et al. Evidence of a third locus in X-linked recessive paraplegia. Hum Genet 1997;100:287–289.
124. Claes S, Devriendt K, Van Goethem G, et al. Novel syndromic form of X-linked complicated spastic paraplegia. Am J Med Genet 2000;94:1–4.
125. Jouet M, Rosenthal A, Armstrong G, et al. X-linked spastic paraplegia (SPG1), MASA syndrome and X-linked hydrocephalus result from mutations in the L1 gene. Nat Genet 1994;7:402–407.
126. Kenwrick S, Ionasescu V, Ionasescu G, et al. Linkage studies of X-linked recessive spastic paraplegia using DNA probes. Hum Genet 1986;73:264–266.
127. Fransen E, Lemmon V, Van Camp G, et al. CRASH syndrome: clinical spectrum of corpus callosum hypoplasia, retardation, adducted thumbs, spastic paraparesis and hydrocephalus due to mutations in one single gene, L1. Eur J Hum Genet 1995;3:273–284.
128. Joosten EA, Gribnau AA. Immunological localization of cell adhesion molecule L1 in developing rat pyramidal tract. Neurosci Lett 1998;100:94–98.
129. Brummendorf T, Rathjen FG. Structure/function relationships of axon-associated adhesion receptors of the immunoglobulin superfamily. Curr Opin Neurobiol 1996;6:584–593.
130. Dahme M, Bartsch U, Martini R, et al. Disruption of the mouse L1 gene leads to malformations of the nervous system. Nat Genet 1997;17:346–349.
131. Cohen NR, Taylor JS, Scott LB, et al. Errors in corticospinal axon guidance in mice lacking the neural cell adhesion molecule L1. Curr Biol 1997;8:26–33.
132. Fransen E, D'Hooge R, Van Camp G, et al. L1 knockout mice show dilated ventricles, vermis hypoplasia and impaired exploration patterns. Hum Mol Genet 1998;7:999–1099.
133. Demyanenko GP, Tsai AY, Maness PF. Abnormalities in neuronal process extension, hippocampal development, and the ventricular system of L1 knockout mice. J Neurosci 1999;19:4907–4920.
134. Castellani V, Chedotal A, Schachner M, et al. Analysis of the L1-deficient mouse phenotype reveals cross-talk between Sema3A and L1 signaling pathways in axonal guidance. Neuron 2000;27:237–249.
135. Johnson AW, McKusick VA. A sex-linked recessive form of spastic paraplegia. Am J Hum Genet 1962;14:83–94.
136. Cambi F, Tang X-M, Cordray P, et al. Refined genetic mapping and proteolipid protein mutation analysis in X-linked pure hereditary spastic paraplegia. Neurology 1996;46:1112–1117.
137. Keppen LD, Leppert MF, O'Connel P, et al. Etiological heterogeneity in X-linked spastic paraplegia. Am J Hum Genet 1987;41:933–943.
138. Bonneau D, Rozet J-M, Bulteau C, et al. X-linked spastic paraplegia (SPG2): clinical heterogeneity at a single locus. J Med Genet 1993;30:381–384.
139. Goldblatt J, Ballo R, Sachs B, Moosa A. X-linked spastic paraplegia: evidence for homogeneity with a variable phenotype. Clin Genet 1989;35:116–120.
140. Saugier-Veber P, Munnich A, Bonneau D, et al. X-linked spastic paraplegia and Pelizaeus-Merzbacher disease are allelic disorders at the proteolipid protein locus. Nat Genet 1994;6:257–261.
141. Renier WO, Gabreels FJ, Hustinx TW, et al. Connatal Pelizaeus-Merzbacher disease with congenital stridor in two maternal cousins. Acta Neuropath 1981;54:11–17.
142. Griffiths I, Klugmann M, Anderson T, et al. Current concepts of PLP and its role in the nervous system. Microscopy research and technique 1998;41:344–358.
143. Boison D, Stoffel W. Disruption of the compacted myelin sheets of axons of the central nervous system in proteolipid protein-deficient mice. Proc Natl Acad Sci USA 1994;91:11709–11713.
144. Kluggmann M, MH S, Puhlhofer A, et al. Assembly of CNS myelin in the absence of proteolipid protein. Neuron 1997;18:59–70.
145. Griffiths I, Kluggmann M, Anderson T, et al. Axonal swellings and degeneration in mice lacking the major proteolipid of myelin. Science 1998;280:1610–1613.
146. Meyer T, Munch C, Volkel H, et al. The EAAT2 (GLT-1) gene in motor neurone disease: absence of mutations in amyotrophic lateral sclerosis and a point mutation in patients with hereditary spastic paraplegia. J Neurol Neurosurg Psychiatry 1998;65:594–596.

147. Giess R, Holtmann B, Braga M, et al. Early onset of severe familial amyotrophic lateral sclero-sis with a SOD-1 mutation: potential impact of CNTF as a candidate modifier gene. Am J Hum Genet 2002;70:1277–1286.
148. Veldink JH, van den Berg LH, Cobben JM, et al. Homozygous deletion of the survival motor neuron 2 gene is a prognostic factor in sporadic ALS. Neurology; 56:749–752.

SECTION 4

THERAPEUTICS OF MOTOR NEURON DISORDERS

19

Quality of Life and Psychosocial Aspects of Care of Patients with Amyotrophic Lateral Sclerosis

Deborah F. Gelinas and Robert G. Miller

This chapter deals with factors contributing to quality of life (QoL), measurement tools of QoL, and psychosocial aspects of the care of patients with amyotrophic lateral sclerosis (ALS) to include depression, anxiety, sexuality, spirituality, and care of the caregiver. Much has been written and published regarding factors that constitute a good QoL. The relationship between health and well-being is being elucidated in a variety of well-designed trials and astute clinical observations. The specific contributions of sexuality and spirituality to well-being and a sense of a good life worth living are still largely a mystery. These aspects of holistic care have not been adequately addressed in the ALS literature, although it is increasingly apparent that they are extremely important to patients. This chapter reviews what presently exists in the literature and sheds light on those areas that have been little studied.

Recently, there has been an increasing interest in understanding the effects of ALS and its potential treatments, not only on quantity of life but also on QoL. In part, this interest is driven by the rising cost of health care and the need for elucidating the costs of alternative treatments, as well as the impact of those interventions on outcomes that are valued by the patient.[1]

The more important reason, however, for understanding the effects of ALS on QoL is the strong prognostic impact that a good QoL has on survival in this still incurable disease.[2]

QUALITY OF LIFE

The need for QoL and quantity-of-life information about treatments in ALS is exemplified in the dilemma about whether riluzole, the only disease-specific treatment for ALS, should be given. Riluzole has been shown to modestly

465

extend survival in patients with ALS,[3] but at a cost of approximately $800 per month. Is it of sufficient value to the patient to justify the expense, especially if that expense is to be paid out of pocket? There are no data to answer this question, because there were no QoL measures incorporated in the original riluzole trials, but one post hoc analysis suggests that patients taking riluzole stay in a milder health state longer.[4] Ideally, QoL measures should be incorporated into all ALS treatment trials. However, because no ALS-specific assessment tool exists, the World Federation of Neurology does not recommend QoL in ALS trials as a primary efficacy variable in clinical trials.

The specific recommendations of the World Federation of Neurology are as follows[4a]:

1. QoL cannot be used as a primary or sole outcome measure at this time.
2. More specific and quality-related scales are needed that should be valid, reliable, sensitive to change, and relevant to the disease. Any ALS-specific measure should be used in conjunction with a recognized generic QoL measure to allow comparisons across disease states.
3. The following generic scales have been used in previous ALS clinical trials:
   Sickness Impact Profile (SIP)
   Short-Form 36 Health Survey (SF-36 Health Survey)
   The SIP has proved difficult to use, and has been reported to cause patient distress. In addition, the SIP is weighted toward functional measures and may partially replicate functional scales, such as the ALS Functional Rating Scale (ALSFRS). A variety of other generic QoL measures could be used such as the Quality of Life Questionnaire, the Nottingham Health profile, and the Quality of Well-Being Scale. These have not been validated in ALS. Generic scales are important because they have been used in many different clinical disorders, both in trials and in the evaluation of the results of clinical practice. Their sensitivity, however, varies in these different clinical contexts.
4. The SF-36 Health Survey is recommended both for screening and for pivotal ALS clinical trials. This generic instrument should be applied in conjunction with an ALS-specific measure, once this has been developed.
5. There is a risk that if questions are isolated from validated and balanced QoL measures, they may replicate data obtained from functional rating scales. This should be avoided.
6. As part of trial design, consideration should be given to the collection of direct and indirect cost data for pharmacoeconomic analysis. This is important in relation to marketing and to decisions made by third-party payers in relation to the availability of the drug once it has been licensed.
7. Consideration should be given to assessment of QoL of caregivers during the trial.
8. The frequency of administration of QoL instruments should be driven by the nature of the specific instrument. In general, current generic measures should not be administered more than four times annually, because of the lack of validated alternative forms of these tests. More frequent administration results in unreliable data because of learning and familiarity effects.
9. Consideration should be given to the use of a depression scale, for example, the Beck Depression Inventory, to recognize treatable factors in

altered QoL. Psychological factors have been shown to influence survival in ALS.[2]

10. Problems of nonlinearity: QoL measures are ordinal and should be treated accordingly in statistical analyses.

By incorporating good QoL data into research trials, we would be better able to maximize responsiveness to change, compare severity of disease states, and influence public policy and resource allocation (Figure 19.1).[1]

Health is defined by the World Health Organization as "a state of complete physical, mental, and social well being and not merely the absence of disease or infirmity."[5] As health is described in holistic terms, so too must illness be described. There is increasing consensus that the personal burden of ALS cannot be described fully by measures of disease severity such as muscle strength testing, functional rating scales, vital capacity, or survival and that psychosocial factors such as restricted mobility, dependency, financial burdens, and the inability to fulfill personal and professional roles must also be encompassed by any meaningful disease measurement, to better understand the various effects that both ALS and its treatments have on daily life and personal satisfaction (Figure 19.2).[6] There are better and worse times in life on which disease may superimpose (Figure 19.2B).[7] The same severity of paralysis in ALS may be expected to have widely varying impacts on a 35-year-old man with a young family and financial responsibilities versus a 75-year-old retired widower in an assisted living facility.

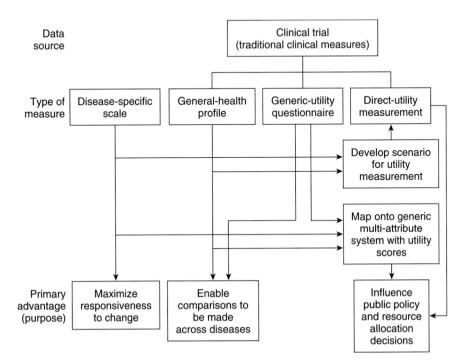

Figure 19.1 Interrelationships between health-related quality-of-life measures.[1]

Although each of us has an inherent belief regarding QoL and thinks he or she knows what constitutes it, there is no universally accepted definition. In fact, definitions of QoL are numerous and inconsistent, as are the methods of assessing it.[8] To the health economist, QoL may be defined in terms of the cost value for certain therapeutic interventions. To the psychologist, QoL is defined in terms of personality traits and past experiences. To the socialist, QoL is defined by community networks and support systems. To the physician, QoL may be defined in terms of the limitations imposed by the disease. All of these definitions are incomplete. The problem with these objective measures is that they tend to define QoL in terms of physical function and well-being, focusing on what patients can and cannot do.

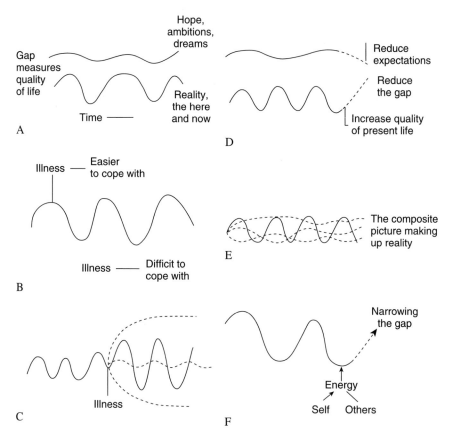

Figure 19.2 **(A)** A representation of the gap between reality and hopes, dreams and ambitions.[7] **(B)** The timing of illness can be related to the ability to cope. **(C)** The impact of illness can have several effects on the quality of life, sometimes enhancing, sometimes diminishing. **(D)** The improvement in the quality of life represents either a reduction in expectations or a change in the present mixture of reality. **(E)** Reality is made up of many components. Even if one aspect, for example, physical illness or mental illness, is limiting, it is still possible to grow in other ways. **(F)** To grow requires energy, from the individual and/or others.

ASSESSING QUALITY OF LIFE

The difficulty with measuring the effects of ALS on the psychosocial aspects of a patient's life becomes a question of what instrument to use. Various QoL instruments exist, each focusing on certain aspects of well-being and yet are inadequate (Table 19.1). QoL instruments may be grouped into two main categories: objective and subjective. The central assumption in objective measures is that a standard set of life circumstances is required for optimal functioning: QoL is an objective characteristic of the person concerned.[33] The problem with these objective measures is that they tend to define QoL in terms of physical function, focusing on what patients can or cannot do. The newer subjective measures state that QoL is perception of life circumstances, dependent on the physiological makeup of the person concerned.[33] When defined subjectively, QoL (unlike beauty) does not rest in the eye of the beholder, but of the "beholdee."[34] Measures such as the SIP[11] and the shortened version designed for patients with ALS, the SIP/ALS-19[14] are examples of objective measures. Although they assess multiple facets of QoL, they are heavily focused on physical functioning and demonstrate a progressive decline as ALS progresses, sometimes in contrast to patients' own assertions about their perceived QoL (Figure 19.3).[14,35,36] Use of the SIP/ALS was found to be associated with a lower QoL than chronic disease or static physical disability (Figure 19.4).[37]

Other measures, such as the McGill Quality of Life (MQOL) instrument, are less weighted toward physical function and include an existential domain.[38] Using the MQOL tool in an ALS population, researchers were able to

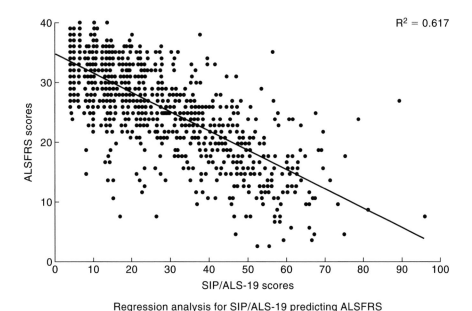

$R^2 = 0.617$

Regression analysis for SIP/ALS-19 predicting ALSFRS

Figure 19.3 Regression analysis for Sickness Impact Profile/Amyotrophic Lateral Sclerosis-19 predicting Amyotrophic Lateral Sclerosis Functional Rating Scale.[36]

Table 19.1 Health-related instruments available and used in patients with amyotrophic lateral sclerosis[a]

Assessment instrument	Key citation (in patients with ALS)	Advantages	Disadvantages	Comments
Instruments that Quantify Health Status				
Health indices: a single, global score of health and well-being				
Euroquality of life	The EuroQoL Group, 1990[9]	Visual analogue scale	—	Not ALS specific
Quality of Well-Being Scale	Kaplan, Bush, and Berry, 1976[10]	—	Requires trained interviewers	Not ALS specific
Health profiles: measurement of multiple domains of health status				
SIP	Bergner et al, 1981[11] Ganzini et al, 1998[12] Cedarbaum et al, 1999[13]	Well validated A "gold standard" for health indices	Depressing effect on patients with ALS Lengthy (136 items) No pain measures	Not ALS specific Used in the BDNF trial
SIP/ALS-19	McGuire et al, 1997[14] Simmons et al, 2000[15]	Short subset of SIP designed for ALS	—	Used in the ALS CARE database
Short-Form 36 Health Survey	Ware and Sherbourne, 1992[16] Shields et al, 1998[17]	Well validated	May lack precision to detect change in clinical setting	Not ALS specific
Short-Form 12 Health Survey	Ware, Kosinski, and Keller, 1995[17a]	—	—	Not ALS specific
ALSFRS ALSFRS-Revised	ACTS Phase I–II Study Group, 1996[18] Cedarbaum et al, 1999[13]	Well validated in patients with ALS Yields prognostic information	Some responses may reflect clinical practice and not stage of ALS (e.g., use of noninvasive intermittent ventilation)	Used in many ALS clinical trials

Instrument	Reference	Characteristics	Limitations	ALS specificity
Nottingham Health Profile	Hunt and McEwen, 1980[19]	Focuses on patient's perception of ill health	May not be sensitive to change over time	Not ALS specific
McMaster Health Index	Kaplan, Bush, and Berry, 1976[20]	—	Not in wide use	Not ALS specific
Quality-of-Life Measurement Instruments				
SEIQoL	O'Boyle, McGee, and Hickey, 1992[21]	Visual analogue scale; Individualized measures of personally important aspects of life	Requires trained interviewers; Time consuming	Not ALS specific
SEIQoL-DW	Hickey, Bury, and O'Boyle, 1996[22]	Individualized measure; Uses colored pie chart for weightings	—	Not ALS specific
McGill Quality of Life	Cohen et al, 1997[23]; Simmons et al, 2000[15]	Individualized measure of physical problems; Well validated	Only limitations on physical functioning are individualized	Not ALS specific
Quality of Life Inventory	Frisch et al, 1992[24]	Well validated	—	Not ALS specific
Patient Generated Index	—	—	—	Not ALS specific
Sendera Quality of Life Index	McMillan and Mahon, 1994[25]	Visual analogue scale; Validated in hospice studies	—	Not ALS specific

Table 19.1   (continued)

Assessment instrument	Key citation (in patients with ALS)	Advantages	Disadvantages	Comments
ALS Quality of Life Index	Gelinas, O'Connor, and Miller, 1998[26]	—	—	—
ALSAQ-40	Jenkinson et al, 1999[27]	ALS-specific scale	Mostly physical functioning	—
ALSAQ-5	Jenkinson and Fitzpatrick, 2001[28]	ALS-specific scale Validated against ALSAQ-40 Shorter version	—	—
MV Quality of Life I-25	Byock and Merriman, 1998[29]	—	—	Not ALS specific
Hospice Index	Donnelly, 2000[30]	Validated for terminal populations	—	Not ALS specific
Spitzer Quality of Life Index	McMillan, 1996[31] Spitzer et al, 1981[32]	Validated for terminal populations	—	Not ALS specific

Adapted with permission from Kasarkis E, Borasio G, Bromberg M. The Robert Wood Johnson Foundation, Promoting Excellence in End-of-Life Care, ALS Peer Workgroup, Project Report by the ALSA Association, 2002.

ALS = amyotrophic lateral sclerosis; ALSAQ = ALS Assessment Questionnaire; ALSFRS = ALS Functional Rating Scale; BDNF = brain-derived neurotrophic factor; SEIQoL = Schedule for the Evaluation of Individual Quality of Life; SEIQoL-DW = Schedule for the Evaluation of Individual Quality of Life-Direct Weighting; SIP = Sickness Impact Profile.

ªNone of these instruments have been used to study quality of life in patients with advanced amyotrophic lateral sclerosis near death.

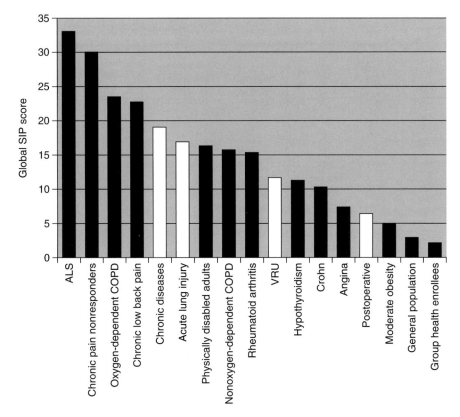

Figure 19.4 Global SIP scores for different previously described patient populations *(black bars)* and for our VRU patients *(white bars)*. ALS = amyotrophic lateral sclerosis; COPD = chronic obstructive pulmonary disease; SIP = Sickness Impact Profile; VRU = ventilator rehabilitation unit.[37]

demonstrate that QoL was maintained as physical function deteriorated and that QoL in ALS may be independent of physical function (Figure 19.5).[39] All of the present QoL instruments have significant shortcomings. The objective measures confuse QoL with functional rating scales and the subjective measurements are neither easily generalizable nor compared with other disease or control populations.

For most of us, good health is not the end to which we aspire as human beings; it is a means of achieving that end. To assign a value to QoL, we must first identify what it is that makes life worth living. QoL in ALS, as in any disease, is inherently subjective and can be assessed only by asking the patient. Outside observers cannot judge a patient's QoL and constantly underestimate the QoL of patients with disabilities. QoL can be described only in individual terms and is dependent on past experiences, present lifestyle, and future hopes. QoL changes with time and circumstances. Calman[7] proposed a working definition of QoL as the difference at a particular moment in time between the hopes and expectations of an individual and that individual's present experience (see Figure 19.2A). A good QoL is said to be present when the hopes of an individual are matched and fulfilled by experience. For one to improve QoL, the gap between aspirations and what actually occurs must narrow (see Figure 19.2D).[7] This concept of QoL helps explain the apparent paradoxes observed in life. Brickman, Coates, and Janoff-Bulman[40] observed that a group of lottery winners (up to $1 million) was not significantly happier than a control group, and that a group of people rendered paraplegic through accidents was not as unhappy as could be expected through objective observation. The fact that QoL may be improved either by improving the present reality or by decreasing the expectations (i.e., making the goals more realistic) helps explain how some patients with ALS are able to have a good QoL despite severe physical disability. In a study of seven ventilator-dependent patients with ALS who were dependent on others for all activities of daily living, who had no ability to speak

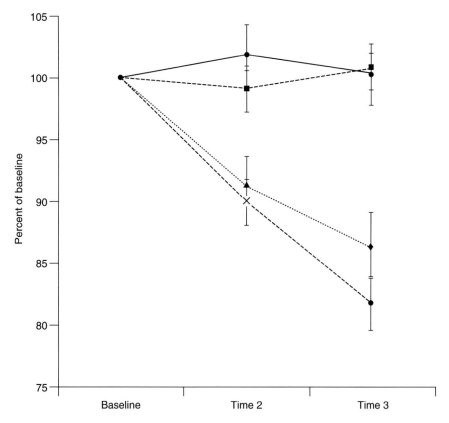

Figure 19.5   Changes over time in the mean scores of 60 patients with amyotrophic lateral sclerosis (ALS) on the McGill Quality of Life (MQOL) questionnaire (♦), the Idler Index of Religiosity (IIR) (■), the Sickness Impact Profile/ALS-19 (SIP/ALS-19) (▲), and the ALS Functional Rating Scale (×).[39]

or to eat by mouth, and who seldom left their beds, it was found that not one of those patients regretted the decision to use the ventilator and that most felt contented and satisfied most of the time.[26] As changes in health occur, life takes on a new form: It narrows, sometimes to a single room, a single bed. Values change such that what was once important may seem inconsequential, and things once ignored take on new significance.[41] In fact, disease may detract from, enhance, or have no effect on QoL (see Figure 19.2C).

QoL is dynamic and changes over time, yet individuals have personal qualities such as optimism and coping skills, which help define their "set point" (Table 19.2). These psychological variables determine the way a given

Table 19.2   Psychological factors influencing quality of life

Trait	Reference	Definition	Implication
Adaptation	Heyink, 1993[42]	Process in which past, present, and future circumstances are given cognitive and emotional meaning, such that an acceptable level of well-being is achieved	Although illness can seriously affect well-being, adaptive processes help achieve a level of well-being "belonging to the person"
Coping	Folkman, 1997[43]	Constantly changing cognitive and behavioral efforts to manage specific external and/or internal demands that exceed the resources of the patient	Problem-focused coping includes information-seeking, help-seeking, and direct action Emotion-focused coping includes humor, detachment, denial
Coping resources	Folkman, 1997[43]	Factors such as health, energy, beliefs, commitments, problem-solving skills, social skills, social support, and materials resources	These tools may enable patients to more effectively engage in both problem and emotion-focused coping
Affect versus cognition	Fischer et al, 1999[44]	Emotions/response to illness versus rational appraisal of illness	Cognitive component of QoL is believed to be less sensitive to change than the affective component
Uncertainty	Mishel[45]	Individual patient's inability to determine the meaning of illness-related events (i.e., opportunity or danger)	In illnesses where conditions progressively worsen, uncertainty helps create the illusion of hope
Self-control	Carver and Scheier, 2000[46]	General approach to self-regulating systems such that change is exerted in a system to achieve a desired outcome, for example, fever → take aspirin → return to health	An individual's "standard" for quality of life is dynamic and may change over time

Table 19.2   (continued)

Trait	Reference	Definition	Implication
Self-concept	Schain[47]	1. Physical function + body image 2. Psychosocial + sexual interaction 3. Job/role function 4. Spiritual + ethical beliefs	Changes in self-concept influence quality of life, through adaptation
Expectancy, optimism self-efficacy	Bandura[48]	The quality of being able to see a desired outcome as attainable	People who are optimistic about an outcome will continue to exert effort to achieve those outcomes, even if the process is difficult; if an outcome is truly unattainable, optimists will disengage from the pursuit and will cope with acceptance/resignation

Adapted with permission from Allison PJ, Locker D, Feine JS. Quality of life: a dynamic construct. Soc Sci Med 1997;45(2):221–230.

individual will perceive self, life circumstance, and the ability to correct factors that inhibit personal happiness. Individuals who are better able to attach meaning to events such as illness and who are better able to seek information and subsequently adapt their cognitive framework are better able to cope with disease. In addition, patients with greater energy to effect change will be more successful (see Figure 19.2F). Ultimately, some individuals are simply more prone to happiness and optimism due to unknown genetic and environmental factors. Not surprisingly, these individual psychological characteristics exert powerful influences over perceived QoL.

A QoL index that can quantify the gap between reality and expectations must allow patients to first specify those areas that have meaning in the context of their everyday lives; second, assess the extent to which reality matches expectation in each of those specified areas; and third, incorporate the patients' own value of the relative importance of these specified areas. QoL is then expressed as a composite of relevant domains (see Figure 19.2E).[50] The difference between reality and expectations reflects QoL (see Figure 19.2A).

The Schedule for the Evaluation of Individual Quality of Life (SEIQoL) is such a measure. Using the SEIQoL in patients with ALS, Bromberg and Forshew[51] found no correlation between physical functional abilities and QoL. However, should the SEIQoL, which is so insensitive to physical functioning, be used to measure the value to a patient for treatment of ALS? In trials, should we be assessing aspects of life that bear no obvious connection to ALS or its treatments, especially because managed care dictates that treatments are rationed according to medical necessity?[52] Would a potential treatment that improved the domain of family relationships have merit as a treatment for ALS? The SEIQoL, though an interesting tool, may have little utility in randomized clinical trials in ALS. Clinically, however, the SEIQoL aptly explains why individuals who come to value less physically dependent domains may have a QoL that is resistant to the ravages of ALS (see Figure 19.2E).[7]

A related, but perhaps more appropriate measure for clinical trials, is the Patient-Generated Index (PGI).[53] In the PGI, patients are asked to identify the five most important areas of life affected by their medical condition. Using this scale, one is able to quantify the effect of a medical condition on patient QoL. The PGI represents the extent to which reality falls short of expectations in those areas of life affected by disease and that are most valued by the patient. A puzzling assumption generated by the PGI is that a high perceived QoL may stem from low expectations. For example, an 80-year-old married man was recently diagnosed with ALS. His wife of 55 years is alive and well. His adult children live nearby and visit him frequently. Although he can no longer walk, he is taken out daily in his wheelchair and is always accompanied by a loved one. He has no physical pain. His brother died 1 year ago of a painful cancer. He had always suspected that he would die in a similar manner. He is satisfied with what he has accomplished in life and his reality (a slow painless death of ALS) is better than his expectation (a painful death from cancer). His QoL is good. Another apparent dilemma is that QoL may be improved (even though external circumstances may have deteriorated) through a reduction in expectations: After 2 years of ALS, a 50-year-old woman has accepted the limitations imposed by her disease. She no longer judges her life in terms of her professional productivity, her tennis game, or her figure. She now enjoys her morning routine with caregivers and daily visits with friends. She is especially looking forward to her oldest daughter's upcoming wedding. Though initially very distressed and depressed after receiving the diagnosis of ALS, 2 years later, she has adjusted and again takes a great deal of satisfaction in her life, as a result of lowering her expectations.

Individuals who have a greater capacity to adapt their expectations to the demands of ALS (i.e., the ability to set reasonable goals) have a greater capacity for life fulfillment and feel less hopeless (see Figure 19.2B).[7] Physicians may feel that some expectations are unrealistically high (denial) or unacceptably low (detachment), yet patients form these expectations by their interpretation of the world around and are subsequently contented or miserable. The perceived reality of the physician has no validity for the patient (misery is misery). QoL is benefited by both increasing quality of present "real" life or decreasing expectations of "ideal" life (see Figure 19.2D). The physician who helps the patient accept the disease (set attainable expectations) is as much a healer as the one who can improve the physical condition of the patient (improve reality). By understanding the patient's hopes and expectations, the physician may suggest management to better achieve patient goals: A 45-year-old man with a diagnosis of ALS ardently desires to see his son graduate from high school. The clinician who understands his patient's aspirations may be able to offer a course of ventilator treatment to help the patient stay healthy and achieve this goal, even though this choice may represent great financial hardship to the patient.

Emerging evidence suggests that improving QoL can also prolong life. Although ALS is a relentlessly progressively paralyzing disease with no known cause or cure and death is inevitable, the disease course and length of survival are highly variable. Natural history studies in ALS report 5-year survival rates ranging from 18 to 42 percent. In a study of 144 patients with ALS, McDonald, Wiedenfeld, and Hillel[2] demonstrated that psychological resiliency, spirituality, and psychological well-being were predictive of long-term survival. After controlling for recognized risk factors for survival such as length of illness, disease severity, and age, the patients with high psychological distress had a 6.8 greater relative risk of mortality than patients with enhanced psychological well-being and a 2.2 greater relative risk of dying in any given time period (Figure 19.6). These data suggest that improvement in psychological well-being extends survival in ALS.[2]

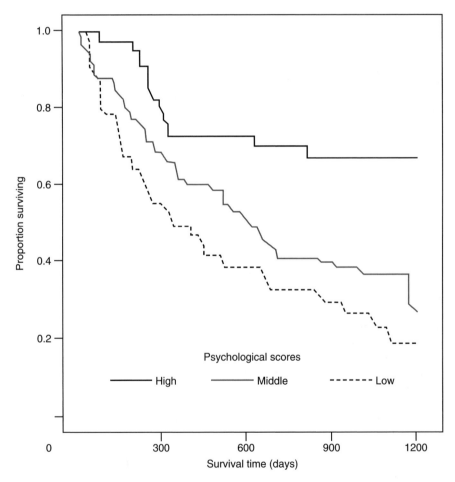

Figure 19.6   Kaplan-Meier survival curves for three levels of psychological status in patients with amyotrophic lateral sclerosis.[2]

PALLIATIVE CARE

Increasingly the importance of psychosocial support and well-being is recognized in palliative and hospice care. Too often, however, treatment strategies are neglected that might improve QoL for patients with ALS early in the course of disease. Treatments for depression, sialorrhea, dysphagia, and hypoventilation are underused.[54] The neglect of palliative measures becomes even harder to understand, given that one of the treatments of hypoventilation, noninvasive ventilatory support, not only benefits QoL[55] but also extends survival.

The World Health Organization defines palliative care as the active total care of patients whose disease is not responsive to curative treatment (when); control of psychological, social, and spiritual problems is paramount.[5] Because ALS today is not a disease that is amenable to cure, palliative care should be incorporated in the patient care plan from the time of diagnosis through and including hospice care. This philosophy enables the active total care of the patient. Attention to the psychosocial and existential aspects of a patient's life is too often lacking, even in our multidisciplinary ALS centers. Few ALS care teams incorporate a chaplain and a psychologist, along with a physical and occupational therapist. Yet emotional needs are as great as the need for wheelchairs. Using various assessment tools, Rabkin, Wagner, and Del Bene[56] the incidence of depression in ALS has been reported to range as high as 44 to 75 percent.

Though not related to symptom severity per se, depression and low self-esteem were related to the impact of motor neuron disease on everyday function.[57] In a recent study of 56 patients with ALS at the Eleanor and Lou Gehrig Clinic in New York, 28 percent of patients had significant depressive symptoms.[8] In addition, depression was positively correlated with other psychological and physical manifestations of distress and was inversely correlated with life satisfaction. Moreover, depressed patients with ALS were more apt to refuse noninvasive ventilatory support. Thus depression interfered with the process of informed decision making. Patients with ALS with a low QoL and hopelessness are also more apt to consider suicide.[12,58] In the Netherlands where physician-assisted suicide is not criminally prosecuted, one in five patients with ALS die this way. Studies show that the choice of euthanasia was not associated with any aspect of disease, patient care, income, or education level but was associated with a greater overall disability and a lack of religious conviction.[59] Depression in ALS, unlike paralysis, is amenable to treatment with a variety of drugs and therapy.

In a study of patients with ALS and their families at the Tufts neuromuscular clinic, the following psychosocial observations were noted:

1. Patients were frustrated over inability to obtain information from the medical community.
2. There was scant provision for continuing medical care.
3. There was minimal involvement by physicians in palliative care.
4. Families who coped well were better able to seek existing support services.
5. The cost of home health care consumed a substantial amount of the life savings of a middle-class family.

6. Feelings of vulnerability and loneliness led to fears of being left alone even for short periods.
7. The impact of ALS was even more profound in families with previously active lifestyles.
8. Difficulties with communication led to increasing patient isolation and decreasing sense of mastery over the environment.

A change in medical practice was advocated to incorporate a greater sharing of information to enhance patients' cognitive mastery and coping skills, as well as providing emotional support to include the upholding of constructive denial systems and validating the range of patient emotions and above all fostering a sense of hope. Without hope, people lose the motivation to live. Without hope, patients are incapable of making life-sustaining choices.

CAREGIVERS

The caregiver is an often overlooked but indispensable member of the care team. Four general themes were common among caregivers:

1. Powerlessness over ALS
2. Guilt over not doing enough for their loved one
3. Resentment over unappreciated and unrecognized efforts in care giving
4. Absence of time to pursue personal interests[6]

Distress in caregivers was not associated so much with increased patient disability but was associated with loss of intimacy with the loved one.[60] Distress levels were highly correlated between patients and caregivers[8] and patients worried about the well-being of their caregivers. Although caregivers felt fulfilled by the care they ministered to patients, they were exhausted. Caregivers also frequently neglected their own health problems.[26] ALS CARE teams must routinely evaluate the well-being of the caregiver and the patient, to ensure maximal QoL for the patient.

SEXUALITY

Perhaps more than any other dimension, the importance of sexuality in ALS remains unelucidated. In a recent U.S. poll of 500 people older than 25 years, 94 percent felt a satisfying sex life was an important component of QoL, 71 percent said they felt their doctors would dismiss any concerns raised about sexual problems, and 68 percent felt that discussing sexuality would embarrass their physicians, but 85 percent indicated that they would discuss sexual problems with their physicians even though they might not receive any help.[61] Patients with ALS, who may be suffering from depression and anxiety, may find they have a loss of libido. In addition, those with diminished respiratory function would be expected to have less energy available for sexual relations. Patients should be instructed in less strenuous (e.g., side-lying) positions and the importance of planning sexual encounters when they are rested. Many of the drugs used in the treatment of ALS symptoms, in particular anticholinergics (for sialorrhea) and antidepressants (especially selective serotonin reuptake inhibitors [SSRIs]) cause impotence. Too few ALS physicians are aware of the fact that bupropion has a much reduced incidence of sexual dysfunction compared with SSRIs (15% compared with 63% of men, and 7% compared with 41% of women). Although very effective, sildenafil is underutilized in combating reduced libido and erectile problems.[62] As with any other medical history taking, the doctor must put the patient at ease, understand the patient's background and history, discover the true nature of the sexual complaint, and work out a plan of management.[63] To do this, physicians must be comfortable with their own sexuality and see sexuality as an important area for medical intervention.[64] An excellent reference is a book by Sipski and Alexander, *Sexual Function in People with Disability and Chronic Illness: A Health Professionals Guide.*

SPIRITUALITY

Hospice considers the religious or spiritual dimension of a patient as independent and not subsumed within social or psychological domains. Historically, hospice care was developed as an adjunct to religious care. Today, the understanding of spirituality has evolved and is no longer seen solely in the traditional framework as a relationship with God or a Greater Power, but in the personal and psychological search for meaning in one's life.[65]

The value of spirituality and the sustaining value of religious conviction benefit the patient in two ways: providing a set of core beliefs about life events and the establishment of an ethical foundation for clinical decision making.[65] In both Oregon and the Netherlands, patients with ALS with strong religious beliefs were less likely to consider assisted suicide.[12,58] Religious belief provides a constant source of strength that helps buffer the changes of ALS. Certain ALS clinicians may not feel comfortable engaging the patient in a personal dialogue about religion and spirituality, but this dialogue must occur. Other team members (e.g., a chaplain) may be better able to explore these beliefs with patients, to help create a supportive framework. Religious congregations may provide assistance in a variety of ways from volunteer hours to financial assistance to eventual acceptance of disability and death.

CONCLUSION

Who is responsible for assessing the psychosocial and spiritual needs of patients with ALS patients: the physicians, nurses, social workers, psychologists, and chaplains? Yes, and the speech, physical, and occupational therapists as well. What happens to patients who are not fully supported? When patients perceive a large discrepancy between reality and expectations and see no way of improving their reality and are incapable or unwilling to lower their expectations, life may become too burdensome. At this point, QoL may be in direct conflict with sanctity of life. Advocates of medically assisted suicide may see this as an acceptable justification for voluntary inducement of death. For those clinicians opposed to the premature inducement of death, the only recourse is to forge a care plan in which better choices for living in comfort and dignity may be offered to patients with ALS until the natural cessation of their lives.[66] The care of a patient with ALS must encompass psychological, social, and spiritual concerns along with the physical needs. Although a cure for ALS is not yet attainable, excellent care is clearly within our grasp.

REFERENCES

1. Drummond M. Introducing economic and quality of life measurements into clinical studies. Ann Med 2001;33:344–349.
2. McDonald ER, Wiedenfeld SA, Hillel A, et al. Survival in amyotrophic lateral sclerosis. The role of psychological factors. Arch Neurol Jan 1994;51:17–23.
3. Miller R, Mitchell J, Moore D. Riluzole for Amyotrophic Lateral Sclerosis/Motor Neuron Disease (Cochrane Review). Oxford: Cochrane Library, 2000.
4. Riviere M, Meininger V, Zeisser P, Munsat T. An analysis of extended survival in patients with amyotrophic lateral sclerosis treated with riluzole. Arch Neurol 1998;55:526–528.
4a. Miller RG, Munsat TL, Swash M, Brooks BR. Consensus guidelines for the design and implementation of clinical trials in ALS. J Neurol Sci 1999;169:2–12.
5. World Health Organization. Constitution of the World Health Organization: Chronicle of the World Health Organization I. Geneva: World Health Organization, 1947.
6. Sebring DL, Moglia P. Amyotrophic lateral sclerosis: psychosocial interventions for patients and their families. Health Social Work 1987;113–120.
7. Calman KC. Quality of life in cancer patients—an hypotheses. J Med Ethics 1984;10:124–127.
8. Muldoon MF, Barger SD, Flory JD, Manujck SB. What are quality of life measurements measuring? Br Med J 1998;316:542–545.
9. EuroQoL—a new facility for the measurement of health-related quality of life. The EuroQoL Group. Health Policy 1990;16:199–208.
10. Kaplan RM, Bush JW, Berry CC. Health status: types of validity and the index of well-being. Health Serv Res 1976;11:478–507.
11. Bergner M, Bobbit RA, Carter WB, Gibson BS. The Sickness Impact Profile: development and final revision of a health status measure. Med Care 1981;19:787–804.
12. Ganzini L, Johnston WS, McFarland BH, et al. Attitudes of patients with amyotrophic lateral sclerosis and their care givers toward assisted suicide. N Engl J Med 1998;339:967–973.
13. Cedarbaum JM, Stambler N, Malta E, et al. The ALSFRS-R: a revised ALS function of rating scale that incorporates assessments of respiratory function. BONF ALS Study Group (Phase III). J Neurol Sci 1999;169:13–21.
14. McGuire D, Garrison L, Armon C, et al. A brief quality of life measure for ALS clinical trials based on a subset of items from the Sickness Impact Profile. J Neurol Sci 1997;152:S18–S22.
15. Simmons Z, Bremmer BA, Robbins RA, et al. Quality of life in ALS depends on factors other than strength and physical function. Neurology 2000;55:388–392.
16. Ware JE, Jr., Sherbourne CD. The MOS 36-item short-form health survey (SF-36). I. Conceptual framework and item selection. Med Care 1992;30:473–483.
17. Shields RK, Ruhland JL, Ross MA, et al. Analysis of health-related quality of life and muscle impairments in individuals without amyotrophic lateral sclerosis using the medical outcome survey and the Tufts Quantitative Neuromuscular Exam. Arch Phys Med Rehabil 1998;79:855–862.
17a. Ware JE, Kosinski M, Keller SD. SF-12: How to score the SF-12 physical and mental status health summary scales (2nd ed). Boston: The Health Institute, New England Medical Center, 1995.
18. The Amyotrophic Lateral Sclerosis Functional Rating Scale. Assessment of activities of daily living in patients with amyotrophic lateral sclerosis. The ALS CNTF treatment study (ACTS) phase I–II Study Group. Arch Neurol 1996;53:141–147.

19. Hunt SM, McEwen J. The development of a subjective health indicator. Sociol Health Illn 1980;2: 231–246.
20. Kaplan RM, Bush JW, Berry CC. Health Status: types of validity and the index of well-being. Health Serv Res 1976;11:478–507.
21. O'Boyle CA, McGee H, Hickey A. Individual quality of life in patients undergoing hip replacement. Cancer 1992;339:1088–1091.
22. Hickey AM, Bury G, O'Boyle CA. A new short form individual quality of life measure (SEIQoL-DW): application in a cohort of individuals with HIV/AIDS. BMJ 1996;313:29–33.
23. Cohen SR, Hassan SA, Lapointe BJ, Mount BH. Quality of life in HIV disease as measured by the McGill quality of life measure questionnaire. AIDS 1996;10:1421–1427.
24. Frisch MB, Cornell J, Villanueva M, Retzlaff PJ. Clinical validation of the quality of life inventory: a measure of life satisfaction for use in treatment planning and outcome assessment. Psychol Assess 1992;4:92–101.
25. McMillan SC, Mahon M. A study of quality of life of hospice patients on admission and at week 3. Cancer Nurs 1994;17:52–60.
26. Gelinas DF, O'Connor P, Miller RG. Quality of life for ventilator-dependent patients with ALS and their caregivers. J Neurol Sci 1998;160:S134–S136.
27. Jenkinson C, Fitzpatrick R, Brennan C, et al. Development and validation of a short measure of health status for individuals with amyotrophic lateral sclerosis/motor neurone disease: the ALSAQ-40. J Neurol 1999;246(suppl 3):III16–21.
28. Jenkinson C, Fitzpatrick R. Reduced item set for the amyotrophic lateral sclerosis assessement questionnaire: development and validation of the ALSAQ-5. J Neurol Neurosurg Psychiatry 2001; 70:70–73.
29. Byock IR, Merriman MP. Measuring quality of life for patients with terminal illness: the Missoula-VITAS quality of life index. Palliat Med 1998;12:231–244.
30. Donnelly S. Quality-of-life assessment in advanced cancer. Curr Oncol Rep 2000;2:338–342.
31. McMillan SC. Quality-of-life assessment in palliative care. Cancer Control 1996;3:223–229.
32. Spitzer WO, Dobson AJ, Hall J, et al. Measuring the quality of life of cancer patients: a concise QL-index for use by physicians. J Chronic Dis 1981;34:585–597.
33. Browne JP, McGee HM, O'Boyle CA. Conceptual approaches to the assessment of quality of life. Psychol Health 1997;12:737–751.
34. Gill TM, Feinstein AR. A critical appraisal of the quality of quality-of-life measurements. JAMA 1994;272:619–626.
35. McGuire D, Garrison L, Armon C, et al. Relationship of the Tufts Quantitative Neuromuscular Exam (TQNE) and the Sickness Impact Profile (SIP) in measuring progression of ALS. Neurology 1996;46:1442–1444.
36. Bromberg M, Anderson F, Davidson M, Miller RG. Assessing health status quality of life in ALS: comparison of the SIP/ALS-19 with the ALS Functional Rating Scale and the Short-Form-12 Health Survey. Amyotroph Lateral Scler Other Motor Neuron Disord 2001;••:31–37.
37. Chatila W, Kreimer DT, Criner GJ. Quality of life in survivors of prolonged mechanical ventilatory support. Crit Care Med 2001;29:737–742.
38. Cohen SF, Mount BM, Strobel MG, et al. The McGill Quality of Life Questionnaire: a measure of quality of life appropriate for people with advanced disease. A preliminary study of validity and acceptability. Palliat Med 1995;9:207–219.
39. Robbins RA, Simmons Z, Bremer BA, et al. Quality of life in ALS is maintained as physical function declines. Neurology 2001;56:442–444.
40. Brickman P, Coates D, Janoff-Bulman R. Lottery winners and accident victims: is happiness relative? J Person Soc Psychol 1978;36:917–927.
41. Farquhar M. Definitions of quality of life: a taxonomy. J Adv Nurs 1995;22:502–508.
42. Heyink J. Adaptation and well-being. Psychol Rep 1993;73(3 Pt. 2):1331–1342.
43. Folkman S. Positive psychological states and coping with severe stress. Soc Sci Med 1997;45: 1207–1221.
44. Fischer JS, La Rocca NG, Miller DM, et al. Recent developments in the assessment of quality of life in multiple sclerosis (MS). Mult Scler 1999;5:251–259.
45. Mishel MH. Uncertainty in illness. J Nurs Scholarsh 1988;20:225–232.
46. Carver CS, Scheier MF. Scaling back goals and recalibration of the affect system are processes in normal adaptive self-regulation: understanding "response shift" phenomenas. Soc Sci Med 2000;50:1715–1722.
47. Schain W. Sexual functioning, self esteem and cancer care. Front Radiation Therapy Oncology 1980;14:29.

48. Bandura A. Self-efficacy mechanism in human agency. Am Psychol 1982;37:47.
49. Allison PJ, Locker D, Feine JS. Quality of life: a dynamic construct. Soc Sci Med 1997;45:221–230.
50. Browne JP, O'Boyle CA, McGee HM, et al. Development of a direct weighting procedure for quality of life domains. Qual Life Res 1997;6:301–309.
51. Bromberg MB, Forshew DA. Comparison of instruments addressing quality of life in patients with ALS and their caregivers. Neurology 2002;58:320–322.
52. Gladis MM, Gosch EA, Dishuk NM, Crits-Christoph P. Quality of life: expanding the scope of clinical significance. J Consult Clin Psychol 1999;67:320–331.
53. Ruta DA, Garratt AM, Mhoira L, et al. A new approach to the measurement of quality of life: the Patient-Generated Index. Med Care 1994;32:1109–1126.
54. Bradley WG, Anderson F, Bromberg M, et al. Current management of ALS: comparison of the ALS CARE database and the AAN Practice Parameter. Neurology 2001;47:500–504.
55. Lyall RA, Donaldson N, Fleming T, et al. A prospective study of quality of life in ALS patients treated with noninvasive ventilation. Neurology 2001;57:153–156.
56. Rabkin JG, Wagner GJ, Del Bene M. Resilience and distress among amyotrophic lateral sclerosis patients and caregivers. Psychol Med 2000;62:271–279.
57. Hogg KE, Goldstein L, Leigh P. The psychological impact of MND. Psychol Med 1994;24:625–632.
58. Ganzini L, Block S. Physician-assisted death—a last resort? N Engl J Med 2002;346:1663–1665.
59. Veldink JH, Wokke JHJ, Van der Wal G, et al. Euthanasia and physician-assisted suicide among patients with amyotrophic lateral sclerosis in the Netherlands. N Engl J Med 2002;346:1638–1644.
60. Goldstein LH, Adamson M, Jeffrey L, et al. The psychological impact of MND on patients and carers. J Neurol Sci 1998;160:S114–S121.
61. Marwick C. Survey says patients expect little physician help on sex. JAMA 1999;281:2173–2174.
62. Seftel A. Sexual function and dysfunction. J Urol 2001;165:707–719.
63. Tomlinson J. ABC of sexual health: taking a sexual history. Br Med J 1998;317:1573–1576.
64. Duldt BW, Pokomy ME. Teaching communication about human sexuality to nurses and other healthcare providers. Nurse Educ 1999;24:27–32.
65. Daaleman TP, VandeCreek L. Placing religion and spirituality in end-of-life care. JAMA 2000;284:2514–2517.
66. Dickens BM. The continuing conflict between sanctity of life and quality of life: from abortion to medically assisted death. Ann N Y Acad Sci 1998;88–104.

20
Symptom Control in Amyotrophic Lateral Sclerosis/Motor Neuron Disease

Johanna Anneser and Gian Domenico Borasio

Amyotrophic lateral sclerosis (ALS) is a relentlessly progressive, incurable disease. Despite our increasing knowledge about genetics, molecular mechanisms, and possible sites of pharmacological interventions of the disease, the many efforts to find a disease-modifying treatment (see Chapter 21) have been mostly disappointing. To date, only a moderate slowing of disease progression can be achieved.

Even if more effective neuroprotective treatments are developed, symptom control will remain the most important task in the care of patients with ALS. To date, standards of palliative treatment in ALS are still largely based on expert opinion and differ between countries.[1] First attempts at establishing evidence-based guidelines have been made, but still more research is needed to optimize symptom control in patients with ALS.[2] However, there is a general consensus that management of the different symptoms occurring during the course of the disease can be accomplished only by a multidisciplinary team (Table 20.1).[3]

DYSPHAGIA

Dysphagia is a common problem in ALS. Because eating and drinking is not only a basic physiological function but also has a great social impact, dysphagia is a very distressing symptom for most patients. The prevalence of swallowing disturbances is generally high but varies depending on the site of onset and stage of the disease. O'Brien, Kelly, and Saunders[4] reported that only 21 percent of patients with ALS in a hospice were able to swallow all foods. Similarly, 90 percent of patients from another hospice described swallowing difficulties.[5] Leighton et al[6] found that 89 percent of patients with bulbar-onset ALS were unable to maintain oral nutrition, compared with only 45 percent of patients with limb-onset ALS.

485

Table 20.1   Palliative care in amyotrophic lateral sclerosis: who is involved?

Chaplain	Physical therapist
Counselor	Physician
Dietitian	Psychologist
Hospice worker	Relatives
Lay associations	Social worker
Nurse	Speech therapist
Occupational therapist	Swallowing therapist

Both upper and lower motor neuron involvement may impair normal swallowing, which occurs in three phases: The *oral phase* comprises mastication and effective transportation of the bolus to the pharynx. In the *pharyngeal phase,* the bolus arrives in the oropharynx and triggers the swallowing reflex. During the *esophageal phase,* the bolus is propelled into the stomach. Weakened tongue and lip function may cause dysphagia and laryngeal dysfunction with the risk of aspiration. Patients complain of fatigue induced by mastication, of difficulties in initiating swallowing, and of choking on food, mainly crumbly food and liquids.

Dysphagia should first be treated by an adjustment in diet consistency (recipe books for patients with ALS are available from patients' associations such as the Muscular Dystrophy Association or the ALS Association in the United States, the Motor Neuron Disease Association in the United Kingdom, and the Deutsche Gesellschaft für Muskelkranke in Germany). Swallowing techniques such as supraglottic swallowing can be taught by specialized speech therapists or physiotherapists and can reduce the risk of aspiration. Moreover, postural changes can improve dysphagic symptoms.[7] As dysphagia becomes more severe and the patient continues to lose weight (>10% of normal body weight before diagnosis) and frequent choking occurs, a percutaneous endoscopic gastrostomy (PEG) should be discussed.

It is generally recommended to make an early decision (before forced vital capacity [FVC] falls below 50% of predicted level) regarding PEG placement, because the procedure has been found to be safer at an earlier stage in the disease.[2,8] A more recent uncontrolled retrospective study, however, reported that FVC did not correlate with postgastrostomy survival.[9] Alternatively, when PEG placement is considered difficult, a radiologically inserted gastrostomy (RIG) may be discussed.[10] The immediate benefit of PEG placement is the maintenance of sufficient food and fluid intake, although PEG does not prevent aspiration.[11]

Even though an early PEG placement may result in an increased life span, this has not been demonstrated convincingly,[12] because patients favoring PEG placement are generally more proactive in the face of the disease.[13] However, as with all other palliative measures, the primary goal is improvement of the quality of life (QoL), rather than prolonging life.

CHRONIC HYPOVENTILATION AND DYSPNEA

Chronic Hypoventilation

Early features of respiratory insufficiency are multifarious (Table 20.2) and can be missed or misdiagnosed. Chronic hypoventilation occurs primarily during sleep and can severely hamper the patients' QoL. It is of paramount importance that respiratory dysfunction is recognized and discussed with patients and their families at an appropriate time.

There is no consensus about which investigation should be used as a reliable indicator for respiratory function in patients with ALS. FVC is often used to detect respiratory dysfunction but correlates poorly with respiratory symptoms.[14] Although recently developed tests like cervical magnetic phrenic nerve stimulation or transdiaphragmatic sniff pressure may be more accurate in assessing ventilatory disturbances,[15] transcutaneous nocturnal oximetry is still the gold standard to diagnose chronic nocturnal hypoventilation.

Noninvasive intermittent ventilation (NIV) via mask is an efficient and cost-effective means of alleviating symptoms of chronic nocturnal hypoventilation: The quality of sleep improves, morning headache is relieved, and even cognitive function may improve.[16,17] To be effective, NIV must be administered for at least 4 hours per day, preferably at night.[18]

Some patients are unable to tolerate NIV. Aboussouan et al[19] reported that about two thirds of patients who did not tolerate this treatment had moderate to severe bulbar involvement. The practicalities and types of NIV have been recently reviewed.[20] The patients and their families should be informed about the temporary nature of the measure, which is primarily directed toward improving QoL rather than prolonging it (as opposed to tracheostomy). The problem with mechanical ventilation is usually not related to cost or technical difficulties, but to the increasing care needs of the ventilated patients. Considerable cross-cultural differences in the use of NIV have been reported.[21] A slow progression, good communication skills, mild bulbar involvement, and above all a motivated patient and a supportive family environment argue in favor of the initiation of NIV.[22]

Table 20.2   Symptoms of chronic respiratory insufficiency

Daytime fatigue and sleepiness, concentration problems
Difficulty falling asleep, disturbed sleep, nightmares
Morning headache
Nervousness, tremor, increased sweating, tachycardia
Depression, anxiety
Tachypnea, dyspnea, phonation difficulties
Visible efforts of accessory respiratory muscles
Reduced appetite, weight loss, recurrent gastritis
Recurrent or chronic upper respiratory tract infections
Cyanosis, edema
Vision disturbances, dizziness, syncope
Diffuse pain in head, neck, and extremities

It is very important to reassure the patients that whenever they decide to stop NIV, all necessary care and appropriate medication will be available to ensure a peaceful death. The physician has a legal and ethical duty to honor a patient's request for discontinuation of mechanical (invasive or noninvasive) ventilation.[23] It is useful that the patient's wishes and ethical and religious attitudes are known and decisions can be made according to the patient's advance directives.[24] Importantly, in a small number of patients, respiratory failure with the need for continuous mechanical ventilation will occur without gross disability of the limbs. In these patients, mechanical ventilation via tracheostomy may ensure a relatively high QoL for several years.

Dyspnea

Dyspnea is a most distressing symptom in ALS. At the beginning of dyspnea, chest physiotherapy is helpful. Dyspneic attacks usually have a pronounced anxiety component and are best managed by anxiolytics (lorazepam 0.5–1.0 mg sublingually) (Table 20.3). Fears of death by choking arise in almost all patients at the onset of dyspneic symptoms and should be met by a frank discussion of the terminal stage of the illness. The latter is characterized by a mostly nocturnal, hypercapnia-induced light coma, that is, most patients die peacefully in their sleep.[25]

In patients not receiving mechanical ventilation, the feeling of shortness of breath can be reduced by the administration of morphine (2.5–5.0 mg orally or 1–2 mg intravenously or subcutaneously every 4 hours). Titration of the morphine dose against the clinical effect will almost never lead to a life-threatening respiratory depression.

OROPHARYNGEAL SECRETIONS

Thick Mucous Secretions

Decreased ability to clear the upper airways because of bulbar weakness and reduced coughing pressure may result in unpleasant thick mucous secretions. Diminished fluid intake may worsen this symptom. Humidifying the atmosphere and improvement of fluid intake may be helpful. *N*-acetylcysteine can be tried but is effective only in a small minority of patients, because it requires a large fluid intake and basically dilutes the secretions, resulting in a higher secretion volume, which does not necessarily ameliorate the problem if the coughing effort is insufficient. In the initial stages, manually assisted coughing techniques may relieve symptoms.

Mechanical insufflation-exsufflation devices have been demonstrated to be helpful in extracting excess mucus from the airways.[26] Similarly, intermittent positive vibration devices are specialized inhalators that deliver a pressurized, intermittent flow of nebulized saline with or without expectorants. They are used for 10 to 15 minutes at a time and can assist in clearing pulmonary and bronchial secretions.[27] However, a satisfactory therapy for

Table 20.3 Symptomatic medication in amyotrophic lateral sclerosis (in order of recommendation)

Symptom/treatment	Dosage[a]
Muscle cramps	
If mild:	
Magnesium	5 mmol qd to tid
Vitamin E	400 IE bid
If severe:	
Quinine sulfate	200 mg bid
Carbamazepine	200 mg bid
Phenytoin	100 mg qd to tid
Spasticity	
Baclofen	10–80 mg
Tizanidine	6–24 mg
Memantine	10–60 mg
Tetrazepam	100–200 mg
Drooling	
Glycopyrrolate	0.1–0.2 mg sc/im tid
Transdermal hyoscine patches	One to two patches
Amitriptyline	10–150 mg
Atropine/benztropine	0.25–0.75/1.0–2.0 mg
Clonidine	0.15–0.3 mg
Pathologic laughing/crying	
Amitriptyline	10–150 mg
Fluvoxamine	100–200 mg
Lithium carbonate	400–800 mg
L-Dopa	500–600 mg
Sedatives	Dosage nocté
Chloral hydrate	250–1000 mg
Diphenhydramine	50–100 mg
Flurazepam (beware of respiratory tract infection)	15–30 mg

bid = twice a day; im = intramuscularly; qd = every day; sc = subcutaneously; tid = three times a day.
[a]Usual range of adult daily dosage; some patients may require higher dosages, for example, of antispastic medication.

thick mucous secretion is still not available and more research is needed in this area.

Mouth Dryness

Mouth dryness is mainly reported from patients with incomplete mouth closure and is most unpleasant during the night. Oxygen administration, which is usually not warranted in ALS, may worsen this symptom significantly. Sips of water or juice, small chunks of ice placed under the tongue, or artificial saliva sprays may relieve this symptom.

Drooling

Anticholinergic drugs can be used, but their effect is often limited by side effects (e.g., constipation and mouth dryness during the night). The most widely used drugs are glycopyrrolate,[28,29] atropine, and amitriptyline (see Table 20.3), although no controlled trials are available for the latter. However, amitriptyline may be useful in cases with accompanying depression. Beta blockers might represent an alternative in severe cases,[30] and hyoscine transdermal patches may be useful in the presence of severe dysphagia. For therapy-refractory cases, salivary gland irradiation[31,32] or topical botulinum toxin (BTX) injections may be considered,[33] although recurrent jaw dislocation following BTX injection has been described in a patient with ALS.[34]

DYSARTHRIA

Progressive dysarthria and eventually a complete loss of the ability to speak results in a reduction in the ability to communicate with other people, to express feelings, wishes, grief, and joy, and to convey the individual's personality and finally a loss of environmental control. Replacement of all these function of speech should be as good as possible. When selecting an appropriate aid for the dysarthric patient, nonverbal communication skills, residual hand mobility, portability, and acceptance of a specific device considered. Pen and paper or more conveniently a magnetic writing board can be sufficient for patients with good hand function. Alphabet boards or picture boards may be useful for patients with upper limb pareses or decreased intellectual capability. For most dysarthric patients, electronic communication devices, preferably with voice output, should be considered, because these devices allow communication via telephone and in groups. It is recommended to test several electronic communication devices before the most suitable one is selected.

MUSCLE WEAKNESS

Progressive muscle weakness is the main symptom in ALS. There is no treatment to improve muscle strength other than temporarily. The most effective way of helping patients is through the *timely* discussion and provision of adequate aids. Walking sticks, foot orthoses, crutches, and walking frames may be helpful in earlier stages, although a wheelchair may be necessary in the later stages. The type of wheelchair should be selected carefully with respect to the individual needs of the patient.[35] A (removable) headrest will be required for almost every patient when disease progresses. For patients with loss of function of the upper extremities, knives, forks, and spoons with a special grip, wrist orthoses, and a pen holder may be helpful

Lack of head control is especially distressing in mobile patients. Soft collars and rigid head supports are available. Because of the risk of additional muscular atrophy resulting from inactivity, head supports should be worn intermittently.

Physiotherapy is of paramount importance in the treatment of muscle weakness. The main purpose of physiotherapy in ALS is to reduce the problems resulting from muscle weakness and to optimize the patient's comfort and mobility.[36] Drory et al[37] demonstrated that regular moderate physical exercise has a temporary positive effect on disability in patients with ALS.

Pharmacologically, acetylcholinesterase inhibitors may have a short-term positive effect on overall muscle strength, especially in patients with bulbar-onset ALS. Because the effect usually lasts only for days to a few weeks, the use of pyridostigmine (up to 40 mg three times per day) can be recommended only for special situations, like a holiday trip. There is no rationale for long-term therapy with pyridostigmine in ALS, and more often than not, patients will have to be taken off this medication to avoid unnecessary side effects.

Creatine monohydrate, which is used by athletes to increase muscle strength, has shown interesting neuroprotective effects in the transgenic copper/zinc superoxide dismutase (SOD1) mouse model.[38] To date, few data are available concerning increases in muscle strength or survival in patients with ALS, although a temporary increase in isometric power has been described.[39]

CRAMPS, SPASTICITY

Painful muscle cramps in ALS may be noticed before the onset of weakness. Cramps may be present at any stage of the disease but very often decrease when the disease progresses. They may appear in unusual locations, such as the abdominal, paraspinal, and finger muscles, and may affect sleep while occurring during unconscious stretching. For mild cramps, magnesium and vitamin E can be helpful, although quinine sulfate is the drug of choice in severe cases (see Table 20.3). Creatine monohydrate may worsen muscle cramps.

Increased muscle tone, exaggerated tendon reflexes, clonus, and muscle spasms are referred to as *spasticity,* which occurs because of involvement of the upper motor neuron.

Baclofen and tizanidine (see Table 20.3) are the drugs of choice. The medication should be given in gradual increments over several days. Generally, with antispasticity drugs, the patient has to titrate the dosage against the subjective clinical effect, because a moderate degree of spasticity is usually better for mobility than a fully flaccid paresis.

When patients fail to respond to oral medication, it may be necessary to deliver baclofen intrathecally via an implanted pump.[40] BTX is effective when injected into selected muscles. However, these more invasive therapies are rarely necessary to treat spasticity in patients with ALS.

Dantrolene, which acts directly on the muscle, has limited applications because it enhances weakness. However, extreme spasticity in the terminal phase, which could be relieved only by high doses of intravenously administered dantrolene, has been reported.[41]

PAIN

Although ALS does not primarily affect sensory nerves other than subclinically, pain is reported by a large proportion of patients with ALS. About 50 to 57 percent of patients with ALS on admission to a hospice were felt to have severe pain.[4] In another ALS population, 19 percent rated their pain as four or greater on a six-point scale.[42]

A careful assessment and medical examination is necessary to diagnose and treat possible causes of pain in ALS including muscle cramps and spasticity, musculoskeletal pain due to atrophy and muscular imbalance, skin pressure pain due to immobility, and possibly other non–ALS-related diseases. Whenever possible, causal treatment should be attempted (e.g., treatment of spasticity with spasmolytics and careful positioning in patients with skin pressure pain). As the disease progresses, regular administration of analgesics may be required. The World Health Organization analgesic ladder (beginning with nonopioid analgesics such as paracetamol, followed by weak opioids such as tramadol or codeine, followed by strong opioids such as morphine can be used as a guideline.[43]

PATHOLOGICAL LAUGHING/CRYING

This symptom is also referred as "pseudobulbar affect" and occurs in up to 50 percent of patients with ALS. It results in the development of uncontrollable bouts of laughter and/or tearfulness when discussing emotive topics or watching touching movies. Because pseudobulbar affect is seldom volunteered by the patients, physicians should carefully ask about this symptom, which can be very disturbing for the patients in social situations.

Physicians should point out that pseudobulbar affect is part of the disease and responds well to medication (see Table 20.3). The point must be made very clearly to the patient and family that this symptom does not imply that the patient has some kind of psychiatric disturbance. The drug of first choice is amitriptyline,[44] but positive effects have also been reported for fluvoxamine,[45] dopamine,[46] and lithium.[47] Because all these medications may also produce side effects, careful discussion with patients is essential so that they are aware of the balance between treatment and side effects.

PSYCHOLOGICAL SYMPTOMS

Anger, fear, hopelessness, and sadness are normal reactions after being told the diagnosis and/or realizing the loss of physical capabilities. However, clinically significant depression requiring medication may also develop. The reported prevalence of depression in ALS varies depending on the assessment method: Self-reported depressive symptoms have been described in 44 to 75 percent of patients,[48] whereas only 11 percent had clinical depression according to the criteria defined in the *Diagnostic and Statistical Manual of Mental Disorders,* fourth edition.[42] It has been demonstrated that depressive symptoms were not related to time from diagnosis, degree of disability, or illness progression.[49] Hence, depressive symptoms should be carefully sought and treated at all stages of the disease. The most widely used drug is amitriptyline (start with 25 mg per day and slowly increase to 100–150 mg per day as tolerated), which may also exert favorable effects on other symptoms such as drooling, pseudobulbar affect, and sleep disturbance. It is important to realize that concordance of depression and distress levels between patients and caregivers is high.[49] Therefore, attention to the caregivers' needs and mental heath is an essential component of symptomatic treatment and may alleviate the patient's distress as well.

LESS COMMON SYMPTOMS

Gastroesophageal reflux disease may occur in ALS as a result of diaphragmatic weakness involving the lower esophageal sphincter. Overfeeding in patients with a PEG may lead to gastroesophageal reflux and even aspiration. Treatment includes prokinetic agents (e.g., metoclopramide) and antacids.

Dependent edema of the hands and feet occurs in weak limbs because of reduced muscle pump activity. Limb elevation, positioning within the wheelchair, physiotherapy, and compression stockings are helpful. If pain develops or swelling persists despite prolonged elevation, a deep venous thrombosis should be ruled out.[50]

Urinary urgency and frequency in the absence of urinary tract infections can be due to spasticity of the bladder and usually responds favorably to oxybutynin (2.5–5.0 mg once or three times per day). However, nocturia with repeated arousals in the absence of daytime symptoms may be the first indicator of chronic hypoventilation.

Jaw quivering or *clenching* may develop in patients with pseudobulbar involvement in response to noxious stimuli and is relieved by benzodiazepines (e.g., lorazepam sublingually).

Laryngospasm (a sudden reflex closure of the vocal cords) can cause panic resulting from a sensation of choking. Several types of stimuli (e.g., emotions, strong flavors or smells, cold air, fluid aspiration, or gastroesophageal reflux) may provoke this symptom, which usually resolves spontaneously within a few seconds. Repeated swallowing while breathing through the nose can accelerate resolution. Antihistamines or antacids may also be helpful.

Nasal congestion in patients with bulbar-onset ALS with a weakening of the nasopharyngeal muscles can be helped by elevating the nasal bridge with nasal tapes and application of topical decongestants.[27]

SPIRITUALITY AND BEREAVEMENT

The role of spiritual care is often underestimated. A recent study indicated that spirituality or religiousness may affect the use of PEG and NIV in ALS and may be a source of comfort to the patients.[51] Cases of patients whose spiritual practice greatly enhanced their ability to cope with ALS have been reported.[52] A simple structured interview to assess the patient's spiritual needs has been recently developed.[53] Spiritual care is not limited to patients and should encompass the whole family as a means of preventing problems during bereavement,[54] which may be particularly severe in ALS families.[55] It is important to acknowledge that the process of bereavement in ALS actually starts immediately after the diagnosis is communicated, in the form of so-called "anticipatory grief," and that callous delivery of the diagnosis may affect the psychological adjustment to bereavement.[56]

TERMINAL PHASE

A retrospective survey of 171 patients with ALS showed that about 90 percent of the patients die peacefully, mostly in their sleep, and none of the patients choked to death.[25] If patients with ALS are not artificially ventilated, the death process usually begins with the patients slipping from sleep into coma due to increasing hypercapnia. If restlessness or signs of dyspnea develop, morphine should be administered beginning with 2.5–5.0 mg subcutaneously or intravenously every 4 hours (if necessary in combination with an antiemetic). Because morphine is not an anxiolytic drug, if anxiety is present, it should be treated with sublingual lorazepam (beginning with 1.0–2.5 mg) or subcutaneously administered midazolam (beginning with 1–2 mg). The dosage of morphine and anxiolytics should be increased until satisfactory symptom control is achieved.[4] The potential of these drugs to induce respiratory depression is usually overestimated and is irrelevant in the terminal phase according to the doctrine of double effect.[24]

Most patients with ALS wish to die at home. This can often best be achieved through enrollment of the patient in a hospice program. It is advisable for the physician to initiate contact with the hospice institution, where available, well in advance of the terminal phase. If death at home is not possible, inpatient hospice or palliative care units should be considered. Hospice teams can also assist the relatives' bereavement after the patient's death.

REFERENCES

1. Borasio GD, Shaw PJ, Hardiman O, et al, for the European ALS Study Group. Standards of palliative care for patients with amyotrophic lateral sclerosis: results of a European survey. Amyotroph Lateral Scler Other Motor Neuron Disord 2001;2:159–164.
2. Miller RG, Rosenberg JA, Gelinas DF, et al. Practice parameter: the care of the patient with amyotrophic lateral sclerosis (an evidence-based review). Neurology 1999;52:1311–1323.
3. Oliver D, Borasio GD, Walsh D (eds). Palliative Care in Amyotrophic Lateral Sclerosis. New York: Oxford University Press, 2000;62–71.
4. O'Brien T, Kelly M, Saunders C. Motor neurone disease: a hospice perspective. Br Med J 1992; 304:471–473.
5. Oliver D. The quality of care and symptom control—the effects on the terminal phase of ALS/MND. J Neurol Sci 1996;139(suppl):134–136.

6. Leighton SEJ, Burton MJ, Lund WS, Cochraine GM. Swallowing in motor neuron disease. J R Soc Med 1994;87:801–805.
7. Wagner-Sonntag E, Allison S, Oliver D, et al. Dysphagia. In D Oliver, GD Borasio, D Walsh D (eds), Palliative Care in Amyotrophic Lateral Sclerosis. New York: Oxford University Press, 2000;62–71.
8. Chiò A, Finocchiaro E, Meineri P, et al. Safety and factors related to survival after percutaneous endoscopic gastrostomy in ALS. ALS Percutaneous Endoscopic Gastrostomy Study Group. Neurology 1999;53:1123–1125.
9. Gregory S, Siderowf A, Golaszewski AL, McCluskey L. Gastrostomy insertion in ALS patients with low vital capacity: respiratory support and survival. Neurology 2002;58:485–487.
10. Woolman BS, D'Agostino HB, Walus-Wigle JR, et al. Radiologic, endoscopic, and surgical gastrostomy: an institutional evaluation and meta-analysis of the literature. Radiology 1995;197:699–704.
11. Kadakia SC, Sullivan HO, Starnes E. Percutaneous endoscopic gastrostomy or jejunostomy and the incidence of aspiration in 79 patients. Am J Surg 1992;164:114–118.
12. Mazzini L, Corra T; Zaccala M, et al. Percutaneous endoscopic gastrostomy and enteral nutrition in amyotrophic lateral sclerosis. J Neurol 1995;242:695–698.
13. Albert SM, Murphy PL, Del Bene M, et al. Incidence and predictors of PEG placement in ALS/MND. J Neurol Sci 2001;191:115–119.
14. Jackson CE, Rosenfeld J, Moore DH, et al. A preliminary evaluation of a prospective study of pulmonary function studies and symptoms of hypoventilation in ALS/MND patients. J Neurol Sci 2001;191:75–78.
15. Lyall RA, Donaldson N, Polkey MI, et al. Respiratory muscle strength and ventilatory failure in amyotrophic lateral sclerosis. Brain 2001;124:2000–2013.
16. Cazzolli PA, Oppenheimer EA. Home mechanical ventilation for amyotrophic lateral sclerosis: nasal compared to tracheostomy-intermittent positive pressure ventilation. J Neurol Sci 1996;139(suppl):123–128.
17. Newsom-Davis IC, Lyall RA, Leigh PN, et al. The effect of non-invasive positive pressure ventilation (NIPPV) on cognitive function in amyotrophic lateral sclerosis (ALS): a prospective study. J Neurol Neurosurg Psychiatry 2001;71:482–487.
18. Kleopa KA, Sherman M, Neal B, et al. BiPAP improves survival and rate of pulmonary function decline in patients with ALS. J Neurol Sci 1999;164:82–88.
19. Aboussouan LS, Khan SU, Meeker DP, et al. Effect of noninvasive positive-pressure ventilation on survival in amyotrophic lateral sclerosis. Ann Intern Med 1997;127:450–453.
20. Lyall R, Moxham, Leigh N. Dyspnea. In D Oliver, GD Borasio, D Walsh (eds), Palliative Care in Amyotrophic Lateral Sclerosis. New York: Oxford University Press, 2000;43–61.
21. Borasio GD, Gelinas DF, Yanagisawa N. Mechanical ventilation in amyotrophic lateral sclerosis: a cross cultural perspective. J Neurol 1998;245:717–722.
22. Oppenheimer EA. Decision-making in the respiratory care of amyotrophic lateral sclerosis patients: should home mechanical ventilation be used? Palliat Med 1993;7(suppl 2):49–64.
23. American Academy of Neurology. Practice advisory on the treatment of amyotrophic lateral sclerosis with riluzole: report of the Quality Standards Subcommittee of the American Academy of Neurology. Neurology 1997;49:657–659.
24. Borasio GD, Voltz R. Discontinuation of mechanical ventilation in patients with ALS. J Neurol 1998;245:717–722.
25. Neudert C, Oliver D, Wasner M, Borasio GD. The course of the terminal phase in patients with amyotrophic lateral sclerosis. J Neurol 2001;248:612–616.
26. Hanayama K, Ishikawa Y, Bach JR. Amyotrophic lateral sclerosis. Successful treatment of mucous plugging by mechanical insufflation-exsufflation. Am J Phys Med Rehabil 1997;76:338–339.
27. Gelinas D, Miller RG. A Treatable Disease: A Guide to the Management of Amyotrophic Lateral Sclerosis. In RH Brown Jr, V Meininger, M Swash (eds), Amyotrophic Lateral Sclerosis. London: Martin Dunitz, 2000;405–421.
28. Blasco PA, Stansbury JCK. Glycopyrrolate treatment of chronic drooling. Arch Pediatr Adolesc Med 1996;150:932–935.
29. Stern LM. Preliminary study of glycopyrrolate in the management of drooling. J Pediatr Child Health 1997;33:52–54.
30. Newall AR, Orser R, Hunt M. The control of oral secretions in bulbar ALS/MND. J Neurol Sci 1996;139(suppl):43–44.
31. Andersen PM, Grönberg H, Franzen L, Funegard U. External radiation of the parotid glands significantly reduces drooling in patients with motor neurone disease with bulbar paresis. J Neurol Sci 2001;191:111–114.

32. Harriman M, Morrison M, Hay J, et al. Use of radiotherapy for control of sialorrhea in patients with amyotrophic lateral sclerosis. J Otolaryngol 2001;30:242–245.
33. Giess R, Naumann M, Werner E, et al. Injections of botulinum toxin A into the salivary glands improve sialorrhea in amyotrophic lateral sclerosis. J Neurol Neurosurg Psychiatry 2000;69:121–123.
34. Tan EK, Lo YL, Seah A, Auchus AP. Recurrent jaw dislocation after botulinum toxin treatment for sialorrhea in amyotrophic lateral sclerosis. J Neurol Sci 2001;190:95–97.
35. Kingsnorth C. Occupational Therapy. In D Oliver, GD Borasio, D Walsh (eds), Palliative Care in Amyotrophic Lateral Sclerosis. New York: Oxford University Press, 2000;111–116.
36. O'Gorman B. Physiotherapy. In D Oliver, GD Borasio, D Walsh (eds), Palliative Care in Amyotrophic Lateral Sclerosis. New York: Oxford University Press, 2000;105–110.
37. Drory VE, Goltsman E, Reznik JG, et al. The value of muscle exercise in patients with amyotrophic lateral sclerosis. J Neurol Sci 2001;191:133–137.
38. Klivenyi P, Ferrante RJ, Matthews RT, et al. Neuroprotective effects of creatine in a transgenic animal model of amyotrophic lateral sclerosis. Nat Med 1999;5:347–350.
39. Mazzini L, Balzarini C, Colombo R, et al. Effects of creatine supplementation on exercise performance and muscular strength in amyotrophic lateral sclerosis: preliminary results. J Neurol Sci 2001;191:139–144.
40. O'Gorman B, Oliver D. Disorders of Nerve I: Motor Neuron Disease. In M Stokes (ed), Neurological Physiotherapy. London: Mosby, 1998;175–176.
41. Raischl J, Hirsch B, Bausewein C, Borasio GD. Hospice Care for ALS Patients in Germany: The Munich Experience. Proceedings of the 9th International Symposium on ALS/MND. Munich: International Alliance of ALS/MND Associations, 1998.
42. Ganzini L, Johnston WS, Hoffmann WF. Correlates of suffering in amyotrophic lateral sclerosis. Neurology 1999;52:1434–1440.
43. World Health Organization. Cancer Pain Relief and Palliative Care. Report of a WHO Expert Committee. Geneva: World Health Organization, 1990.
44. Schiffer RB, Herndon RM, Rudick RA. Treatment of pathologic laughing and weeping with amitriptyline. N Engl J Med 1985;312:1480–1482.
45. Iannaccone S, Ferini-Strambi L. Pharmacologic treatment of emotional lability. Clin Neuropharmacol 1996;19:532–535.
46. Udaka F, Yamao S, Nagata H, et al. Pathologic laughing and crying treated with levodopa. Arch Neurol 1984;41:1095–1096.
47. Norris FH, Smith RA, Denis EH. Motor neurone disease: towards better care. Br Med J 1985;291:259–262.
48. Ganzini L, Johnston WS, McFarland BH, et al. Attitudes of patients with amyotrophic lateral sclerosis and their care givers towards assisted suicide. N Engl J Med 1998;38:967–973.
49. Rabkin G, Wagner GJ, Del Bene M. Resilience and distress among amyotrophic lateral sclerosis patients and caregivers. Psychosom Med 2000;62:271–279.
50. Gelinas DF, O'Connor P, Miller RG. Deep Vein Thrombosis/Pulmonary Embolism in Amyotrophic Lateral Sclerosis. Proceedings of the 12th International Symposium on ALS/MND. Oakland: International Alliance of ALS/MND Associations, 2001.
51. Murphy PL, Albert SM, Weber C, et al. Impact of spirituality and religiousness on outcomes in patients with ALS. Neurology 2000;55:1581–1584.
52. Borasio GD. Meditation and ALS. In H Mitsumoto, T Munsat (eds), Amyotrophic Lateral Sclerosis: A Comprehensive Guide to Management. New York: Demos Medical Publishing, 2001.
53. Puchalski C, Romer AL. Taking a spiritual history allows clinicians to understand patients more fully. J Palliat Med 2000;3:129–137.
54. McMurray A. Bereavement. In D Oliver, GD Borasio, D Walsh (eds), Palliative Care in Amyotrophic Lateral Sclerosis Oxford: Oxford University Press, 2000;169–181.
55. Martin J, Turnbull J. Lasting impact, and ongoing needs, in families months to years after death from ALS. Amyotroph Lateral Scler 2000;1(suppl 3):S14–S15.
56. Ackerman GM, Oliver D. Psychosocial support in an outpatient clinic. Palliat Med 1997;11:167–168.

21
Disease-Modifying Therapies in Motor Neuron Disorders: The Present Position and Potential Future Developments

Martin R. Turner and P. Nigel Leigh

It is more than 135 years since the original descriptions of amyotrophic lateral sclerosis (ALS) by Jean-Martin Charcot.[1] ALS today remains a devastating condition. This chapter focuses primarily on the current state of therapeutics in ALS, including predictions for future developments. There are of course other motor neuron disorders, and attempts to develop new treatment strategies in these is also addressed in this chapter.

Clinical trials in ALS have been systematically documented for half a century now.[2] From Charcot's era to the 1960s, these were essentially anecdotal reports, and over the next 20 years, small, usually inadequately powered, trials were carried out. The development of standardized clinical measures and clinical endpoints beyond simply survival, with parallel improvements in statistical methodology and global communications, has resulted in several large multicenter international trials, involving many hundreds of patients (Table 21.1). The results of these trials are discussed in greater detail.

A cure (by which is meant complete arrest of disease and the ability to prevent disease developing in people known to be at risk) remains an elusive goal, but there is agreement that the goal is to halt disease progression as early as possible, certainly before the patient has developed significant disability. The key question is which mechanisms should be targeted. There are many choices (see Section 2 in this book). Until the molecular cascade that leads to motor neuron death is fully understood, it will be difficult to target the most fruitful therapeutic strategies. Effective interventions could act on events some distance upstream of cell death, although the key target may prove to be the cell death pathway itself, for example, agents that inhibit key aspects of caspase activation or cytochrome c release from mitochondria.

For now we are limited to identifying agents for therapeutic trials that are hypothesized to act on some or many of the numerous potential targets. The

497

Table 21.1   Development of clinical trials in amyotrophic lateral sclerosis

Dates	Details	Examples
Charcot–1960s	Anecdotal reports	Glycosamine/betaine
1960s–1980s	Small trials, inadequate power	Isoprinosine
		Guanidine
		Ribonucleotides
1980s–1990s	More systematic trials, still largely underpowered	TRH
		Gangliosides
	Development of endpoints, largely functional	Branched-chain amino acids
1990s–present	1994—El Escorial criteria[3]	Riluzole
	1995, 1998—Airlie House ALS trial recommendations (see Table 21.2)[4,5]	CNTF
		IGF-I
	1998—Revised El Escorial criteria[6]	BDNF
	Large-scale, double-blind, randomized, placebo-controlled trials	Xaliproden
	Survival included as an endpoint	

ALS = amyotrophic lateral sclerosis; BDNF = brain-derived neurotrophic factor; CNTF = ciliary neurotrophic factor; IGF-I = insulin-like growth factor I; TRH = thyroid releasing hormone.

entry of candidate drugs into clinical trials depends largely on the vagaries of the pharmaceutical industry, although a few wholly or partly academic-led trials have been carried out. Sadly, most therapeutic agents tried in motor neuron disorders have failed. However, these trials have provided crucial information on the natural history of motor neuron disorders and on clinical trial design.

CLINICAL TRIAL METHODOLOGY

The design and conduct of clinical trials in ALS is not without scientific and ethical controversy. Debates on methodology and ethics led to the formulation of updated consensus guidelines from the World Federation of Neurology ALS Research Group Subcommittee (Table 21.2).[4,6] This group looked at all aspects of trial design and implementation including disclosure of information, publication of results and detailed statistical considerations, in addition to a review of the suitability of various clinical measures and quality-of-life (QoL) concerns.

A key issue in clinical trial design is how to measure disease progression. The choice of measure determines the structure and size of the study. Equally as important is an accurate understanding of how the variables chosen behave in a typical ALS population. Specifically, we need to know the natural history of the disease and characteristics of the measures chosen in a population identical to that we intend to recruit into a trial. This ideal is never realized completely but can be approximated by pilot studies and through information from previous randomized trials.

Table 21.2 Summary of consensus guidelines for the design and implementation of clinical trials in amyotrophic lateral sclerosis; second Airlie House Workshop, 1998

Guidelines
 1. Diagnosis must conform to WFN criteria.
 2. Trials can include sporadic and familial ALS cases.
 3. Age limit 18 to 85 years.
 4. Onset of disease minimum 6 months and maximum 5 years.
 5. Exclusion criteria—significant concurrent medical/psychiatric conditions or other trial medications.
 6. Clearly defined 1-degree (Δmuscle strength, survival, PAV) and 2-degree endpoints.
 7. QoL scales mandatory outcome measure.
 8. Detailed statistical analysis and planning.
 9. Provision for "compassionate release" and provision of drug after trial to all pending final analysis.
10. Clear protocol for release of trial results.
11. Independence of trial investigators from commercial interests.
12. Standard clinical trial phases I, II and III.
13. Phase I should incorporate placebo and ideally run for minimum 6 months.
14. Phase II may be use placebo or historical controls, or a crossover design. If endpoints expected to improve, trial should last at least 6 months; if expected to deteriorate more slower than for 12 months. Interim analysis to be performed beyond 9 months.
15. Phase III to be appropriately controlled and include analysis of muscle strength, pulmonary/bulbar function and time to death +/− survival.
16. Trials conform to statements of Declaration of Helsinki.
17. Trials to take account of treatments already available of proven efficacy.
18. Independent Data & Safety Monitoring Committee for all trials to act on patients' behalf.
19. Steering Committee to be established by mutual agreement between investigators and sponsor.
20. Publications Committee to be established with full access to database and in accordance with CONSORT guidelines on reporting of clinical trials.

ALS = amyotrophic lateral sclerosis; PAV = permanent assisted ventilation; QoL = quality of life; WFN = World Federation of Neurology.

Treatments tested in ALS have been aimed at slowing disease progression rather than arrest, although this remains the goal of disease-modifying treatment. Robust, reproducible, and practical measures of disease progression are required, as in any clinical trial. ALS is a heterogeneous disorder in molecular pathogenesis, presentation, and course. Thus, demonstrating beyond doubt a small (but clinically significant) effect may be difficult even with agents that target specific disease mechanisms. The definition of what amount of functional change is clinically significant is also problematic.

Markers of Disease Progression and Endpoint Selection

Table 21.3 summarizes some of the possible markers of disease progression in ALS. Not all have been used or have practical potential for use in clinical trials, for example, imaging studies (see Chapter 4).

Table 21.3　Endpoints and potential surrogate markers for clinical trials in amyotrophic lateral sclerosis

Measure	Subcategories	Parameter
Survival	Possible caveats, such as tracheostomy-free survival only	Date of death (or tracheostomy if applicable)
Motor function	Muscle strength	Quantitative myometry (MVIC); manual testing (e.g., MRC)
	Respiratory function	FVC; nasal sniff pressure test
	Bulbar function	SaLT quantitative assessments, for example, Frenchay Dysarthria Assessment
	UMN function	Clinical measures; neurophysiological measures (e.g., PSTHs); imaging studies[7] (e.g., MRS, DTI, PET?)
	AHC function	Motor unit estimates; neurophysiological measures
Disability/dysfunction	May contain qualitative elements of the above subcategories	For example, the Schwab & England scale; Norris, TQNE and Appel scales; ALSFRS-R
Quality of life	—	For example, SF-36; SIP; ALSAQ-40; SEIQOL-DW

Adapted and reprinted with permission from Turner MR, Parton MJ, Leigh PN. Clinical trials in ALS: an overview. Semin Neurol 2001;21(2):167–175.

AHC = anterior horn cell; ALS = amyotrophic lateral sclerosis; ALSFRS-R = ALS Functional Rating Scale (Revised)[8]; ALSAQ-40 = the 40-item ALS Assessment Questionnaire[49]; FVC = forced vital capacity; MRC = Medical Research Council; MRS = magnetic resonance spectroscopy[9]; MVIC = maximal voluntary isometric contraction; PET = positron emission tomography[10]; PSTHs = peristimulus time histograms[11]; SaLT = speech and language therapy; SEIQoL-DW = Schedule for the Evaluation of Individual Quality of Life, Direct Weighting[12,13]; SIP = Sickness Impact Profile[12,14]; TQNE = Tufts Quantitative Neuromuscular Exam[15]; UMN = upper motor neuron.

Survival

Death can be used as a primary endpoint for a clinical trial in ALS. It is an unambiguous outcome. The precise time and date of death can be recorded and verified. In most countries, obtaining a death certificate is possible. However, its use carries a requirement for longer studies, usually at least 18 months— about half the length of the natural disease course. Of course, power depends on the event rate, so the size of the trial cohort depends on the interaction of size (numbers of patients randomized) and duration. One must choose between a short but very large study and a smaller but longer study. For example, in the trial of riluzole,[16] power calculations indicated that a minimum of 150 subjects would be needed in each group to detect a hazard ratio of 0.67 with 85 percent power and an alpha of 0.05 (one sided) at 18 months. This calculation was based on an assumed 35-percent survival rate in the placebo group at 18 months. Survival rates differ among ALS populations and ALS Care Centers, so these assumptions can be misleading. In the riluzole trial, more than 200 subjects were randomized to each of the four limbs, yet the reduction in absolute survival (6.4% at 18 months) and the relative risk reduction (0.79) for the 100-milligram dose were not statistically significant using an unadjusted (log-rank) analysis. The differences at 12 months were, however, significant. Using an analysis adjusting for known prognostic factors (the Cox model), the relative risk reduction at 12 and 18 months was statistically significant. The Cox proportional hazards model allows one to adjust for prognostic factors that may not, despite randomization and large numbers of patients, be equally distributed in the trial population. The Cox model makes the assumption that the hazards are proportional, which may not be true for ALS trial populations. Nevertheless, the trend is clear and indicates a biological effect, although the methodology remains controversial.[17]

Various factors make survival as a primary endpoint more complex than appears at first sight.[18] Interventions such as ventilatory support (invasive or not) or percutaneous endoscopic gastrostomy (PEG) influence survival and therefore must be controlled for in some way. Noninvasive ventilation (NIV) and tracheostomy, in particular, pose problems for trial design using survival as a primary endpoint. In the riluzole trial,[16] tracheostomy was included so the final endpoint was death and/or tracheostomy. For the Xaliproden trial, the solution was to consider "permanent" NIV, tracheostomy (permanent assisted ventilation [PAV]), and death as a single endpoint. PAV was defined as continuous NIV for more than 23 hours per day, for 14 days, or permanent tracheostomy. Such definitions are somewhat cumbersome to use and difficult to validate through source documents. No universally accepted criteria for initiating NIV have been agreed. There may be relatively little loss of power in restricting the survival endpoint to death alone.

NIV prolongs survival in ALS[19–21] by about 6 months. At present NIV is used only in a minority of patients with ALS. In our experience, patients considered suitable for NIV who after a trial of treatment decline ongoing treatment with NIV die within 4 to 6 weeks. This reflects the fact that they are usually in early respiratory failure when NIV is started. If, as seems likely, the use of NIV becomes more widespread and is started earlier, the assumption that the timing of NIV is equivalent to the time of death (had NIV not been started) may not be valid, implying that the combined endpoint of death and PAV may be unsatisfactory.

A treatment may influence survival by a mechanism other than slowing the rate of motor neuron death, for example, by reducing salivary secretions or by altering mood. Not only may better (and possibly more inexpensive) alternative treatments already be available that achieve the same result, but such effects may also lead to involuntary unblinding in a trial.[22]

Functional Measures

Techniques used to measure functional change in ALS must, in addition to having validity, be reliable between assessors (inter-rater reliability), be reproducible by a single tester, and be adequately sensitive to small changes. The aim must be to reduce the variance attributable to the measurement technique to a minimum. A technique is of little use if it is unacceptable to patients in the later stages of the disease, leading to a high drop-out rate. Indeed, missing data due to death and whether a particular measure is unpleasant, tiring, or difficult pose major problems for all clinical trials in ALS. It is, of course, particularly problematic for trials in which the primary endpoint is some aspect of function. Except in brief trials (e.g., those lasting less than 6 months), which exclude more severely affected patients, there will always be some missing data, whether the analysis of functional change is based on time to event (e.g., time to reach a forced vital capacity [FVC] 50% of predicted) or slope (comparison of rate of change over time). When such functional measures are used as a *primary* outcome measure, missing data can seriously weaken the assessment of efficacy. Various imputations can be made (e.g., the last value carried forward, or assuming that death is equivalent to a zero score), but none of these provide a perfect solution compared to an analysis of a complete data set. It must also be recognized that missing data are associated with poor prognosis, so the final analysis will be based on a population of less severely affected individuals. Thus although the ALS population recruited to the study may have been representative, the population available for a full analysis will not be. Of key importance is to define clearly the hypothesis to be tested, to ensure that power calculations are based on reliable natural history data in a comparable population of patients, and to use measures that will keep missing data to a minimum. Other concerns include the practicality and safety of testing, as well as cost. If functional measures are to be treated as surrogate markers of disease progression, they must be easily and consistently quantifiable and have a clear relationship to ALS across the whole range of patients.

Muscle Strength

Muscle strength is related to disease progression in ALS, but its measurement can present difficulties.[23–25] Not all muscle groups can be reliably assessed. For bulbar muscles, functional scales rather than muscle strength are used. Limb testing, either manually or mechanically, raises issues about interassessor and intra-assessor variability and reproducibility, as well as practicality and cost. Manual muscle testing (MMT) using the Medical Research Council scale has the advantage of standardization and is reasonably reproducible, but the difference between categories and thus the significance of observed change is not equivalent. Muscle strength testing using a strain gauge and transducer attached to a metal frame inside which the patient is positioned allows measurement of maximal voluntary isometric contraction (MVIC). MVIC requires careful standardization if results between centers are to be combined.[25] Results are expressed as megascores for groups of muscles (e.g., arm or leg megascores).[26] The megascores are derived from the mean of Z-scores for each muscle tested. The predicted force and standard deviation are normalized for age, sex, weight, and height:

$$Z = \frac{\text{Muscle force (kg)} - \text{predicted force (kg)}}{\text{Standard deviation of predicted force}}$$

Direct comparison of MMT and MVIC in a multicenter study suggests that although MVIC is somewhat more reproducible than MMT, the latter has greater sensitivity for detecting progressive weakness, mainly because more muscles can be sampled.[23,25,27] Most studies with MVIC have sampled fewer than ten muscles, for practical reasons. With MMT, more than 30 muscles can be assessed within 10 to 15 minutes. The coefficient of variation falls below 2 if more than ten muscles are assessed with MMT. It is desirable to test at least 12 muscles. MMT is easy for investigators to perform and most patients tolerate it well. MVIC is time consuming and requires specialized equipment and staff. It can be tiring for patients, and the frequency of missing data is higher for MVIC than MMT.

Thus although MVIC is a sensitive and reliable technique for measuring change in muscle strength over time, in practice (and certainly in large studies) it does not have clear advantages over MMT, providing that MMT training is thorough and that enough muscles are tested.

Respiratory Function

Vital capacity (VC) is commonly used as a measure of disease progression. It is recorded as FVC or slow vital capacity (SVC) and can be measured simply and reliably using standard spirometers. The result is expressed as a percentage of the value predicted for a subject of the same sex, age, and weight. VC is an independent prognostic factor for survival[23,28] and is correlated with QoL measures.[29,30] Not surprisingly, the coefficient of variation of VC increases as absolute values decrease, but (with adequate training) test-retest reliability and reproducibility is excellent[23] and inter-rater reliability is good.

There are, however, problems with VC. First, patients with significant bulbar symptoms perform the test poorly. Indeed, VC is not predictive of respiratory failure in patients with bulbar-onset ALS, although it does have predictive power in patients with limb (spinal)-spinal onset ALS.[21] Second, VC is a relatively weak predictor of respiratory function or death compared to other (noninvasive) measures of respiratory muscle weakness such as sniff nasal inspiratory pressure or mouth inspiratory pressure.[21,31] No tests of respiratory muscle weakness are entirely satisfactory in patients with bulbar-onset ALS. The use of VC (FVC or SVC) as a primary outcome measure is an attractive option for ALS trials in view of its simplicity, acceptability to patients and investigators, and relative cheapness, but it is still not ideal for definitive phase III studies. For phase II trials, focusing on a selected patient population (perhaps excluding patients with bulbar-onset ALS and those with more severe spinal-onset ALS), VC is an acceptable and useful outcome measure.

Functional Scales

Functional scales attempt to produce a score reflecting the patient's condition, calculated from the summation of individual category scores (often weighted according to importance) in several areas felt to be relevant to ALS. Attempts have been made in some cases to validate such scales by comparing them to measures of muscle strength.

The Norris scale comprises a series of questions on function[32] and can be broken into limb and bulbar components. The Appel ALS rating scale includes assessment, both subjective and objective, of elements of bulbar and respiratory function, muscle strength, and upper and lower extremity function.[28,33] The Appel scale is thus a hybrid of measures obtained by examination and questions related to function, but slopes of deterioration are linear.[28,34,35]

Currently the most widely used functional rating scale in ALS trials is the ALS Functional Rating Scale (ALSFRS). It is sensitive and reliable.[36] The ALSFRS comprises questions relating to bulbar and limb function. It has been validated in ALS and modified to incorporate questions on respiratory function (the ALSFRS-R).[8]

The fact that so many smaller trials using functional measures as primary endpoints have proven negative is not surprising, because most could only have detected a huge effect. These authors point out that the key factors determining whether a drug effect will be detected are the standard deviation (SD) of the slope of deterioration and the number of patients. Because the SD of the slope of decline of most functional measures is large (between 0.7 and 1.5 of the mean), and because small numbers of patients (about 20 subjects per arm) have been included in more than half the trials reported, such trials could only detect a difference between active drug and placebo for MMT or FVC of 80 to 90 percent.[37] Nevertheless, even a large study, for example, the phase III riluzole trial, which showed survival benefit revealed only trends toward efficacy for functional measures. Rigorous training to reduce intraobserver and interobserver variability is now recognized as essential. However, it is probably impossible to reduce the coefficient of variation below 1.5 to 2.0 for functional outcomes relevant to ALS in multicenter studies.

Prognostic Matching

Another suggestion, given the heterogeneity in ALS cases, is to match and stratify patients at the start of clinical trials according to known prognostic factors, for example, site of disease onset (bulbar versus limb), age at onset, El Escorial category at presentation, and even referral delay (in itself a surrogate marker for rapid disease progression).[38,39] A prognostic model can be created for patients with ALS that has robust predictive power in terms of survival, despite heterogeneity in disease presentation and course.[40]

Assessment of Quality of Life

The absence of health-related QoL data has been a major criticism of past trials (see Chapter 19). QoL is not easy to define but implies a relationship between expectations and reality. Used in the medical context, the term embraces physical and mental health and the ability to fulfill individual aspirations. The latter will be different for each individual. Generally, measures of QoL correlate poorly with physical impairment.[12,41] QoL as a measurement of disease

Table 21.4 Potential quality-of-life measures in amyotrophic lateral sclerosis

Category	Measures
Individual or existential	Schedule for the Evaluation of Individual Quality of Life-Direct Weighting
Health related or generic	SIP; Functional Limitations Profile; SIP/ALS-19[a]
	SF-36 Health Survey/SF-12 Health Survey; Mental Component and Physical Component Scores[a]
	SF Mental Health Index (MHI-5)[a]
	ALSAQ-40/5[a]
	Psychological General Well-Being Index[a]
	MND Coping Scale
	Nottingham Health Profile
	COOP charts
	EuroQoL EQ-5D
	McGill Quality-of-Life Questionnaire
	Respiratory Quality-of-Life Questionnaires (e.g., Chronic Respiratory Disease Questionnaire)

ALSAQ = Amyotrophic Lateral Sclerosis Assessment Questionnaire; ALS = amyotrophic lateral sclerosis; MND = motor neuron disease; SF-12 Health Survey = Short-Form 12 Health Survey; SIP = Sickness Impact Profile.
[a]Formally validated in ALS studies.

progression is unsatisfactory, although it may be the key issue in interventions such as NIV. Measures of QoL should fulfill various criteria.[42,43]

The options for QoL measures in ALS are summarized in Table 21.4. Generic scales such as the Short-Form 36 Health Survey (SF-36 Health Survey) are useful because they have been incorporated and validated in studies covering a wide range of other clinical disorders.[44] Their relevance varies between conditions however, and recent years have seen the development of disease-specific scales that reflect the particular problems seen in ALS. A scale that is to be useful must be sensitive to clinically significant change.

The Sickness Impact Profile (SIP) is a lengthy questionnaire in which patients report health-related dysfunction both in physical and in psychosocial aspects of daily life on the specific day of attendance.[14] Many patients find it distressing.[45] It also has a strong functional element that may have unnecessary overlap with functional scales such as the ALSFRS, although it correlates well with the latter.[46] Attempts have also been made to correlate the SIP with disease progression as measured by MVIC, but this does not hold true for all categories.[47,48] There is a shorter form of the SIP specifically designed for ALS—the SIP/ALS-19. This is more convenient to use, has been validated, and correlates well with other QoL measures.[12,46]

The 40-item ALS Assessment Questionnaire (ALSAQ-40) is a recent addition to QoL measurement, developed on the basis of interviews with patients with ALS. It has good reliability and validity.[49–51] A short form, the ALSAQ-5, has also been validated.[52]

The Schedule for the Evaluation of Individual Quality of Life-Direct Weighting (SEIQoL-DW) is a tool incorporating relevant areas of experience chosen by subjects. These can vary over time and are weighted by subject, so that a weighted index is then calculated, score 0 to 100. The advantages of this measure are that it is preferred by patients over the SIP and the SF-36 Health Survey.[45] Areas selected and the scoring reflect the patient's real priorities at the time of questioning, and it is useful for communication between patients, caregivers, and health providers. It is complex rather than simplistic. The disadvantages are that areas selected change over time; there are "response shifts" during course of disease. It is also complicated, time consuming (15 to 20 minutes), and requires a trained interviewer. There is a poor correlation with functional scales (including the ALSFRS).[53] It has not been used in ALS clinical trials.

QoL assessment will be an increasingly important addition for future studies but should not be used as the primary or sole outcome measure. The consensus document on ALS trial design also suggests consideration be given to assessing QoL of caregivers too and the incorporation of depression scales for patients.[4]

THERAPEUTIC MECHANISMS

Research into the pathogenesis of ALS and other motor neuron disorders has rapidly increased over the last 20 years, and there are numerous theories with variable evidence to support them (see Section 2 in this book, also references 54 through 58). These theories and the resulting therapeutics—past, present and future—are now outlined and summarized in Table 21.5.

Table 21.5 Summary of therapeutic strategies by mechanism of action in amyotrophic lateral sclerosis

Therapeutic category	Human trials	Laboratory-only studies at present
Excitotoxicity	Dextromethorphan	—
	Branched-chain amino acids	
	L-Threonine	
	Riluzole	
	Lamotrigine	
	Gabapentin	
	Topiramate	
Neuroprotection	Verapamil	RPR-119990
	Nimodipine	Memantine
	Pimozide	ONO-2506
Neurotrophic agents	TRH	VEGF
	Thymic factor	Cardiotropin-1
	Ribonucleotides	GDNF
	Phthalazinol	
	Growth hormone	
	CNTF	
	IGF-I	
	BDNF	
	Xaliproden	

Table 21.5   (continued)

Therapeutic category	Human trials	Laboratory-only studies at present
Immunomodulatory therapy	Plasmapheresis	—
	Interferon-α	
	Cyclophosphamide	
	Cyclosporin	
	Prednisone	
	Azathioprine	
	Interferon-β	
	Total lymphoid irradiation	
	Gangliosides	
	Levamisole	
	Immunoglobulin	
Oxidative stress	Acetylcysteine	MnSOD
	Procysteine	D-Penicillamine
	Bromocriptine	Trientine
	Selegiline	
	Superoxide dismutase	
	Dithiothreitol, vitamin C and 2,3-Dimercaptosuccinic acid	
	Celecoxib	
	Tamoxifen	
	Pentoxifylline	
Antiapoptotics	—	Minocycline
Nutritional supplements	Vitamin E	Selenium
	Glycocyamine and betaine	Coenzyme Q_{10}
	Octacosanol	Lipoic acid
	Methylcobalamin	
	Creatine	
Antimicrobial agents	Ceftriaxone	—
	Isoprinosine	
	Guanidine	
	Amantadine	
	Tilorone	
	Transfer factor	
	Indinavir	
	Pleconaril	
Neuromuscular potentiation	Electrical stimulation	—
	Baclofen	
	Physostigmine	
	Neostigmine	
	3,4-Diaminopyridine	
	Tetrahydroaminoacridine	
	L-Dopa	

ALS = amyotrophic lateral sclerosis; BDNF = brain-derived neurotrophic factor; CNTF = ciliary neurotrophic factor; GDNF = glial-derived neurotrophic factor; IGF-I = insulin-like growth factor I; MnSOD = manganese superoxide dismutase; TRH = thyrotropin-releasing hormone; VEGF = vascular endothelial growth factor.

Excitotoxicity

Excitotoxicity may contribute to the mechanism of neuronal damage in several neurodegenerative conditions,[59] including ALS (see Chapter 10).[60,61] Several strands of circumstantial evidence suggest this as a potential mechanism in motor neuronal cell death in ALS. Early reports of the finding of increased levels of glutamate in the plasma[62] and cerebrospinal fluid (CSF) of patients with ALS compared with controls,[63,64] though not consistently reproduced, seemed to support the hypothesis and have been recently confirmed.[65] Reduced functional transport by the excitatory amino acid transporter type 2 is described,[66] notably in the ALS brain[67] and transgenic rat model,[68] and more controversially aberrant messenger RNA (mRNA) splicing as evidenced by the finding of abnormal transcripts in patient CSF by some groups,[69] but not others.[70,71]

A variety of drugs thought to modify glutamate neurotransmission have therefore been used in an attempt to treat ALS, including dextromethorphan unsuccessfully.[72] Trials of branched-chain amino acids[73–79] were very variable in terms of statistical power, and a recent meta-analysis of these trials concluded no overall benefit.[80] L-Threonine was tested separately in other studies, with the rationale that it would increase levels of the glycine, itself a glutamate inhibitor.[81–85] These were without success however.

Riluzole

Originally developed unsuccessfully as an anticonvulsant, riluzole stands out as a drug with clear, though modest, benefit in the treatment of ALS (Figure 21.1). Its exact mode of action is not known, but there are several possibilities (Table 21.6).

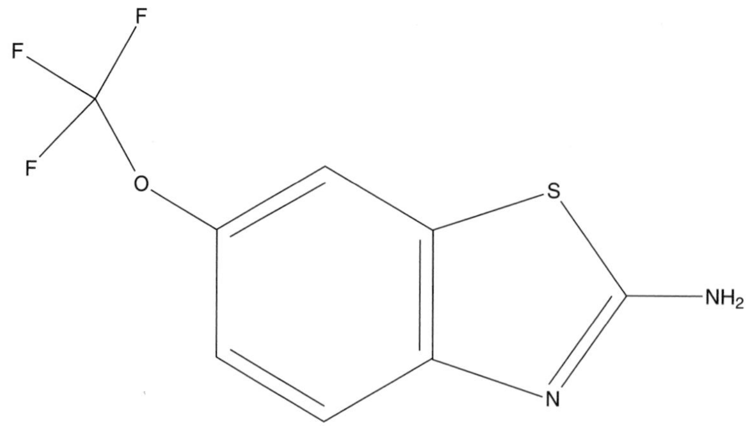

Figure 21.1 Chemical structure of riluzole.

Table 21.6 Potential therapeutic mechanisms of riluzole

Category	Effect	Mechanism
Likely effects[86]	Blockade of presynaptic glutamate release	Uncertain: ?effects on Na$^+$ channels; activation of G-protein–linked signal transduction
	NMDA receptor antagonism	Direct, noncompetitive receptor blockade
	Inhibition of glutamate-evoked Ca^{2+} entry	Activation of G-protein–mediated signal transduction
Possible additional or primary mechanisms	Inhibition of apoptosis	Inhibition of stress-activated protein kinase
	Inhibition of protein aggregation[87]	Uncertain

NMDA = *N*-methyl-D-aspartate.

Two large randomized, double-blind, placebo-controlled trials were carried out. The first of these examined 155 patients using a dose of 100 milligrams per day for up to 21 months.[88] Primary efficacy outcomes used were death and tracheostomy. Secondary efficacy outcomes included the rate of decline of a functional status score, which included limb/bulbar function measured using the Norris scales, clinical examination and reported symptoms, MMT (22 muscles), FVC as a percentage of expected value (%FVC), scores on the Clinical Global Impression of Change (CGIC) scale, and patient's evaluation of symptoms on visual analogue scales. Scores were documented at entry and every other month thereafter, except respiratory function, which was at entry and every 6 months. At 12 and 21 months, there was a significant difference in survival in the whole patient group, and a significantly slower deterioration in muscle strength, both in favor of those treated with riluzole. The apparent benefit for patients with bulbar-onset ALS is almost certainly attributable to small sample size.

The second study tested three doses against placebo and involved 959 patients receiving either 50, 100, or 200 mg per day over 18 months.[16] The primary efficacy outcome was tracheostomy-free survival, with secondary outcomes being identical measures of functional status, muscle strength, respiratory function, CGIC score, and visual analogue score of symptoms, to those in the previous trial (and at the same intervals). The outcome was a trend toward increased survival with riluzole at 18 months (the end of the double-blind phase), with significant improvement in survival at 1 year. There was a clear dose-response effect, with 100 milligrams daily having the optimal adverse effect profile. The difference in survival and/or tracheostomy between placebo and riluzole (100 milligrams daily) was 6.4 percent at 18 months, with a gain in survival with riluzole of about 3 months (though only an estimate, as the Kaplan-Meier plot did not reach the median by 18 months). The Cox proportional hazards model was then used to adjust for differences in known prognostic factors between patients, particularly as the expected number of events at 18 months was less than expected and so included patients less severely affected than initial power calculations had anticipated. In this analysis, the relative risk of riluzole versus placebo was more profound, being 0.65 (confidence interval, [CI] 0.50 to 0.85) at 18 months, although the methodology has been challenged.[17] Riviere et al[89] developed a model in which the disease burden in ALS was stratified and studied the transition times between these strata. Their finding was a significant difference in the time to transit between the riluzole-treated and the placebo-treated group in the less severely affected cases. However, the question of the benefit of riluzole in advanced cases of ALS remains controversial.[101]

The recently updated systematic review of riluzole therapy in ALS in the Cochrane Database examined data on 876 riluzole-treated patients and 406 placebo-treated patients,[90] which included these two trials, but also a third carried out using 168 patients who were not eligible for the trial by Meininger, Lacomblez, and Bensimon[91] on grounds of either age, length of time since disease onset, or FVC. Here the primary endpoint was also survival without PAV, with muscle strength, functional, and respiratory scales as secondary endpoints. Other more recent trials were excluded from the meta-analysis mostly on the basis of lack of randomization.[89,92–101]

For the primary outcome measures, Miller et al[90] found that for the three trials at all time points, there was a 16-percent reduction in the hazard ratio for those taking 100 milligrams of riluzole daily, which did not quite reach statistical significance ($p = 0.056$). This represents a 9% absolute increase in the probability of surviving for 1 year (57% in the placebo and 66% in the riluzole group), corresponding to an increase in median survival of the riluzole group of only 2 months. However, the significant heterogeneity of patients in the third trial by Meininger and colleagues[81] (more elderly patients with more advanced disease), compared to the homogeneity of the two trials by Bensimon and Lacomblez and colleagues,[5,78] was noted and this was felt to have diluted the benefit to some extent. The relatively small number of patients in the negative study by Meininger and colleagues[81] was also probably insufficient to adequately answer the question of benefit in this particular sub-group of patients.

Turning to secondary outcome measures, the combined results in terms of relative risk from all three trials based on percent mortality at 12 months for riluzole (100 milligrams) versus placebo were nearly the same as those based on the previous analysis of only the two published trials by Bensimon and colleagues.[5,78] The hazard ratio for the combined data from all three studies was 0.78 (95% CI, 0.65 to 0.92) at 12 months (Figure 21.2). In secondary analyses of survival at separate times, there was a significant survival advantage with riluzole (100 milligrams) at 6, 9, 12, and 15 months, but not at 3 or 18 months. There was a small beneficial effect noted in both bulbar and limb function, but not in muscle strength. There were no data on QoL. Significant side effects were noted in the riluzole-treated versus the placebo-treated group, including nausea and asthenia, and the potentially more serious threefold or greater increase of serum alanine transferase level (overall combined relative risk for all three trials 2.62, 95% CI, 1.59 to 4.31). Overall, 100 milligrams is accepted as the dose with the most favorable benefit-to-risk ratio.

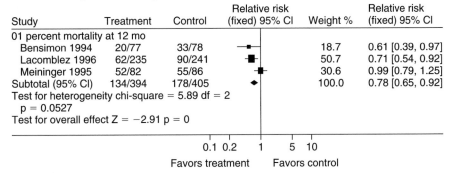

Review: Riluzole for amyotrophic lateral sclerosis/motor neuron disease
Comparison: 1 riluzole 100 mg vs placebo
Outcome: 1 percent mortality at 12 mo

Study	Treatment	Control	Relative risk (fixed) 95% CI	Weight %	Relative risk (fixed) 95% CI
01 percent mortality at 12 mo					
Bensimon 1994	20/77	33/78		18.7	0.61 [0.39, 0.97]
Lacomblez 1996	62/235	90/241		50.7	0.71 [0.54, 0.92]
Meininger 1995	52/82	55/86		30.6	0.99 [0.79, 1.25]
Subtotal (95% CI)	134/394	178/405		100.0	0.78 [0.65, 0.92]

Test for heterogeneity chi-square = 5.89 df = 2
   p = 0.0527
Test for overall effect Z = −2.91 p = 0

0.1 0.2   1   5 10

Favors treatment   Favors control

Figure 21.2 Forest plot resulting from meta-analysis of three randomized placebo-controlled trials, showing combined effect on mortality of 100 mg of riluzole versus placebo at 12 months.[90] The result favors treatment with an overall relative risk of 0.78. (Reprinted with permission from Miller RG, Mitchell JD, Lyon M, Moore DH. Riluzole for amyotrophic lateral sclerosis [ALS]/motor neuron disease [MND]. Cochrane Database Syst Rev 2002;[2]:CD001447.)

More controversial evidence from a large and importantly retrospective database of patients with ALS not only confirmed the improved survival in riluzole-treated patients but suggested an increased benefit over an extended treatment period.[40] Using the Cox proportional hazards model to control for other known prognostic factors, the authors carried out an analysis of the effect on survival of those patients given riluzole at any time during their disease course, compared with those who never received the drug. The retrospective data compared well with those of the prospective randomized trials for increase in survival probability at 12 months (about 4 months in the riluzole-treated group) (Figure 21.3). Furthermore, the benefit appeared to increase over an extended period, so at 60 months, exposure to riluzole resulted in about a 24-percent improvement in survival probability at the covariate mean (Figure 21.4). There was also limited evidence of benefit in patients diagnosed by El Escorial criteria as "suspected" or "possible" at presentation, although the assumption that treatment with riluzole earlier in the course of the disease remains controversial.[102] Other groups have carried out similar database analyses.[98–98b,103,104] Turner et al[40] clearly point out the limitations of this methodology, particularly in adequately controlling for all potentially confounding factors and therefore the need for caution in interpretation. These concerns are echoed by others,[105] but given that further randomized placebo-controlled trials with riluzole are now generally regarded as unethical, alternative methods for answering important questions about drug efficacy must be explored.

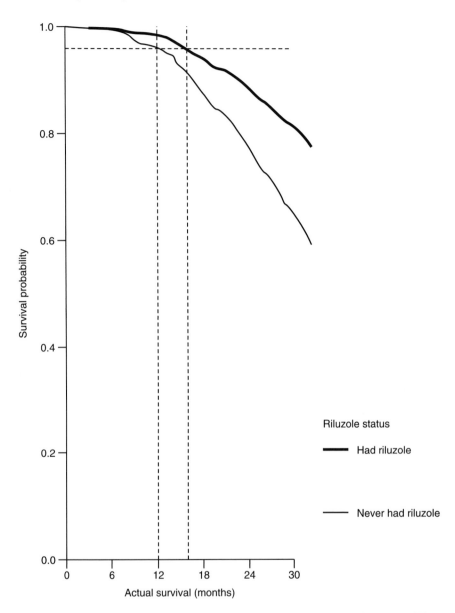

Figure 21.3 Survival probability plot by riluzole therapy status from the King's Amyotrophic Lateral Sclerosis Database of more than 800 patients.[40] Other prognostic factors are fixed at their covariate means by Cox regression and so "controlled" for. At 12 months, the riluzole-treated group survival is on average about 4 months longer than the untreated group. (Reprinted with permission from Turner MR, Bakker M, Sham P, et al. Prognostic modeling of therapeutic interventions in amyotrophic lateral sclerosis. Amyotroph Lateral Scler Other Motor Neuron Disord 2002;3[1]:15–21.)

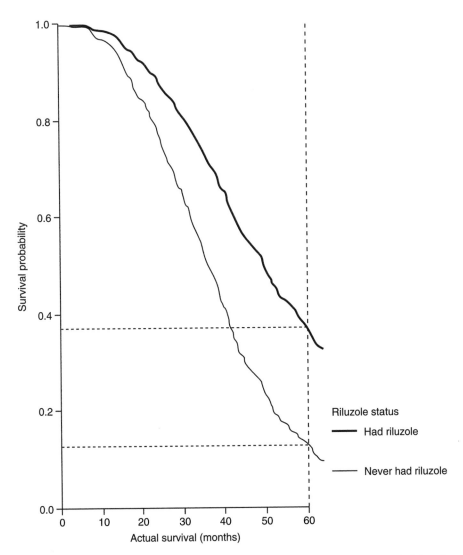

Figure 21.4 Expansion of Figure 21.3 from the King's Amyotrophic Lateral Sclerosis Database,[40] showing about a 24 percent difference in cumulative survival between riluzole-treated and untreated groups for a theoretical average individual at 5 years. (Reprinted with permission from Turner MR, Bakker M, Sham P, et al. Prognostic modeling of therapeutic interventions in amyotrophic lateral sclerosis. Amyotroph Lateral Scler Other Motor Neuron Disord 2002;3[1]:15–21.)

Cost-Effectiveness Issues with Riluzole

In view of the relatively modest benefits demonstrated and its significant cost, riluzole remains controversial in clinical use and has been refused therapeutic license in some countries, including Canada and Australia. Guidelines for its use are established in the United States,[106] and these are summarized in Table 21.7.

In United Kingdom, with a nationally funded health service (NHS) provided to all free of charge at the point of delivery, the issue of cost-effectiveness has been felt more acutely. In a report to the Development and Evaluation Committee of the Wessex Institute for Health Research and Development,[107] the concept of the "number needed to treat" (NNT) was introduced into the riluzole debate. Using data from the study by Lacomblez and colleagues, the authors calculated that for every six (95% CI, 4 to 13) patients treated with riluzole, one death or tracheostomy at 18 months was delayed, which in cost terms was estimated at £33,500 (95% CI £22,500 for 4 patients; £72,000 for 13 patients). Overall the authors of this report felt that the case for riluzole was "not proven." In another analysis based in Israel, the cost-benefit ratio of the additional 3 months survival provided by riluzole therapy was felt to be clearly favorable.[108] In a United Kingdom–based study looking at several doses, the incremental cost per life-year gained with riluzole therapy was estimated at ~£45,000 based on 100 mg per day, noted to be "well in excess of the range that is normally considered to be acceptable in U.K. health technology assessment."[109] Other studies of cost-effectiveness have been conducted,[110,111] including one with a more favorable estimate of cost per life-year gained at about £27,000 (currency equivalent).[112]

Table 21.7   Summary of practice advisory on the treatment of amyotrophic lateral sclerosis with riluzole: report of the Quality Standards Subcommittee of the American Academy of Neurology

Category	*Inclusion criteria*
ALS patients for whom class I evidence suggests riluzole may prolong survival	Definite or probable ALS by original WFN criteria (other causes for PMA have been excluded)
	Symptoms present for less than 5 years
	FVC > 60 percent of predicted value
	No tracheostomy
ALS patients for whom no class I evidence supports the use of riluzole, but expert opinion suggests potential benefit	Suspected or possible ALS by original WFN criteria
	Symptoms present for more than 5 years
	FVC < 60 percent of predicted value
	Tracheostomy for prevention of aspiration only (ventilator independent)
Expert consensus suggests riluzole is of uncertain benefit in patients with	Tracheostomy required for ventilation
	Other incurable life-threatening disorders
	Other forms of anterior horn cell disease

ALS = amyotrophic lateral sclerosis; FVC = forced vital capacity; PMA = progressive muscular atrophy; WFN = World Federation of Neurology.

Tavakoli and colleagues used the disease burden stratification method described by Riviere et al[89] to develop a Markov model of cost-effectiveness for riluzole therapy versus best supportive care.[113,114] The later model contained probability data for transition between the disease strata based on 954 patients from a previous randomized drug trial in ALS, in association with patient reported utility data for each health state derived from structured interviews with 77 patients.[115] The cost per life-year gained in this analysis was more favorable at about £14,000, and the corresponding cost per quality-adjusted life-year (QALY) was about £20,000. The authors, however, acknowledge the omission of potentially significant indirect costs to caregivers, their families, and the community, which were not accounted for by this study.

To assign priority to the funding of new drugs in the United Kingdom, a body—the National Institute of Clinical Excellence (NICE)—was set up to examine all the available evidence for a given drug, including cost-effectiveness analyses, and to decide whether its prescription would remain within the NHS framework. NICE conducted a rigorous review of the evidence for riluzole.[116] Four studies were considered, including a negative one,[92] in addition to the three used in the Cochrane Database discussed earlier. It concluded the cost per QALY to be £34,000 to £43,500, although long-term data submitted to the committee suggested a value nearer £20,000.[117] The estimated cost of making riluzole available to all individuals with ALS in England and Wales was about £5,000,000 per annum. Overall, it was decided that riluzole would be recommended, within strict clinical parameters, for NHS prescription. The NICE guidelines are summarized in Table 21.8. In a commentary on the NICE

Table 21.8 Summary of National Institute of Clinical Excellence guidance on the use of riluzole for the treatment of motor neuron disease

Category	Guidance
Guidance	Riluzole is recommended for the ALS form of MND. Therapy should be initiated by a neurologist with MND expertise, with routine supervision through locally agreed shared care protocols.
Clinical need	Definition of MND: MND is clinically heterogeneous. Specific MND variants include ALS, PMA, and PBP. Riluzole has been used to treat all of the above. There is no test for MND and often diagnostic delay. The prevalence of ALS in England and Wales is about 2000. There are numerous options, both medical and surgical (e.g., PEG), for symptomatic treatment. There is a need for multidisciplinary care, community services, including palliative care in the later stages.
Technology	Riluzole is currently the only licensed drug for ALS, designed to delay time to mechanical ventilation. The SPC recommends riluzole should not be used for any other form of MND. Riluzole inhibits the release of glutamate thought to be toxic to motor neurons.

Table 21.8   (continued)

Category	Guidance
	The major side effect of riluzole is abnormal hepatic function and blood should be checked monthly for the first 3 months, then every 3 months for a further 9 months, then annually.
	Dosage is 50 milligrams twice daily. The total annual cost of treatment is estimated as at £3742.
Evidence	Four randomized controlled trials (1477 patients).
	All trials used tracheostomy-free survival as primary outcome.
	Overall relative reduction in hazard ratio at 18 months of 17 percent (0.88, 95% confidence interval: 0.75 to 1.02) with heterogeneity across trials.
	Small reduction in rate of deterioration of functional status observed, but statistical methods "questionable."
	Few adverse affects.
	Strong clinical support for riluzole use in forms of MND other than ALS, but trials used ALS only.
	Current estimates of cost-effectiveness must be viewed cautiously. Key uncertainties about which stage of disease the survival gain is experienced. Mean gain in survival estimated at 2 to 4 months.
	Conservative estimate of cost per QALY £34,000 to £43,500.
	The committee took short life span of ALS patients into consideration when assessing cost-effectiveness.
Implications for the NHS	Estimated additional cost to NHS for provision of riluzole to all ALS patients in England and Wales ~£5,000,000.
	Diagnosis of MND to be made by specialist, and monitoring of therapy to be either by specialist or general practitioner.
	In latter stages of disease, patients may wish to review continued use of riluzole.
Further research	Further trials of riluzole at different dosing regimes are needed.
	Methods for earlier diagnosis, and so treatment, are needed.
Implementation	NHS trusts with MND patients should enable neurologists to consider option of riluzole.
	Neurologists' practice should be reviewed in light of NICE guidance.
	Patient information leaflet provided.
Clinical audit advice	Treatment plans to be recorded for each patient.
	Information to be incorporated into local audit systems.
	Multidisciplinary care protocols to be reviewed in light of NICE guidance.
	Prospective clinical audit programs should be initiated to record adherence to guidelines.
Review of guidance	January 2004

ALS = amyotrophic lateral sclerosis; MND = motor neuron disease; NHS = nationally funded health service; NICE = National Institute of Clinical Excellence; PMA = progressive muscular atrophy; PBP = progressive bulbar palsy; PEG = percutaneous endoscopic gastrostomy; QALY = quality-adjusted life-year; SPC = summary of product characteristics.

decision,[118] the author acknowledges that the evidence continues to be challenged by many and laments the lack of QoL data for the riluzole studies, which are now seen as vital to future therapeutic studies in ALS.

Other Anticonvulsants

Other anticonvulsants with effects on the glutamatergic transmitter system, including lamotrigine[119] and gabapentin,[120] have been tried in patients with ALS without success.[121] Publication of the results from a trial of topiramate is awaited, although these have been presented in abstract form with an overall negative conclusion and substantial unwanted drug effects also noted.

Neuroprotection

Glutamate toxicity is thought to be mediated through a pathway, common to many neurodegenerative states as well as stroke, involving unregulated flow of calcium into cells.[122] This provided the rationale for the trial of general calcium antagonists such as verapamil,[123] nimodipine,[124] and pimozide[125] to treat ALS, though without success. The ongoing work characterizing the specific transmembrane cellular channels through which calcium flows—N-methyl-D-aspartate (NMDA) and α-amino-3-hydroxy-5-methyl-4-isoxazole propionic acid—provides the hope of new neuroprotective channel-blocking drugs, and RPR 119990[126] and memantine[127,128] are two potential candidates. The propyl octanoic acid derivative ONO-2506 demonstrates neuroprotective activity in rats[129] and is the subject of ongoing trials in stroke. There are plans for a trial in ALS.

Neurotrophic Factors

Neurotrophic substances have a well-established place in both the development and the maintenance of the healthy human nervous system, and it is reasonable to conclude that they may also therefore have a beneficial effect in either preventing or delaying neurodegenerative processes. A range of candidate substances with neurotrophic potential have therefore been put forward. Early suggestions tried in human ALS studies included thymic factor,[130] ribonucleotides,[131] phthalazinol,[132] and growth hormone,[133] although none were successful. A disproportionately large number of clinical studies using thyroid releasing hormone (TRH), through various delivery routes, have been reported in ALS.[134–155] Overall analysis is generally considered to be negative however.[156–158]

Ciliary neurotrophic factor (CNTF), insulin-like growth factor I (IGF-I), brain-derived neurotrophic factor (BDNF), and most recently Xaliproden (formerly SR 57746A) have all been studied in large, well-organized, multicenter randomized controlled trials (Table 21.9).

Table 21.9   History of neurotrophic factors as therapeutic agents in amyotrophic lateral sclerosis

NTF	Route	No. of Patient nos.	Outcome measures	Comments
TRH	sc im iv it	~35 ~50 ~90 ~40	Muscle strength, spasticity, respiratory and disability scales, EMG measures	Overall negative
CNTF	sc	1300	Rate of decline of muscle strength and vital capacity (1 degree); isometric muscle strength, pulmonary function (including VC), functional scales (Schwab, England, ALSFRS, CGIC), survival, SIP (2 degrees)	Negative; double death rate in 5-microgram group
IGF-I	sc	449	Rate of change of Appel ALS score (1 degree); change in score, time to defined failure point, change in VC or SIP (2 degrees)	Negative; further studies planned
BDNF	sc it	1135 + ~200 281	Change in baseline %FVC at 6 months and survival at 9 months (1 degree); syllable repetition, walking speed, ALSFRS, SIP, and spasticity (2 degrees)	Overall negative (one sc and it study results unpublished); marked central a/e of it BDNF
Xaliproden	po	2077	Survival (time to PAV or death) (1 degree); manual muscle testing, VC, ALSFRS, CGIC, and spasticity scales, SIP (2 degrees)	Trial arms with and without concurrent riluzole; "positive trends only" —formal results awaited

a/e = adverse effects; ALS = amyotrophic lateral sclerosis; ALSFRS = ALS Functional Rating Scale; BDNF = brain-derived neurotrophic factor; CGIC = Clinical Global Impression of Change scale; CNTF = ciliary neurotrophic factor; EMG = electromyographic; IGF-I = insulin-like growth factor I; im = intramuscular; it = intrathecal; iv = intravenous; NTF = neurotrophic factor; PAV = permanent assisted ventilation; po = per os; s.c. = subcutaneous; SIP = Sickness Impact Profile; TRH = thyroid releasing hormone; VC = vital capacity.

Ciliary Neurotrophic Factor

Two large studies have been conducted on CNTF, both using subcutaneous injections of recombinant human CNTF, which was shown to prolong survival of motor neurons in vitro[159] and in mouse models of ALS.[160] The first of these trials involved 730 patients over 9 months, with three arms including 15 or

30 µg/kg three times a week and a placebo group.[161] Outcome measures included isometric muscle strength (muscles not specified), pulmonary function (including VC) and scores on functional scales including the ALSFRS, a modified Schwab and England scale, and the CGIC. Rate of decline in muscle strength was taken as the primary endpoint, with all other parameters being secondary. Results were not significant comparing both all CNTF patients versus placebo and with subgroup analysis of just the 30-microgram group versus placebo. Death rates were also identical. The ALSFRS was validated during this CNTF study,[36,162] and the later revised form accommodating respiratory function measures has become a standard tool.[8]

The other trial had four treatment arms with CNTF at doses of 0.5, 2.0, and 5.0 µg/kg per day and placebo, using 570 randomized patients.[163] The primary endpoint was the decline (from baseline) of a megascore calculated from the MVIC of 18 muscles and pulmonary function (i.e., VC). Secondary endpoints included individual limb megascores, pulmonary function, survival, and the SIP score. Tests were carried out monthly over 6 months. Analysis, including survival in both the intention-to-treat group and a group composed of only those who actually completed the study, produced no significantly positive results compared with placebo. Indeed the death rate was doubled in the 5-microgram group.

In a study of the prognostic indicators of survival from the ALS CNTF Treatment Study group,[164] shorter survival was associated with older age, lower %FVC, lower serum chloride level at study entry (reflecting degree of respiratory acidosis), shorter interval from symptom onset to diagnosis, or greater weight loss in the 2 months before enrollment, but not rate of muscle strength loss before study entry. CNTF has not been licensed for use as a treatment for ALS.

More recently, CNTF was delivered intrathecally in a small randomized trial.[165] Although the trial results were negative, they demonstrated that this method of delivery could produce high levels of drug within the central nervous system (CNS) with few complications, thereby paving the way for later studies using other neurotrophic factors.

Insulin-Like Growth Factor I

IGF-I is a polypeptide discovered to have neurotrophic actions on the motor unit[166] and promote the survival of motor neurons in an excitotoxic model of neurodegeneration.[167] Subcutaneous recombinant human IGF-I was tested in a three-arm trial including 266 patients with ALS receiving either 0.05 or 0.1 mg/kg per day or placebo.[34] The Appel ALS rating scale total score was used as the measure of disease progression. The SIP score was also used, along with VC, all measured monthly. Treatment failure was classed as an Appel score of more than 115 or VC of less than 39 percent of the predicted value. The primary endpoint was defined as the rate of change of the Appel ALS rating scale score after the period of randomization. Secondary endpoints included a change in the score from baseline, time to failure (as defined), and change in SIP score or VC.

A significant result was found in the group of patients receiving 0.1 mg/kg per day, whose progression of functional impairment was 26 percent slower than that in patients receiving placebo and exhibited slower decline in QoL (as measured by the SIP). In contrast, a later European study of 183 patients randomized to 0.1 mg/kg per day or placebo for 9 months,[35] again using change in disease progression as measured by the Appel rating scale, showed no significant difference between treatment groups. A cost-effectiveness analysis[168] judged IGF-I to be most favorable for patients with ALS either in the earlier stages of the disease or in a rapidly progressing stage.

A Cochrane Database meta-analysis concluded that although the results of the North American trial suggested slowing in decline of functional health status, this was not reproduced to the same extent in the European study. For the primary outcome measure of change in disease progression using the Appel scale at 9 months using 0.1 mg/kg per day subcutaneously, the combined analysis from both randomized clinical trials showed a weighted mean difference of −4.75 (95% CI, −8.41 to −1.09) favoring the treated group (Figure 21.5). Survival was not a prime focus of study in either trial, so no meaningful conclusions could be drawn pending further trials.[169] Overall it was felt that the use of IGF-I could not be recommended. Further trials have been started in the United States.

Brain-Derived Neurotrophic Factor

BDNF has been shown to support the survival and growth of developing motor neurons in vitro,[170] as well as to slow the loss of motor neurons and function in

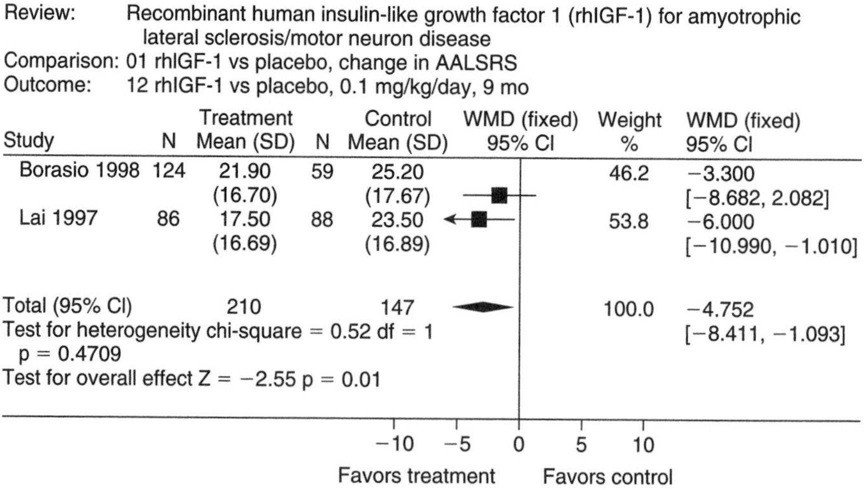

Review: Recombinant human insulin-like growth factor 1 (rhIGF-1) for amyotrophic
            lateral sclerosis/motor neuron disease
Comparison: 01 rhIGF-1 vs placebo, change in AALSRS
Outcome: 12 rhIGF-1 vs placebo, 0.1 mg/kg/day, 9 mo

Study	N	Treatment Mean (SD)	N	Control Mean (SD)	WMD (fixed) 95% CI	Weight %	WMD (fixed) 95% CI
Borasio 1998	124	21.90 (16.70)	59	25.20 (17.67)		46.2	−3.300 [−8.682, 2.082]
Lai 1997	86	17.50 (16.69)	88	23.50 (16.89)		53.8	−6.000 [−10.990, −1.010]
Total (95% CI)	210		147			100.0	−4.752 [−8.411, −1.093]

Test for heterogeneity chi-square = 0.52 df = 1
p = 0.4709
Test for overall effect Z = −2.55 p = 0.01

−10   −5   0   5   10
Favors treatment   Favors control

Figure 21.5 Forest plot, resulting from meta-analysis of two randomized placebo-controlled trials, showing the effect on disease progression in amyotrophic lateral sclerosis of 0.1 mg/kg per day of insulin-like growth factor I versus placebo at 9 months.[169] The result favors treatment with a weighted mean difference of −4.752. (Reprinted with permission from Mitchell JD, Wokke JH, Borasio GD. Recombinant human insulin-like growth factor I (rhIGF-I) for amyotrophic lateral sclerosis/motor neuron disease. Cochrane Database Syst Rev 2002;[3]:CD002064.)

the mouse model of ALS.[160,171] In a randomized, placebo-controlled, parallel-group phase III study, 1135 patients were assigned either to 25 or 100 μg/kg per day subcutaneously or to placebo.[172] Baseline assessment of disease (carried out monthly thereafter) included %FVC, syllable repetition, walking speed over 15 feet, and the ALSFRS score. The SIP (physical dimension) and the spasticity score (Ashworth Scale) were measured at 3, 6, and 9 months. The two primary endpoints were change from baseline of 6-month %FVC and 9-month survival. Other parameters were considered secondary endpoints.

In the primary endpoint analysis, the study failed to show any significant benefit of drug over placebo. Subgroup analysis demonstrated that patients with early respiratory impairment did show a statistically significant benefit. The authors comment that the unexpectedly high 9-month survival across all groups (85%) reduced the power of the study to detect significant change.

A pilot study using an intrathecal delivery method for BDNF proved feasible, although clear reversible central side effects were noted at higher doses.[173] Two further multicenter placebo-controlled trials, one studying high-dose subcutaneously administered BDNF and the other intrathecal delivery of drug, have taken place. The results of these studies were negative (unpublished data).

Xaliproden

Sanofi Recherche is currently studying the first orally active drug with neurotrophic activity to be used in patients with ALS—Xaliproden (formerly SR57746A). The drug itself has affinity for serotonin (5-hydroxytryptamine [5-HT]) 1A receptors and has observed neurotrophic actions in rodent and primate models of neurodegeneration.[174] A total of 23 clinical studies have been initiated with xaliproden in healthy volunteers, patients with ALS, Alzheimer's disease and chemotherapy-induced peripheral neuropathy. The first double-blind phase II trial in ALS involved 77 patients, receiving 2 milligrams per day of Xaliproden or placebo. It is reported that Xaliproden-treated patients had lower rates of decline at 32 weeks than placebo-treated patients in all measured functional ratings (Sanofi Recherche, unpublished data). More than 2000 patients with ALS were recruited, with treatment arms including patients with and without concurrent riluzole therapy. The parameters being monitored included muscle testing (MMT), VC, limb and bulbar functional scales (including ALSFRS, CGIC, and a spasticity scale), and QoL measures (including the SIP). Although the original trial is now complete and final results awaited, a long-term safety study remains in progress pending full assessment of the results so far by the U.S. Food and Drug Administration.

Although the precise mechanism of action of Xaliproden is not clear, other drugs with 5-HT$_{1A}$ activity such as buspirone have also been reported to have in vitro neurotrophic effects,[175] and there is independent evidence for serotonergic systems having a neurotrophic role more generally.[176] Pilot work by the authors studying cerebral binding of the 5-HT$_{1A}$ positron emission tomography ligand WAY100635, demonstrates a marked deficit in nondepressed patients with ALS compared to controls,[177] suggesting that serotonergic systems may be a novel area of increasing interest, possibly with therapeutic implications.

Other Potential Neurotrophic Agents

Finally another recent development and new potential therapeutic target is the finding that deletion of the hypoxia-responsive element in the vascular endothelial growth factor (VEGF) leads to reduced hypoxic VEGF expression in the spinal cord, possibly through reduced neural perfusion, causing an ALS-like syndrome.[178] Two other neurotrophic gene products—cardiotropin-1 and glial-derived neurotrophic factor (GDNF)—appear to demonstrate neuroprotective properties in the transgenic mouse model of ALS,[179–182] both of which may have similar potential.

Immunomodulation

A variety of evidence for an autoimmune pathogenesis in ALS has been suggested (see Chapter 13).[183] Briefly, this stems from work with animal models of the disease created by immunization with motor neuronal components[184] and the finding of immunoglobulin reactivity in the spinal cords of patients with ALS.[185] Several published articles report the finding of a variety of antibodies in ALS. Gangliosides have been of particular interest because of their presence in high concentration in neuronal cell membrane terminals, although therapeutic administration failed to show benefit.[186] Antibodies to these molecules were originally ascribed to ALS pathogenesis.[187,188] However, their more consistent finding, specifically anti-G_{M1} antibodies, in the condition of multifocal motor neuropathy (MMN) with conduction block[189,190] has led to more targeted and successful immunomodulatory therapy for these latter patients (see later discussion). More controversially, antibodies to motor neurons directly, as well as to calcium channels, have been described in ALS.[191,192] The description of an inflammatory infiltrate in the spinal cords of postmortem patients with ALS pathologically[193] and a report of CSF antibodies to macrophages[194] have also lent support to an immune role in the pathogenesis of ALS.

However, despite this evidence, none of the numerous immunomodulatory agents tried for the treatment of ALS have been successful. These have included plasmapheresis,[195] interferon-α (IFN-α),[196] cyclophosphamide with and without prednisone,[197,198] cyclosporin,[199] azathioprine,[200] IFN-β,[201] total lymphoid irradiation,[202] and levamisole.[203]

Immunoglobulin

Pooled donor intravenous immune globulin (IVIG) is now established for the treatment of many diseases that are thought to have an autoimmune basis for pathogenesis and has gained numerous applications within the field of neurology.[204] Its mechanism of action is not fully understood but may be through an anti-idiotype action, Fc receptor modulation or blockade, regulation of B-cell or T-cell function, or complement inhibition to name a few of the hypotheses.

Although trials of IVIG in ALS proved unsuccessful,[205] it now has an accepted place in the treatment of MMN with conduction block. This relatively rare group of patients with solely lower motor neuron clinical features, conduction block on neurophysiological testing, and often with anti-G_{M1} ganglioside antibodies were previously labeled as very slowly progressive or even "plateaued" ALS cases. However, neurophysiological and clinical diagnostic criteria are now firmly established.[190,206–208] Furthermore, several randomized studies of IVIG therapy in MMN have established it firmly as the treatment of choice.[208–212] The response can be variable,[213–215] but there is also evidence that patients without demonstrable conduction block but who have relatively slowly progressive lower motor neuron syndromes may also benefit from a trial of treatment.[216] A meta-analysis of all randomized controlled trials is planned as part of the Cochrane Database.

A Cochrane Database meta-analysis of trials of immunosuppressive agents other than IVIG has been attempted for MMN,[217] although no randomized controlled studies were found and so the conclusions are limited. The authors' overall conclusion from the numerous uncontrolled trials of cyclophosphamide in MMN was of some reported benefit, but also of serious adverse events, when used either as a primary agent or for patients who do not respond to IVIG, lose their responsiveness to IVIG, or require frequent infusions. With those studies that looked at corticosteroids as a treatment option in MMN, many reported a detrimental effect. There is felt to be little evidence currently about less toxic immunosuppressive agents such as azathioprine, IFN-β, or plasma exchange.

Oxidative Stress, Apoptosis, and Inflammation

The single most important discovery in ALS in terms of providing a window on pathogenesis was the finding of genetic linkage in some familial ALS cases to chromosome 21,[218,219] and the subsequent characterization of more than 100 mutations within the copper/zinc superoxide dismutase (SOD1) gene.[220–223] Although such mutations are present in only about 20% of familial cases and 3 percent of sporadic cases, it is nonetheless of pivotal interest in terms of mechanisms and future therapeutic targeting (see Chapter 9). It has also been invaluable in the development of transgenic mouse models of ALS,[224,225] which show remarkable similarity in many ways to the human condition and have allowed the testing of many potentially disease-modifying agents.

The SOD1 gene codes for a 153 amino acid, copper-containing metalloenzyme dimer. It is ubiquitously expressed in human cells but constitutes nearly 1 percent of the total protein of motor neurons. It is thought to have a critical role in the neutralization of superoxide and other free radicals, preventing cellular damage[226] (see Chapter 9). In ALS cases with mutations of the gene, there is thought to be a toxic gain of function, that is, an aberrantly functioning SOD1 molecule, rather than a total loss of function.[54] Certainly "knockout" mice without any expression of SOD1 show normal development.[227] Exogenous supplementation with SOD in humans failed as a therapy for ALS,[228] although increased expression of a manganese-containing SOD seems to be protective in human cell culture models of disease.[229] The nature of this toxic function is still not fully understood, and broadly speaking, there are two main hypotheses: catalysis and aggregation.[230] In the former, the mutant SOD protein is thought to catalyze the formation of peroxidase[231] or peroxinitrite,[232,233] resulting in free-radical–mediated cell damage. The latter hypothesis arose from the finding of cellular aggregates of SOD in transgenic animal models of ALS.[234,235] Furthermore, the finding that a knockout mouse model lacking the copper chaperone for the enzyme still develops disease[236] is more evidence that the gain of function is independent of a catalytic role. There may also be a role for copper chelation to disable the aberrant SOD in ALS and possibilities for the future here include D-penicillamine[237] and trientine.[238,239]

Despite the competing theories, numerous compounds with antioxidant activity have been used in mouse models and occasionally in humans in an attempt to compensate for this proposed free-radical damage. Acetylcysteine,[240] procysteine,[241] selegiline,[242] bromocriptine,[243] and "an array of antioxidants" including dithiothreitol, vitamin C, and 2,3-dimercaptosuccinic acid[244] were all however unsuccessful.

In terms of new developments, the recent report of benefit from coenzyme Q_{10} in Parkinson's disease[245] has raised the possibility of a trial of this in other neurodegenerative conditions, including ALS,[246] where mitochondrial dysfunction is a developing concept[247,248] (see Chapter 11).

The concept of programmed cell death in neurodegenerative diseases, termed *apoptosis,* is an attractive concept and there is already a large body of evidence for this process occurring in ALS (see Chapter 14), possibly triggered by excitotoxic mechanisms or under conditions of increased oxidative stress.[249] The evidence that the process occurs as part of ALS pathogenesis has been derived from neuropathological studies,[250,251] and improved understanding of the wider molecular details of the apoptotic pathway using transgenic mouse models has revealed the key players likely to be involved in ALS pathogenesis and so become potential targets for intervention. These include the Par-4 protein[252] alteration in expression of the regulatory oncoprotein Bcl-2 family members,[251,253] and caspases 1 and 3.[251,254,255]

In terms of possible therapeutic agents, minocycline has been shown to have anti-caspase activity[256,257] and appears to slow disease progression in mouse models.[258,259] There has also been increasing interest recently in the use of nonsteroidal anti-inflammatory drugs as neuroprotective agents, through a proposed mechanism of free-radical scavenging[260] and the inhibition of cyclooxygenase (COX). COXs are found throughout the CNS.[261] COX-2 is involved in the synthesis of prostaglandin E_2 and possibly the regulation of glutamate release. Marked increases in COX-2 have been demonstrated in ALS spinal cord.[262] Celecoxib, an inhibitor of COX-2, has been shown to have neuroprotective effects in animal models of ALS,[263] and clinical trials are in progress.

An increasingly prominent role is being found for the ubiquitous cellular enzyme protein kinase C (PKC), and there is evidence for a role in both NMDA-mediated excitotoxicity[264] and oxidative stress. Riluzole has been suggested to have an additional antioxidant role through PKC inhibition,[265] and recently the breast cancer drug tamoxifen has also been shown to have PKC inhibitory activity,[266] with the potential for future trials in ALS. Finally, pentoxifylline is a methylxanthine derivative and phosphodiesterase inhibitor. Although its mechanism of action is not fully characterized, it may have antioxidant activity,[267] and a multicenter randomized clinical trial is recruiting patients with ALS at the time of writing.

Nutritional Supplements

One of the first human trials ever published in ALS involved nutritional supplementation with presumed "building blocks" for muscle regrowth betaine and glycocyamine.[268] More recently, based mainly on results from animal models,[269,270] creatine has found a place in the treatment of ALS, but substantial human data on its benefit are lacking.[271–274] Vitamin E supplementation has been suggested for the treatment of a variety of neurodegenerative conditions, including ALS,[275] because of its presumed antioxidant activity,[276–278] but once again there is a lack of human data available to support this indication. Similarly selenium supplementation is suggested to be beneficial by reducing aberrant SOD peroxidase activity.[279] Octacosanol[280] and methylcobalamin[281] have been tried as nutritional supplements without success in ALS, and lipoic acid is a more recent suggestion,[239] although a formal human trial has not yet been carried out.

Antimicrobial Agents

Aside from trials of the broad-spectrum antibiotic ceftriaxone,[282,283] attention has really focused on antiviral agents and their role, if any, in ALS treatment. The evidence for a viral origin to ALS, though an attractive idea and recurrent theme over the last 25 years, remains highly controversial.[55,284–288] The basis of the debate includes the detection, or not, of a variety of viral signatures in ALS tissue samples.[289–300]

As a result, a variety of antiviral agents have been tried in human studies over the years, although none has demonstrated any convincing benefit. They included isoprinosine,[301] guanidine,[32] amantadine,[302] tilorone,[303] transfer factor,[304] and in the case of an ALS-like syndrome associated with the human immunodeficiency virus, indinavir.[305,306] Finally, there is a case report of a single patients with ALS treated with pleconaril who showed limited unsustained benefit.[307]

Neuromuscular Potentiation

Finally, there is a rather mixed bag of therapeutic trials all aimed, sometimes rather tenuously, at neuromuscular potentiation in ALS in an unsuccessful attempt to modify the disease course. They have included L-dopa,[308] electrical stimulation,[309] baclofen,[310] physostigmine and neostigmine,[311] 3,4-diaminopyridine,[312] and tetrahydroaminoacridine.[313]

POTENTIAL FUTURE DEVELOPMENTS

With the development of gene therapy techniques, many already showing some clinical success in other diseases, it is possible to envisage a range of potential therapeutic targets at a genetic level for the full range of motor neuron disorders. Replacement of mutant genes for healthy copies, deletion of aberrantly processed gene products (e.g., antisense mRNA), or enhancement through increased expression of neuroprotective gene products are all possible strategies that could be applied, although all of the motor neuron disorders are thought to have highly complex polygenetic etiologies. Other advances in disease-modifying therapies for motor neuron disorders may come from the development of high-throughput drug screening, proteomics, improved drug targeting, and stem cell technology.

GENETICALLY GUIDED THERAPEUTICS

The discovery of the SOD1 gene was an important step in understanding pathogenesis in ALS and developing therapeutic targets, although mutations in this gene alone clearly cannot account for the whole story in most patients. Understanding of the influence of genetics on disease incidence and expression generally has expanded enormously. Early human leukocyte antigen (HLA) associations have given way for more complex polygenetic models, involving haplotype and single nucleotide polymorphisms. Moreover, these developments are not restricted to ALS and now extend to the wider range of motor neuron disorders with great implications for therapeutic developments.[314] The main potential focuses for future genetic and therapeutic research in the motor neuron disorders are summarized in Table 21.10.

Amyotrophic Lateral Sclerosis

Within the field of ALS research new genetic loci associated with familial forms of the disease are now being increasingly described, and it is hoped these will

Table 21.10   Potential genetic targets in motor neuron disorders

Disease	Genetic targets
ALS	SOD1, alsin, APEX nuclease gene mutations
	Glutamate transporter—EAAT2 messenger RNA expression
	Neurofilament dysfunction—NF-L, NF-H, peripherin, kinases
	Mitochondrial DNA mutations
	Neurotrophin gene delivery—VEGF deletion, GDNF, cardiotropin-1
	Apoptosis modulation—Bcl-2 expression
SMA	SMN, NAIP gene mutations
HSP	Spastin, paraplegin, L1CAM, proteolipid protein mutations
SBMA	Androgen receptor trinucleotide repeat

ALS = amyotrophic lateral sclerosis; APEX = apurinic endonuclease; EAAT = excitatory amino acid transporter; GDNF = glial-derived neurotrophic factor; HSP = hereditary spastic paraparesis; L1CAM = L1 cell adhesion molecule; NF = neurofilament (L- light; H- heavy); NAIP = neuronal inhibitor of apoptosis; SBMA = spinobulbar muscular atrophy (Kennedy's disease); SMA = spinal muscular atrophy; SMN = survival motor neuron; SOD = superoxide dismutase; VEGF = vascular endothelial growth factor.

continue to lead the way in shedding further light on molecular mechanisms.[315] An international database of ALS mutations has also been established.[316] The finding of a recessive mutation in the "alsin" or ALS2 gene on chromosome 2, which seems to code for a guanosine triphosphatase (GTPase), regulator may be a significant development.[317–319a] The mutation leads to protein truncation and is therefore likely to represent a loss of function. Linkage has also been established on chromosomes 15,[320] 9,[321,322] 18,[323] and 16.[324] The finding of mutations in the APEX nuclease gene in patients with ALS compared with controls may provide a novel genetic target.[325]

The early finding of axonal enlargement[326] and subsequently of accumulations of neurofilaments (NFs) in the cell bodies of patients with sporadic and familial ALS[327,328] focused attention on a possible role of NF dysfunction in motor neuron disorders (see Chapter 12),[329] possibly in part through deranged axonal transport.[330] Transgenic mouse models,[331] combined with more recent genetic advances characterizing NF mutations involved in ALS,[332,333] are beginning to shed light at the very heart of selective vulnerability in ALS,[334] and overexpression of certain NF genes may be one therapeutic strategy.[335,336] Genetic expression of another NF protein peripherin, which is associated with degenerating motor neurons in mouse models, is another potential target for future therapeutic intervention.[337] NF phosphorylation and function is tightly regulated and controlled by various kinases in a complex cascade of events, which is slowly being unraveled. The "alsin" gene, discussed earlier, may have a direct role in NF phosphorylation/transport, for example.

Finally, the developing appreciation of mitochondrial dysfunction in the pathogenesis of ALS (see Chapter 11),[338,339] with the finding of mutations in mitochondrial DNA in ALS,[340,341] provides another potential route for genetic manipulation in the future.

Spinal Muscular Atrophy

The lower motor neuron disease spinal muscular atrophy (SMA) is now undergoing the same sort of rapid increase in pathogenetic understanding experienced by those in the field of ALS research[342] (see Chapter 16). The discovery of mutations in the survival motor neuron gene, now SMN1,[343] and the neuronal inhibitor of apoptosis gene,[344] in close proximity on chromosome 5, was the major first step in unraveling what is a clinically and pathologically complex disease.[345] In terms of the molecular mechanisms, a role for these genes in the processing of RNA has emerged,[346,347] as well as links to apoptotic mechanisms,[348] with Bcl-2 gene expression surfacing once more as a potential therapeutic target. More controversially, there may be evidence linking the genetics of SMA to ALS.[349–351]

Hereditary Spastic Paraparesis

Hereditary spastic paraparesis (HSP) is a diagnosis encompassing a spectrum of conditions unified by the presence of lower extremity weakness and spasticity (see Chapter 18). Autosomal dominant, autosomal recessive, and X-linked pedigrees are all described at a variety of genetic loci, and in one series, approximately 20 percent of cases were apparently sporadic.[352] The most common type of inherited HSP involves autosomal dominant mutations in the spastin gene located on chromosome 2. It codes for a nuclear adenosine triphosphate cleavage protein of uncertain function, and no one mutation seems to be more common than another.[353] In X-linked forms, mutations of myelin proteolipid protein (PLP),[354] and in the L1 cell adhesion molecule (L1CAM) have been identified.[355] In some autosomal recessive cases, mutations in the paraplegin gene on chromosome 16, a nuclear-encoded mitochondrial metalloproteinase, are described.[356] Overall, in what is undoubtedly a vastly heterogeneous clinical condition, the molecular pathology of HSP is complex and remains unclear.[357] Clinically, there is a mild loss of anterior horn and Betz cells on pathological study of HSP cases,[358] but whether this has a major clinical manifestation in most cases remains controversial. The potential clinical overlap of HSP with ALS is therefore mainly through the presence of a corticospinal tract lesion, and spastin mutations are now being sought in familial ALS pedigrees.[359]

X-Linked Spinobulbar Muscular Atrophy

Kennedy's disease (X-linked spinobulbar muscular atrophy [SBMA]) was first described in 1968[360] (see Chapter 17). This solely lower motor neuron syndrome is usually markedly slower in progression than ALS and is associated with gynecomastia and other endocrine abnormalities. The specific gene abnormality is known to be a trinucleotide (CTG) repeat expansion within the androgen receptor gene.[361]

High-Throughput Drug Screening

High-throughput drug screening is an effective strategy, developed by the pharmaceutical industry to identify new drugs, in which robotics are used to simultaneously test thousands of distinct chemical compounds in miniaturized versions of disease models. Assays may involve proteins, cells, or model organisms. The National Institute for Neurological Disorders and Stroke (NINDS) Neurodegeneration Drug Screening Consortium is currently studying more than 1000 candidate drugs using these techniques. It is hoped this method will rapidly identify a range of drugs that can then progress to phase I studies.

Proteomics

With the prospect of a full map of the human genome now a reality, attention has turned to the study of the protein products of these genes. Serum or CSF proteins, for example, can be separated as "spots" according to both their pH level and mass across a two-dimensional gel by electrophoresis. By comparing samples from patients with those of healthy controls, individual spots underexpressed, overexpressed, or absent in one sample can be individually removed and characterized into constituent amino acids, after tryptic digestion, using mass spectroscopy. This technique has great potential to reveal novel molecular mechanisms and therapeutic targets across the whole range of human disease, including motor neuron disorders.

Therapeutic Targeting: "The Magic Bullet"

The exquisitely accurate delivery of viral particles to the intracellular space, in some cases with subsequent seamless incorporation of their genetic material into that of the host, offers the potential for "magic bullet" therapies in many diseases. Adenovirus-mediated gene transfer has already been used to beneficial effect in ALS mouse models, delivering neurotrophic genes for GDNF and cardiotropin-1.[179–182] There is already potential to extend this to interfere with apoptotic mechanisms, for example, through Bcl-2 expression.[362] Lentiviruses are another potential candidate as vectors for gene transfer.[363] Returning to motor neuron disorders specifically, one can envisage that in the future it might be possible to employ an attenuated poliovirus, tagged with a therapeutic agent to directly target the spinal anterior horn.

Stem Cells

Although the discovery of stem cells—circulating progenitor cells able to differentiate into the full range of tissue—is not all that recent, it is the ability to isolate and therefore begin to manipulate such cells for the first time that has sparked great interest and genuine hope. The "new cells for old ones" idea is simple and attractive, with obvious applications for the whole range of neurodegenerative conditions.[364] In the normal mammalian brain, neuronal cells of the olfactory bulb, hippocampus, and parts of the neocortex are known to undergo stem cell replacement.[365–368]

The obstacles in the treatment of ALS with stem cells however are significant, not the least of which is the type of cell to use—embryonic, adult, neural, blood, or embryoid body derived. Where and how to insert the cells so that they survive within the particularly hostile environment of the CNS; what factors are required to stimulate appropriate and importantly controlled differentiation, as well as how to prevent immune rejection and local tissue damage, are also key issues. How these cells will work is not clear—replacing motor neurons directly or perhaps in a supportive role to surrounding cells.

It has already been possible, using developmentally relevant signaling factors, to induce mouse embryonic stem (ES) cells to differentiate into spinal progenitor cells and subsequently into motor neurons.[369] Neuronal cells derived from fetal human neural stem cells and transplanted into adult rat CNS have been successfully developed,[257] and neuronal cells derived from tumor cell lines have shown some modest benefit in the mouse model of ALS.[370,371] Early stem cell work in rats may appear promising[372] but also highlights the challenges ahead before human trials can be responsibly undertaken.

CONCLUSION

This chapter has attempted to review the full range of potentially disease-modifying therapies in motor neuron disorders, focusing mainly on the enormous gains in our understanding of molecular mechanisms, which have prompted the trial of more than 60 compounds and in turn shaped clinical trial methodology in ALS. Clearly most of drugs tried have failed, but parallel advances in high-throughput screening of novel compounds can only increase the chance of better results in the future. The authors favor a two-stage model for a cure in ALS (a view expressed by others in the field too[57]), likely to be a mixture of drugs aimed at various molecular targets such as those already outlined, to arrest the disease process at least. In parallel, it may be that advances in genetic engineering will contribute to this arrest. Given that most diseases seem to have polygenetic influences however, a single gene therapy seems unlikely. The second and much longer term stage would then involve regeneration of motor pathways, and stem cells seem to be the most likely candidate for this task, if significant scientific hurdles can be overcome.

REFERENCES

1. Charcot JM. Sclerose des cordons lateraux de la moelle epiniere chez une femme hysterique atteinte de contracture permanente des quatre membres. Bull Soc Med Hopit Paris 1865;24–35.
2. Turner MR, Parton MJ, Leigh PN. Clinical trials in ALS: an overview. Semin Neurol 2001;21: 167–175.
3. Brooks BR. El Escorial World Federation of Neurology criteria for the diagnosis of amyotrophic lateral sclerosis. Subcommittee on Motor Neuron Diseases/Amyotrophic Lateral Sclerosis of the World Federation of Neurology Research Group on Neuromuscular Diseases and the El Escorial "Clinical limits of amyotrophic lateral sclerosis" workshop contributors. J Neurol Sci 1994; 124(suppl):96–107.
4. Miller RG, Munsat TL, Swash M, Brooks BR. Consensus guidelines for the design and implementation of clinical trials in ALS. World Federation of Neurology Committee on Research. J Neurol Sci 1999;169:2–12.
5. World Federation of Neurology Research Group on Neuromuscular Diseases Subcommittee on Motor Neuron Disease. Airlie House guidelines. Therapeutic trials in amyotrophic lateral sclerosis. Airlie House "Therapeutic Trials in ALS" Workshop Contributors. J Neurol Sci 1995; 129(suppl):1–10.
6. Brooks BR, Miller RG, Swash M, Munsat TL. El Escorial Revisited: Revised Criteria for the Diagnosis of Amyotrophic Lateral Sclerosis. London, UK: World Federation of Neurology, 1998. Available at: www.wfnals.org/guidelines/1998elescorial/elescorial1998.htm.
7. Leigh PN, Simmons A, Williams SCR, et al. Imaging: MRS/MRI/PET/SPECT: Summary. Amyotroph Lateral Scler Other Motor Neuron Disord 2002;3(suppl 1):S75–S80.
8. Cedarbaum JM, Stambler N, Malta E, et al. The ALSFRS-R: a revised ALS functional rating scale that incorporates assessments of respiratory function. BDNF ALS Study Group (Phase III). J Neurol Sci 1999;169:13–21.
9. Pioro EP. Proton magnetic resonance spectroscopy (^{1}H-MRS) in ALS. Amyotroph Lateral Scler Other Motor Neuron Disord 2000;1(suppl 2):S7–S16.
10. Turner MR, Leigh PN. Positron emission tomography (PET)—its potential to provide surrogate markers in ALS. Amyotroph Lateral Scler Other Motor Neuron Disord 2000;1(suppl 2): S17–S22.
11. Mills KR. Motor neuron disease. Studies of the corticospinal excitation of single motor neurons by magnetic brain stimulation. Brain 1995;118(pt 4):971–982.
12. Goldstein LH, Atkins L, Leigh PN. Correlates of quality of life in people with motor neuron disease (MND). Amyotroph Lateral Scler Other Motor Neuron Disord 2002;3:123–129.

13. Hickey AM, Bury G, O'Boyle CA, et al. A new short form individual quality of life measure (SEIQoL-DW): application in a cohort of individuals with HIV/AIDS. BMJ 1996;313:29–33.
14. Bergner M, Bobbitt RA, Carter WB, Gilson BS. The Sickness Impact Profile: development and final revision of a health status measure. Med Care 1981;19:787–805.
15. Andres PL, Hedlund W, Finison L, et al. Quantitative motor assessment in amyotrophic lateral sclerosis. Neurology 1986;36:937–941.
16. Lacomblez L, Bensimon G, Leigh PN, et al. Dose-ranging study of riluzole in amyotrophic lateral sclerosis. Amyotrophic Lateral Sclerosis/Riluzole Study Group II. Lancet 1996;347:1425–1431.
17. Guiloff RJ, Goonetilleke A, Emami J. Riluzole and amyotrophic lateral sclerosis. Lancet 1996;348: 336–337.
18. Eisen A, Krieger C. ALS Therapy, Therapeutic Trials, and Neuroprotection. Amyotrophic Lateral Sclerosis—A Synthesis of Research and Clinical Practice. Cambridge University Press, 1998;209–237.
19. Pinto AC, Evangelista T, Carvalho M, et al. Respiratory assistance with a non-invasive ventilator (BiPAP) in MND/ALS patients: survival rates in a controlled trial. J Neurol Sci 1995;129(suppl): 19–26.
20. Aboussouan LS, Khan SU, Banerjee M, et al. Objective measures of the efficacy of noninvasive positive-pressure ventilation in amyotrophic lateral sclerosis. Muscle Nerve 2001;24:403–409.
21. Lyall RA, Donaldson N, Polkey MI, et al. Respiratory muscle strength and ventilatory failure in amyotrophic lateral sclerosis. Brain 2001;124(pt 10):2000–2013.
22. Armon C. How can physicians and their patients with ALS decide to use the newly-available treatments to slow disease progression? ALS and other motor neuron disorders 1999;1:3–14.
23. Brooks BR, Sanjak M, Belden D, Waclawik A. Motor Neurone Disease: Basic Designs, Sample Sizes and Pitfalls. In Guiloff RJ (ed), Clinical Trials in Neurology. New York: Springer, 2001; 427–450.
24. Miller RG. Measurement of strength: summary. Amyotroph Lateral Scler Other Motor Neuron Disord 2002;3(suppl 1):S51–S53.
25. Sorenson E. Measurement of strength: Con. Amyotroph Lateral Scler Other Motor Neuron Disord 2002;3(suppl 1):S49–S50.
26. Andres PL, Finison LJ, Conlon T, et al. Use of composite scores (megascores) to measure deficit in amyotrophic lateral sclerosis. Neurology 1988;38:405–408.
27. Andres PL, Skerry LM, Thornell B, et al. A comparison of three measures of disease progression in ALS. J Neurol Sci 1996;139(suppl):64–70.
28. Haverkamp LJ, Appel V, Appel SH. Natural history of amyotrophic lateral sclerosis in a database population. Validation of a scoring system and a model for survival prediction. Brain 1995; 118(pt 3):707–719.
29. Bourke SC, Shaw PJ, Gibson GJ. Respiratory function vs sleep-disordered breathing as predictors of QOL in ALS. Neurology 2001;57:2040–2044.
30. Lyall RA, Donaldson N, Fleming T, et al. A prospective study of quality of life in ALS patients treated with noninvasive ventilation. Neurology 2001;57:153–156.
31. Fitting JW, Paillex R, Hirt L, et al. Sniff nasal pressure: a sensitive respiratory test to assess progression of amyotrophic lateral sclerosis. Ann Neurol 1999;46:887–893.
32. Norris FH Jr, Calanchini PR, Fallat RJ, et al. The administration of guanidine in amyotrophic lateral sclerosis. Neurology 1974;24:721–728.
33. Appel V, Stewart SS, Smith G, Appel SH. A rating scale for amyotrophic lateral sclerosis: description and preliminary experience. Ann Neurol 1987;22:328–333.
34. Lai EC, Felice KJ, Festoff BW, et al. Effect of recombinant human insulin-like growth factor-I on progression of ALS. A placebo-controlled study. The North America ALS/IGF-I Study Group. Neurology 1997;49:1621–1630.
35. Borasio GD, Robberecht W, Leigh PN, et al. A placebo-controlled trial of insulin-like growth factor-I in amyotrophic lateral sclerosis. European ALS/IGF-I Study Group. Neurology 1998;51: 583–586.
36. The ALS CNTF Treatment Study (ACTS) Phase I–II Study Group. The Amyotrophic Lateral Sclerosis Functional Rating Scale. Assessment of activities of daily living in patients with amyotrophic lateral sclerosis. The ALS CNTF treatment study (ACTS) phase I–II Study Group. Arch Neurol 1996;53:141–147.
37. Meininger V, Salachas F. Review of Clinical Trials. In V Meininger, M Swash, RH Brown Jr (eds), Amyotrophic Lateral Sclerosis. London: Martin Dunitz, 2000;389–402.
38. Iwasaki Y, Ikeda K, Ichikawa Y, et al. The diagnostic interval in amyotrophic lateral sclerosis. Clin Neurol Neurosurg 2002;104:87–89.

39. Turner M, Al Chalabi A. Early symptom progression rate is related to ALS outcome: a prospective population-based study. Neurology 2002;59:2012–2013.
40. Turner MR, Bakker M, Sham P, et al. Prognostic modeling of therapeutic interventions in amyotrophic lateral sclerosis. Amyotroph Lateral Scler Other Motor Neuron Disord 2002;3: 15–21.
41. Simmons Z, Bremer BA, Robbins RA, et al. Quality of life in ALS depends on factors other than strength and physical function. Neurology 2000;55:388–392.
42. Jenkinson C, Fitzpatrick R, Swash M, Peto V. The ALS Health Profile Study: quality of life of amyotrophic lateral sclerosis patients and carers in Europe. J Neurol 2000;247:835–840.
43. Jenkinson C. Quality of life in ALS. Amyotroph Lateral Scler Other Motor Neuron Disord 2000;1: 223–224.
44. Coulthard-Morris L, Burks JS, Herndon RM. Rehabilitation Outcome Measures. In RM Herndon (ed), Handbook of Neurologic Rating Scales. New York: Demos Vermande, 1997;225–264.
45. Neudert C, Wasner M, Borasio GD. Patients' assessment of quality of life instruments: a randomized study of SIP, SF-36 and SEIQoL-DW in patients with amyotrophic lateral sclerosis. J Neurol Sci 2001;191:103–109.
46. Bromberg MB, Anderson F, Davidson M, Miller RG. Assessing health status quality of life in ALS: comparison of the SIP/ALS-19 with the ALS Functional Rating Scale and the Short Form-12 Health Survey. ALS C.A.R.E. Study Group. Clinical Assessement, Research, and Education. Amyotroph Lateral Scler Other Motor Neuron Disord 2001;2:31–37.
47. McGuire D, Garrison L, Armon C, et al. Relationship of the Tufts Quantitative Neuromuscular Exam (TQNE) and the Sickness Impact Profile (SIP) in measuring progression of ALS. SSNJV/ CNTF ALS Study Group. Neurology 1996;46:1442–1444.
48. McGuire D, Garrison L, Armon C, et al. A brief quality-of-life measure for ALS clinical trials based on a subset of items from the sickness impact profile. The Syntex-Synergen ALS/CNTF Study Group. J Neurol Sci 1997;152(suppl 1):S18–S22.
49. Jenkinson C, Fitzpatrick R, Brennan C, et al. Development and validation of a short measure of health status for individuals with amyotrophic lateral sclerosis/motor neurone disease: the ALSAQ-40. J Neurol 1999;246(suppl 3):III16–III21.
50. Jenkinson C, Fitzpatrick R, Brennan C, Swash M. Evidence for the validity and reliability of the ALS assessment questionnaire: the ALSQ-40. Amytroph Lateral Scler Other Motor Neuron Disord 1999;1:33–40.
51. Jenkinson C, Levvy G, Fitzpatrick R, Garratt A. The amyotrophic lateral sclerosis assessment questionnaire (ALSAQ-40): tests of data quality, score reliability and response rate in a survey of patients. J Neurol Sci 2000;180:94–100.
52. Jenkinson C, Fitzpatrick R. Reduced item set for the amyotrophic lateral sclerosis assessment questionnaire: development and validation of the ALSAQ-5. J Neurol Neurosurg Psychiatry 2001;70: 70–73.
53. Bromberg MB, Forshew DA. Comparison of instruments addressing quality of life in patients with ALS and their caregivers. Neurology 2002;58:320–322.
54. Al-Chalabi A, Leigh PN. Recent advances in amyotrophic lateral sclerosis. Curr Opin Neurol 2000;13:397–405.
55. Shaw CE, Al Chalabi A, Leigh N. Progress in the pathogenesis of amyotrophic lateral sclerosis. Curr Neurol Neurosci Rep 2001;1:69–76.
56. Rowland LP, Shneider NA. Amyotrophic lateral sclerosis. N Engl J Med 2001;344:1688–1700.
57. Cleveland DW, Rothstein JD. From Charcot to Lou Gehrig: deciphering selective motor neuron death in ALS. Nat Rev Neurosci 2001;2:806–819.
58. Morrison KE. Therapies in amyotrophic lateral sclerosis-beyond riluzole. Curr Opin Pharmacol 2002;2:302–309.
59. Doble A. The role of excitotoxicity in neurodegenerative disease: implications for therapy. Pharmacol Ther 1999;81:163–221.
60. Leigh PN, Meldrum BS. Excitotoxicity in ALS. Neurology 1996;47(6, suppl 4):S221–S227.
61. Heath PR, Shaw PJ. Update on the glutamatergic neurotransmitter system and the role of excitotoxicity in amyotrophic lateral sclerosis. Muscle Nerve 2002;26:438–458.
62. Plaitakis A, Caroscio JT. Abnormal glutamate metabolism in amyotrophic lateral sclerosis. Ann Neurol 1987;22:575–579.
63. Rothstein JD, Tsai G, Kuncl RW, et al. Abnormal excitatory amino acid metabolism in amyotrophic lateral sclerosis. Ann Neurol 1990;28:18–25.
64. Shaw PJ, Forrest V, Ince PG, et al. CSF and plasma amino acid levels in motor neuron disease: elevation of CSF glutamate in a subset of patients. Neurodegeneration 1995;4:209–216.

65. Spreux-Varoquaux O, Bensimon G, Lacomblez L, et al. Glutamate levels in cerebrospinal fluid in amyotrophic lateral sclerosis: a reappraisal using a new HPLC method with coulometric detection in a large cohort of patients. J Neurol Sci 2002;193:73–78.

66. Maragakis NJ, Rothstein JD. Glutamate transporters in neurologic disease. Arch Neurol 2001;58: 365–370.

67. Rothstein JD, Van Kammen M, Levey AI, et al. Selective loss of glial glutamate transporter GLT-1 in amyotrophic lateral sclerosis. Ann Neurol 1995;38:73–84.

68. Howland DS, Liu J, She Y, et al. Focal loss of the glutamate transporter EAAT2 in a transgenic rat model of SOD1 mutant–mediated amyotrophic lateral sclerosis (ALS). Proc Natl Acad Sci USA 2002;99:1604–1609.

69. Lin CL, Bristol LA, Jin L, et al. Aberrant RNA processing in a neurodegenerative disease: the cause for absent EAAT2, a glutamate transporter, in amyotrophic lateral sclerosis. Neuron 1998;20: 589–602.

70. Meyer T, Fromm A, Munch C, et al. The RNA of the glutamate transporter EAAT2 is variably spliced in amyotrophic lateral sclerosis and normal individuals. J Neurol Sci 1999;170:45–50.

71. Flowers JM, Powell JF, Leigh PN, et al. Intron 7 retention and exon 9 skipping EAAT2 mRNA variants are not associated with amyotrophic lateral sclerosis. Ann Neurol 2001;49:643–649.

72. Askmark H, Aquilonius SM, Gillberg PG, et al. A pilot trial of dextromethorphan in amyotrophic lateral sclerosis. J Neurol Neurosurg Psychiatry 1993;56:197–200.

73. Plaitakis A, Smith J, Mandeli J, Yahr MD. Pilot trial of branched-chain aminoacids in amyotrophic lateral sclerosis. Lancet 1988;1:1015–1018.

74. Testa D, Caraceni T, Fetoni V. Branched-chain amino acids in the treatment of amyotrophic lateral sclerosis. J Neurol 1989;236:445–447.

75. Gil R, Neau JP, et al. A double-blind placebo-controlled study of branched chain amino acids and L-threonine for the short-term treatment of signs and symptoms of amyotrophic lateral sclerosis. La Semaine des Hôpitaux (Paris) 1992;68:1472–1475.

76. Plaitakis A, Sivak M, et al. Treatment of amyotrophic lateral sclerosis with branched chain amino acids (BCAA): results of a second study. Neurology 1992;42(suppl 3):454.

77. The Italian ALS Study Group. Branched-chain amino acids and amyotrophic lateral sclerosis: a treatment failure? Neurology 1993;43:2466–2470.

78. Steiner TJ. Multinational trial of branched-chain amino acids in amyotrophic lateral sclerosis. Muscle Nerve 1994;(suppl 1):S166.

79. Tandan R, Bromberg MB, Forshew D, et al. A controlled trial of amino acid therapy in amyotrophic lateral sclerosis, I: clinical, functional, and maximum isometric torque data. Neurology 1996;47: 1220–1226.

80. Amino Acids for Amyotrophic Lateral Sclerosis (ALS)/Motor Neuron Disease (MND) (Protocol for a Cochrane Review). Oxford: Update Software, 2002.

81. Patten BM, Klein LM. L-Threonine and the modification of ALS. Neurology 1988;38(suppl 1): 354–355.

82. Blin O, Serratrice G, Pouget J, et al. Short-term double-blind vs placebo trial of L-threonine in amyotrophic lateral sclerosis [in French]. Presse Med 1989;18:1469–1470.

83. Blin O, Pouget J, Aubrespy G, et al. A double-blind placebo-controlled trial of L-threonine in amyotrophic lateral sclerosis. J Neurol 1992;239:79–81.

84. Hugon J, Preux PM. Glycine and L-threonine therapeutic trials in amyotrophic lateral sclerosis (ALS). Neurology 1992;42(suppl 3):454.

85. Testa D, Caraceni T, Fetoni V, Girotti F. Chronic treatment with L-threonine in amyotrophic lateral sclerosis: a pilot study. Clin Neurol Neurosurg 1992;94:7–9.

86. Doble A. The pharmacology and mechanism of action of riluzole. Neurology 1996;47(6, suppl 4): S233–S241.

87. Schiefer J, Landwehrmeyer GB, Luesse HG, et al. Riluzole prolongs survival time and alters nuclear inclusion formation in a transgenic mouse model of Huntington's disease. Mov Disord 2002;17:748–757.

88. Bensimon G, Lacomblez L, Meininger V. A controlled trial of riluzole in amyotrophic lateral sclerosis. ALS/Riluzole Study Group. N Engl J Med 1994;330:585–591.

89. Riviere M, Meininger V, Zeisser P, Munsat T. An analysis of extended survival in patients with amyotrophic lateral sclerosis treated with riluzole. Arch Neurol 1998;55:526–528.

90. Miller RG, Mitchell JD, Lyon M, Moore DH. Riluzole for amyotrophic lateral sclerosis (ALS)/ motor neuron disease (MND). Cochrane Database Syst Rev 2002;CD001447.

91. Meininger V, Lacomblez L, Bensimon G. Unpublished report: Controlled Trial of Riluzole in Patients with Advanced ALS. RP 54272-302 1995. 1995.

92. Yanagisawa N, Tashirao K, Tohgi H, et al. Efficacy and safety of riluzole in patients with amyotrophic lateral sclerosis: double-blind placebo controlled study in Japan. Igakuno Ayumi 1997; 182:851–866.

93. Sojka P, Andersen PM, Forsgren L. Effects of riluzole on symptom progression in amyotrophic lateral sclerosis. Lancet 1997;349:176–177.

94. Kalra S, Cashman NR, Genge A, Arnold DL. Recovery of *N*-acetylaspartate in corticomotor neurons of patients with ALS after riluzole therapy. Neuroreport 1998;9:1757–1761.

95. Pongratz D, Neundorfer B, Fischer W. German open label trial of riluzole 50 mg b.i.d. in treatment of amyotrophic lateral sclerosis (ALS). J Neurol Sci 2000;180:82–85.

96. Desiato MT, Palmieri MG, Giacomini P, et al. The effect of riluzole in amyotrophic lateral sclerosis: a study with cortical stimulation. J Neurol Sci 1999;169:98–107.

97. Arriada-Mendicoa N, Otero-Siliceo E, Burbano G, Corona-Vazquez T. Open label study of riluzole for the treatment of amyotrophic lateral sclerosis. Revista Ecuatoriana Neurol 1999;8:33–36.

98. Couratier P, Druet-Cabanac M, Truong CT, et al. Interest of a computerized ALS database in the diagnosis and follow-up of patients with ALS [in French]. Rev Neurol (Paris) 2000;156:357–363.

98a. Brooks BR, Belden DS, Roelke K, et al. Survival in non-riluzole treated amyotrophic lateral sclerosis (ALS)/motor neuron disease (MND) patients with disease onset before and since 1996 is identical: a clinic-based epidemiologic study. Amyotroph Lateral Scler Other Motor Neuron Disord 2001;2(suppl 2):60–61.

98b. Traynor BJ, Alexander M, Corr B, et al. An outcome study of riluzole in amyotrophic lateral sclerosis. A population-based study in Ireland 1996–2000. J Neurol 2003;250:473–479.

99. Debove C, Zeisser P, Salzman PM, et al. The Rilutek (riluzole) Global Early Access Programme: an open-label safety evaluation in the treatment of amyotrophic lateral sclerosis. Amyotroph Lateral Scler Other Motor Neuron Disord 2001;2:153–158.

100. Lacomblez L, Bensimon G, Leigh PN, et al. Long-term safety of riluzole in amyotrophic lateral sclerosis. Amyotroph Lateral Scler Other Motor Neuron Disord 2002;3:23–29.

101. Bensimon G, Lacomblez L, Delumeau JC, et al. A study of riluzole in the treatment of advanced stage or elderly patients with amyotrophic lateral sclerosis. J Neurol 2002;249:609–615.

102. Ludolph AC, Riepe MW. Do the benefits of currently available treatments justify early diagnosis and treatment of amyotrophic lateral sclerosis? Arguments against. Neurology 1999;53(8, suppl 5):S46–S49.

103. Meininger V, Lacomblez L, Salachas F. What has changed with riluzole? J Neurol 2000;246(suppl 6):19–22.

104. Chio A, Mora G, Leone M, et al. Early symptom progression rate is related to ALS outcome: a prospective population-based study. Neurology 2002;59:99–103.

105. Armon C, Guiloff RJ, Bedlack R. Limitations of inferences from observational databases in amyotrophic lateral sclerosis: all that glitters is not gold. Amyotroph Lateral Scler Other Motor Neuron Disord 2002;3:109–112.

106. Practice advisory on the treatment of amyotrophic lateral sclerosis with riluzole: report of the Quality Standards Subcommittee of the American Academy of Neurology. Neurology 1997;49: 657–659.

107. Booth-Clibborn N, Best L, Stein K. Riluzole for motor neurone disease. In L Best, R Milne, K Stein (eds), The Wessex Institute for Health Research & Development. Development & Evaluation Committee Report. 1997;73:1–21.

108. Ginsberg GM, Lev B. Cost-benefit analysis of riluzole for the treatment of amyotrophic lateral sclerosis. Pharmacoeconomics 1997;12:578–584.

109. Gray AM. ALS/MND and the perspective of health economics. J Neurol Sci 1998;160(suppl 1): S2–S5.

110. Chilcott J, Golightly P, Jefferson D, et al. The Use of Riluzole in the Treatment of Amyotrophic Lateral Sclerosis (Motor Neurone Disease). Sheffield: Trent Institute for Health Services Research, University of Leicester, Nottingham and Sheffield, 1997;1–37.

111. Munsat TM, Riviere M, Swash M, Leclerc C. Economic burden of amyotrophic lateral sclerosis in the United Kingdom. J Med Econ 1998;1:235–245.

112. Messori A, Trippoli S, Becagli P, Zaccara G. Cost effectiveness of riluzole in amyotrophic lateral sclerosis. Italian Cooperative Group for the Study of Meta-Analysis and the Osservatorio SIFO sui Farmaci. Pharmacoeconomics 1999;16:153–163.

113. Tavakoli M, Davies HTO, Malek M. Modelling the long-term cost-effectiveness of riluzole for the treatment of amyotrophic lateral sclerosis. J Med Econ 1999;2:1–14.

114. Tavakoli M, Malek M. The cost utility analysis of riluzole for the treatment of amyotrophic lateral sclerosis in the UK. J Neurol Sci 2001;191:95–102.

115. Kiebert GM, Green C, Murphy C, et al. Patients' health-related quality of life and utilities associated with different stages of amyotrophic lateral sclerosis. J Neurol Sci 2001;191:87–93.
116. National Institute of Clinical Excellence. Guidance on the Use of Riluzole (Rilutek) for the Treatment of Motor Neurone Disease. National Institute of Clinical Excellence, 2001.
117. Bryan S, Barton P, Burls A. The Clinical Effectiveness and Cost-Effectiveness of Riluzole for Motor Neurone Disease—An Update. West Midland Development and Evaluation Service, Full Document and Summary of Evidence Submitted to NICE. Update Assessment Report. 2000.
118. Leigh N. NICE recommends riluzole for the treatment of ALS. Adv Clin Neurosci Rehabil 2001;1: 9–12.
119. Eisen A, Stewart H, Schulzer M, Cameron D. Anti-glutamate therapy in amyotrophic lateral sclerosis: a trial using lamotrigine. Can J Neurol Sci 1993;20:297–301.
120. Miller RG, Moore D, Young LA, et al. Placebo-controlled trial of gabapentin in patients with amyotrophic lateral sclerosis. WALS Study Group. Western Amyotrophic Lateral Sclerosis Study Group. Neurology 1996;47:1383–1388.
121. McDermott MP, Rowland LP. ALS defeats gabapentin: reflections on another failed treatment. Neurology 2001;56:826–827.
122. Simpson EP, Mosier D, Appel SH. Mechanisms of disease pathogenesis in amyotrophic lateral sclerosis. A central role for calcium. Adv Neurol 2002;88:1–19.
123. Miller RG, Smith SA, Murphy JR, et al. A clinical trial of verapamil in amyotrophic lateral sclerosis. Muscle Nerve 1996;19:511–515.
124. Miller RG, Shepherd R, Dao H, et al. Controlled trial of nimodipine in amyotrophic lateral sclerosis. Neuromusc Disord 1996;6:101–104.
125. Szczudlik A, Tomik B, Slowik A, Kasprzyk K. Assessment of the efficacy of treatment with pimozide in patients with amyotrophic lateral sclerosis. Introductory notes [in Polish]. Neurol Neurochir Pol 1998;32:821–829.
126. Canton T, Bohme GA, Boireau A, et al. RPR 119990, a novel alpha-amino-3-hydroxy-5-methyl-4-isoxazolepropionic acid antagonist: synthesis, pharmacological properties, and activity in an animal model of amyotrophic lateral sclerosis. J Pharmacol Exp Ther 2001;299:314–322.
127. Jain KK. Evaluation of memantine for neuroprotection in dementia. Expert Opin Investig Drugs 2000;9:1397–1406.
128. Parsons CG, Danysz W, Quack G. Memantine is a clinically well tolerated N-methyl-D-aspartate (NMDA) receptor antagonist—a review of preclinical data. Neuropharmacology 1999;38:735–767.
129. Tateishi N, Mori T, Kagamiishi Y, et al. Astrocytic activation and delayed infarct expansion after permanent focal ischemia in rats. Part II: suppression of astrocytic activation by a novel agent (R)-(–)-2-propyloctanoic acid (ONO-2506) leads to mitigation of delayed infarct expansion and early improvement of neurologic deficits. J Cereb Blood Flow Metab 2002;22:723–734.
130. Provinciali L, Giovagnoli AR, Di Bella P, et al. A therapeutic trial of thymic factor in amyotrophic lateral sclerosis (ALS). Adv Exp Med Biol 1987;209:293–296.
131. Bunina TL, Khondkarian OA, Korshunova TS, et al. Treatment of amyotrophic lateral sclerosis with ribonucleotides [in Russian]. Zh Nevropatol Psikhiatr Im S S Korsakova 1976;76:166–174.
132. Majkowski J. Long-term treatment of amyotrophic lateral sclerosis with phthalazinol. Adv Second Messenger Phosphoprotein Res 1992;25:409–416.
133. Smith RA, Melmed S, Sherman B, et al. Recombinant growth hormone treatment of amyotrophic lateral sclerosis. Muscle Nerve 1993;16:624–633.
134. Engel WK, Siddique T, Nicoloff JT. Effect on weakness and spasticity in amyotrophic lateral sclerosis of thyrotropin-releasing hormone. Lancet 1983;2:73–75.
135. Imoto K, Saida K, Iwamura K, et al. Amyotrophic lateral sclerosis: a double-blind crossover trial of thyrotropin-releasing hormone. J Neurol Neurosurg Psychiatry 1984;47:1332–1334.
136. Braun SR, Sufit RL, Brooks BR. Pulmonary effects of thyrotropin-releasing hormone in amyotrophic lateral sclerosis. Lancet 1984;2:529–530.
137. Stober T, Schimrigk K, Dietzsch S, Thielen T. Intrathecal thyrotropin-releasing hormone therapy of amyotrophic lateral sclerosis. J Neurol 1985;232:13–14.
138. Serratrice G, Desnuelle C, Guelton C, et al. Trial of thyrotropin-releasing factor in amyotrophic lateral sclerosis [in French]. Presse Med 1985;14:487–488.
139. Caroscio JT, Cohen JA, Zawodniak J, et al. A double-blind, placebo-controlled trial of TRH in amyotrophic lateral sclerosis. Neurology 1986;36:141–145.
140. Brooke MH, Florence JM, Heller SL, et al. Controlled trial of thyrotropin releasing hormone in amyotrophic lateral sclerosis. Neurology 1986;36:146–151.

141. Mitsumoto H, Salgado ED, Negroski D, et al. Amyotrophic lateral sclerosis: effects of acute intravenous and chronic subcutaneous administration of thyrotropin-releasing hormone in controlled trials. Neurology 1986;36:152–159.
142. Serratrice G, Desnuelle C, Crevat A, et al. Treatment of amyotrophic lateral sclerosis with thyrotropin releasing hormone [in French]. Rev Neurol (Paris) 1986;142:133–139.
143. Yamane K, Osawa M, Kobayashi I, Maruyama S. Treatment of amyotrophic lateral sclerosis with thyrotropin-releasing hormone (TRH). Jpn J Psychiatry Neurol 1986;40:179–187.
144. Formisano R, Antonini G, Bove R, et al. Preliminary clinical study on the treatment of amyotrophic lateral sclerosis with TRH [in Italian]. Clin Ter 1986;119:479–481.
145. Brooks BR, Sufit RL, Montgomery GK, et al. Intravenous thyrotropin-releasing hormone in patients with amyotrophic lateral sclerosis. Dose-response and randomized concurrent placebo-controlled pilot studies. Neurol Clin 1987;5:143–158.
146. Thielen T, Stober T, Schimrigk K. Therapeutic trial of intrathecal thyrotropin-releasing hormone (TRH) and a TRH-analogue in amyotrophic lateral sclerosis (ALS). Adv Exp Med Biol 1987;209: 305–308.
147. Hawley RJ, Kratz R, Goodman RR, et al. Treatment of amyotrophic lateral sclerosis with the TRH analog DN-1417. Neurology 1987;37:715–717.
148. Munsat TL, Taft J, Kasdon D. Intrathecal thyrotropin-releasing hormone in amyotrophic lateral sclerosis. Neurol Clin 1987;5:159–170.
149. Munsat TL, Taft J, Kasdon D, Jackson IM. Prolonged intrathecal infusion of thyrotropin releasing hormone in amyotrophic lateral sclerosis. Ann N Y Acad Sci 1988;531:187–193.
150. Gueguen B, Puymirat J, Grouselle D, et al. Clinical, electrophysiologic and endocrine effects of the perfusion of high doses of TRH in amyotrophic lateral sclerosis [in French]. Rev Neurol (Paris) 1988;144:704–709.
151. Klimek A, Szulc-Kuberska J, Czernielewska-Rutkowska I, Gluszcz-Zielinska A. Treatment of amyotrophic lateral sclerosis with TRH [in Polish]. Neurol Neurochir Pol 1988;22:206–210.
152. Testa D, Chiodini PG, Girotti F, Attanasio R. Amyotrophic lateral sclerosis: thyroid and prolactin hormone changes in thyrotropin-releasing hormone therapy. Ital J Neurol Sci 1990;11:601–603.
153. Klimek A, Szulc-Kuberska J, Stepien H. Effect of thyroliberin treatment on the thyrotropin and prolactin levels in patients with amyotrophic lateral sclerosis [in Polish]. Neurol Neurochir Pol 1990;24:31–36.
154. Munsat TL, Taft J, Jackson IM, et al. Intrathecal thyrotropin-releasing hormone does not alter the progressive course of ALS: experience with an intrathecal drug delivery system. Neurology 1992; 42:1049–1053.
155. Patrignani J, Proano J, Morales MD. Treatment of amyotrophic lateral sclerosis with daily intrathecal TRH. A year's experience. Pilot study II [in Spanish]. Neurologia 1992;7:4–9.
156. Current status of thyrotropin-releasing hormone therapy in amyotrophic lateral sclerosis. Committee on Health Care Issues, American Neurological Association. Ann Neurol 1987;22: 541–543.
157. Brooke MH. Thyrotropin-releasing hormone in ALS. Are the results of clinical studies inconsistent? Ann N Y Acad Sci 1989;553:422–430.
158. Miller SC, Warnick JE. Protirelin (thyrotropin-releasing hormone) in amyotrophic lateral sclerosis. The role of androgens. Arch Neurol 1989;46:330–335.
159. Martinou JC, Martinou I, Kato AC. Cholinergic differentiation factor (CDF/LIF) promotes survival of isolated rat embryonic motoneurons in vitro. Neuron 1992;8:737–744.
160. Mitsumoto H, Ikeda K, Klinkosz B, et al. Arrest of motor neuron disease in wobbler mice cotreated with CNTF and BDNF. Science 1994;265:1107–1110.
161. The ALS CNTF Treatment Study Group. A double-blind placebo-controlled clinical trial of subcutaneous recombinant human ciliary neurotrophic factor (rHCNTF) in amyotrophic lateral sclerosis. ALS CNTF Treatment Study Group. Neurology 1996;46:1244–1249.
162. Cedarbaum JM, Stambler N. Performance of the Amyotrophic Lateral Sclerosis Functional Rating Scale (ALSFRS) in multicenter clinical trials. J Neurol Sci 1997;152(suppl 1):S1–S9.
163. Miller RG, Bryan WW, Dietz MA, et al. Toxicity and tolerability of recombinant human ciliary neurotrophic factor in patients with amyotrophic lateral sclerosis. Neurology 1996;47:1329–1331.
164. Stambler N, Charatan M, Cedarbaum JM. Prognostic indicators of survival in ALS. ALS CNTF Treatment Study Group. Neurology 1998;50:66–72.
165. Penn RD, Kroin JS, York MM, Cedarbaum JM. Intrathecal ciliary neurotrophic factor delivery for treatment of amyotrophic lateral sclerosis (phase I trial). Neurosurgery 1997;40:94–99.
166. Lewis ME, Neff NT, Contreras PC, et al. Insulin-like growth factor-I: potential for treatment of motor neuronal disorders. Exp Neurol 1993;124:73–88.

167. Neff NT, Prevette D, Houenou LJ, et al. Insulin-like growth factors: putative muscle-derived trophic agents that promote motoneuron survival. J Neurobiol 1993;24:1578–1588.
168. Ackerman SJ, Sullivan EM, Beusterien KM, et al. Cost effectiveness of recombinant human insulin-like growth factor I therapy in patients with ALS. Pharmacoeconomics 1999;15:179–195.
169. Mitchell JD, Wokke JH, Borasio GD. Recombinant human insulin-like growth factor I (rhIGF-I) for amyotrophic lateral sclerosis/motor neuron disease. Cochrane Database Syst Rev 2002; CD002064.
170. Henderson CE, Bloch-Gallego E, Camu W, et al. Motoneuron survival factors: biological roles and therapeutic potential. Neuromusc Disord 1993;3:455–458.
171. Ikeda K, Klinkosz B, Greene T, et al. Effects of brain-derived neurotrophic factor on motor dysfunction in wobbler mouse motor neuron disease. Ann Neurol 1995;37:505–511.
172. The BDNF Study Group (Phase III). A controlled trial of recombinant methionyl human BDNF in ALS: The BDNF Study Group (Phase III). Neurology 1999;52:1427–1433.
173. Ochs G, Penn RD, York M, et al. A phase I/II trial of recombinant methionyl human brain derived neurotrophic factor administered by intrathecal infusion to patients with amyotrophic lateral sclerosis. Amyotroph Lateral Scler Other Motor Neuron Disord 2000;1:201–206.
174. Fournier J, Steinberg R, Gauthier T, et al. Protective effects of SR 57746A in central and peripheral models of neurodegenerative disorders in rodents and primates. Neuroscience 1993;55:629–641.
175. Lechtzin N, Cudkowicz ME, Clawson LL, et al. Clinical trial of buspirone in patients with amyotrophic lateral sclerosis. Amyotroph Lateral Scler Other Motor Neuron Disord 2001;2(suppl 2):162–162(abst).
176. Yan W, Wilson CC, Haring JH. 5-HT1a receptors mediate the neurotrophic effect of serotonin on developing dentate granule cells. Brain Res Dev Brain Res 1997;98:185–190.
177. Turner MR, Rabiner EA, Grasby P, et al. [^{11}C]-WAY100635 PET: A potential in vivo marker for ALS? Neurology 2002;58(7 suppl 3):A413.
178. Oosthuyse B, Moons L, Storkebaum E, et al. Deletion of the hypoxia-response element in the vascular endothelial growth factor promoter causes motor neuron degeneration. Nat Genet 2001;28:131–138.
179. Bordet T, Lesbordes JC, Rouhani S, et al. Protective effects of cardiotrophin-1 adenoviral gene transfer on neuromuscular degeneration in transgenic ALS mice. Hum Mol Genet 2001;10:1925–1933.
180. Acsadi G, Anguelov RA, Yang H, et al. Increased survival and function of SOD1 mice after glial cell-derived neurotrophic factor gene therapy. Hum Gene Ther 2002;13:1047–1059.
181. Wang LJ, Lu YY, Muramatsu S, et al. Neuroprotective effects of glial cell line-derived neurotrophic factor mediated by an adeno-associated virus vector in a transgenic animal model of amyotrophic lateral sclerosis. J Neurosci 2002;22:6920–6928.
182. Manabe Y, Nagano I, Gazi MS, et al. Adenovirus-mediated gene transfer of glial cell line-derived neurotrophic factor prevents motor neuron loss of transgenic model mice for amyotrophic lateral sclerosis. Apoptosis 2002;7:329–334.
183. Drachman DB, Fishman PS, Rothstein JD, et al. Amyotrophic lateral sclerosis. An autoimmune disease? Adv Neurol 1995;68:59–65.
184. Engelhardt JI, Appel SH, Killian JM. Experimental auto-immune motoneuron disease. Ann Neurol 1989;26:368–376.
185. Engelhardt JI, Appel SH. IgG reactivity in the spinal cord and motor cortex in amyotrophic lateral sclerosis. Arch Neurol 1990;47:1210–1216.
186. Bradley WG, Hedlund W, Cooper C, et al. A double-blind controlled trial of bovine brain gangliosides in amyotrophic lateral sclerosis. Neurology 1984;34:1079–1082.
187. Pestronk A, Adams RN, Clawson L, et al. Serum antibodies to G_{M1} ganglioside in amyotrophic lateral sclerosis. Neurology 1988;38:1457–1461.
188. Pestronk A, Adams RN, Cornblath D, et al. Patterns of serum IgM antibodies to G_{M1} and G_{D1a} gangliosides in amyotrophic lateral sclerosis. Ann Neurol 1989;25:98–102.
189. Pestronk A, Cornblath DR, Ilyas AA, et al. A treatable multifocal motor neuropathy with antibodies to G_{M1} ganglioside. Ann Neurol 1988;24:73–78.
190. Pestronk A. Multifocal motor neuropathy: diagnosis and treatment. Neurology 1998;51(6, suppl 5):S22–S24.
191. Wolfgram F, Myers L. Amyotrophic lateral sclerosis: effect of serum on anterior horn cells in tissue culture. Science 1973;179:579–580.
192. Smith RG, Hamilton S, Hofmann F, et al. Serum antibodies to L-type calcium channels in patients with amyotrophic lateral sclerosis. N Engl J Med 1992;327:1721–1728.

193. Troost D, Van den Oord JJ, Vianney de Jong JM. Immunohistochemical characterization of the inflammatory infiltrate in amyotrophic lateral sclerosis. Neuropathol Appl Neurobiol 1990;16: 401–410.
194. Banati RB, Gehrmann J, Kellner M, Holsboer F. Antibodies against microglia/brain macrophages in the cerebrospinal fluid of a patient with acute amyotrophic lateral sclerosis and presenile dementia. Clin Neuropathol 1995;14:197–200.
195. Kelemen J, Hedlund W, Orlin JB, et al. Plasmapheresis with immunosuppression in amyotrophic lateral sclerosis. Arch Neurol 1983;40:752–753.
196. Mora JS, Munsat TL, Kao KP, et al. Intrathecal administration of natural human interferon alpha in amyotrophic lateral sclerosis. Neurology 1986;36:1137–1140.
197. Brown RH Jr, Hauser SL, Harrington H, Weiner HL. Failure of immunosuppression with a ten- to 14-day course of high-dose intravenous cyclophosphamide to alter the progression of amyotrophic lateral sclerosis. Arch Neurol 1986;43:383–384.
198. Tan E, Lynn DJ, Amato AA, et al. Immunosuppressive treatment of motor neuron syndromes. Attempts to distinguish a treatable disorder. Arch Neurol 1994;51:194–200.
199. Appel SH, Stewart SS, Appel V, et al. A double-blind study of the effectiveness of cyclosporine in amyotrophic lateral sclerosis. Arch Neurol 1988;45:381–386.
200. Werdelin L, Boysen G, Jensen TS, Mogensen P. Immunosuppressive treatment of patients with amyotrophic lateral sclerosis. Acta Neurol Scand 1990;82:132–134.
201. Westarp ME, Westphal KP, Kolde G, et al. Dermal, serological and CSF changes in amyotrophic lateral sclerosis with and without intrathecal interferon beta treatment. Int J Clin Pharmacol Ther Toxicol 1992;30:81–93.
202. Drachman DB, Chaudhry V, Cornblath D, et al. Trial of immunosuppression in amyotrophic lateral sclerosis using total lymphoid irradiation. Ann Neurol 1994;35:142–150.
203. Olarte MR, Shafer SQ. Levamisole is ineffective in the treatment of amyotrophic lateral sclerosis. Neurology 1985;35:1063–1066.
204. Otten A, Vermeulen M, Bossuyt PM, Otten A. Intravenous immunoglobulin treatment in neurological diseases. J Neurol Neurosurg Psychiatry 1996;60:359–361.
205. Meucci N, Nobile-Orazio E, Scarlato G. Intravenous immunoglobulin therapy in amyotrophic lateral sclerosis. J Neurol 1996;243:117–120.
206. Chaudhry V, Corse AM, Cornblath DR, et al. Multifocal motor neuropathy: electrodiagnostic features. Muscle Nerve 1994;17:198–205.
207. Taylor BV, Wright RA, Harper CM, Dyck PJ. Natural history of 46 patients with multifocal motor neuropathy with conduction block. Muscle Nerve 2000;23:900–908.
208. Nobile-Orazio E. Multifocal motor neuropathy. J Neuroimmunol 2001;115:4–18.
209. Azulay JP, Blin O, Pouget J, et al. Intravenous immunoglobulin treatment in patients with motor neuron syndromes associated with anti-G_{M1} antibodies: a double-blind, placebo-controlled study. Neurology 1994;44(3, pt 1):429–432.
210. Van den Berg LH, Kerkhoff H, Oey PL, et al. Treatment of multifocal motor neuropathy with high dose intravenous immunoglobulins: a double blind, placebo controlled study. J Neurol Neurosurg Psychiatry 1995;59:248–252.
211. Federico P, Zochodne DW, Hahn AF, et al. Multifocal motor neuropathy improved by IVIg: randomized, double-blind, placebo-controlled study. Neurology 2000;55:1256–1262.
212. Leger JM, Chassande B, Musset L, et al. Intravenous immunoglobulin therapy in multifocal motor neuropathy: a double-blind, placebo-controlled study. Brain 2001;124(pt 1):145–153.
213. Azulay JP, Rihet P, Pouget J, et al. Long term follow up of multifocal motor neuropathy with conduction block under treatment. J Neurol Neurosurg Psychiatry 1997;62:391–394.
214. Berg-Vos RM, Franssen H, Wokke JH, et al. Multifocal motor neuropathy: diagnostic criteria that predict the response to immunoglobulin treatment. Ann Neurol 2000;48:919–926.
215. Nobile-Orazio E, Cappellari A, Meucci N, et al. Multifocal motor neuropathy: clinical and immunological features and response to IVIg in relation to the presence and degree of motor conduction block. J Neurol Neurosurg Psychiatry 2002;72:761–766.
216. Ellis CM, Leary S, Payan J, et al. Use of human intravenous immunoglobulin in lower motor neuron syndromes. J Neurol Neurosurg Psychiatry 1999;67:15–19.
217. Umapathi T, Hughes RA, Nobile-Orazio E, Leger JM. Immunosuppressive treatment for multifocal motor neuropathy. Cochrane Database Syst Rev 2002;CD003217.
218. Siddique T, Figlewicz DA, Pericak-Vance MA, et al. Linkage of a gene causing familial amyotrophic lateral sclerosis to chromosome 21 and evidence of genetic-locus heterogeneity. N Engl J Med 1991;324:1381–1384.
219. Rosen DR, Siddique T, Patterson D, et al. Mutations in Cu/Zn superoxide dismutase gene are associated with familial amyotrophic lateral sclerosis. Nature 1993;362:59–62.

220. Radunovic A, Leigh PN. Cu/Zn superoxide dismutase gene mutations in amyotrophic lateral sclerosis: correlation between genotype and clinical features. J Neurol Neurosurg Psychiatry 1996;61:565–572.
221. Cudkowicz ME, McKenna-Yasek D, Sapp PE, et al. Epidemiology of mutations in superoxide dismutase in amyotrophic lateral sclerosis. Ann Neurol 1997;41:210–221.
222. Orrell RW, Habgood JJ, Malaspina A, et al. Clinical characteristics of SOD1 gene mutations in UK families with ALS. J Neurol Sci 1999;169:56–60.
223. Gaudette M, Hirano M, Siddique T. Current status of SOD1 mutations in familial ALS. ALS and other motor neuron disorders 2000;1:83–90.
224. Gurney ME, Pu H, Chiu AY, et al. Motor neuron degeneration in mice that express a human Cu, Zn superoxide dismutase mutation [published erratum in Science 1995;269:149]. Science 1994; 264:1772–1775.
225. Newbery HJ, Abbott CM. Of mice, men and motor neurons. Trends Mol Med 2002;8:88–92.
226. Noor R, Mittal S, Iqbal J. Superoxide dismutase. Med Sci Monit 2002;8:RA210–RA216.
227. Reaume AG, Elliott JL, Hoffman EK, et al. Motor neurons in Cu/Zn superoxide dismutase-deficient mice develop normally but exhibit enhanced cell death after axonal injury. Nat Genet 1996;13: 43–47.
228. Cudkowicz ME, Warren L, Francis JW, et al. Intrathecal administration of recombinant human superoxide dismutase 1 in amyotrophic lateral sclerosis: a preliminary safety and pharmacokinetic study. Neurology 1997;49:213–222.
229. Flanagan SW, Anderson RD, Ross MA, Oberley LW. Overexpression of manganese superoxide dismutase attenuates neuronal death in human cells expressing mutant (G37R) Cu/Zn-superoxide dismutase. J Neurochem 2002;81:170–177.
230. Valentine JS. Do oxidatively modified proteins cause ALS? Free Radic Biol Med 2002;33: 1314–1320.
231. Wiedau-Pazos M, Goto JJ, Rabizadeh S, et al. Altered reactivity of superoxide dismutase in familial amyotrophic lateral sclerosis. Science 1996;271:515–518.
232. Estevez AG, Spear N, Manuel SM, et al. Role of endogenous nitric oxide and peroxynitrite formation in the survival and death of motor neurons in culture. Prog Brain Res 1998;118:269–280.
233. Beckman JS, Estevez AG, Crow JP, Barbeito L. Superoxide dismutase and the death of motoneurons in ALS. Trends Neurosci 2001;24(11 suppl):S15–S20.
234. Stieber A, Gonatas JO, Gonatas NK. Aggregates of mutant protein appear progressively in dendrites, in periaxonal processes of oligodendrocytes, and in neuronal and astrocytic perikarya of mice expressing the SOD1(G93A) mutation of familial amyotrophic lateral sclerosis. J Neurol Sci 2000;177:114–123.
235. Watanabe M, Dykes-Hoberg M, Culotta VC, et al. Histological evidence of protein aggregation in mutant SOD1 transgenic mice and in amyotrophic lateral sclerosis neural tissues. Neurobiol Dis 2001;8:933–941.
236. Subramaniam JR, Lyons WE, Liu J, et al. Mutant SOD1 causes motor neuron disease independent of copper chaperone-mediated copper loading. Nat Neurosci 2002;5:301–307.
237. Hottinger AF, Fine EG, Gurney ME, et al. The copper chelator D-penicillamine delays onset of disease and extends survival in a transgenic mouse model of familial amyotrophic lateral sclerosis. Eur J Neurosci 1997;9:1548–1551.
238. Nagano S, Ogawa Y, Yanagihara T, Sakoda S. Benefit of a combined treatment with trientine and ascorbate in familial amyotrophic lateral sclerosis model mice. Neurosci Lett 1999;265:159–162.
239. Andreassen OA, Dedeoglu A, Friedlich A, et al. Effects of an inhibitor of poly(ADP-ribose) polymerase, desmethylselegiline, trientine, and lipoic acid in transgenic ALS mice. Exp Neurol 2001; 168:419–424.
240. Louwerse ES, Weverling GJ, Bossuyt PM, et al. Randomized, double-blind, controlled trial of acetylcysteine in amyotrophic lateral sclerosis. Arch Neurol 1995;52:559–564.
241. Cudkowicz ME, Sexton PM, Ellis T, et al. The pharmacokinetics and pharmaco-dynamics of Procysteine in amyotrophic lateral sclerosis. Neurology 1999;52:1492–1494.
242. Mazzini L, Testa D, Balzarini C, Mora G. An open-randomized clinical trial of selegiline in amyotrophic lateral sclerosis. J Neurol 1994;241:223–227.
243. Szulc-Kuberska J, Klimek A, Stepien H, Woszczak M. Clinical trial of the treatment of amyotrophic lateral sclerosis with bromocriptine [in Polish]. Neurol Neurochir Pol 1990;24:37–41.
244. Vyth A, Timmer JG, Bossuyt PM, et al. Survival in patients with amyotrophic lateral sclerosis, treated with an array of antioxidants. J Neurol Sci 1996;139(suppl):99–103.
245. Shults CW, Oakes D, Kieburtz K, et al. Effects of coenzyme Q_{10} in early Parkinson disease: evidence of slowing of the functional decline. Arch Neurol 2002;59:1541–1550.

246. Beal MF. Coenzyme Q_{10} as a possible treatment for neurodegenerative diseases. Free Radic Res 2002;36:455–460.
247. Bowling AC, Schulz JB, Brown RH Jr, Beal MF. Superoxide dismutase activity, oxidative damage, and mitochondrial energy metabolism in familial and sporadic amyotrophic lateral sclerosis. J Neurochem 1993;61:2322–2325.
248. Albers DS, Beal MF. Mitochondrial dysfunction and oxidative stress in aging and neurodegenerative disease. J Neural Transm Suppl 2000;59:133–154.
249. Sathasivam S, Ince PG, Shaw PJ. Apoptosis in amyotrophic lateral sclerosis: a review of the evidence. Neuropathol Appl Neurobiol 2001;27:257–274.
250. Troost D, Aten J, Morsink F, de Jong JM. Apoptosis in amyotrophic lateral sclerosis is not restricted to motor neurons. Bcl-2 expression is increased in unaffected post-central gyrus. Neuropathol Appl Neurobiol 1995;21:498–504.
251. Martin LJ. Neuronal death in amyotrophic lateral sclerosis is apoptosis: possible contribution of a programmed cell death mechanism. J Neuropathol Exp Neurol 1999;58:459–471.
252. Pedersen WA, Luo H, Kruman I, et al. The prostate apoptosis response-4 protein participates in motor neuron degeneration in amyotrophic lateral sclerosis. FASEB J 2000;14:913–924.
253. Kostic V, Jackson-Lewis V, de Bilbao F, et al. Bcl-2: prolonging life in a transgenic mouse model of familial amyotrophic lateral sclerosis. Science 1997;277:559–562.
254. Pasinelli P, Borchelt DR, Houseweart MK, et al. Caspase-1 is activated in neural cells and tissue with amyotrophic lateral sclerosis-associated mutations in copper-zinc superoxide dismutase. Proc Natl Acad Sci USA 1998;95:15763–15768.
255. Li M, Ona VO, Guegan C, et al. Functional role of caspase-1 and caspase-3 in an ALS transgenic mouse model. Science 2000;288:335–339.
256. Sanchez Mejia RO, Ona VO, Li M, Friedlander RM. Minocycline reduces traumatic brain injury-mediated caspase-1 activation, tissue damage, and neurological dysfunction. Neurosurgery 2001; 48:1393–1399.
257. Zhu S, Stavrovskaya IG, Drozda M, et al. Minocycline inhibits cytochrome *c* release and delays progression of amyotrophic lateral sclerosis in mice. Nature 2002;417:74–78.
258. Kriz J, Nguyen M, Julien J. Minocycline slows disease progression in a mouse model of amyotrophic lateral sclerosis. Neurobiol Dis 2002;10:268.
259. Van Den BL, Tilkin P, Lemmens G, Robberecht W. Minocycline delays disease onset and mortality in a transgenic model of ALS. Neuroreport 2002;13:1067–1070.
260. Asanuma M, Nishibayashi-Asanuma S, Miyazaki I, et al. Neuroprotective effects of non-steroidal anti-inflammatory drugs by direct scavenging of nitric oxide radicals. J Neurochem 2001;76: 1895–1904.
261. Yermakova A, O'Banion MK. Cyclooxygenases in the central nervous system: implications for treatment of neurological disorders. Curr Pharm Des 2000;6:1755–1776.
262. Yasojima K, Tourtellotte WW, McGeer EG, McGeer PL. Marked increase in cyclooxygenase-2 in ALS spinal cord: implications for therapy. Neurology 2001;57:952–956.
263. Drachman DB, Rothstein JD. Inhibition of cyclooxygenase-2 protects motor neurons in an organotypic model of amyotrophic lateral sclerosis. Ann Neurol 2000;48:792–795.
264. Wagey R, Hu J, Pelech SL, et al. Modulation of NMDA-mediated excitotoxicity by protein kinase C. J Neurochem 2001;78:715–726.
265. Noh KM, Hwang JY, Shin HC, Koh JY. A novel neuroprotective mechanism of riluzole: direct inhibition of protein kinase C. Neurobiol Dis 2000;7:375–383.
266. Schwartz Z, Sylvia VL, Guinee T, et al. Tamoxifen elicits its anti-estrogen effects in growth plate chondrocytes by inhibiting protein kinase C. J Steroid Biochem Mol Biol 2002;80:401–410.
267. Savas S, Delibas N, Savas C, et al. Pentoxifylline reduces biochemical markers of ischemia-reperfusion induced spinal cord injury in rabbits. Spinal Cord 2002;40:224–229.
268. Liversedge LA. Glycocyamine and betaine in motor-neurone disease. Lancet 1956;1136–1138.
269. Klivenyi P, Ferrante RJ, Matthews RT, et al. Neuroprotective effects of creatine in a transgenic animal model of amyotrophic lateral sclerosis. Nat Med 1999;5:347–350.
270. Ikeda K, Iwasaki Y, Kinoshita M. Oral administration of creatine monohydrate retards progression of motor neuron disease in the wobbler mouse. Amyotroph Lateral Scler Other Motor Neuron Disord 2000;1:207–212.
271. Earnest CP, Snell PG, Rodriguez R, et al. The effect of creatine monohydrate ingestion on anaerobic power indices, muscular strength and body composition. Acta Physiol Scand 1995;153: 207–209.
272. Tarnopolsky M, Martin J. Creatine monohydrate increases strength in patients with neuromuscular disease. Neurology 1999;52:854–857.

273. Rosenfeld J, Jackson CE, Smith J, et al. A pilot trial of ultrapure creatine in amyotrophic lateral sclerosis. Amyotroph Lateral Scler Other Motor Neuron Disord 2001;2(suppl 2):20.
274. Drory VE, Gross D. No effect of creatine on respiratory distress in amyotrophic lateral sclerosis. Amyotroph Lateral Scler Other Motor Neuron Disord 2002;3:43–46.
275. Denker PG, Scheinman L. Treatment of amyotrophic lateral sclerosis with vitamin E (alpha-tocopherol). JAMA 1941;116:1893–1895.
276. Desnuelle C, Dib M, Garrel C, Favier A. A double-blind, placebo-controlled randomized clinical trial of alpha-tocopherol (vitamin E) in the treatment of amyotrophic lateral sclerosis. ALS riluzole-tocopherol Study Group. Amyotroph Lateral Scler Other Motor Neuron Disord 2001;2:9–18.
277. Esposito E, Rotilio D, Di M, et al. A review of specific dietary antioxidants and the effects on biochemical mechanisms related to neurodegenerative processes. Neurobiol Aging 2002;23:719.
278. Butterfield DA, Castegna A, Drake J, et al. Vitamin E and neurodegenerative disorders associated with oxidative stress. Nutr Neurosci 2002;5:229–239.
279. Apostolski S, Marinkovic Z, Nikolic A, et al. Glutathione peroxidase in amyotrophic lateral sclerosis: the effects of selenium supplementation. J Environ Pathol Toxicol Oncol 1998;17:325–329.
280. Norris FH, Denys EH, Fallat RJ. Trial of octacosanol in amyotrophic lateral sclerosis. Neurology 1986;36:1263–1264.
281. Kaji R, Kodama M, Imamura A, et al. Effect of ultrahigh-dose methylcobalamin on compound muscle action potentials in amyotrophic lateral sclerosis: a double-blind controlled study. Muscle Nerve 1998;21:1775–1778.
282. Norris FH. Ceftriaxone in amyotrophic lateral sclerosis. Arch Neurol 1994;51:447.
283. Couratier P, Vallat JM, Merle L, et al. Report of six sporadic cases of ALS patients receiving ceftriaxone. Therapie 1994;49:146.
284. Johnson RT. Virological studies of amyotrophic lateral sclerosis: an overview. UCLA Forum Med Sci 1976;173–180.
285. Smith RA, Norris FH. Antiviral therapy. Adv Exp Med Biol 1987;209:297–304.
286. Jubelt B. Motor neuron diseases and viruses: poliovirus, retroviruses, and lymphomas. Curr Opin Neurol Neurosurg 1992;5:655–658.
287. Karpati G, Dalakas MC. Viral hide-and-seek in sporadic ALS: a new challenge. Neurology 2000;54:6–7.
288. Jubelt B, Berger JR. Does viral disease underlie ALS? Lessons from the AIDS pandemic. Neurology 2001;57:945–946.
289. Viola MV, Myers JC, Gann KL, et al. Failure to detect poliovirus genetic information in amyotrophic lateral sclerosis. Ann Neurol 1979;5:402–403.
290. Miller JR, Guntaka RV, Myers JC. Amyotrophic lateral sclerosis: search for poliovirus by nucleic acid hybridization. Neurology 1980;30:884–886.
291. Kohne DE, Gibbs CJ, White L, et al. Virus detection by nucleic acid hybridization: examination of normal and ALS tissues for the presence of poliovirus. J Gen Virol 1981;56(pt 2):223–233.
292. Brahic M, Smith RA, Gibbs CJ Jr, et al. Detection of picornavirus sequences in nervous tissue of amyotrophic lateral sclerosis and control patients. Ann Neurol 1985;18:337–343.
293. Bartfeld H, Dham C, Donnenfeld H, et al. Enteroviral-related antigen in circulating immune complexes of amyotrophic lateral sclerosis patients. Intervirology 1989;30:202–212.
294. Swanson NR, Fox SA, Mastaglia FL. Search for persistent infection with poliovirus or other enteroviruses in amyotrophic lateral sclerosis-motor neurone disease. Neuromusc Disord 1995;5:457–465.
295. Berger MM, Kopp N, Vital C, et al. Detection and cellular localization of enterovirus RNA sequences in spinal cord of patients with ALS. Neurology 2000;54:20–25.
296. Andrews WD, Tuke PW, Al Chalabi A, et al. Detection of reverse transcriptase activity in the serum of patients with motor neurone disease. J Med Virol 2000;61:527–532.
297. Pamphlett R. Detection and cellular localization of enterovirus RNA sequences in spinal cord of patients with ALS. Neurology 2000;55:1420–1421.
298. Walker MP, Schlaberg R, Hays AP, et al. Absence of echovirus sequences in brain and spinal cord of amyotrophic lateral sclerosis patients. Ann Neurol 2001;49:249–253.
299. Giraud P, Beaulieux F, Ono S, et al. Detection of enteroviral sequences from frozen spinal cord samples of Japanese ALS patients. Neurology 2001;56:1777–1778.
300. Sola P, Bedin R, Casoni F, et al. New insights into the viral theory of amyotrophic lateral sclerosis: study on the possible role of Kaposi's sarcoma-associated virus/human herpesvirus 8. Eur Neurol 2002;47:108–112.
301. Fareed GC, Tyler HR. The use of isoprinosine in patients with amyotrophic lateral sclerosis. Neurology 1971;21:937–940.

302. Munsat TL, Easterday CS, Levy S, et al. Amantadine and guanidine are ineffective in ALS. Neurology 1981;31:1054–1055.
303. Olson WH, Simons JA, Halaas GW. Therapeutic trial of tilorone in ALS: lack of benefit in a double-blind, placebo-controlled study. Neurology 1978;28:1293–1295.
304. Nevsimal O, Pekarek J, Koubek K, et al. Low-molecular transfer factor and its use in the treatment of amyotrophic lateral sclerosis [in Czech]. Cesk Neurol Neurochir 1991;54:220–222.
305. Moulignier A, Moulonguet A, Pialoux G, Rozenbaum W. Reversible ALS-like disorder in HIV infection. Neurology 2001;57:995–1001.
306. MacGowan DJ, Scelsa SN, Waldron M. An ALS-like syndrome with new HIV infection and complete response to antiretroviral therapy. Neurology 2001;57:1094–1097.
307. Ansevin CF. Treatment of ALS with pleconaril. Neurology 2001;56:691–692.
308. Mendell JR, Chase TN, Engel WK. Amyotrophic lateral sclerosis: metabolism of central monoamines and treatment with L-dopa. Trans Am Neurol Assoc 1971;96:284–286.
309. Handa I, Matsushita N, Ihashi K, et al. A clinical trial of therapeutic electrical stimulation for amyotrophic lateral sclerosis. Tohoku J Exp Med 1995;175:123–134.
310. Norris FH Jr, KS U, Sachais B, Carey M. Trial of baclofen in amyotrophic lateral sclerosis. Arch Neurol 1979;36:715–716.
311. Aquilonius SM, Askmark H, Eckernas SA, et al. Cholinesterase inhibitors lack therapeutic effect in amyotrophic lateral sclerosis. A controlled study of physostigmine versus neostigmine. Acta Neurol Scand 1986;73:628–632.
312. Aisen ML, Sevilla D, Edelstein L, Blass J. A double-blind placebo-controlled study of 3,4-diaminopyridine in amyotrophic lateral sclerosis patients on a rehabilitation unit. J Neurol Sci 1996;138:93–96.
313. Askmark H, Aquilonius SM, Gillberg PG, et al. Functional and pharmacokinetic studies of tetrahydroaminoacridine in patients with amyotrophic lateral sclerosis. Acta Neurol Scand 1990;82:253–258.
314. Orrell RW, Figlewicz DA. Clinical implications of the genetics of ALS and other motor neuron diseases. Neurology 2001;57:9–17.
315. Shaw PJ. Genetic inroads in familial ALS. Nat Genet 2001;29:103–104.
316. Radunovic A, Leigh PN. ALS Database: database of SOD1 (and other) gene mutations in ALS on the Internet. European FALS Group and ALSOD Consortium. Amyotroph Lateral Scler Other Motor Neuron Disord 1999;1:45–49.
317. Hadano S, Hand CK, Osuga H, et al. A gene encoding a putative GTPase regulator is mutated in familial amyotrophic lateral sclerosis 2. Nat Genet 2001;29:166–173.
318. Yang Y, Hentati A, Deng HX, et al. The gene encoding alsin, a protein with three guanine-nucleotide exchange factor domains, is mutated in a form of recessive amyotrophic lateral sclerosis. Nat Genet 2001;29:160–165.
319. Leavitt B. Hereditary motor neuron disease caused by mutations in the ALS2 gene: "The long and the short of it." Clin Genet 2002;62:265.
319a. A1-Chalabi A, Hansen VK, Simpson CL, et al. Variants in the ALS2 gene are not associated with sporadic amyotrophic lateral sclerosis. Neurogenetics 2003 (in press).
320. Hentati A, Ouahchi K, Pericak-Vance MA, et al. Linkage of a commoner form of recessive amyotrophic lateral sclerosis to chromosome 15q15–q22 markers. Neurogenetics 1998;2:55–60.
321. Chance PF, Rabin BA, Ryan SG, et al. Linkage of the gene for an autosomal dominant form of juvenile amyotrophic lateral sclerosis to chromosome 9q34. Am J Hum Genet 1998;62:633–640.
322. Hosler BA, Siddique T, Sapp PC, et al. Linkage of familial amyotrophic lateral sclerosis with frontotemporal dementia to chromosome 9q21–q22. JAMA 2000;284:1664–1669.
323. Hand CK, Khoris J, Salachas F, et al. A novel locus for familial amyotrophic lateral sclerosis, on chromosome 18q. Am J Hum Genet 2002;70:251–256.
324. Ruddy DM, Parton MJ, Al-Chalabi A, et al. Two families with familial amyotrophic lateral sclerosis are linked to a novel locus on chromosome 16q. Am J Hum Genet 2003 (in press).
325. Hayward C, Colville S, Swingler RJ, Brock DJ. Molecular genetic analysis of the APEX nuclease gene in amyotrophic lateral sclerosis. Neurology 1999;52:1899–1901.
326. Carpenter S. Proximal axonal enlargement in motor neuron disease. Neurology 1968;18:841–851.
327. Hirano A, Donnenfeld H, Sasaki S, Nakano I. Fine structural observations of neurofilamentous changes in amyotrophic lateral sclerosis. J Neuropathol Exp Neurol 1984;43:461–470.
328. Hirano A, Nakano I, Kurland LT, et al. Fine structural study of neurofibrillary changes in a family with amyotrophic lateral sclerosis. J Neuropathol Exp Neurol 1984;43:471–480.

329. Xu Z, Cork LC, Griffin JW, Cleveland DW. Increased expression of neurofilament subunit NF-L produces morphological alterations that resemble the pathology of human motor neuron disease. Cell 1993;73:23–33.

330. Williamson TL, Cleveland DW. Slowing of axonal transport is a very early event in the toxicity of ALS-linked SOD1 mutants to motor neurons. Nat Neurosci 1999;2:50–56.

331. Cote F, Collard JF, Julien JP. Progressive neuronopathy in transgenic mice expressing the human neurofilament heavy gene: a mouse model of amyotrophic lateral sclerosis. Cell 1993;73:35–46.

332. Figlewicz DA, Krizus A, Martinoli MG, et al. Variants of the heavy neurofilament subunit are associated with the development of amyotrophic lateral sclerosis. Hum Mol Genet 1994;3: 1757–1761.

333. Al-Chalabi A, Andersen PM, Nilsson P, et al. Deletions of the heavy neurofilament subunit tail in amyotrophic lateral sclerosis. Hum Mol Genet 1999;8:157–164.

334. Williamson TL, Bruijn LI, Zhu Q, Anderson KL, et al. Absence of neurofilaments reduces the selective vulnerability of motor neurons and slows disease caused by a familial amyotrophic lateral sclerosis-linked superoxide dismutase 1 mutant. Proc Natl Acad Sci USA 1998;95:9631–9636.

335. Couillard-Despres S, Zhu Q, Wong PC, et al. Protective effect of neurofilament heavy gene overexpression in motor neuron disease induced by mutant superoxide dismutase. Proc Natl Acad Sci USA 1998;95:9626–9630.

336. Kong J, Xu Z. Overexpression of neurofilament subunit NF-L and NF-H extends survival of a mouse model for amyotrophic lateral sclerosis. Neurosci Lett 2000;281:72–74.

337. Beaulieu JM, Nguyen MD, Julien JP. Late onset death of motor neurons in mice overexpressing wild-type peripherin. J Cell Biol 1999;147:531–544.

338. Menzies FM, Cookson MR, Taylor RW, et al. Mitochondrial dysfunction in a cell culture model of familial amyotrophic lateral sclerosis. Brain 2002;125(pt 7):1522–1533.

339. Menzies FM, Ince PG, Shaw PJ. Mitochondrial involvement in amyotrophic lateral sclerosis. Neurochem Int 2002;40:543–551.

340. Vielhaber S, Kunz D, Winkler K, et al. Mitochondrial DNA abnormalities in skeletal muscle of patients with sporadic amyotrophic lateral sclerosis. Brain 2000;123(pt 7):1339–1348.

341. Dhaliwal GK, Grewal RP. Mitochondrial DNA deletion mutation levels are elevated in ALS brains. Neuroreport 2000;11:2507–2509.

342. Talbot K, Davies KE. Spinal muscular atrophy. Semin Neurol 2001;21:189–197.

343. Lefebvre S, Burglen L, Reboullet S, et al. Identification and characterization of a spinal muscular atrophy-determining gene. Cell 1995;80:155–165.

344. Roy N, Mahadevan MS, McLean M, et al. The gene for neuronal apoptosis inhibitory protein is partially deleted in individuals with spinal muscular atrophy. Cell 1995;80:167–178.

345. Nicole S, Diaz CC, Frugier T, Melki J. Spinal muscular atrophy: recent advances and future prospects. Muscle Nerve 2002;26:4–13.

346. Talbot K, Ponting CP, Theodosiou AM, et al. Missense mutation clustering in the survival motor neuron gene: a role for a conserved tyrosine and glycine rich region of the protein in RNA metabolism? Hum Mol Genet 1997;6:497–500.

347. Talbot K, Miguel-Aliaga I, Mohaghegh P, et al. Characterization of a gene encoding survival motor neuron (SMN)-related protein, a constituent of the spliceosome complex. Hum Mol Genet 1998; 7:2149–2156.

348. Iwahashi H, Eguchi Y, Yasuhara N, et al. Synergistic anti-apoptotic activity between Bcl-2 and SMN implicated in spinal muscular atrophy. Nature 1997;390:413–417.

349. Orrell RW, Habgood JJ, de Belleroche JS, Lane RJ. The relationship of spinal muscular atrophy to motor neuron disease: investigation of SMN and NAIP gene deletions in sporadic and familial ALS. J Neurol Sci 1997;145:55–61.

350. Parboosingh JS, Meininger V, McKenna-Yasek D, et al. Deletions causing spinal muscular atrophy do not predispose to amyotrophic lateral sclerosis. Arch Neurol 1999;56:710–712.

351. Veldink JH, Van den Berg LH, Cobben JM, et al. Homozygous deletion of the survival motor neuron 2 gene is a prognostic factor in sporadic ALS. Neurology 2001;56:749–752.

352. Fink JK. Progressive spastic paraparesis: hereditary spastic paraplegia and its relation to primary and amyotrophic lateral sclerosis. Semin Neurol 2001;21:199–207.

353. Hazan J, Fonknechten N, Mavel D, et al. Spastin, a new AAA protein, is altered in the most frequent form of autosomal dominant spastic paraplegia. Nat Genet 1999;23:296–303.

354. Saugier-Veber P, Munnich A, Bonneau D, et al. X-linked spastic paraplegia and Pelizaeus-Merzbacher disease are allelic disorders at the proteolipid protein locus. Nat Genet 1994;6: 257–262.

355. Saugier-Veber P, Martin C, Le Meur N, et al. Identification of novel L1CAM mutations using fluorescence-assisted mismatch analysis. Hum Mutat 1998;12:259–266.
356. Casari G, De Fusco M, Ciarmatori S, et al. Spastic paraplegia and OXPHOS impairment caused by mutations in paraplegin, a nuclear-encoded mitochondrial metalloprotease. Cell 1998;93: 973–983.
357. Casari G, Rugarli E. Molecular basis of inherited spastic paraplegias. Curr Opin Genet Dev 2001; 11:336–342.
358. Schwartz GA, Lui CN. Hereditary (familial) spastic paraplegia: further clinical and pathological observations. AMA Arch Neurol Psychiatry. 1956;75:144–162.
359. Smith BN, Shaw CE. Screening of FALS patients with wild-type SOD1 for mutations in the SPG4 gene that is linked to autosomal dominant hereditary spastic paraplegia. Amyotroph Lateral Scler Other Motor Neuron Disord 2002;3(suppl 2):64.
360. Kennedy WR, Alter M, Sung JH. Progressive proximal spinal and bulbar muscular atrophy of late onset: a sex-linked recessive trait. Neurology 1968;18:671–680.
361. La Spada AR, Wilson EM, Lubahn DB, et al. Androgen receptor gene mutations in X-linked spinal and bulbar muscular atrophy. Nature 1991;352:77–79.
362. Yamashita S, Mita S, Kato S, et al. Effect on motor neuron survival in mutant SOD1 (G93A) transgenic mice by Bcl-2 expression using retrograde axonal transport of adenoviral vectors. Neurosci Lett 2002;328:289–293.
363. Martin-Rendon E, Azzouz M, Mazarakis ND. Lentiviral vectors for the treatment of neurodegenerative diseases. Curr Opin Mol Ther 2001;3:476–481.
364. Holden C. Neuroscience. Versatile cells against intractable diseases. Science 2002;297:500–502.
365. Johansson CB, Svensson M, Wallstedt L, et al. Neural stem cells in the adult human brain. Exp Cell Res 1999;253:733–736.
366. Magavi SS, Macklis JD. Manipulation of neural precursors in situ: induction of neurogenesis in the neocortex of adult mice. Neuropsychopharmacology 2001;25:816–835.
367. Song HJ, Stevens CF, Gage FH. Neural stem cells from adult hippocampus develop essential properties of functional CNS neurons. Nat Neurosci 2002;5:438–445.
368. Gritti A, Bonfanti L, Doetsch F, et al. Multipotent neural stem cells reside into the rostral extension and olfactory bulb of adult rodents. J Neurosci 2002;22:437–445.
369. Wichterle H, Lieberam I, Porter JA, Jessell TM. Directed differentiation of embryonic stem cells into motor neurons. Cell 2002;110:385–397.
370. Maragakis NJ, et al. Transplanted neural stem cells are capable of engraftment and differentiation in transgenic mutant SOD1 mice. Soc Neurosci Abstracts 2000;26:668.3.
371. Garbuzova-Davis S, Willing AE, Milliken M, et al. Positive effect of transplantation of hNT neurons (NTera 2/D1 cell-line) in a model of familial amyotrophic lateral sclerosis. Exp Neurol 2002;174:169–180.
372. Vastag B. Stem cells step closer to the clinic: paralysis partially reversed in rats with ALS-like disease. JAMA 2001;285:1691–1693.

Index

Page numbers followed by f indicate figures; t, tables.